# CHARTING NURSING'S FUTURE

*Agenda for the 1990s*

# CHARTING NURSING'S FUTURE

*Agenda for the 1990s*

LINDA H. AIKEN, Ph.D.

CLAIRE M. FAGIN, Ph.D.

 J. B. LIPPINCOTT COMPANY · *Philadelphia*

NEW YORK · LONDON · HAGERSTOWN

Acquisitions Editor: Diana Intenzo
Production Supervisor: Robert D. Bartleson
Production: P. M. Gordon Associates
Compositor: Achorn Graphic Services
Printer/Binder: R. R. Donnelley & Sons

6  5  4  3  2

**Library of Congress Cataloging-in-Publication Data**

Charting nursing's future : agenda for the 1990s / Linda H. Aiken,
    Claire M. Fagin, [editors].
        p.  cm.
    Includes bibliographical references and index.
    ISBN 0–397–54800–1
    1. Nursing.  I. Aiken, Linda H.   II. Fagin, Claire M.
RT41.C49  1991
610.73—dc20                                        91–19193
                                                        CIP

Any procedure or practice described in this book should be applied by the health-care
practitioner under appropriate supervision in accordance with professional standards of care
used with regard to the unique circumstances that apply in each practice situation. Care
has been taken to confirm the accuracy of information presented and to describe generally
accepted practices. However, the authors, editors, and publisher cannot accept any
responsibility for errors or omissions or for consequences from application of the
information in this book and make no warranty, express or implied, with respect to the
contents of the book.

Every effort has been made to ensure drug selection and dosages are in accordance with
current recommendations and practice. Because of ongoing research, changes in
government regulations, and the constant flow of information on drug therapy, reactions,
and interactions, the reader is cautioned to check the package insert for each drug for
indications, dosages, warnings, and precautions, particularly if the drug is new or
infrequently used.

# Contributors

LINDA H. AIKEN, PH.D., is Trustee Professor of Nursing, Professor of Sociology, Director of the Center for Health Services and Policy Research, and Associate Director of the Leonard Davis Institute of Health Economics at the University of Pennsylvania, Philadelphia. Dr. Aiken is a past President of the American Academy of Nursing and a member of the Institute of Medicine of the National Academy of Sciences. Dr. Aiken is nationally known for her research on the nursing shortage and served as a member of the 1989 Secretary's Commission on Nursing as well as the 1983 Institute of Medicine Study of Nursing. She was a member of the Advisory Council on Social Security chaired by Otis Bowen and a member of the Wyden Commission on long-term care insurance. While Vice President of the Robert Wood Johnson Foundation, she designed a $100 million demonstration to improve care for the chronically mentally ill for which she received an unusual Joint Secretarial Commendation from the Secretary of the U.S. Department of Health and Human Services and the Secretary of the U.S. Department of Housing and Urban Development. She chaired the Governor's Mental Health Advisory Council in New Jersey in 1989–1990, a group that developed a 10-year mental health services plan for the state. Her funded research initiatives include a national study of dedicated AIDS units and research on the outcomes of hospital nursing care. She is a member of the National Advisory Council of the Agency for Health Care Policy and Research (AHCPR) and the Physician Payment Reform Commission.

CLAIRE M. FAGIN, PH.D., F.A.A.N., is Margaret Bond Simon Dean and Professor at the University of Pennsylvania School of Nursing. She directs one of the three WHO Global Collaborating Centers in Nursing. Dr. Fagin is a fellow in the American Academy of Nursing, a fellow of the College of Physicians of Philadelphia, and a member of the Institute of Medicine. She is also an advisor to the World Health Organization and on the Board of Directors of the Provident Mutual Life Insurance Company and the Daltex Company, Inc. She is a former member of the National Advisory Council of the National Institute of Mental Health and past President of

v

the American Orthopsychiatric Association. She received the first Distinguished Scholar Award from the American Nurses Foundation in 1988, and in 1990 she was named a "Woman of Courage" by Philadelphia's WOMEN'S WAY, in honor of her contributions to the physical and mental well-being of women. In recognition of her contribution to nursing education and leadership and her influence on health care policy, in June 1988 Dr. Fagin received the Honorary Recognition Award of the American Nurses' Association, the most prestigious honor awarded in the nursing profession.

LAUREN S. ARNOLD, PH.D., R.N., is Clinical Director, Obstetrical/Neonatal Nursing, at the Hospital of the University of Pennsylvania in Philadelphia. She is also a Project Consultant with the National Commission to Prevent Infant Mortality, a bipartisan Congressional commission charged with designing a plan to reduce infant mortality. Dr. Arnold has served as the chairperson of the Council of Perinatal Nurses of the American Nurses' Association, and on numerous other national and regional committees that address issues related to maternal and child health.

MYRTLE K. AYDELOTTE, PH.D., R.N., is Dean Emeritus of the University of Iowa College of Nursing, where she was the school's first Dean from 1957 to 1962. A distinguished and still productive scholar, Dr. Aydelotte continues to teach at the College and is a valuable resource to faculty and graduate students. She has held positions as Associate Chief Nurse and Chief of Nursing Research at Iowa City Veterans Hospital, Director of Nursing at the University of Iowa Hospitals and Clinics, and was Executive Director of the 1.6 million member American Nurses' Association from 1977 to 1981. An accomplished consultant, researcher, writer, and lecturer, her career has been dedicated to seeing that the public is better served by the practice of nursing.

ROSEMARY A. BOWMAN, M.B.A., R.N., is President of Trimark Health Services, Inc., a nursing service in Atlanta, GA. A co-founder of Trimark, Bowman has been a nurse entrepreneur in home health care since 1981. She received her MBA from the University of Denver. Bowman has been Executive Director of the Tennessee Nurses' Association. She has held appointive positions in the American Nurses' Association and has served two years in work groups for the National Commission on Nursing Implementation Project. Bowman maintains an active clinical practice in addition to her responsibilities as chief executive officer of Trimark.

JEANNE BROOKS-GUNN, PH.D., is Senior Research Scientist in the Division of Education Policy Research at Educational Testing Service. In addition, she is the Virginia and Leonard Marx Professor in Child and Parent Development and Education; Director, Center for the Development and Education of Young Children and Their Parents, Teachers College, Columbia University; the Director of the Adolescent Study at Educational Testing Service and the St. Luke's Roosevelt Hospital Center in New York City; and Adjunct Associate Professor of Pediatrics at the University of Pennsylvania. A development psychologist, she received her Master's degree from Harvard University and her Ph.D. from the University of Pennsylvania. Her specialty is policy-oriented research focusing on familial influences upon children's development (achievement, psychological well-being, school and behavioral problems) and intervention efforts aimed at ameliorating the developmental delays seen in poor children. She recently completed a year at the Russell Sage Foundation as a Visiting Scholar, studying poor children and their families. Dr. Brooks-Gunn is studying the long-term consequences of unplanned pregnancies on teenage girls, their children, and their children's children in a 20-year intergenerational investigation and is investigating cognitive, academic, and behavioral consequences of low birth weight in elementary school children.

DOROTHY BROOTEN, R.N., PH.D., F.A.A.N., is Professor and Chair, Health Care of Women & Childbearing, University of Pennsylvania, School of Nursing. She is also Director of the Graduate Perinatal Nursing Program and Director of the Center for Low Birthweight Research at the same school. Dr. Brooten has served on numerous national panels in the area of low birth weight prevention and care. Her longstanding program of research centers on delivery of health services to childbearing families and the prevention and care of low birth weight infants. She is the author of several books in the area of nursing leadership and childbearing and the author of numerous articles in the same area.

ANN WOLBERT BURGESS, R.N., D.N.SC., is the van Amerigen Professor of Psychiatric Mental Health Nursing at the University of Pennsylvania School of Nursing. She, with Lynda Lytle Holmstrom, co-founded one of the first hospital-based crisis intervention programs for rape victims at Boston City Hospital in 1972. She served as chair of the first Advisory Council to the National Center for the Prevention and Control of Rape of the National Institute of Mental Health, 1976–1980. She was a member of the 1984 U.S. Attorney General's Task Force on Family Violence and on the planning committee for the Surgeon General's Symposium on Violence in October 1985, and served on the National Institutes of Health National Advisory Council of the Adolescent Health Advisory Panel to the Congress of the United States Office of Technology Assessment. She has been principal investigator of research projects on the use of children in pornography; heart attack victims and return to work; sexual homicide and patterns of crime scenes; possible linkages between sexual abuse and exploitation of children; juvenile delinquency and criminal behavior; children as witnesses in child sexual abuse trials; and AIDS, ethics, and sexual assault.

LUTHER CHRISTMAN, PH.D., R.N., Dean Emeritus, College of Nursing, Rush University, is now a nurse consultant in private practice. Christman is also a medical sociologist, as well as a member of the Institute of Medicine of the National Academy of Sciences; a Fellow in the American Academy of Nursing; a Fellow, Society for Applied Anthropology; Fellow, American Association for the Advancement of Science; Honorary Member, Alpha Omega Alpha; Distinguished Practitioner, National Academies of Practice; and Old Master, Purdue University. He was awarded a Doctor of Humane Letters, Thomas Jefferson University; the Editor Moore Copeland Founders Award for Creativity, Sigma Theta Tau; the Jesse M. Scott Award, American Nurses' Association; and the Honorary Recognition Award, Illinois Nurses' Association.

JOYCE C. CLIFFORD, R.N., M.S.N., F.A.A.N., is the Vice President for Nursing and Nurse-in-Chief at Boston's Beth Israel Hospital. A graduate of St. Anselm College, she received her Master's in nursing from the University of Alabama and is presently a Ph.D. candidate in the field of Health Planning and Policy Analysis at the Heller School of Brandeis University. She is a fellow of the American Academy of Nursing and is a former President of the American Organization of Nurse Executives. In addition, she is a trustee for her alma mater, St. Anselm College, and is the first nurse to be a member of Harvard Medical School's Admissions Committee. Clifford is an established author and consultant on the subject of primary nursing care and the development of a professional practice model and has spoken both nationally and internationally in countries such as Norway, Finland, and Japan. She is co-editor of the book *Advancing Professional Nursing Practice: Innovations at Boston's Beth Israel Hospital.*

DONNA DIERS, R.N., M.S.N., F.A.A.N., is the Annie W. Goodrich Professor of Nursing, Yale University School of Nursing, New Haven, CT, where she teaches nursing and policy as well as health policy and management. She is a member of the Institute of Medicine of the National Academy of Sciences and a former Dean of the School of Nursing at Yale. She has published widely on topics in nursing research, policy, and general issues in nursing, and she is editor of *Image—Journal of Nursing Scholarship,* the official publication of Sigma Theta Tau International, the nursing honorary society.

BARBARA A. DONAHO, R.N., M.A., F.A.A.N., joined Strengthening Hospital Nursing Program staff as Director in August 1989. She joined St. Anthony's Hospital, St. Petersburg, FL, as Senior Vice President, Patient Services, in November 1990, having held executive level positions in Shands Hospital at the University of Florida and the Sisters of Mercy Health Corporation since 1979. She just completed a term as a member of the American Hospital Association Board of Directors, and she received their Trustees Award in 1988. She has served as a Commissioner of the Joint Commission on Accreditation of Hospitals (JCAH) since 1979 (the first nurse to be so appointed) and chaired the Accreditation Committee from 1983 to 1987. She has also chaired the American Hospital Association's Council on Nursing, and is past President of the Midwest Alliance in Nursing and the American Organization of Nurse Executives. She holds a BSN degree from the Johns Hopkins University and an MA from the University of Chicago. She has held faculty appointments at the University of Florida, the University of Michigan, the University of Minnesota, and Boston University.

LORETTA C. FORD, ED.D., R.N., F.A.A.N., is Professor and Dean Emeritus, School of Nursing, University of Rochester, Rochester, NY. An internationally known nursing leader, Ford's career was devoted to practice, education, consultation and influencing health services inquiry, and innovation. Her numerous publications and awards cite her for major contributions: the development of the nurse practitioner program at the University of Colorado and the Unification of Nursing Practice, Education and Research at the University of Rochester.

JEANNE C. FOX, R.N., PH.D., former Galt Visiting Scholar for the Commonwealth of Virginia, is an Associate Professor of Nursing and Professor of Behavioral Medicine and Psychiatry at the University of Virginia, Charlottesville, VA. Fox, a psychiatric nurse and sociologist, is a past President of the Society for Education and Research in Psychiatric Nursing and member of the NIMH Task Force on Nursing. She is the principal investigator of an Institute on Community Integration of the Seriously Mentally Ill and a multidisciplinary graduate training grant in chronic mental illness and psychogeriatrics. Her research interests include living environments and recidivism in schizophrenic clients, mental health-psychiatric manpower, and alternative care delivery systems.

RAE K. GRAD, PH.D., who received her B.S.N. from Cornell University; MA in Parent/Child Nursing from New York University; and Ph.D. from the University of Maryland, began her career as a labor and delivery nurse in a small, community hospital in Northern Virginia. During that time, she also taught Maternal and Child Health Nursing at George Mason University in Fairfax, VA, as well as lamaze classes. After obtaining her Ph.D., she started a consulting firm (Alliance for Perinatal Research and Services), wrote a book (*The Father Book: Pregnancy and Beyond*), and published a national newsletter ("The Federal Monitor"), which discussed national legislative and regulatory issues affecting mothers and infants. In 1982, she founded the Virginia Perinatal Association, a statewide advocacy group for mothers and babies. Her work was recognized by former Governor Charles Robb, who asked that she head up a project to develop a Southern Regional Project on Infant Mortality. Dr. Grad directed that project for four years before being asked to serve in her present position as Executive Director of the National Commission to Prevent Infant Mortality, a Congressional Commission formed to develop a national strategy to reduce infant mortality. She was recently awarded a three-year Fellowship in leadership by the Kellogg Foundation.

CHARLENE HARRINGTON, PH.D., is a professor in the Department of Social and Behavioral Sciences and an Associate Director of the Institute for Health and Aging at the University of California, San Francisco, CA. She is a medical sociologist and a nurse whose primary interests are in health care policy and financing systems. She is currently the principal investigator on a study of the nursing home and home health care markets and a co-principal investigator on the national evaluation of the social health maintenance organization demonstrations. As a former California state director of licensing and certification, she served on the Institute of Medicine's Committee on Nursing Home Regulation in 1984–1986, which resulted in federal legislation to improve nursing home regulation.

CAROL R. HARTMAN, R.N., D.N.SC., is Professor and Chair of the Psychiatric Mental Health Nursing Program at Boston College School of Nursing. Her research interests have been diverse, starting with a clinical intervention study of joint admission of mentally disturbed mothers and their babies, following them with home nursing visits. She has studied the rural health needs of women and children and consulted with the Appalachian Regional Hospital, Beckley, WV. Her work with Dr. Burgess in the area of rape victimization has expanded to studying the neuropsychosocial processes of trauma that underlie responses to sexual abuse and the implications for therapeutic nursing intervention. Dr. Hartman has served on the American Psychiatric Association's revision of its Diagnostic and Statistical Manual (DSM-IIIR), the Task Force on Post-Traumatic Stress Disorder, and she serves on the Board of Directors for Nurses United for Responsible Services (NURS) and Child Safe.

ADA SUE HINSHAW, PH.D., R.N., F.A.A.N., nationally recognized for her contributions in the field of nursing research, assumed the position of Director of the National Center for Nursing Research at the National Institutes of Health in June 1987. She assumed this position following 12 years with the University of Arizona in Tucson, where she served concurrently as Professor and Director of Research at the University of Arizona College of Nursing and Director of Nursing Research in the Nursing Department, University Medical Center, located in the Arizona Health Sciences Center. In acknowledgment of her contributions to the field of nursing research, Dr. Hinshaw received the American Nurses' Association's Nurse Scientist of the Year award in 1985. Among numerous other honors, she also received the Distinguished Alumnus Award from Yale University's School of Nursing and the Alumnus of the Year Award from the University of Kansas School of Nursing. Most recently she received the Elizabeth McWilliams Miller Award for Excellence in Nursing Research from Sigma Theta Tau International. Dr. Hinshaw received her Ph.D. in sociology from the University of Arizona and holds two master's degrees—in sociology from the University of Arizona and in nursing from Yale University. She received her undergraduate degree in nursing from the University of Kansas. Dr. Hinshaw has published widely and given numerous presentations. Her honorary and professional affiliations include the American Nurses' Association, Council of Nurse Researchers, Maryland Nurses' Association, Sigma Xi, Western Society for Research in Nursing, American Academy of Nursing, Sigma Theta Tau, and the National Academies of Practice.

JUDITH B. IGOE, R.N., M.S., F.A.A.N., is an associate professor at the University of Colorado Health Sciences Center with appointments in the Schools of Nursing and Medicine. She is director of School Health Programs at the University of Colorado and was involved in the development of the School Nurse Practitioner role and other teaching programs for school health personnel. She is currently a doctoral student at the University of Colorado Graduate School of Public Affairs.

ADA K. JACOX, R.N., PH.D., F.A.A.N., is Independence Professor of Health Policy at the Johns Hopkins University School of Nursing. Her present research is focused on determinants of nursing care costs and patient outcomes in hospitals. Her interest in technology assessment reflects her concern for using research findings to influence policy.

HELEN S. KNAPP, M.S.N., B.S.N., P.N.P., is a lecturer in the University of Pennsylvania School of Nursing. She received her Bachelor's Degree in Nursing from Indiana University of Pennsylvania and her Master's Degree from the University of Pennsylvania Perinatal Nursing Program. Prior to her appointment as a lecturer in the School of Nursing she was a Clinical Nurse Specialist in the grant, Early Hospital Discharge and Nurse Specialist Follow-up of Women Following Cesarean Birth Program.

MARY KAY KOHLES, R.N., M.S.W., is the Deputy Director of the Strengthening Hospital Nursing Program. Kohles has held nursing management and administrative positions in university and community hospitals in Wisconsin and Nebraska before joining the national Program. Kohles' clinical practice interest is in critical care nursing.

EILEEN V.T. LAKE, R.N., M.P.P., is assistant director of the Center for Health Services and Policy Research and research associate at the School of Nursing, University of Pennsylvania. Presently, she directs a national study of the impact of innovation in AIDS nursing care on nurse retention and patient outcomes. Lake came to Penn from the staff of the Prospective Payment Assessment Commission, which advises the Secretary of Health and Human Services and the Congress on the maintenance and updating of the Medicare prospective payment system. While at ProPAC, she assessed the relation between DRGs and nursing intensity, and analyzed trends in hospital use and mortality of frail Medicare beneficiaries. While practicing as a nurse, Lake received her Master's in public policy studies at Georgetown University. Her research interests include nursing services and health policy, patient outcomes of nursing care, and innovation in hospital nursing organization and practice.

ADA M. LINDSEY, R.N., PH.D., is Dean and Professor at the School of Nursing, University of California, Los Angeles. Lindsey has had administrative responsibility for the School of Nursing's nurse-managed health centers located in the Skid Row area of downtown Los Angeles since 1986. One clinic primarily serves homeless adult men and a second was established primarily to provide primary health care to homeless children and families. In addition to studying issues pertinent to the provision of health care to this very needy population, Lindsey has authored a number of publications concerning the health problems of breast and lung cancer patients, and co-edited *Pathophysiological Phenomena: Human Responses to Illness.* Lindsey has served on the governing council of the American Academy of Nursing, and as chair of the research committees of the Oncology Nursing Society and currently for Sigma Theta Tau, International.

CAROL ANN LOCKHART, R.N., PH.D., is founder of C. Lockhart Associates of Tempe, AZ, a health-systems relations and policy consulting firm. She was formerly Executive Director of the Greater Phoenix Affordable Health Care Foundation, Phoenix, AZ, a business and health coalition working to provide community information, dialogue, and action toward private (or necessary public) sector solutions to issues confronting the health care system. Lockhart has served on the Physician Payment Review Commission (1986–1991) as the only nurse member of the Commission since its creation in 1986. She has held positions in public health at both local and state levels and was appointed Acting Director of Arizona Health Care Cost Containment System (AHCCCS) during the initial months of the newly created indigent care program. Dr. Lockhart serves on the faculty of the Arizona State University College of Business Administration, School of Health Administration and Policy, and has taught at schools of nursing and public health. She has co-authored two books on labor relations in health care and writes and speaks in the area of public health and health administration and policy. A Fellow of the American Academy of Nursing, she received her Ph.D. from the Florence Heller Graduate School for Social Policy, Brandeis University.

JOAN E. LYNAUGH, PH.D., F.A.A.N., is Associate Professor, School of Nursing, University of Pennsylvania, and Director, Center for the Study of the History of Nursing. Lynaugh is a nurse and historian whose interests include the history of health care and the health professions in the United States, health care delivery, especially for the aged and chronically ill, and specialty preparation for nursing practice in primary care. She serves on the Board of the American Association for the History of Nursing, the Shryock Medal Committee of the American Association for the History of Medicine, and the Executive Committee for Community Home Health Services, successor to the Visiting Nurse Society of Philadelphia.

PAMELA J. MARALDO, PH.D., R.N., F.A.A.N., has served as Executive Director of the National League for Nursing, a coalition of individual and agency members that promotes quality nursing care to the public, since 1983. During this time, she has led a programmatic and financial revitalization of the organization. Prior to assuming this post, she established and administered the NLN Office of Public Policy, which has become an authoritative source on health policy issues, especially those related to quality in the areas of home health and long term care. Active in many organizations, Dr. Maraldo is a Fellow of the American Academy of Nursing, a member of the American Express Health Care Faculty, and a member of the New York City Board of Health. She is listed in *Who's Who,* and was named one of the nation's top 12 nonprofit executives by *Savvy* magazine. After receiving a Bachelor of Science in Nursing Degree from Adelphi University, Dr. Maraldo went on to earn her Master's Degree and Doctor of Philosophy in Nursing at New York University.

MATHY MEZEY, R.N., ED.D., F.A.A.N., is the Independence Chair Professor of Nursing Education in the Division of Nursing, SEHNAA, New York University. She is past Director of the Robert Wood Johnson Foundation Teaching Nursing Home Program, a five-million dollar initiative that sought to improve care to nursing home patients and entice nurses to work in long-term care by linking 11 schools of nursing to 12 nursing homes. Dr. Mezey's research interests focus on the role of geriatric nurse specialists in nursing homes, assessment in the elderly, and recovery following hip fracture.

ANN O'SULLIVAN, PH.D., is Associate Professor of Pediatric Nursing at the University of Pennsylvania School of Nursing and Associate Professor in the Department of Pediatrics of the School of Medicine. She received her pediatric nurse practitioner credentials while a Robert Wood Johnson Nurse Faculty Fellow at the University of Maryland and the Johns Hopkins Hospital. Her special area of research focuses on teenage parents and their infants.

PATRICIA A. PRESCOTT, PH.D., is Professor and Chair, Department of Psycho Physiological Nursing, University of Maryland. Prescott is a sociologist and nurse whose research interests include health services research and health manpower issues. She has been actively involved in studying various aspects of nurse shortage for the past ten years and now is working with the federal government and professional associations to improve methods of forecasting requirements for health professionals. She has authored numerous articles on nurse shortage and other personnel related issues.

LOUISE B. RUSSELL, PH.D., is Research Professor of Economics in the Institute for Health, Health Care Policy, and Aging Research, Rutgers University, and Professor in the Department of Economics. Her major area of research is the economics of medical care. Dr. Russell is a member of the Institute of Medicine of the National Academy of Sciences and serves on its Board on Health Sciences Policy. She was also a member of the Institute's Committee for the Study of the Future of Public Health (1986–1987) and of the U.S. Preventive Services Task Force of the Department of Health and Human Services (1984–1988). Before joining Rutgers in August 1987, Dr. Russell was a senior Fellow at the Brookings Institution. Her Brookings books include *Medicare's New Hospital Payment System: Is It Working?* (1989); *Is Prevention Better Than Cure?* (1986); and *Technology in Hospitals: Medical Advances and Their Diffusion* (1979).

DONALD F. SCHWARZ, M.D., M.B.A., is Assistant Professor of Pediatrics at the University of Pennsylvania School of Medicine and Attending Physician in Adolescent Medicine at the Children's Hospital of Philadelphia. In addition, he is an Adjunct Assistant Professor in the University of Pennsylvania School of Nursing. Dr. Schwarz was a Robert Wood Johnson Foundation Clinical Scholar and General Academic Pediatrics Fellow at the University of Pennsylvania. Dr. Schwarz's research has focused on the development and evaluation of preventive health programs for adolescents-at-risk in urban areas. With Ann O'Sullivan, he is conducting a randomized, clinical trial of a family model of intensive education with outreach and follow-up to improve the outcomes of teenage mothers, their siblings, and infants. Dr. Schwarz is a founder of the West Philadelphia Collaborative Program for Child Health, a geographically based, multifaceted program to coordinate urban resources to improve adolescent and child health.

PAULINE M. (POLLY) SEITZ, R.N., M.S., M.P.A., is a Program Officer for the Robert Wood Johnson Foundation. Seitz is the Program Officer for the Strengthening Hospital Nursing Program. Seitz, a certified nurse-midwife, is a member of the American Nurses' Association, the National League for Nursing, the American College of Nurse-Midwives, the American Public Health Association, and Sigma Theta Tau.

CATHERINE M. STEVENSON, M.S.N., R.N.,C., C.R.N.P., is a Geriatric Nurse Practitioner at the Veterans Administration Medical Center Nursing Home, Philadelphia, and an adjunct clinical preceptor at the University of Pennsylvania.

NEVILLE E. STRUMPF, PH.D., R.N.,C., F.A.A.N., is Associate Professor and Director, Gerontological Nurse Clinician Program at the University of Pennsylvania. Her scholarly and research interests include older women, ethics and long-term care, and problems of frail elders in nursing homes, most notably overuse of physical restraints. Dr. Strumpf has consulted widely on gerontological nursing education, was a member of the ANA Task Force to Revise *A Statement of the Scope of Gerontological Nursing Practice*, and is a Fellow in the American Academy of Nursing.

MARGRETTA M. STYLES, R.N., ED.D., is Livingston Professor of Nursing at the University of California, San Francisco, where she teaches professional issues and nursing administration. She has for some years been interested in professional credentialing and regulation and has been involved in national and international studies and policy development in this area. Specifically, she chaired the National Study of

Credentialing in Nursing; she was project director for the International Council of Nurses (ICN) Study on Nursing Regulation and author of the ICN's position paper on the subject; she studied nursing specialty development and regulation as American Nurses' Foundation Distinguished Scholar, the study cited in her chapter in this volume. Styles is immediate past President of the American Nurses' Association and is currently on the ICN Board of Directors and chairperson of the Professional Services Committee. She is a member of the Institute of Medicine of the National Academy of Sciences.

GWEN VAN SERVELLEN, PH.D., R.N., is Associate Professor and Vice-Chair of the Psychiatric Mental Health Nursing and Administration section of the School of Nursing, University of California at Los Angeles. Dr. van Servellen's research interests include AIDS education, nursing care modalities, and variables affecting distress in persons with AIDS and their caregivers. Her funded studies here have been targeted at the stresses of hospitalization in persons with AIDS, the cost and quality of hospital care to persons with AIDS, job-related stress in nurses caring for HIV infected persons, and hope and psychological adversity in persons with AIDS and their supportive others. She is a member of the American Academy of Nursing; a member of the Scientific Advisory Committee of the American Foundation for AIDS Research; and she serves on the California Nurses' Association AIDS Education and Training Project Advisory Board.

CAROLYN A. WILLIAMS, R.N., PH.D., is Dean and Professor at the College of Nursing at the University of Kentucky in Lexington. She received a Master's Degree in Public Health Nursing Education from the University of North Carolina in 1965 and obtained a Ph.D. in Epidemiology from the University of North Carolina in 1969. Prior to appointment to the faculty at the University of Kentucky, she held several positions, including Staff Public Health Nurse, Associate Professor of Epidemiology in the School of Public Health, and Associate Professor of Nursing in the School of Nursing at the University of North Carolina in Chapel Hill; and Professor and Director of Graduate Programs and Research at the Neil Hodgson Woodruff School of Nursing, Emory University. Since 1968, she has been actively involved in educational and practice activities through her teaching appointments and her role as a consultant to a number of educational and service institutions, including the World Health Organization. She has held a number of national appointments, including membership on the President's Commission for the Study of Ethical Problems in Medicine and Biomedical and Behavioral Research, Washington, DC (1980–1982), and most recently served as a member of the U.S. Preventive Services Task Force, Office of the Assistant Secretary of Health, Washington, DC. She is a fellow of the American Public Health Association and the American Academy of Nursing, for which she served as President from 1983 to 1985.

# Preface

*C*HARTING NURSING'S FUTURE: *Agenda for the 1990s* is a book that contains many parts but is a cohesive whole. Its cohesion lies in the fact that it tells a story. The story is of accomplishment, achievement, innovation, passion, caring, and advocacy. Each chapter defines an area of concern that is directly tied to the needs of the public, sick or well. Tracing the past, describing the present, and outlining the future, the book frames the development of the profession in societal terms. The authors show, with clarity, the work of nursing in the public interest.

We wanted the book to represent the leading edge of thought on nursing. The authors included are pacesetters and pioneers in the field. We intended to be provocative, and to stimulate thought and action, but not necessarily agreement. The views expressed in each chapter, as should be expected from authors such as we have selected, are distinctly their own.

While there is considerable diversity in the subject matter, there is a pervasive theme underlying the content. This theme can best be expressed by the phrase "working in the public interest." All of the chapters deal with one or another area of serving the public, whether dealing with prevention, Medicare, hospital nursing, community health, or education; vulnerable populations such as the elderly, people with AIDS, the homeless, or the chronically mentally ill; or policy issues. The authors' concerns for their topics are within the broader perspective of meeting people's needs for health care.

The 1990s present challenges and opportunities for energetic, people-centered action—fueled by new ideas. Each chapter in the book presents such ideas, and we hope the book's story will be energizing to nurses, nursing students, policy makers, and others interested in the broad health world, of which nursing is a vital part.

We are indebted to our colleagues who took time out from busy schedules to write chapters for the volume. We would also like to acknowledge the assistance of Pamela Barry and Mariea Williams in managing the many details associated with editing a volume of this magnitude. Finally, we thank Diana Intenzo at Lippincott for encouraging us to take on this project.

Linda H. Aiken, Ph.D.
Claire M. Fagin, Ph.D.

# Contents

## PART III CHALLENGES AND OPPORTUNITIES ACROSS PRACTICE SETTINGS

PART IV   CARING FOR VULNERABLE GROUPS

PART V   SHAPING THE FUTURE

# CHARTING NURSING'S FUTURE

*Agenda for the 1990s*

# PART I

## Policy and Practice Debates

## Chapter 1

# Charting Nursing's Future

LINDA H. AIKEN

*T*HE BEGINNING of a new decade, the last in this century, presents an opportunity for reflection on past accomplishments, anticipation of future challenges, development of new agendas, and identification of strategies for achieving the unfinished agenda of the last decade in the next one. The purpose of this volume is to contribute to a productive dialogue on how nursing should position itself to be most effective as an advocate for the health of the American public, assuming that what is good for the public is also good for nursing. This introductory chapter reviews selected opportunities and dilemmas that will or have already surfaced to challenge the future directions and priorities of nursing. The following chapters examine each of these issues in greater depth and collectively point out an agenda for nursing in the decade of the 1990s.

## The Unfinished Agenda of the Eighties

The decade of the 1990s began on a negative note with a loud chorus of voices raised in criticism of American health care. Although the majority of Americans reported satisfaction with their own health care arrangements, a majority also agreed with the statement that so much was wrong with American health care that major system reform was needed (Freeman et al., 1987). Two thirds of the American public believe that people are beginning to lose faith in doctors; paradoxically, the growth of disillusionment with physicians has accompanied dramatic medical advances (Mechanic, 1985). Even hospitals, institutions that have enjoyed great community support over the years (Stevens, 1989), have suffered a decline in prestige. Consumers report that hospitals put too much emphasis on the financial aspects of their institution and too little on the reason for their existence—the care of sick people. Public opinion polls suggest that the more "businesslike" hospitals have become in the public's mind, the lower the public's level of trust and confidence in them. As a result, the quality of the nation's hospital care is ranked somewhat higher than that of automotive repair shops but lower than that of supermarkets and airlines (Blendon, 1988).

Even the continued impressive successes of biomedical research have been overshadowed by the inadequacies of the health care delivery system in bringing these advances to those most in need. A poignant but by no means unique illustration of the growing gap between what we know and what we do is the appalling tragedy of the inability of many of those infected with the human immunodeficiency virus to obtain needed care and access to the promising drugs developed by the nation's biomedical enterprise.

The decade of the eighties is remembered not in terms of the successes and accomplishments in health care but by the erosion of gains made in earlier decades. Topping the list of failures was the 25 percent increase in the number of Americans without health insurance, totaling 37 million people by the end of the decade (Congressional Research Service, 1988). This was a major reversal of a long-standing trend toward incrementally better insurance coverage for the American public that had been associated with better health. Access to health care deteriorated for the poor and minorities over the decade of the 1980s, particularly those in poor health (Freeman et al., 1987). Despite spending more on health care than any other country in the world, the United States ranks 17th among the world's nations with respect to infant mortality and 15th in life expectancy (Hiatt, 1987).

The average employed, insured American was not exempt from the chaos in health services. Consumers' out-of-pocket costs increased substantially as employers tried to control their escalating health insurance expenses by reducing coverage and increasing employee cost sharing. Among the memorable statistics of the 1980s, by 1987, employers' direct health care spending grew to 94 percent of net after-tax profits, and the total liabilities represented by health benefits promised by employers to their retirees totaled more than the net worth of many corporations (Levit, Freeland, & Waldo, 1989). Not surprisingly, health benefits became a contentious issue between unions and management, overshadowing wages as a reason for work stoppages and strikes.

Amidst all of the turmoil, nursing was the focus of unprecedented levels of public attention. Although the public's confidence in physicians, hospitals, and nursing homes eroded over the decade, nurses continued to be held in positive regard. A nationwide survey of public attitudes toward health care and nurses conducted in the late 1980s showed that the public admired nurses and that most people were willing to receive more of their health care from nurses (Hart, 1990). Three blue-ribbon panels on nursing were commissioned during the decade of the eighties, primarily in response to continuing reports of shortages of nurses (Institute of Medicine, 1983; National Commission on Nursing, 1983; U.S. Department of Health and Human Services Secretary's Commission on Nursing, 1988). At the request of the Congress, the Office of Technology Assessment undertook a major review of the evidence of the effectiveness of nurse practitioners. The review found overwhelming evidence that nurse practitioners practicing within their areas of expertise provide as good as or better quality of care than physicians and at lower overall costs (Office of Technology Assessment, 1986). Although serious impediments to their practices persist, nurse practitioners, nurse midwives, and nurse anesthetists were successful in achieving improved third-party reimbursement over the decade of the eighties.

Nurses also gained a foothold in national, state, and local public policy arenas during the 1980s. Using their voting strength, they effectively lobbied for the establishment of the National Center for Nursing Research within the National Institutes of Health, bringing nursing research into the mainstream of scientific inquiry. More nurses were elected or appointed to influential positions in public policy, including the chief of staff to the Senate Minority Leader of the United States Senate, Administrator of the Health Care Financing Administration (the agency that administers Medicare and Medicaid), and state health commissioner positions.

## Public Policy and Nursing

Given its recent victories, nursing enters the decade of the nineties ever more optimistic about public policy as a vehicle to advance its professional agenda and to improve health care. Thus, it is worth pausing here at the beginning of a volume that identifies a rich public policy agenda for nursing to focus on the public policy process.

The United States federal government owns and operates an insignificant portion of the health care system. Most of the approximately 6000 hospitals, 18,000 nursing homes, 570,000 physicians, and thousands of other health care facilities and businesses operate as private enterprises. Thus, the "health care system" in the United States is highly decentralized, as compared with many other Western democracies such as Canada and the United Kingdom. It is not possible, then, for the federal government to directly "legislate" many changes in health services delivery because health care providers are free to conduct their businesses as they choose. Moreover, in a federal form of government such as ours, the constituent units are separate and to a large extent independent financing powers. Under the Federal Constitution, the states retain for themselves all powers not specifically conferred upon the federal government. Thus, the central or federal United States government has limited powers to mandate national health policy. In fact, over the decade of the eighties, the political ideology of the executive branch of the federal government was to give the states greater discretion in establishing health policies and in allocating resources, including federal funds.

Federal health policy as we know it today grew out of the collapse of local governments and the American economy, in the Great Depression of 1929. The federal government not only assumed a larger role in public spending, which undercut the pre-eminence of local governments, but also moved toward centrally defined goals and standardized programs across the states (Hofferbert, 1974). The historic report of the Committee on Economic Security, which led to the Social Security Act of 1935, endorsed the principle of national health insurance. While more than 55 years have passed and we still do not have national health insurance, the stage was set for incremental federal steps toward greater involvement in health care (Somers & Somers, 1977).

Between 1935 and 1965, the federal government gradually assumed greater and greater responsibility for financing health services. Federal health policy became explicit in 1965 with the passage of Medicare and Medicaid. Since 1965, 68 million

Americans have been covered by Medicare, and the number of Medicaid recipients served annually has grown from 11.5 million in 1968 to 25 million in 1990. Medicare has paid more than $800 billion in benefits during its 25-year history; Medicaid has paid more than $500 billion (Firshein, 1990).

Once the federal government began to pay for health care for so many Americans, it necessarily became a federal commitment to ensure that adequate health resources were available. Thus, the federal government provided subsidies to expand the number of hospital beds and the supply of both physicians and nurses.

Because of the decentralized, highly private nature of health care in the United States, the federal and the state governments exert their influence on the organization and delivery of health care primarily through their purchasing power as the agents for almost 60 million Medicare and Medicaid beneficiaries. Together the federal and state governments account for 42 percent of all health care expenditures. Federal health spending alone in 1988 totaled $158 billion and accounted for 14 percent of all federal expenditures (Levit et al., 1990). The federal government can affect medical practice patterns by the "conditions" it attaches to reimbursement within its own programs. Moreover, since the federal government is the largest single purchaser of health care, its reimbursement decisions are often followed by private third-party payers, thus extending its influence throughout the health care system. Thus, the major vehicle government has to shape the contours of health care delivery is the use of financial incentives, particularly through reimbursement policies in federal health care programs.

Nursing has been effective in obtaining federal funding for nursing education and nursing research, and these funds have been critical in building a strong nursing infrastructure and leadership group. Only recently have nurses begun to pursue with vigor the possibilities of changing federal health care reimbursement policies to provide a more stable financial base for the expansion of nursing services.

## Nursing's Agenda for the Nineties

The prime challenges for nursing in the policy arena over this new decade are to effectively advocate expansion of health insurance coverage to those who are uninsured or underinsured at present *and* in the process to bring about a better match between services that are covered and the needs of the American public. Extending the existing insurance system to the 37 million uninsured would help improve access to care and add a measure of financial stability to nursing services in all settings. However, nursing should also advocate modifications in the structure of the existing insurance system to include better coverage of primary care, chronic illness care, and long-term care, which are all seriously neglected in the existing health insurance system. The Nurses' National Health Plan, discussed by Maraldo and Fagin in the final section of this volume, has as its objectives both universal insurance coverage and changes in benefit structure that recognize that the burden of illness and disability in the United States is increasingly of a more chronic, long-term nature requiring more than acute, episodic medical care.

Public policy changes usually require either a broad-based consensus on the key issues under debate or a narrow consensus among a recognized elite on highly technical issues of a less controversial nature or issues about which the public appears unconcerned. Timing is often of key importance. One of the purposes of this volume is to explore some of the issues currently under debate that have a chance of resulting in significant policy and/or organizational change over the next decade that could substantially affect nurses and nursing care. The following discussion highlights a few of the possibilities that are discussed in greater detail in the chapters that follow.

## Health Insurance

Opinion poll trends suggest that public support for a national health program that is totally government financed is now at the highest point since World War II and approximates the level of support for Medicare in the year before its enactment (Blendon & Donelan, 1990). What is lacking at this point is consensus about the particulars of such a program and how it should be financed. Several themes dominate public concern. Although many informed Americans recognize that health care is overly expensive and inefficient, they appear to reject the compromises made by other countries such as Canada and the United Kingdom that have achieved universal access to health care, namely, waiting periods for access to some expensive diagnostic and therapeutic technologies or limits to the public's freedom of choice of health care provider. Additionally, Americans seem to be much more adverse to solving some of these problems via taxation than people in other industrialized countries. In fact, despite popular opinion that taxes in this country are very burdensome, the United States has one of the lowest levels of taxation among the industrialized countries of the world (Estes & Newcomer, 1983). Another major stumbling block in extending health care coverage to the poor is the present linkage of Medicaid with welfare and the distaste of Americans for expanding welfare benefits. Ultimately, health care will probably have to be disentangled from welfare policy in order to implement universal coverage.

Given the ferment and continuing debate about universal entitlement to health care, it makes considerable sense for nursing to put forth its own proposals as well as participate in the ongoing debate. Although any expansion of insurance coverage will yield benefits to nurses because care of the populations they serve will be better financed than before, some of the services that nurses value most will still be without financing unless the benefit structure is changed. No other stakeholder in the current debate except nursing is seriously focusing on the need to reshape the benefit structure in an expanded insurance system except advocates for long-term care insurance benefits.

## Third-Party Reimbursement for Nurses

Many of the chapters in this volume present data documenting the cost-effectiveness of nursing care. In a context of national concern about rising health care costs, the track record of nurses for delivering care of high quality at lower costs will become an increasingly powerful lever to promote expansion of third-party reimbursement for nurses. The physician payment reform policies currently under development for the Medicare program and discussed in the chapter by Carol Lockhart open the door for debate about nurses' payment as well. On the surface, it would seem smart for nurses to accept a reimbursement rate set at some percentage of that received by physicians for the same service. Such a move might make direct reimbursement more palatable to policy makers, who fear that opening the door to a potentially large group of additional persons billing Medicare for services will only increase overall expenditures. There is a downside risk, however, in nurses' accepting only a percentage of the physician's fee for the same service. Most nurses are employed in organizations and group practices rather than self-employed. Lower reimbursement rates for nurses could discourage employers from hiring nurses or result in the use by employers of a physician's billing number rather than the nurse's, which defeats the rationale for direct third-party reimbursement for nurses.

A missing ingredient thus far in the debate over payment for nursing services is whether nurses' practice patterns vary significantly enough from those of physicians to result in patient utilization patterns with very different cost implications. Professional fees account for only about 20 percent of health expenditures, but the decisions professionals make account for most of the remainder. Thus, provider decision making is a much more important matter than provider fees from a cost perspective.

An impressive body of data is beginning to accumulate documenting that patients cared for by nurses have very different and less costly service utilization patterns. For example, nurse-midwives can be credited with providing care at substantially lower costs because of less use of inpatient care services and substantially fewer patients having cesarean sections (see Chapter 12 for a complete review of these data). A second less well-known example is the recent evidence from three multisite demonstrations (Aiken, 1990b) showing that the introduction of nurse practitioners into nursing homes results in substantial savings to the Medicare program because nursing home residents are much less likely to be hospitalized as a result of this additional care (see Chapter 14 for additional information).

The strongest position of nurses in the debate over professional fees is their ability to achieve good patient outcomes at lower costs because their practice patterns are different from those of physicians. Researchers should continue to amass data comparing nurse and physician practice patterns and outcomes to ensure that sufficient evidence is available to move nursing's professional agenda into the political arena. The recent expansion of Medicare Part B to reimburse for the services of nurse practitioners in nursing homes was achieved, in large part, by the availability of evaluation research results documenting reduced hospital use and cost savings.

## Nursing Shortage

Cyclical shortages of nurses since World War II have provided leverage in the policy arena to obtain nursing education subsidies, nursing research support, and sometimes special supportive legislative action, as in recent changes in immigration policy establishing priority for nurses from abroad seeking work visas. Yet, as Ginzberg (1990) notes, nursing has chosen to play both sides of the nursing shortage issue, advocating higher wages on the one hand and expansion of the supply of nurses on the other. These are contradictory positions. The greater the supply of nurses, the lower the market wage is likely to be.

The evidence strongly points to unbridled demand fueled by low relative wages and inappropriate deployment of nurses, particularly in hospitals, as the driving forces behind cyclical shortages (Aiken & Mullinix, 1987). It is difficult to identify a public policy strategy to intervene in a process that is largely dependent on the functioning of the labor market. This may explain why nursing continues to support initiatives to increase supply, since one of the things the Federal and state governments can do is to provide educational subsidies to expand educational opportunities in a given field (see Chapter 4 for more extensive discussion of the causes of nursing shortages).

Although there appears to be a sufficient supply of nurses in the aggregate to meet national needs now and in the near term (Aiken, 1990a), nursing still needs educational subsidies to meet its goal of upgrading the educational qualifications of the nurse pool. Close to 90 percent of nurses now receive their basic education in an institution of higher education compared with 20 percent in 1960. Although nurses with baccalaureate degrees or higher education are still in the minority, representing approximately one third of nurses, the numerical count is more impressive. More than 650,000 nurses have baccalaureate or higher degrees and one in every ten nurses is working on an advanced degree. Although nursing leaders were widely criticized for many years for promoting the baccalaureate degree as the entry credential for professional practice, the educational revolution has clearly taken root.

Aydelotte's chapter (Chapter 29) in this volume reviews the history of this revolution and concludes that nursing should set its sights higher—at the professional doctorate level to gain parity with other health professionals. Many will decide that this is an idea whose time has not yet come and may never arrive for a variety of reasons. But, even though only two schools have adopted the professional nurse doctorate and few of nursing's leaders support movement to the professional doctorate, the debate itself is further evidence of how far the educational revolution in nursing has advanced in a 30-year period.

The educational revolution in nursing was aided substantially by federal and state educational subsidies. The challenge for the future will be whether nursing can sell policy makers on the idea of targeting subsidies and student aid to baccalaureate and graduate level programs, which is where the need is given the very large existing supply of nurses. (The United States now has one nurse for every 145 Americans, most of whom are well most of the time.) The targeting of baccalaureate and higher education could be a "hard sell," as it can easily be seen as an elite strategy. Moreover, nursing has traditionally been a career offering its members upward mobility. Indeed, many nursing education programs still garner substantial local support because they target an applicant pool that is unlikely to enter a four-year college or university.

The educational revolution could be significantly slowed without public educational subsidies and student aid. Nursing students are significantly more likely than other college first-year students to come from families with parental income under $25,000 a year. Nursing students are more likely to have received Federal grants and loans based on economic need to finance their education, and more than twice as likely to work full time while attending college (unpublished data from the American Council of Education–UCLA Cooperative Institutional Research Program, 1989). Black and Hispanic students report greater dependence on loans, a higher average debt at graduation, and greater sensitivity to financial factors in deciding whether to attend college than do white students (Morhman, 1987). Blacks continue to be under-represented in the nursing profession relative to their numbers in the general population.

In this coming decade nursing needs to develop a more consistent policy with regard to nursing shortage. On the one hand, public subsidies are needed to continue to upgrade the educational level of the nurse pool and to provide opportunities for minority recruitment in order to redress current imbalances. On the other hand, there is ample evidence that further increases in the aggregate supply of nurses, whether through educational expansion or recruitment of foreign nurses, is not in the interests of meeting nurses' wage expectations.

## Opportunities for Change

Sometimes catastrophes present unusual opportunities to change the status quo. The acquired immunodeficiency syndrome (AIDS) is one example. This terrible epidemic has resulted in perhaps the largest "natural experiment" in hospital restructuring in recent memory. In a context in which the hospital industry had been relatively unresponsive to ample evidence from blue-ribbon expert panels and a number of studies of model hospital programs all suggesting that similar strategies would work to attract and retain nurses, the AIDS epidemic has actually been a catalyst for major experimentation in health services, particularly in hospitals (Fox, Aiken, & Messikomer, 1990).

Apparently motivated by concerns that insufficient numbers of nurses would be available to care for the expected increase in AIDS patients requiring hospitalization, some hospitals in large urban areas granted their nurses unusual latitude in designing and managing new specialized AIDS units. In late 1988, there were over 40 dedicated AIDS units nationwide (Taravella, 1989). There is little empirical evidence yet to confirm whether dedicated AIDS units are better or worse than scattering AIDS patients throughout the hospital. Yet, at the heart of the debate is whether dedicated AIDS units can attract and retain nurses.

Testimonials and descriptive information on some existing dedicated AIDS units suggest that not only can dedicated AIDS units attract nurses but some have waiting lists of nurses wanting to work in them. Although final judgment must be withheld until empirical research has been completed, including a national evaluation of dedicated AIDS units currently being conducted by the Center for Health Services and Policy Research at the University of Pennsylvania School of Nursing, published descriptions of successful AIDS units suggest that they have incorporated the dimensions of care long advocated by nurses but rarely seen in actual hospital settings (see, for example, Morrison, 1987; Gross, 1988; Fox et al., 1990).

In many ways, AIDS care is a worst case scenario for attracting nurses: the disease is potentially infectious and fatal; those likely to have AIDS belong to groups that are highly stigmatized; and forming close interpersonal relationships with people who will inevitably die soon is painful. If hospital units can be restructured to be so attractive to nurses that all of these potential negative aspects are overshadowed by the intrinsic rewards of professional nursing practice, the principal dimensions of the restructuring should also result in a positive outcome in other kinds of hospital units.

As unfortunate as the AIDS epidemic is, nursing care is key to the nation's response. The epidemic can be used as an opportunity to help people with AIDS and to solve some of nursing's long-standing problems.

## Concluding Comments

The ferment in all aspects of health care can only be positive for nursing because it is resulting in numerous innovations that offer nursing a plethora of opportunities for repositioning and strengthening the profession's power base. The purpose of this volume is to highlight some of the opportunities that could be seized and turned to nursing's advantage over the decade of the nineties, and to demonstrate forcefully that what is good for nursing is also good for the American public.

REFERENCES

Aiken, L.H. (1990a). Charting the future of hospital nursing. *Image: The Journal of Nursing Scholarship, 22*(2), 72–78.
Aiken, L.H. (1990b). *Educational innovations in gerontology: Teaching nursing homes and gerontological nurse practitioners.* The Beverly Lecture on Gerontology and Geriatrics Education, No. 5. Washington, DC: Association for Gerontology in Higher Education.
Aiken, L.H., & Mullinix, C.F. (1987). The nurse shortage: Myth or reality? *New England Journal of Medicine, 317,* 641–646.
American Council on Education (1989). [UCLA Cooperative Institutional Research Program]. Unpublished data.
Blendon, R.J. (1988). The public's view of the future of health care. *Journal of the American Medical Association, 259,* 3587–3593.
Blendon, R.J., & Donelan, K. (1990). The public and emerging debate over national health insurance. *New England Journal of Medicine, 323,* 208–212.
Congressional Research Service, Library of Congress (1988). *Health insurance and the uninsured: Background data and analysis.* Special Committee on Aging, Serial No. 100-1. Washington, DC: U.S. Government Printing Office.
Estes, C.L., & Newcomer, R.J. (1983). *Fiscal austerity and aging.* Beverly Hills, CA: Sage Library of Social Research, vol. 152.
Firshein, J. (1990). Medicare and Medicaid Turn 25. *Medicine and Health, 44*(30), July 30.
Freeman, H.E., Blendon, R.J., Aiken, L.H., Sudman, S., Mullinix, C., & Corey, C. (1987). Americans report on their access to care. *Health Affairs, 6,* 6–18.
Fox, R., Aiken, L.H., & Messikomer, C. (1990). The culture of caring: AIDS and the nursing profession. *Milbank Memorial Fund Quarterly, 68* (Suppl. 2), 226–256.

Ginzberg, E. (1990). *The medical triangle: Physicians, politicians and the public.* Cambridge, MA: Harvard University Press.

Gross, J. (1988, August 22). Mission of an AIDS unit is not to cure, but to care. *New York Times,* p. 1.

Hart, P.D. (1990). *A nationwide survey of attitudes toward health care and nurses.* Washington, DC: P.D. Hart Research Associates, Inc.

Hiatt, H.H. (1987). *America's health in the balance: Choice or chance?* New York: Harper & Row.

Hofferbert, R.I. (1974). *The study of public policy.* Indianapolis: Bobbs-Merrill.

Institute of Medicine (1983). *Nursing and nursing education: Public policies and private actions.* Washington, DC: National Academy Press.

Levit, K.R., Freeland, M.S., & Waldo, D.R. (1989). Health spending and ability to pay: Business, individuals, and government. *Health Care Financing Review, 10*(3), 1–11.

Levit, K.R., Freeland, M.S., & Waldo, R.R. (1990). National health care spending trends: 1988. *Health Affairs, 9*(2), 171–183.

Mechanic, D. (1985). Public perceptions of medicine. *New England Journal of Medicine, 312,* 181–183.

Mohrman, K. (1987). Unintended consequences of federal student aid policies. *The Brookings Review, 5,* 24–30.

Morrison, C. (1987). Establishing a therapeutic environment: Institutional resources. In J.D. Durham and F.L. Cohen (Eds.), *The person with AIDS: Nursing perspectives* (pp. 110–125). New York: Springer Publishing Co.

National Commission on Nursing (1983). *Summary report and recommendations.* Chicago: Hospital Research and Hospital Trust.

Office of Technology Assessment (1986). *Study of the effectiveness of nurse practitioners, nurse midwives, and physician assistants.* Washington, DC: U.S. Congress.

Somers, A.R., & Somers, H.M. (1977). *Health and health care: Policies in perspective.* Germantown, MD: Aspen Systems Corporation.

Stevens, R. (1989). *In sickness and in wealth: American hospitals in the twentieth century.* New York: Basic Books.

Taravella, S. (1989). Reserving a place to treat AIDS patients in the hospital. *Modern Healthcare, 19,* 32–39.

U.S. Department of Health and Human Services (1988). *Secretary's Commission on Nursing: Final report.* Washington, DC: U.S. Department of Health and Human Services.

## Chapter 2

# Cost-Effectiveness of Nursing Care Revisited: 1981–1990

CLAIRE M. FAGIN

*D*ESPITE INCREASINGLY AGGRESSIVE efforts to contain health care costs over the decade of the 1980s, expenditures continue to increase at rates well over the growth in the general economy. Mounting concern on the part of government, employers, and insurers suggests that the 1990s may lead to more powerful efforts to examine alternatives for quality health care at reduced cost. Nursing is in a unique position among health care providers to respond to these efforts and is ready to provide evidence of its cost-effectiveness.

In earlier articles (Fagin, 1982a,b; Fagin & Jacobsen, 1985) I discussed the pro-competition environment of the early 1980s. The cumulative evidence showed that nurses provided cost-effective care that substituted for physician services in many situations and new and important services in long-term care and nursing homes. These findings led me to call for increased third-party reimbursement for nurses in areas where efficacy had been proved. There has been considerable progress in the reimbursement of nurses over this decade, but not nearly enough in view of the growing evidence from research that nurses achieve outcomes as good as or better than physicians in broad areas of primary care and midwifery, and at lower overall costs.

The purpose of this chapter is to update my previous synthesis of research on the cost-effectiveness of nursing care. It focuses on research published in the 1980s and re-examines the issues of costs and outcomes from professional and policy perspectives.

## Nursing in Hospitals

Hospital care is the largest health care expenditure. Thus cost containment pressures have and will continue to focus on inpatient care. Quality and cost tradeoffs in hospitals dominate the literature, with concerns about diminished quality resulting from cost constraints, early discharge, the nursing shortage, and managed care expressed by professionals and consumers alike.

There is a growing body of research linking surgical volume (hence experience) with lower inpatient mortality (Bennett et al., 1989; Hannan et al., 1989). Similarly, a comparative study of 30 hospital emergency departments showed a positive correlation between hospital size and the quality of both medical and nursing care (Georgopoulos, 1985).

Several studies have pointed to the importance of nurses or nurse-physician relationships in patient outcome. One study found "significant associations between higher mortality rates among inpatients and the stringency of state programs to review hospital rates . . . the stringency of certificate-of-need legislation . . . and the intensity of competition in the marketplace, as measured by enrollment in health maintenance organizations" (Shortell & Hughes, 1988). The higher the percentage of registered nurses, the lower the mortality rates were. This finding is substantiated by other studies showing that hospitals with a high proportion of registered nurses provide a better quality of care, as measured by lower mortality rates (Hartz, Krakauer, & Kuhn, 1989).

These studies suggest that the greater the experience of the "medical" team, the better the patient outcomes. The specific contributions of nurses to these improved outcomes have not been well documented. Nor is it clear what specific impact nurses' experience or level of education has on improved outcomes. More targeted research is necessary to clarify the relationships.

In addition, more recent publications often document cost savings resulting from a higher productivity of registered nurses in institutions employing a large number of registered nurses. For example, in one hospital, researchers compared the changes in dependency needs of patients between 1969 and 1985 and the percentage of registered nurses during the same time periods. The study showed that although there was a 13 percent decrease in occupancy on medical units in the two time periods, acuity had indeed risen sharply. "In 1972, the nursing salary budget supported 1169 full-time equivalents (FTEs), of whom 36% were registered nurses. In 1985, the nursing salary budget supported 1618 FTEs, of whom 94 percent were registered nurses (approximately 15 percent with master's or doctoral degrees). In 1972 the nursing salary budget represented 17.8 percent of the corporate budget; in 1985, however, nursing accounted for only 14.7 percent of the corporate budget" (Donovan & Lewis, 1987). Nursing productivity increased sharply between the two time periods in that more than twice the amount of patient care was given in the same amount of time during the second period. Other studies support the same conclusion and indicate that lower turnover among nurses results from increased job satisfaction derived from the more professional work force with concomitant increases in autonomy and flexibility (Dahlen & Gregor, 1985; Wolf et al., 1986).

Concern regarding collaboration between physicians and nurses continues. Whether real progress has been made in further developing the relationships between nurses and physicians is not clear; however, there are indications that in certain areas the collaborative relationship is vital and thriving. Many authors show positive results when nurses and physicians collaborate in care of the elderly, in discovering ameliorative procedures for managing pressure sores, in the administration of analgesia, and in other inpatient and out of hospital health and medical care activities. Further exploration is needed of the dynamics of the nurse-physician relationship in the areas of the barriers to collaboration and the outcome of successful and unsuccessful interactions (DeFede et al., 1989; Kitz et al., 1989).

One of the most important recent studies on the impact of nurse-physician collaboration was an evaluation of mortality in intensive care units in 13 tertiary care hospitals. The researchers compared actual and predicted death rates for 5030 patients in intensive care units and found significant differences in mortality among the hospitals. Taking into account the severity of illness of patients across these hospitals, the most important factor contributing to differences in mortality rates was physician-nurse communication. This factor was even more important than teaching status or the presence of an intensive care unit medical director (Knaus, Draper, Wagner, & Zimmerman, 1986).

Many articles were published during the 1980s that described specific and new nursing interventions. Some have evaluated the cost-effectiveness of these nursing interventions. Nurse investigators have discussed the use of restraints and ways to improve the individual's capacity for daily living (Evans, Stumpf, & Williams, 1991). Numerous papers have been published describing nursing programs to help patients with cancer and their families deal with the illness and treatment. Many of these studies show positive outcomes with regard to patient attitude, compliance, and tension reduction.

One interesting study reports the implementation of a surgical nurse coordinator program utilizing operating room nurses to improve communication for patients and their families during the perioperative period (Watson & Hickey, 1984). Since the program did not require additions of nursing staff, it was viewed as "cost-effective." The quality outcomes are clear: ". . . the families now gather in one area to await information instead of being scattered throughout the hospital. . . . The recovery room notes fewer calls from patient units, and anxious parents or spouses seldom wait outside the doors to catch a glimpse of the patient. . . . The time spent by floor nurses and evening supervisors in pacifying angry relatives is virtually eliminated" (Watson & Hickey, 1984).

Other innovative nursing interventions that have been evaluated include programs of shorter stays for patients, with heavy reliance on nursing care and observation (Balik et al., 1988; Boland, 1985); competitive programs with monetary incentives; and alternative nursing schedules or flextime, which contributed to increased productivity and cost-effective outcomes (Elliott, 1989).

Several studies examine nursing costs from the standpoint of diagnostic related groups (DRGs) or other patient classification systems. These studies indicate the extreme cost-effectiveness of nursing personnel and, in some instances, suggest that nursing care is far less costly than nurses themselves might think (Bailie, 1986; McKibben, 1982; Mitchell et al., 1984; Riley & Schaefers, 1983; Sovie et al., 1985; Walker, 1985; "What's the cost," 1986; Wilson et al., 1988).

Far fewer articles about the benefits of primary nursing and all registered nursing staffs were found in this current review than in the review 10 years ago. Some nursing administrators believe that a staff of all registered nurses has become almost a luxury in this time of nursing shortage.

A larger study using the data base of the Medicus Nursing Productivity and Quality system found productivity and quality improvement, even in the face of staff cutting and cost reduction. They attribute this finding to the "widespread increase in the use of RNs. Every nursing manager . . . cited this as a significant factor in improved quality in their institution" (Helt & Jelinek, 1988). The hospitals in the study were mostly large, urban, teaching facilities using the Medicus Nursing Productivity and Quality system, whose "production-unit-based information systems" are reported to receive high marks from the users at all levels. Other studies support these findings and suggest that cost savings are demonstrated in staff turnover, low sick time, length of patient hospital stay, and overtime (LaForme, 1982; Hinshaw et al., 1981).

Over this decade considerable interest has been shown in the concept of primary nursing in many parts of the world. Research in this area has been reported in all English language nursing journals. Although results of studies of primary nursing are somewhat mixed as to cost-effectiveness, there appears to be a sizable body of literature supporting the view that primary nursing is worth trying, that its implementation is a worthwhile experience for both patients and nurses, and that the outcomes may be significantly better than for other forms of nursing organization (MacDonald, 1988; Sellick et al., 1983).

Overall, these studies of organization of nursing services have revealed important outcomes in quality and cost resulting from volume of care, experience of providers, collaboration between nurses and physicians, and the cost-effectiveness of nursing care in hospitals (as a portion of hospital charges); they have also expressed an overall positive view of an all registered nurse staff and of primary nursing and the positive effects of schedule flexibility, autonomy, and monetary incentives. Further research is necessary to quantify and evaluate the clinical efficacy of nursing interventions, the value of experience and education of nurses in improving patient outcomes, and the organizational designs that work best to facilitate nursing and patient satisfaction. These kinds of studies will greatly strengthen nursing's participation in technology assessment.

The lack of uniform standards for outcome evaluation is interesting to consider in light of the need to quantify nursing's contributions to health care. The Nursing Minimum Data Set (NMDS) was an initial effort to establish such standards and "draws on the documentation of the nursing process that occurs whenever nurses provide care to people in any setting" (Werley & Zorn, 1989). The NMDS includes specific items used on a regular basis by the majority of nurses involved in health care delivery. Its purposes are "(1) to establish comparability of nursing across clinical populations, settings, geographic areas, and time; (2) to describe the nursing care of patients or clients and their families in a variety of settings; . . . (3) to demonstrate or project trends regarding nursing care needs and allocation of nursing resources . . . ; and (4) to stimulate nursing research through links to the detailed data existing in nursing information systems . . ." (Werley & Zorn, 1989). Werley has been engaged in the process of developing and testing the concept of the NMDS for over 10 years and there is, currently, considerable interest in the method in the United States and internationally.

The NMDS includes nursing care, patient or client demographics, and service elements. There is not yet an acceptable scheme for categorizing nursing interventions, and research and development are urgently recommended by Werley and associates. Germane to this chapter is the view that an NMDS would provide improved data for quality assurance and costing of nursing services. Health policy debates frequently do not include nursing concerns and recommendations because data on nursing are incomplete.

The NMDS is said to be invaluable to nurse researchers interested in the "broad areas of the process, outcome or cost of nursing care." A review of the literature did not reveal studies that utilized the NMDS in the way proposed by Werley and others interested in this method. It may be that NMDS is what is needed to give similarity of form to outcome studies, but work is needed to determine the efficacy of this method for this purpose.

## Substitution of Nurses for Other Providers

Two major reviews of the practice and cost-effectiveness of nurse practitioners were published during the decade. In 1983, the American Nurses Association (ANA) published a review of the literature on the impact of nurse practitioners (NPs), and in 1986 the Office of Technology Assessment published its review of the work of NPs and other nonphysician providers. The OTA concluded that NPs, physician assistants, and certified nurse-midwives (CNMs) provide care of quality comparable to physician care, and that "NPs and CNMs are more adept than physicians at providing services that depend on communication with patients and preventive actions." The Office of Technology Assessment report recommends extending reimbursement to these nurses and believes that in some settings this "could benefit the health status of . . . segments of the population currently not receiving appropriate care [and that among the] long term effects could be a decrease in total costs."

The results of the ANA (1983) review of the literature on NPs indicated consistent findings of cost-effectiveness, evidence of better control of obesity and hypertension among clients of NPs as compared with clients of physicians, relief of symptoms, compliance with appointments and treatment regimen, and continuity of care. Further, the review indicated that clients of NPs had fewer emergency room visits and documented an increase in clients returning to work and better results in a variety of other areas. Other studies carried out during the decade support these data. For example, one study showed that nurses provide more health education than physician providers and more follow-up care (Bibb, 1982), whereas others documented reductions in health-related costs, diagnostic tests, and medication use while maintaining quality of care. The latter studies also refuted a commonly held assumption that NPs take more time with patients, thus eliminating the cost differential between nurses and physicians. Indeed, in one study it was found that physicians' initial visit times were shorter than those of NPs but follow-up visit times were similar for both. Per episode, costs when NPs were the initial providers were 20 to 50 percent lower than when physicians were the initial providers (Salkever, Skinner, Steinwachs, & Katz, 1982).

In a review of evaluation research on nurse practitioners, Prescott and Driscoll concluded that the majority of studies reported no difference between nurse practitioners and physicians on many measures but that "the findings which indicated nurse practitioners score higher than physicians have been frequently overlooked." These included such areas as discussion about child care, preventive health, amount of advice offered, therapeutic listening and support, completeness of history taken, interviewing skills, and patients' knowledge about their management plan (Prescott & Driscoll, 1980). Wanting to understand whether and why such differences occur, the study compared outcomes in two groups of patients attending a hypertension clinic (Ramsay, McKenzie, & Fish, 1986). One group was seen by physicians and the other by nurses. Treatment outcome variables and patient compliance were compared, and the findings indicated superior outcomes in the nurse-staffed clinic for weight reduction, blood pressure reduction, and patient attrition. It is interesting to note that even though physicians referred nearly half of their patients to dietitians, weight control was poorer in this group.

During the 1980s, Ginsberg, Marks, and Waters continued their comparative studies of the use of nurse psychotherapists. Their most recent work was a randomized, controlled trial of behavioral psychotherapy provided by nurse therapists compared with routine management by the patient's general practitioner. Most of the patients had phobic disorders. At the end of one year, clinical outcomes "were significantly better in patients cared for by the nurse therapist" (Ginsberg et al., 1984). Economic outcomes were also better for the nursing group because the general practitioners prescribed more drugs and hospital treatment.

Studies that examined the use of NPs in occupational health settings also documented improved outcomes at lower costs. Annual cost savings were achieved by more effective handling of employee health problems and reductions in related health care utilization. One study reported a benefit/cost ratio of 2.1:1.0 for in-house primary care delivered by NPs as compared with physicians (Scharon & Bernacki, 1984).

There is no need to repeat the strong conclusions regarding the cost-effectiveness and quality of care of nurse-midwives reported in earlier articles. Suffice it to say that over 25 years of study of the practice of nurse-midwives has revealed excellent results for both cost and quality (Diers, 1982). The latest survey of maternity care costs makes the argument for midwife care of healthy maternal patients even more compelling. This report of findings of a 1989 survey of 173 community hospitals, 70 childbirth centers, and 153 licensed midwives reveals that the average cost of a nurse-midwife's services is $994 compared with physicians' fees for a normal pregnancy and delivery of $1492. The cost of a cesarean section averages $7186 (Minor, 1989).

Sufficient evidence is available to conclude that the NP is a provider who can maintain or increase quality of care at lower cost than physicians in a number of areas of vital importance. In this section I have discussed NPs as replacements for physicians in care traditionally provided in our health care system. I will discuss NPs further in terms of new and alternative modes of care in the section that follows.

## Alternative Models of Practice

The studies relating to alternative modes of practice deal with innovative practices of care of the elderly and with home or community care. Early patient discharge from the hospital with nurse follow-up, home nursing care with a variety of populations, and care of teen-aged mothers and their children are also included in this survey. Nurses are engaged in solving the most pressing health problems of our society, and their work is exemplary in cost and outcome. In addition to reviewing individual studies, I will discuss three large-scale, systematic studies and several review articles about the cost-effectiveness of home care. In addition, I have included here a study that describes a system of nursing care management that implements a nursing network of all care services.

### Nursing Homes and Geriatric Nurse Practitioners

The evaluation of the Robert Wood Johnson National Teaching Nursing Home (TNH) Program offers important insights about the value of professional nursing. The evaluation of this experiment at 11 sites, which tested the outcomes of affiliation between nursing homes and university schools of nursing, found that the TNH approach reduced hospitalization rates for nursing home patients and fostered an environment conducive to maximizing patients' physical and cognitive functioning (Shaughnessy, Kramer, & Hittle, 1988). These accomplishments occurred at no additional cost, and reductions in hospitalization created substantial savings for Medicare. The evaluators recommended that the teaching nursing home approach be encouraged on a more widespread basis by Medicare and Medicaid. Specifically, they recommended reimbursement for the cost of nurse clinicians, education for aides, and selected educational programs, since these resulted in lower hospitalization rates for TNH patients in contrast with those in the comparison nursing homes (Shaughnessy et al., 1988).

Another comparative study examined quality of care and health services utilization in 30 nursing homes employing geriatric nurse practitioners versus those in 30 matched control homes (Kane et al., 1989). There were a number of quality improvements in the geriatric nurse practitioner group, including reduction in hospital admissions, reduction in use of restraints, and increase in the number of patients discharged to their homes. The potential to reduce total costs of care "is suggested by the data on hospital utilization, especially the reduction in hospital days. The savings occur through fewer hospitalizations and less emergency room use" (Kane et al., 1989).

An interesting analysis modeled outcomes of nursing home care by demonstrating that use of resources, as measured by minutes of nursing time, is associated with patient outcomes (Rohrer & Hogan, 1987). The results of this study indicated that care given by nurses, psychosocial care, and physician care were related to future functional status. The study does not differentiate among nurses offering "basic services" and does not investigate the cost/quality possibilities of upgrading nursing credentials versus adding other providers, such as physicians or others offering psychosocial care.

### Community and Home Care

The effectiveness of a team approach to outpatient geriatric care was established through a randomized controlled clinical trial. The experimental group was cared for by a team that included physicians, nurses, social workers, and nutritionists. The control group was cared for by physicians alone. The team assessed the patients' physical, mental, and social functioning and provided counseling and family support to the experimental group as compared with the control intervention of only physician care. Hospital lengths of stay were 39 percent shorter for the experimental group over a 12-month period. The net result was a 25 percent reduction in cost for the treatment group. There was no reduction in satisfaction or functional level of the patient.

The literature has been greatly enriched during this decade by a number of studies of the cost-effectiveness of community and home care. The weakness in most of the series reviewed was that community care did not substitute for nursing home or hospital care but rather added to existing care. Thus, costs were increased overall (Berkeley Planning Associates, 1987). The Channeling Demonstration is an example of this phenomenon. It was ". . . a rigorous test of the effectiveness of comprehensive case management and expanded community services . . . as a way to contain the costs of long-term care of the elderly and to improve the quality of life of elderly clients . . . " and their caretakers (Carcagno & Kemper, 1988). Ten sites were included in the final evaluation. The evaluation found that average costs of caring for these patients increased because the cost of expanding case management and formal community services was not offset by reductions in nursing home or other types of care. The Channeling Demonstration did produce some increase in the measured well-being of clients and caretakers (Thornton, Dunston, & Kramer, 1988).

Weissert's review of a decade of research on home and community-based care concludes that "Community care rarely reduces nursing home or hospital use; it provides only limited outcome benefits; and to this point, it has usually raised overall use of health services as well as total expenditures" (Weissert, 1985).

The questions about cost in these studies appears conclusive. However, the assumption that community care would reduce cost was, in my opinion, erroneous in the first place because the demonstrations did not mandate specific populations where such care would more likely be substitutive. Further, at this time, there is considerable interest in community services for all functionally dependent people, including the elderly. Recognition that services to this population should not be compared with costs for a nursing home alternative is proposed by Weissert and others. Other writers examining the same or additional information stress the "need for additional methodologically rigorous research to assess the effectiveness of home care" (Green, 1989; Hedrick & Inui, 1986).

Besides cost reduction, there are important reasons for providing home care and other forms of community care. The outcry on the part of some of the public in response to Medicare's Catastrophic Care Coverage was, in part, related to a correct perception that this coverage would not provide for long-term or chronic care in the home and community. There are programs that have demonstrated considerable savings when community care is *substituted* for institutional long-term care. The OnLok Senior Health Services Community Care Organization, which manages and delivers all long-term care services to its clients, finds community care 26 percent lower in costs than institutional care (Berkeley Planning Associates, 1987). The Nursing Home Without Walls Program in New York State has shown that it can provide care for patients in the community at 50 percent of the cost of institutional care. Thus, despite the negative conclusions reported by many of the studies cited above and in other reviews (General Accounting Office Report, 1983), many private and state payers draw different conclusions from their experiences.

The Health Insurance Association of America, Blue Cross and Blue Shield Association, Aetna Life and Casualty, and others appear convinced that home care is a cost-effective offering. Several states and counties and Visiting Nurse Associations have instituted and studied programs offering community care and have found them to be uniformly successful in reducing costs *if they have served as an alternative for other care.* Such services to the chronically ill and the functionally impaired appear to private and governmental payers to be cost-effective alternatives (Cabin, 1985). Kramer and coworkers provide data to support the views of the payers. After assessing the mix of patients currently treated in nursing homes and home health agencies, they drew inferences about the cost-effectiveness of the two modalities (Kramer, Shaughnessy, & Pettigrew, 1985). They concluded that home health care is a cost-effective alternative to acute care hospital use at the end of a hospital stay and may prevent exacerbations of medical problems resulting in rehospitalization (Kramer et al., 1985). Also, home health care might be a more viable option in the care of patients who are neither severely disabled nor have profound functional problems.

It is important to note here that these studies are not nursing studies per se; however, any study of home care or community care of a functionally impaired population at risk must be presumed to lean heavily on nursing because these are the services this population requires directly from nurses or services that are managed by nurses.

Nurses have done important research on home and community care during this decade. Most of these studies utilized clinical nurse specialists working with a variety of populations in innovative ways to shorten hospitalization, improve outcomes of care, or both.

McCorkle (McCorkle et al., 1989) studied home nursing care follow-up of a group of patients with progressive lung cancer by master's-prepared oncology nurses. The results of this study indicated that patients receiving home care had less symptom distress and social dependency than a group receiving only office care. The total length of hospital stays was lower among the specialized home care group as compared with the control groups. The quality outcomes are clear and obviously resulted in cost reductions because of decreased rates of complications and hospitalizations.

Another study of home follow-up services by clinical nurse specialists was done by Burgess (Burgess et al., 1987). When master's-prepared nurse specialists followed up postmyocardial infarction patients at home, the patients suffered less psychological distress and were less dependent on family supports than the control group.

The aforementioned populations are particularly amenable to innovative nursing interventions, and more recent studies can be expected to examine cost directly rather than by implication of outcome. For example, Naylor's (Naylor, 1990) randomized clinical trial compared the effects of a comprehensive discharge planning protocol implemented by a gerontologic nurse specialist with the hospital's standard discharge planning procedure. Rehospitalizations and total costs were reduced in the experimental group. Naylor's current research involves a large sample of elderly patients and addresses the cost issues in more detail and more extensively.

Teen-aged pregnancy and low birth weight infants are problems of great concern to American society and to health care providers. Nurses are making major contributions in these important areas through practice and research. O'Sullivan's (O'Sullivan & Jacobsen, unpublished) randomized trial of a health care program for infants of first-time adolescent mothers demonstrated that this comprehensive program reduced dropout rates from school, repeat pregnancies, and emergency room use. The number of fully immunized infants increased. The experimental group received routine and additional services, including counseling about returning to school, use of family planning methods, and extra health care teaching from pediatric nurse practitioners and trained volunteers. The public cost of teenage childbearing has been estimated at $15,620 per child (Burt, 1986). Thus the 18 prevented pregnancies in this group could be said to have resulted in savings of $281,160. The most interesting factor of the special program was that it not only reduced system costs by the outcome, but the program itself was less expensive by $16.00 per client per visit than routine care for the following reasons: volunteer teaching of self-care for certain procedures; the pediatric nurse practitioner and the physician gave the immunizations rather than an additional registered nurse; less space was needed per provider; and no teaching of residents was involved. Clearly, even with teaching costs added, the program would be less costly than routine care because of the change in style of health care delivery. The effectiveness of this program in cost and quality is impressive even without attempting to quantify the increase in accountability among volunteers and clients.

A recent study of women in a rural area near Elmira, New York, showed that home visits by nurses to low-income women during and after pregnancy to teach them the basics of childrearing resulted in less child abuse, healthier babies, and better employment and educational achievements by the mothers. The vast majority of the women were teenagers and unmarried (Olds, Henderson, Tatelbaum, & Chamberlin, 1988). As in the O'Sullivan study, the subsequent pregnancies were 43 percent lower than in the control group, and the young women in the experimental group returned to school more rapidly. Both of these studies reveal the weaknesses in our current reimbursement policies, in which these nurse practitioners must be "hidden" in the system rather than accessed directly by clients for their valuable services of health promotion, counseling, direct care, and education.

The definitive work in cost and quality during this decade is that of Brooten (Brooten et al., 1986) dealing with early discharge of very low birth weight infants, with home follow-up by nurse specialists. In this study, very low birth weight infants were discharged from the hospital early and received home follow-up services from a master's-prepared perinatal nurse specialist. The group of infants was discharged a mean of 11 days earlier, 200 g less in weight, and 2 weeks younger than the control group. There was a mean saving of $18,560 per infant over conventional care.

Brooten's work highlights the need for randomized clinical trials of nursing interventions and alternatives to traditional practices. She provides a useful model for study using master's-prepared clinical specialists with advanced practice skills. Although there is a growing body of literature on home care using similar models, there is a paucity of such work attesting to the cost-effective practice of in-hospital clinical specialists. Many writers believe that clinical specialists with advanced practice skills are cost-effective providers in hospitals. Others report positive results in influencing care delivery through nurse specialists' interaction with staff. Despite a consensus on the high value of clinical nurse specialists among nurses, additional research is crucial for understanding and providing a rationale for the support of clinical nurse specialists during an era of cost containment.

## Case Management

Many articles during this decade discuss case management as an organizational strategy for improving the cost-effectiveness of nursing in hospitals. However, the authors do not present their work in a way that allows us to draw conclusions as to cost-effectiveness or quality outcomes. Some articles describe case management as an organizational structure for hospital patient care. Others define case management as "a set of logical steps and a process of interaction with service networks, which assures that a client receives needed services in a supportive, effective, efficient, and cost-effective manner" (Weil & Karls, 1985). Concerned about the increased number of patients with complicated care needs, one ambulatory care center established a case management system using registered nurses to make primary care more accessible. Preliminary findings show improved quality of care and cost reduction through reduced hospitalization. There was also an increase in patient counseling and health education and promotion activities (Winder, 1988).

One article offers an interesting model that has implications for the future world of health care delivery. It describes a nursing network that includes acute care inpatient services, extended care/long-term services, home care, hospice, and ambulatory care services. The last group includes both traditional physician services and nurse-managed community based clinics (Ethridge & Lamb, 1989). Preliminary analysis of data indicates that "nurse case managers appear to exert a financial impact through decreased length of stay . . . even though case-managed patients had a higher average acuity . . . than non-case-managed patients."

The alternative care models identified during this decade and summarized here have important benefits for patients and have been shown to be cost-effective additions or alternatives to traditional care.

## Summary and Conclusion

During the decade of the 1980s, nurses and others have examined many aspects of nursing interventions from the perspective of cost and quality. This work has covered the gamut of clinical care integral to the broadest definition of nursing and dealt with patient populations from the neonate and the pregnant woman to the extreme elderly. Stimulated by the changes in hospital reimbursement, a great deal of attention has been paid to the organization and cost of nursing services within hospitals. This chapter has summarized the papers reviewed in three categories: (1) those dealing with nursing care in hospitals; (2) those dealing with nurse practitioners substituting for other providers; and (3) alternatives to traditional modes of care.

There are some areas where more work is needed to flesh out strong impressions and beginning data. This is particularly the case in relation to the clinical nurse specialist, community care, and organization of nursing services in nursing homes. However, even in these areas, the data are accumulating to attest to the powerful contribution nurses are making to enhancing the quality of care, promoting health, and lowering total system costs. What is very clear is that nursing is a bargain, in and out of hospitals. We need to make the results of these studies available to policy makers and the public, since they strongly support nursing's political agenda and provide a solution to the cost problems plaguing our country.

Many believe the myth that increasing nursing compensation is not affordable given cost constraints. Yet, a cursory glance at the many articles examining cost of nursing care in this chapter and others in the book will debunk that myth and force exploration of where the money for health care is currently going. It is not going to nursing care. Nurse administrators in hospitals have shown both their accountability and loyalty as they have worked diligently to contain costs without sacrificing quality. However, hospital boards need to be familiar with the facts about nursing's small share of the hospital dollar as they plan and implement hospital policy for spending and saving.

Reviewing the data on nurse practitioners and nurse midwives gives rise to the reaction: Enough! There is no excuse for the perpetuation of policies that restrict the practices of NPs. Although there has been progress on a state-by-state basis in reimbursement for NPs, the limited public awareness of nursing's unique contribution has not been much improved in this decade.

As was said earlier, "Lack of public access to nursing outcome data . . . nursing's reluctance to make their contributions known, [and] . . . the way payment for institutional nursing services is handled in most settings" support nursing's low profile in all areas but the nursing shortage in hospitals. It is ironic that the extreme shortage of registered nurses in nursing homes is barely mentioned in the press.

The invisibility of nursing is causing problems more serious than those affecting the individual nurse's image. It is creating a dangerous situation with regard to the future pool of nurses, since fewer young people want a career in which practitioners appear unappreciated and unable to practice at their full potential. Nurses have the knowledge and skill to act independently, cost-effectively, and accountably in a vast array of services needed by the American people. The articles reviewed in this chapter attest to this fact.

In *Poor Richard's Almanac*, Benjamin Franklin wrote:

> Hide not your talents
> They for use were made
> What's a sundial in the shade?

## REFERENCES

American Nurses' Association (1983). *Nurse practitioners: A review of the literature (1965–1982)*. Kansas City, MO: American Nurses' Association.

Bailie, J.S. (1986). *Determining nursing costs: The nursing intensity index* (pp. 199–211). New York: National League for Nursing Publication, No. 20–2155.

Balik, B., Seitz, C.H., & Gilliam, T. (1988). When the patient requires observation not hospitalization. *Journal of Nursing Administration, 18*(10), 20–23.

Bennett, C.L., Garfinkle, J.B., Greenfield, S., Draper, D., Williams, R., Matthews, W.C., & Kanouse, D.E. (Eds.) (1989). The relation between hospital experience and in-hospital mortality for patients for AIDS-related PCP. *Journal of the American Medical Association, 261*, 2975–2979.

Berkeley Planning Associates (1987). *Evaluation of community-oriented long-term care demonstration projects.* Health Care Financing Extramural Report. Health Care Financing Administration Pub. No. 0342, Washington, DC: U.S. Government Printing Office.

Bibb, B. (1982). Comparing nurse practitioners and physicians on processes of care. *Evaluation and Health Professions, 6*(3), 28–42.

Boland, L.S. (1985). An interim stay unit reduces costs. *Journal of Nursing Administration, 18*, 42–45.

Brooten, D., Kumar, S., Brown, L., Butts, P., Finkler, S.A., Bakewell-Sachs, J., Gibbons, A., & Delivoria-Papadopoulos, M. (1986). A randomized clinical trial of early hospital discharge and home follow up of very low birthweight infants. *New England Journal of Medicine, 315*(15), 934–939.

Burgess, A.W., Lerner, D.J., D'Agostino, R.B., Vokonas, P.S., Hartman, C.R., & Gaccione, P. (1987). A randomized control trial of cardiac rehabilitation. *Social Science and Medicine, 24*, 359–370.

Burt, M.R. (1986). *Estimates of public costs of teenage childbearing: A review of recent studies and estimates of 1985 public cost.* Washington, DC: Center for Population Options.

Cabin, W. (1985, May). Some evidence of the cost-effectiveness of home care. *Caring, 4*, 62–67, 70.

Carcagno, G.J., & Kemper, P. (1988). The evaluation of the national long-term care demonstration 1: An overview of the channeling demonstration and its evaluation. *Health Services Research, 23*(1), 2.

Dahlen, A.L., & Gregor, J.R. (1985). Nursing costs by DRG with an all-RN staff. In F.A. Shaffer, (Ed.), *Costing out nursing: Pricing our Product* (pp. 113–122). New York: National League for Nursing Publication, No. 20–1982.

DeFede, J.P., Dhanens, B.E., & Keltner, N.L. (1989). Cost benefits of patient-controlled analgesia. *Nursing Management, 20*, 5.

Diers, D. (1982). Future of nurse-midwives in American health care. In L. Aiken, (Ed.), *Nursing in the 1980s: Crises, opportunities, challenges* (pp. 267–295). Philadelphia: J.B. Lippincott.

Donovan, M.I., & Lewis, G. (1987). Increasing productivity and decreasing costs: The value of RNs. *Journal of Nursing Administration, 17*(9), 17.

Elliott, T.L. (1989). Cost analysis of alternative scheduling. *Nursing Management, 20*, 4.

Ethridge, P., & Lamb, G.S. (1989). Professional nursing case management improves quality, access and costs. *Nursing Management, 20*(3), 33.

Evans, L., Strumpf, N., & Williams, C. (1991). Re-defining a standard of care for frail older people: Alternatives to reduce routine physical restraint. In P. Katz, R. Kane, & M. Mezey (Eds.), *Advances in long term care*, vol. 1 (pp. 81–108). New York: Springer.

Fagin, C.M. (1982a). Nursing's pivotal role in American health care. In L. Aiken (Ed.), *Nursing in the 1980s: Crises, opportunities, challenges* (pp. 459–475). Philadelphia: J.B. Lippincott.

Fagin, C.M. (1982b). The economic value of nursing research. *American Journal of Nursing*, 82(12), 1844–1849.

Fagin, C.M., & Jacobsen, B.J. (1985). The economic value of nursing research: A critical review. In H. Werley (Ed.), *Annual review of nursing research*, 3 (pp. 215–238). New York: Springer.

General Accounting Office Report (May, 1983). GAO/IPE 83, 1: Washington, DC, December 7, 1982. *Health policy alternatives: Expansion of cost-effective home health care.* Washington, DC: Government Printing Office.

Georgopoulos, B.S. (1985). Organization structure and the performance of hospital emergency services. *Annals of Emergency Medicine 14*(7): 677–684.

Ginsberg, G., Marks, I., & Waters, H. (1984). Cost-benefit analysis of a controlled trial of nurse therapy for neuroses in primary care. *Psychiatric Medicine 14*, 683–690.

Green, J.H. (1989). Long-term care research. *Nursing and Health Care, 10*(3), 139–144.

Hannan, E.L., O'Donnell, J.F., Kilburn, H., Jr., Bernard, H.R., & Yazici, A. (1989). Investigation of the relationship between volume and mortality for surgical procedures performed in New York state hospitals. *Journal of the American Medical Association, 262*(4), 503–510.

Hartz, A.J., Krakauer, H., & Kuhn, E.M. (1989). Hospital characteristics and mortality rates. *New England Journal of Medicine, 321*, 1720–1725.

Hedrick, S.C., & Inui, T.S. (1986). The effectiveness and cost of home care: An information synthesis. *Health Services Research, 20*(6), part II, 876.

Helt, E.H., & Jelinek, R.C. (1988). In the wake of cost cutting, nursing productivity and quality improve. *Nursing Management, 19*(6), 42.

Hinshaw, A.S., Scofield, R., & Atwood, J.R. (1981, November/December). Staff, patient, and cost outcomes of all-registered nurse staffing. *Journal of Nursing Administration, 11*(11,12), 30–36.

Kane, R.L., Garrard, J., Skay, C.L., Radosevich, D.M., Buchanon, J.L., McDermott, S.M., Arnold, S.B., & Kepferle, L. (1989). Effects of a geriatric nurse practitioner on process and outcome of nursing home care. *American Journal of Public Health*, 79(9), 1271–1277.

Kitz, D.S., McCartney, M., Kissick, J.E., & Townsend, R. (1989). Examining nursing personnel costs: Controlled versus noncontrolled oral analgesic agents. *Journal of Nursing Administration, 19*(1), 10–14.

Knaus, W.A., Draper, E.A., Wagner, D.P., & Zimmerman, J.E. (1986). An evaluation of outcome from intensive care in major medical centers. *Annals of Internal Medicine, 104*(3), 410–418.

Kramer, A.M., Shaughnessy, P.W., & Pettigrew, M.L. (1985). Cost-effectiveness implications based on a comparison of nursing home and home health care mix. *Health Services Research, 20*(4), 387–405.

LaForme, S. (1982, April). Primary nursing. Does good care cost more? *The Canadian Nurse*, 74(4), a46–47; b47–49.

MacDonald, M. (1988). Primary nursing: Is it worth it? *Journal of Advanced Nursing, 13*, 797–806.

McCorkle, R., Benoliel, J.Q., Donaldson, G., Georgiadou, F., Moinpour, C., & Goodell, B. (1989). A randomized clinical trial of home nursing care for lung cancer patients. *Cancer, 66*, 1375–1382.

McKibben, R. (1982). Registered nurses' wages have minor effects on total hospital costs. *American Journal of Nursing, 12.*

Minor, A.F. (1989). The cost of maternity care and childbirth in the United States 1989. Washington, DC: *Health Insurance Administration of America.*

Mitchell, M., Miller, J., Welches, L., & Walker, D. (1984). Determining cost of direct nursing care by DRGs. *Nursing Management, 15*(4), 29–32.

Naylor, M. (1990, May/June). Comprehensive discharge planning for hospitalized elderly: A pilot study. *Nursing Research, 39*(3), 156–160.

O'Sullivan, A.L., & Jacobsen, B.S. *A randomized trial of a health care program of first-time adolescent mothers.* Philadelphia: University of Pennsylvania School of Nursing, unpublished.

Office of Technology Assessment (1986). *Physicians assistants and certified nurse-midwives: A policy analysis* (a, p6; b, p66). Washington, DC: U.S. Government Printing Office.

Olds, D.L., Henderson, C.R., Tatelbaum, R., & Chamberlin, R. (1988). Improving the life-course development of socially disadvantaged mothers: A randomized trial of nurse home visitation. *American Journal of Public Health, 78*(11), 1436–1445.

Prescott, P.A., & Driscoll, L. (1980, July-August). Evaluating nurse practitioner performance. *The Nurse Practitioner, 5*(4), 28–29, 31–32.

Ramsay, J.A., McKenzie, J.K., & Fish, D.G. (1986). Physicians and nurse practitioners: Do they provide equivalent health care? *American Journal of Public Health, 72*(1), 55–56.

Riley, W., & Schaefers, V. (1983, December). Costing nursing services. *Nursing Management, 14*(12), 40.

Rohrer, J.E., & Hogan, A.J. (1987). Modeling the outcomes of nursing home care. *Social Science and Medicine, 24*(3), 219–223.

Salkever, D.S., Skinner, E.A., Steinwachs, D.M., & Katz, H. (1982). Episode based efficiency comparisons for physicians and nurse practitioners. *Medical Care, 20*(2), 143–153.

Scharon, G.M., & Bernacki, E.J. (1984). A corporate role for nurse practitioners. *Business and Health, 1*(9), 26–27.

Sellick, K.J., Russell, S., & Beckmann, J.L. (1983). Primary nursing: An evaluation of its effects on patient perception of care and staff satisfaction. *International Journal of Nursing Studies, 20*(4), 265–273.

Shaughnessy, P.W., Kramer, A.M., & Hittle, D.F. (1988). *The teaching nursing home experiment: Its effects and implications.* Study Paper 6, December 1988. Denver: Center for Health Services Research, University of Colorado Health Sciences Center, unpublished paper.

Shortell, S.M., & Hughes, F.X. (1988). The effects of regulation, competition, and ownership on mortality rates among hospital inpatients. *New England Journal of Medicine, 318,* 1100–1107.

Sovie, M.D., Tarcinale, M.A., Vanputee, A.W., & Stunden, A.E. (1985, March). Amalgam of nursing acuity DRGs and costs. *Nursing Management, 16*(3), a, p22; b, p34; c, p38; d, p42.

Stevenson, B. (1948). *The home book of proverbs, maxims, and familiar phrases* (p. 2275). New York: Macmillan.

Thornton, C., Dunstan, S.M., & Kemper, P. (1988). The evaluation of the national long-term care demonstration 8: The effect of channeling on health and long-term care costs. *Health Services Research, 23,* 130.

Walker, D. (1985). The cost of nursing care in hospitals. *Journal of Nursing Administration,* *13,* 13–18.

Watson, S., & Hickey, P. (1984). Help for the family in waiting. *American Journal of Nursing,* *84*(5), 604–607.

Weil, M., & Karls, J. (1985). Historical origins and recent developments. In M. Weil, & J. Karls (Eds.), *Case management in human service practice* (p. 2). San Francisco: Jossey-Bass.

Weissert, W.G. (1985). Seven reasons why it is so difficult to make community-based long-term care cost-effective. *Health Services Research, 20*(4), 424.

Werley, H.H., & Zorn, C.R. (1989). The nursing minimum data set: Benefits and implications. *Perspectives in nursing—1987–1989* (pp. 105–114). New York: National League for Nursing Publication, No. 19–229.

What's the cost of nursing care? (1986, November 5). *Hospitals,* p. 49.

Wilson, L., Prescott, P.A., & Aleksandrowicz, L. (1988). Nursing: A major hospital cost component. *Health Services Research, 22*(6), 773–796.

Winder, P.G. (1988, July). Case management by nurse at a county facility. *QRB, 14*(7), 215–219.

Wolf, G.A., Lesic, L.K., & Leak, A.G. (1986). Primary nursing. The impact on nursing costs within DRGs. [Financial Management Services]. *Journal of Nursing Administration,* *16*(3), 9–11.

# Chapter 3

# Specialization and Credentialing*

## MARGRETTA M. STYLES

*I*N A 1986 comparison of approaches to the study of health professions, Dag Hofoss, a Norwegian health services researcher, reported how he looks at specialization from three different disciplines.

> First, I assume the view of the sociologist (Specialization certainly is a reflection of the selfish interest of the professions, who strive for job monopoly), then, that of the physician (Specialization is the natural response to medical and technological progress) and, finally, that of the economist (Specialization is a result of increased market demand for health services) (Hofoss, 1986, p. 201).

When I was invited to study nursing specialization in the 1980s as an American Nurses' Foundation Distinguished Scholar, I chose the social systems perspective as that most useful in examining the "profession-building" behavior of a profession and its subgroups as they continue to evolve.

Power, of course, is essential for social systems, such as professions, to fulfill their missions. As such systems grow and undergo differentiation into specialty subsystems, at least three characteristics are necessary for them to acquire and maintain the power to function effectively: legitimacy, homogeneity, and unity. In brief, in order for the whole system and its specialty subsystems to be empowered to get the job done, there must be some recognized authority and accepted principles and rules of order, adequate comparability and compatibility among the parts, and unity of purpose and standard throughout.

A study of the contemporary scene in nursing specialization discloses that it is one of the most dramatic movements in the profession today, that the above essentials are considerably lacking, and that the consequences of this deficit are evident in the

---

* This chapter is based on the book *On Specialization in Nursing: Toward a New Empowerment* by the author, American Nurses' Foundation, 1989.

struggle of the movement to achieve its full potential for health care, for nursing, and for nurses. Other health professions—medicine in particular—face similar and mounting problems. Specialization is unquestionably a nursing and health policy issue in the 1990s. It is also apparent, and most encouraging, that nursing organizations intend to confront the issue and find solutions.

## Nursing Specialization

### The Status

Counting nursing specialties and specialists today would be to aim at a moving target, at best. The situation, however, is worse because the target is not only moving but poorly defined as well.

There is no recognized authority for defining nursing specialties, as is true for medicine and other professions. To compile such a list one must search from among a number of sources, such as specialty organizations, national certifying bodies, state regulatory agencies, postlicensure nursing programs, and institutional credentials. No coherent pattern emerges from such an exercise; therefore, a sampling from these sources must suffice.

In terms of certifying bodies, nursing is in the anomalous situation of being the only profession that conducts certification both internal and external to the professional association. A 1988 survey of national specialty nursing certifying organizations and organizations planning to certify in the future listed 25 such groups (Styles, 1988). The total number of specialists certified by these groups at that time was 149,127. The range of certificatees was from 229 to 35,000. Three groups had certified over 20,000 nurses; two between 10,000 and 20,000; ten between 1000 and 10,000; and five below 1000. Three groups were just planning their certification programs (Styles, 1989) (Table 3–1).

The American Nurses' Association (ANA) offered nine "generalist" certifications, five practitioner certifications, three clinical specialist certifications, and two levels of nursing administration certifications—a total of 19 certification programs. The total number certified by the ANA was 56,476; the range of certificatees was from 356 to 10,329, with two programs still under development (Styles, 1989) (Table 3–2).

As for statutory credentialing, in 1986 state boards of nursing reported that 39 states were recognizing advanced nurse practitioners and/or specialists through some form of title or practice protection. Titles encompassed the very broad (e.g., nurse specialist, nurse clinician, nurse practitioner) to the very specific (e.g., neonatal nurse practitioner, family planning nurse practitioner, nurse-midwife, nurse anesthetist). Some of the smallest states designated the largest number of categories, the greatest number for one state being 13. Some of the largest states designated few or no categories. These discrepancies point out that the statutory regulation of nurse specialists is an area of considerable uncertainty and controversy. Such a practice is anathema to the other health fields that have zealously guarded the right and responsibility of specialty development as a professional prerogative.

**TABLE 3–1 Organizations Outside of the American Nurses' Association That Certify Nurses***

| Organization | Number Certified (as of 1988) |
|---|---|
| American Association of Critical Care Nurses Certification Corporation | 28,563 |
| American Board of Neuroscience Nursing | 767 |
| American Board for Occupational Health Nurses, Inc. | approx. 3700 |
| American Board of Urologic Allied Health Professionals, Inc. | 1200 |
| American College of Nurse-Midwives Division of Competency Assessment | 3000 |
| Association of Rehabilitation Nurses—Certification Board | 1325 |
| Board of Certification for Emergency Nursing | 16,153 |
| Board of Nephrology Examiners, Nursing and Technology | approx. 2250 |
| Certification Board on Infection Control | 2000 |
| Certifying Council for Gastroenterology Clinicians, Inc. | approx. 700 |
| Council on Certification of Nurse Anesthetists | 35,000 |
| Council on Recertification of Nurse Anesthetists | 21,000 |
| Enterostomal Therapy Nursing Certification Board | 1200 |
| Intravenous Nurses Society Certification Corporation | 1100 |
| Nursing Association of the American College of Obstetrics and Gynecology Certification Corporation | 13,274 |
| National Board for Certification of School Nurses/National Association of School Nurses, Inc. | 0 |
| National Board of Nutrition Support Certification | 229 |
| National Board of Pediatric Nurse Practitioners and Associates | 3550 |
| National Certification Board for Diabetes Educators | N/A |
| National Certifying Board for Ophthalmic Registered Nurses | 0 |
| National Certification Board: Perioperative Nursing, Inc. | 9077 |
| National Nurses Society on Addiction | 0 |
| Nephrology Nursing Certification Board | 850 |
| Oncology Nursing Certification Corporation | 3639 |
| Orthopaedic Nurses Certification Board | 550 |
| Total | 149,127 |

* Source: Styles, M.M.: *A Directory of Information on National Specialty Nursing Certifying Organizations and Organizations Planning to Certify,* November, 1988 (mimeographed). New York, American Board of Neuroscience Nursing, 1988.

It would be unconvincing, also, to argue that the more than 300 graduate programs in nursing, some offering up to 30 "majors" or "areas of concentration," either define or correspond to the profession's areas of specialty practice, as is essentially the case for postgraduate education in medicine and other health fields. In the first place, of the 23 specialty organizations responding to the American Nurses' Foundation (ANF) survey in 1985, only two required graduation from accredited specialty education programs for certification (Styles, 1989). These are certificate programs, not graduate degree programs, and they do not necessarily require the Bachelor of Science in Nursing for admission. The requirement of a master's degree in nursing is only just becoming established for the ANA clinical nurse specialist certifications (Styles, 1989). Second, the curricula of graduate programs are more divergent than consistent, ranging from the very generic to the very idiosyncratic. There are, how-

**TABLE 3–2 American Nurses' Association Certification Programs***

| Program | Number Certified (as of 10/88) |
|---|---|
| Generalist certification programs | |
| Medical-surgical nurse | 9135 |
| Gerontological nurse | 5884 |
| Psychiatric and mental health nurse | 10,329 |
| Child and adolescent/pediatric nurse | 988 |
| School nurse | 0 |
| High-risk perinatal nurse | 591 |
| Community health nurse | 2741 |
| General nursing practice | 0 |
| Maternal and child health nurse | 503 |
| Practitioner certification programs | |
| Gerontological nurse practitioner | 961 |
| Pediatric nurse practitioner | 1426 |
| Adult nurse practitioner | 4645 |
| Family nurse practitioner | 5700 |
| School nurse practitioner | 469 |
| Specialist certification programs | |
| Clinical specialist in medical-surgical nursing | 785 |
| Clinical specialist in adult psychiatric and mental health nursing | 3141 |
| Clinical specialist in child and adolescent psychiatric and mental health nursing | 356 |
| Nursing administration certification programs | |
| Nursing administration | 7541 |
| Nursing administration, advanced | 1281 |
| Total | 56,476 |

* Source: Styles, M.M.: *The Career Credential: Professional Certification*. Kansas City, Missouri, American Nurses' Association, 1988.

ever, some discernible patterns, perhaps most closely related to the ANA broader areas of generalist, practitioner, and clinical specialist certification (Styles, 1989).

A survey of job descriptions and independent roles would be necessary to identify those nursing specialties recognized and emerging in the practice environment and the extent to which they reflect the ones identified through the above sources. Lacking such a survey, it is worth noting that it is the exception rather than the rule that specialty certification is required for such positions and roles, except for those specialties in which statutory regulation has most often intervened, specifically nurse midwifery and nurse anesthesia.

The endless and growing list of practice branches, specialties, arguable subspecialties, and hybrids generated from these multiple and sometimes competing sources ranges in scope from procedures to populations. These "specialties" represent a combination of technologies, functions or roles, loci or systems of care, developmental stages or gender of clients, acuity of care, anatomic or functional systems or processes, and diseases or pathologic conditions.

To the degree it is acknowledged that new areas of practice should be defined or accompanied by new knowledge, it is enlightening to see how specialties support and disseminate research. Among the specialty organizations surveyed, many had research committees, a few sponsored research symposia, some had set aside limited resources for researchers, and one presented an annual research award. Peer-reviewed journals, a hallmark of scholarship, were just beginning to emerge.

From this overview it can be seen that (1) professional, practice, and market forces are accelerating the development of specialties in nursing; (2) this proliferation is not occurring in an orderly manner overall; and (3) there are no universally recognized specialties, no accepted standards, and no common principle or authority. Two futures are possible. This teeming, growing edge of nursing either can mesh and reinforce the borders of nursing practice or pull loose and unravel the fabric of the profession.

## The Consequences

To assess the consequences to nursing's specialty development as described above, it is useful to look first at the proposed benefits to specialization.

Schnaps and Sales, in a paper entitled "Specialization in Psychology: Lessons from Other Professions," traced specialization from the crafts and guilds of the Middle Ages to modern-day medicine, dentistry, nursing, law, and psychology. From a review of the literature, they identified several advantages to specialization in the professions, having to do with (1) professional competence, (2) quality of services, (3) cost of services, and (4) professional satisfaction (Schnaps & Sales, 1986). Some of these benefits are summarized below.

Most fields have become too vast and complex for any one person to master the full range of information and skills encompassed within them. Specialization enables practitioners to concentrate in one area of knowledge and technique, contributing to the best possible service for clients with particular problems. It can be argued that specialty standards and certification procedures lead to better prepared practitioners. Moreover, through the increased interaction of practitioners with similar preparation and interests, the exchange of ideas and discoveries is augmented.

Specialty certification is said to facilitate public recognition of practitioners with special qualifications and thus to improve access to their expert care. Quality of services is also enhanced through external controls, for example, by having third-party payers link reimbursement for specialized and complex care to specialist certification. Schnaps and Sales also argue that efficiency, economies of scale, and cost containment are possible through "standardized mass operations" and lend themselves to higher quality care.

Advantages of specialization to the practitioner are found to be both intrinsic and extrinsic in nature. Satisfaction often accompanies mastery of a branch of service and the ability to concentrate interests and energies, as well as the sense of close affiliation with a peer group. Increased professional stature accrues to specialists, along with increased income potential . . . (Schnaps & Sales, 1986). Differential rewards accompany different roles to ensure an adequacy of trained, talented people (Duke, 1976).

In relation to these benefits of specialization, the question should be asked: How are specialty credentials in nursing recognized as a mark of professional competence, as an essential for quality control, as a tool for achieving efficiency and economy in managing health services, as a means of public communication, and as an avenue to professional satisfaction and reward (Styles, 1989)? What are some key indicators of specialty nursing empowerment, as compared with those in medical specialization? Some of these are cited below.

First, as to *professional competence*, in the modest survey conducted for the ANF project, 86.4 percent of respondents identified themselves as "specialists," but only 46.2 percent claimed specialty certification. How can specialized professional competence be recognized and assessed if not through some form of credentialing?

Second, as to *quality control*—a major initiative for the 1990s—federal and state health care regulations and Joint Commission on Accreditation of Health Care Organizations guidelines repeatedly refer to board-certified medical specialists. References to nurses seldom, if ever, acknowledge such specialty credentials as indicators of quality or as essential to achieving a specified standard.

Third, as to *practice entitlements and institutional privileges*, nurses have reported that certification is generally not a requirement for their positions in specialty areas in hospitals and other settings, as opposed to the case for medical practice privileges. Direct third-party reimbursement for nurses has been an important goal of the nursing profession for more than 40 years. In addition to being a source of autonomy and revenue to nurses, direct reimbursement has important cost, access, and quality implications for the public. Over time some progress has been made in securing such payments to nurses through social security, rural health clinics, and military-dependent health programs legislation (Griffith, 1987). Numerous bills have been and continue to be introduced in Congress to increase the nursing services that would be covered by external payment mechanisms.

Although progress in this effort has been very slow, the mere existence of the legislation underscores the potential for society's recognition of the nurse specialist as a professional health caregiver who provides distinct services worthy of distinct compensation. Nonetheless, nursing has far to go to achieve medicine's success in securing direct reimbursement and recognition for its services (Styles, 1989).

Fourth, as to *professional satisfaction and reward*, studies have found that the rewards of nursing certification are largely intangible, including such nonmaterial rewards as the increase in personal satisfaction, the bolstering of self-esteem, and better working relations with nurse colleagues (Styles, 1979; Collins, 1987). Whereas the average income for the physician specialist may be double or triple that of the generalist, the average salary for the clinical nurse specialist is about 18 percent higher than that of the staff nurse (Styles, 1987).

Fifth, as to *public recognition and consumer choice*, it is apparent that although there is public awareness of what it means to be cared for by specialists in other fields, consumers do not seem to think of nurses as specialists. In one informal survey, only 6 percent of the respondents could name one nursing specialty (Kalish, 1988). In view of these circumstances, it seems unlikely that consumers can make informed choices about nursing care or that they will come to demand nurse specialists for their particular needs. Related access, cost savings, and quality benefits are thus being denied to them.

Sixth, in terms of *recruitment into the profession,* it is possible that an ill-defined image of the diverse and complex jobs nurses do has dampened interest in the field. Thus the prospects of a more well-defined field and its enhanced opportunities could attract more recruits into nursing, especially those more likely to pursue higher education and specialized career pathways.

These points would support the contention that the public and the profession have more to gain from nursing specialization than is currently realized. Quality, access, efficiency, and cost of health care would be better served (1) if nursing specialties were better developed to match health care need and more consistently governed to ensure a standard of preparation and performance, and (2) if nurses were motivated to gain and maintain specialized expertise and were recognized and rewarded for doing so.

## *The Issues*

*For external stakeholders*—i.e., payers, regulators, providers, consumers—the issues relative to nursing specialization must be as follows:

1. How do nursing specialties correspond to patient care needs and to work environments and their requirements?
2. What does specialty certification stand for in terms of education, experience, and competence?
3. What is the relationship of specialty competence to quality, access, and cost and efficiency of health care?

*For the profession* the issues regarding specialization are complex and involved. Also they are fundamental in that the profession's responses will establish the outcomes of the public issues. To circle back to the beginning of this chapter, these questions reflect the developmental tasks to be addressed if accepted principles and rules of order are to be brought to bear on the development of nursing's practice field—that is, if we are to be fully functioning as a profession fulfilling a social mandate and we are to be fair to our present and future members.

1. *Defining specialties:* What are the parameters and the characteristics of nursing specialties? Through what mechanisms and processes should specialties and subspecialties be identified by the profession? What criteria should be applied in making such determinations?

2. *Defining specialist:* Is a nurse specialist a nurse who practices in a specialty area of the work environment and/or a nurse who is prepared through advanced education and experience to develop the knowledge and skill base for the area of practice? Are there two levels of specialists? Should the two be differentiated in titles, certification, and practice roles? Does the first (i.e., the generalist practicing in a specialty environment) represent a transitional phase for the profession in defining specialist and in the evolution of practice roles and qualifications, or does this "level" of specialization represent an ongoing need? What are the proposed and the actual distinctions between a nurse practitioner and a clinical nurse specialist?

3. *Defining standards:* What are the appropriate educational, experience, and performance standards for nurse specialists? What is necessary for the profession

and for nurses to achieve those standards? Do standards represent basic competence or excellence/mastery in the specialty? What means are essential to ensure that performance standards are maintained by certified specialists after initial certification?

4. *Defining regulatory mechanisms:* What are the purposes of credentialing nurse specialists—for public protection, for public information, for professional reimbursement, and for professional development and recognition? Who should be the agent(s) of regulation—the profession or the state or both? What is the role of each in setting standards for and in certifying or recognizing nurse specialists?

Intense action on the quality assurance front at the federal, state, and institutional levels makes this an ideal time for nursing to address these issues and put into place standards and processes for the development of specialty practice. Technologic advances are occurring with breathtaking speed and causing sweeping changes in nursing practice. The health care financing and delivery systems are in a state of flux, bordering on chaos, and some dramatic improvements must soon be made. Payers and consumers alike are seeking alternatives to the costly and fragmented medically-centered care prevailing today. These developments create both challenges and opportunities for organized nursing in this country.

In other parts of the world, nurses also are facing these same issues with respect to defining specialty practice. Heretofore, in most countries the development of specialties has largely been under the control of a centralized authority such as the professional association and/or the ministry of health. However, pressures for re-examination of specialties and their standards of practice are occurring with the development of international societies of nurse specialists, with the movement of nursing and postbasic education into the universities, and with the emergence of new groups of technicians are forcing redefinition or reinforcement of nursing practice roles and functions. The creation of the 12-member European Community, with the free movement of workers across national boundaries, has also served as an impetus for nurses from all of Western Europe to develop guidelines regarding the nature of nursing specialties and the qualifications of specialists upon which international directives for the region will be based.

The International Council of Nurses, through its position paper (Styles, 1985) and workshops on nursing regulation and the ongoing work of its Professional Services Committee, is addressing the definition, titling, and credentialing of nurse specialists on a global basis. Also, an organizational self-study is under way to examine and propose the relationship of the International Council of Nurses and its member national nurses' associations to specialty organizations. Thus, it is apparent that American nurses are not alone in confronting these issues and challenges.

## Solutions

Through a number of mechanisms, the nursing profession in this country is recognizing problems surrounding the development of nursing specialties and is seeking solutions to them. Specialty organizations meet together under the aegis of the National Federation of Specialty Nursing Organizations and the ANA Nursing Organization Liaison Forum. The National Specialty Nursing Certifying Organizations also meet informally. As yet, these groups have not developed into policy-making bodies, although they do provide opportunities for discussion of a wide range of issues regarding nursing and the specialties.

Within the past year a Committee for the National Board of Nursing Specialties has been formed, with a grant from the Josiah Macy Jr. Foundation, to explore and stimulate the development of a board made up primarily of nursing certifying bodies, established for the purpose of recognizing specialties and approving their certification standards and processes. Much discussion is occurring around the concept and design of such an organization. It is largely through the American Board of Medical Specialties and its liaison relationships with the American Medical Association, the Association of American Medical Colleges, and other groups that specialty boards in medicine are recognized and coordinated.

After studying nursing specialization today from the social science perspective, I have concluded that nursing needs to achieve greater authority, homogeneity, and unity of its specialty subsystems if it is to attain its goals as a profession. First and foremost, the responsibility of the profession for its own development must be accepted. It must be acknowledged that, although it is the responsibility of the state to license registered nurses for the broad field of nursing for the purpose of safeguarding the public, it is the responsibility of the profession to ensure the orderly development and recognition of its internal branches for the purpose of refining, advancing, and organizing nursing practice.

Based on these conclusions and the issues identified in the previous section, there would seem to be at least three essential elements for empowering nursing as an increasingly complex and differentiated profession:

- An authoritative, criterion-based professional review mechanism for the recognition and sanction of specialties and subspecialties and the approval of their certification standards and procedures.
- A conceptual schema within which unity of purpose and fit among the specialties and subspecialties can be determined.
- A plan for promoting specialist credentials in order to achieve their maximum effect on health care quality, access, and economy and on nurse recognition and satisfaction (Styles, 1989).

As to the criteria for a specialty, it would seem that the following conditions must be met:

1. The specialty defines itself as nursing and subscribes to the overall purpose and functions of nursing.
2. The specialty subscribes to the overall education, practice, and ethical standards of the profession.
3. There is both demand and need for the services of the specialty.
4. The specialty is national in its geographic scope.
5. The specialty is clearly defined in relationship to and differentiated from other specialties.

6. The specialty is sufficiently complex and advanced that it is beyond the qualifications for general practice.
7. Practice standards have been developed for the specialty.
8. The specialty knowledge base is well developed and is concerned with phenomena and problems within the discipline and practice of nursing.
9. Mechanisms exist for supporting, reviewing, and disseminating research in the specialty.
10. Advanced education programs, leading to a certificate or graduate degree in nursing, prepare specialists in the field.
11. The area of specialization includes a substantial number of practitioners who devote most of their practice to the specialty.
12. Practitioners of the specialty are licensed as registered nurses.
13. A peer review certification program exists to evaluate candidates to ensure initial and continued competence in the specialty.
14. Practitioners are organized and represented within a specialty association or branch of a parent organization (Styles, 1989).

Viewed in the aggregate, these directions are sound beginnings to the profession's renewed effort to be responsibly self-governing as its practice evolves to higher levels of public service along differentiated yet holistic lines.

## Summary and Summons

This chapter has provided an overview of activities, issues, and proposals in the rapidly growing nursing specialization movement. It was concluded that, although this movement is both necessary and promising, the differentiation of nursing as a complex health service can at this stage be better characterized as discrete, vigorous, and proliferative than as organic, orderly, and progressive. Developments in nursing specialization must occur as a result of a variety of professional, practice, and market forces and within the broad background of health care, the spectrum of health professions, and worldwide nursing. These contexts have only been touched upon.

It is incumbent upon a profession to adopt essential principles and rules of order to fulfill its social mission and to be fair to its members who are committed to that mission. It may be appropriate to experiment with lines of development for a period. However, the time of decision must come and, in fact, has arrived.

REFERENCES

Collins, H.L. (1987, July). Certification: Is the payoff worth the price? RN, *50*(7), 36–44.
Duke, J.T. (1976). *Conflict and power in social life.* Provo, UT: Brigham Young University Press.

Griffith, H.M. (1987). Direct third party reimbursement for nursing service: A review of legislation and implementation. *Nursing Administration Quarterly, 12,* 19–23.

Hofoss, D. (1986). Health professions: The origin of species. *Social Science and Medicine, 22,* 201–209.

Kalish, P. (1988). Personal communication.

Schnaps, L.S., & Sales, B. (1986). *Specialization in psychology: Lessons from other professions.* Report to the Subcommittee on Specialization of the American Psychological Association's Board of Professional Affairs.

Styles, M.M. (1979). *The study of credentialing in nursing: A new approach,* vol. II. Kansas City, MO: American Nurses' Association.

Styles, M.M. (1985). *Report on the regulation of nursing.* Geneva, Switzerland: International Council of Nurses.

Styles, M.M. (1987). *Facts about nursing 86–87.* Kansas City, MO: American Nurses' Association.

Styles, M.M. (1988). *A directory of information on national specialty nursing certifying organizations and organizations planning to certify.* New York: American Board of Neuroscience Nursing.

Styles, M.M. (1989). *On specialization in nursing: Toward a new empowerment.* Kansas City, MO: American Nurses' Foundation.

## Chapter 4

# The Nurse Labor Market: Considerations for the 1990s*

PATRICIA A. PRESCOTT

*U*NDERSTANDING DISEQUILIBRIUM in health personnel markets is a difficult undertaking because of the complexity and rapidly changing nature of the health care industry, substitution among types of health care workers, and a variety of conceptual and methodologic issues associated with definition and measurement of shortage. This chapter explores the concept of workforce shortage from economic and nursing perspectives. Data relevant to the current supply of nurses, demand for nursing service, and wages are examined in light of past trends, and selected issues related to interpreting data and determining health workforce requirements are discussed.

## Economic Perspectives on Shortage

The three basic concepts central to economic discussions of shortage are supply, demand, and wage. Supply refers to the amount of labor available for work, and it is usually measured by the number of people licensed as registered nurses. Demand is the amount of labor that employers are able and willing to purchase at a specific price or wage. Demand differs from want and need, which are terms found in nursing discussions of shortage. The number of nurses wanted or needed is usually a clinically derived expression devoid of economic constraint. Thus, hospitals may want or need many more hours of nursing care than they demand.

A labor market is in equilibrium when the supply of labor available at a given wage is equal to the services or labor demanded by employers. A labor shortage exists when the demand for nursing services exceeds the supply available at a specific

* I wish to express my appreciation and thanks to Dr. Ada Jacox for her assistance in the analysis of the aging of the registered nurse work force and its effect on the future supply of nurses.

market price, and conversely a surplus exists when the number of people willing to work at a specified wage is greater than that demanded by employers. Economic theory indicates that price is inversely related to supply, and supply, demand, price, and employment are constantly adjusting toward equilibrium in a competitive market place.

How well has economic theory been able to explain behavior in the nurse labor market? Not very well according to some economists, who argue that the nurse labor market is constrained by monopsony or oligopsony. Monopsonistic or oligoponistic markets exist when there are too few employers to stimulate meaningful wage competition. This exists in the United States, where hospitals employ 69 percent of all nurses, and in many communities there is only a single hospital or a small group of hospitals. Under these conditions, wages are not free to rise and serve as the equilibrator of supply and demand. As Yett (1975) has argued, in such circumstances employers will express demand in excess of the supply that the current wage will purchase, that is, they would like to hire more nurses, but they are not willing to raise wages sufficiently to attract more nurses into the market. Raising wages sufficiently to attract more nurses means that employers must raise wages for all existing staff as well as for those they wish to recruit. Thus, raising wages increases the marginal labor costs of hospitals, and even relatively small wage increases can have substantial effects on hospital budgets.

The type of shortage that results from restricted markets has been described as a static or equilibrium shortage, and this contrasts with a dynamic shortage, which results from imbalances between supply and demand in competitive markets (Yett, 1975). The distinction between types of shortage is important. In an equilibrium shortage, the logical solution is to remove wage constraints so that wages can rise to the level needed to balance supply with demand. The traditional approach to solving the nursing shortage in the United States has been to increase the nurse supply. This strategy actually may have worsened the problem by preventing wages from rising (Aiken & Blendon, 1981; Edgren, 1976; Yett, 1975). On the other hand, when faced with a dynamic shortage where wages are freely rising but unable to balance supply and demand, remedial actions to increase the supply and/or decrease demand are appropriate.

There is no general agreement among economists about the nature of the nurse labor market. Some have argued that the nursing shortage is not the result of depressed wages. Instead, they point to geographic maldistribution, the functioning of local rather than national markets, demographic variables predictive of labor force participation, and the insensitivity of the nurse labor market to wage changes (Bognanno et al., 1974; Sloan & Richupan, 1975). Despite the lack of agreement within the economic community, this general perspective is useful for understanding changes in supply and demand at an aggregate national or regional level.

The theories and models used at one level of analysis do not necessarily transfer directly to other levels (Burnstein, 1980; Hannan, 1971; Herman & Hulin, 1972; Roberts & Burnstein, 1980; Rousseau, 1982). This means that predictors of shortage or labor force participation at the level of individual institutions, such as hospitals, may not be predictors at an aggregate national level. To illustrate, nurse turnover is frequently mentioned as a cause of nursing shortage. This is true at the level of individual institutions because, by definition, a nurse who resigns, that is, "turns over," creates a vacant position at that institution. At the aggregate level, however, turnover is not a cause of shortage unless the nurse who leaves her position also leaves the active labor force either for retirement or another occupation. Existing data on nurse turnover indicate that the majority of nurses do not leave nursing. Instead they take another, often parallel, job in a different institution. Hence, turnover operates much like a revolving door at the aggregate market level and is not a cause of shortage at this level as it is at the level of individual institutions (Prescott, 1987; Prescott & Bowen, 1987).

The distinction between the institutional and aggregate levels of analysis is important because policy makers and administrators attempting to deal with shortage often have tried to transfer ideas directly from one level of analysis to another. For example, using ideas from the aggregate macrolevel analyses, many hospital and nursing administrators have assumed that turnover is inevitable and beyond hospital control because economic studies indicate that participation of nurses in the labor force is determined by demographic factors outside an institution's control. This has led to the belief that because turnover is inevitable, hospitals should focus on recruitment of new nurses rather than retention of existing staff. Data from recent nursing studies of turnover at an institutional level, however, indicate that there are many things that hospitals can do to prevent or decrease turnover among the nursing staff. In a study conducted between 1980 and 1984, nurses cited many work-related reasons for resignations, including scheduling of work, problems with administrators (especially head nurses), lack of stimulation and dissatisfaction with nursing practice, inadequate salary, poor nurse staffing, desire for new experiences, and problems in interpersonal relationships among staff (Prescott & Bowen, 1987).

## Nursing Perspectives on Shortage

Nursing descriptions of shortage generally express the concepts of need or want, and they are derived from a clinical perspective of how many nurses it takes to provide care for patients at some professionally determined level of adequacy. Nursing takes a broad view of shortage and attributes it to a variety of factors related to job dissatisfaction. There are four general categories of job dissatisfiers found in the nursing literature: (1) salary and fringe benefits; (2) control over hours, days, shifts, and basic conditions of work; (3) professional issues related to respect from others, freedom to control nursing practice, and opportunities for growth and promotion; and (4) increased hospital demand for nursing services as a result of increasing patient acuity, decreased lengths of stay associated with the prospective payment system, and aging of the patient population (Aiken, 1982; Aiken & Mullinex, 1987; American Academy of Nursing, 1983; Diers, 1988; Department of Health and Human Services, 1988; Jacox, 1982; Prescott et al., 1985; Roberts et al., 1989).

In general, the nursing literature has focused on shortage at the institutional

**TABLE 4–1  Employed Nurses by Year**

| Year | Employed Nurses | Nurses per 100,000 Population | FTEs* per 100,000 Population |
| --- | --- | --- | --- |
| 1988 | 1,627,036 | 668 | 560 |
| 1985 | 1,531,200 | 641 | 533 |
| 1980 | 1,272,900 | 560 | 470 |
| 1978 | 1,123,200 | 506 | 425 |

\* Full Time Equivalents

Source: Division of Nursing, U.S. Department of Health and Human Services. (1978, 1980, 1985, 1988). *National Sample Surveys of Registered Nurses.* Washington, DC: U.S. Department of Health and Human Services. Bureau of Health Professions, Health Resources Services Administration, Public Health Services.

level as opposed to at the aggregate market level. Job dissatisfiers are linked to institutional shortage via turnover as dissatisfied nurses resign their positions and go elsewhere. However, as long as nurses simply move around among employers, job dissatisfiers do not explain shortage at the aggregate level. Whereas the professional literature has focused on factors relevant to job satisfaction and retention of staff, many institutions have focused primarily on recruitment and only secondarily, if at all, on issues of retention. The reason is economic, that is, it has been, and may still be, less costly for hospitals to replace nurses than it is to build serious retention programs (Sloan, 1975). Salary compression has been a major indicator that employers have not valued the long-term nurse employee. In 1985, for example, staff nurses in practice 5 years or less averaged $22,000 per year, whereas nurses with 6 to 10 years of experience averaged only $25,000 and gained very little thereafter (Nursing Pay, 1985). The current picture of nursing wages is more thoroughly discussed after data on supply and demand are examined.

## Supply, Demand, and Wages

### Supply

Comparing the supply of nurses in 1988 with that in the past decade, it is evident that the number of employed nurses has increased dramatically to the current estimated all-time high of 1,627,035 (Division of Nursing, 1989). Not only has the number of nurses increased 65 percent over what it was in 1977, but from Table 4–1 it can be seen that the supply has increased faster than the general population.

These large increases have been discounted by some, who argue that although there are more nurses, they are not working in nursing. Data do not support this belief; in fact, the labor force participation rate of nurses has steadily increased from 73 percent in 1977 to 80 percent in 1988. Although it is true that large numbers of nurses work part time as opposed to full time, the labor force participation of nurses is high relative to that of other female-dominated occupations. Furthermore, as seen

**TABLE 4–2 Percentage of Registered Nurses Employed Outside Nursing and Unemployed**

| Year | Nurse Seeking Nursing Position Employed Outside Nursing | Not Employed But Seeking Nursing Position | Not Employed Not Looking | Average Registered Nurse Unemployment Rate | Average Unemployment Rate Women 25–54 Years |
|------|------|------|------|------|------|
| 1977 | 4.4 | 3.0 | 27.2 | 2.6 | 6.4 |
| 1984 | 4.6 | 1.9 | 14.6 | 2.0 | 6.3 |
| 1988 | 5.1 | 1.4 | 18.6 | 1.2 | 4.5 |

Source: Division of Nursing U.S. Department of Health and Human Services. (1977, 1984, 1988). *National Sample Surveys of Registered Nurses* [unemployment rates for health fields]. Washington, DC: U.S. Department of Health and Human Services, Bureau of Health Professions.

in Table 4–2, few nurses are employed outside nursing, and a large number of these in the inactive pool are over the age of 60 years (30 percent).

In summary, the current supply of registered nurses is at historically high levels. Unless there is evidence of even larger increases in demand for nurses on the part of employers, there is little reason to attribute the shortage of nurses experienced during the 1980s to inadequacies of supply. Also it is not supportable to attribute the perceived shortage to large numbers of inactive nurses or large numbers of nurses leaving nursing for other occupations.

The future supply of nurses is likely to grow at a slower rate than in the recent past. As seen in Table 4–3, nursing school enrollment decreased from 1983 to 1987. However, this decline now appears to be leveling off and actually reversing. If the increase of nursing school students experienced between 1988 and 1989 is indicative of things to come, the declines of the mid-1980s will have only a short-term effect on the supply of nurses in the first half of this decade.

An additional impact on the future supply of nurses, and one that has not received a great deal of attention, is related to the age of the registered nurse work force. Given that the average age of registered nurses is 39 years, and given that labor force participation rates decline steadily with age, in the next 20 years there will be a substantial decline in the rate of growth in the supply of nurses based on aging of

**TABLE 4–3 Nursing School Enrollments by Year**

| Year | Nursing School Enrollments % Change | Number |
|------|------|------|
| 1983 | +3.5 | 250,553 |
| 1984 | −5.3 | 237,232 |
| 1985 | −8.1 | 217,955 |
| 1986 | −11.1 | 193,712 |
| 1987 | −5.6 | 182,947 |
| 1988 | +1.0 | 184,924 |
| 1989 | — | — |

Source: National League for Nursing, *Nursing Data Review 1988* (1988). New York: National League for Nursing, Publication No. 19-2290.

**TABLE 4–4  Estimates of Number of Employed Registered Nurses in the Future by Age Groups**

| Age Group | LFPRs* | 1988† | 1993‡ | 1998‡ |
|---|---|---|---|---|
| <25 yr. | .975 | 76,592 | 84,811 | 75,159 |
| 25–29 | .922 | 219,047 | 158,590 | 161,787 |
| 30–34 | .874 | 322,490 | 265,480 | 204,911 |
| 35–39 | .865 | 287,318 | 385,924 | 309,699 |
| 40–44 | .843 | 225,568 | 305,711 | 413,260 |
| 45–49 | .826 | 175,811 | 233,827 | 319,443 |
| 50–54 | .787 | 136,803 | 170,764 | 226,273 |
| 55–59 | .698 | 97,853 | 120,361 | 150,240 |
| 60–64 | .501 | 54,619 | 69,725 | 85,763 |
| 65+ | .209 | 21,122 | 22,660 | 28,927 |
| | | 1,617,223 | 1,817,853 | 1,975,462 |
| | | <———> | <———> | |
| | | 12.0% | 8.7% | |

* Labor Force Participation Rates (LFPRs) used throughout this analysis are based on those obtained in the 1988 National Sample Survey of Registered Nurses, Division of Nursing. Washington, DC: U.S. Department of Health and Human Services, Bureau of Health Professions, Health Resources Services Administration, Public Health Services.

† Number of employed nurses by age group based on data from 1988 National Sample Survey, Division of Nursing. Washington, DC: U.S. Department of Health and Human Services, Bureau of Health Professions, Health Resources Services Administration, Public Health Services.

‡ Estimates are based on number of new graduates entering the work force during the time interval (assuming 70,561 per year as in 1987), the number of new graduates who moved into an age category during the interval, and the number of people from the original 1988 pool who remain in the interval. All estimates were adjusted by a median annual death rate for working women (0.0015) and by age category labor force participation rates (Division of Nursing, 1989).

the registered nurse work force. Overall, the supply of nurses will continue to increase, but the rate of growth will slow. This slowed growth will impact on the supply of nurses in all settings but will have the greatest impact on hospitals as the percentage of nurses working in staff nurse positions declines sharply with age (Division of Nursing, 1989).

To estimate the effects of age on the replacement needs for the nurse supply, the data from the National Sample Survey were "aged" 10 years. Then new graduates were added to the aged population of nurses based on the assumption that the number graduating in future years would be unchanged from that in 1988. The 70,561 new nurses per year were added to the aged population using the age distribution of 1987 graduates found in the 1988 National Sample Survey (Division of Nursing, 1989).

This age distribution was assumed to change at 25 percent of the rate of change that occurred between 1977 and 1988. That is, it was assumed that the new graduates entering the work force would continue to be older than in previous years but they would age at a slower rate than that observed in the 1977 to 1988 interval.

Next the data were adjusted using a median death rate for working women and the labor force participation rates for age groups based on the 1988 sample survey data (Division of Nursing, 1989; United States Bureau of Census, 1987). The resulting estimated distribution of employed nurses by age groups for 10 years in the future is seen in Table 4–4.

**TABLE 4–5 Estimated Number of Employed Nurses by Age Groups Working in Hospitals**

| Age Group | % Working in Hospitals | 1988 | 1998 |
|---|---|---|---|
| <25 | 92.3 | 70,694 | 69,371 |
| 25–29 | 88.7 | 194,294 | 143,505 |
| 30–34 | 83.2 | 268,311 | 170,485 |
| 35–39 | 78.2 | 224,682 | 242,184 |
| 40–44 | 70.5 | 159,025 | 291,348 |
| 45–49 | 64.0 | 112,519 | 204,443 |
| 50–54 | 60.1 | 82,218 | 135,990 |
| 55–59 | 57.0 | 57,776 | 85,636 |
| 60–64 | 49.6 | 27,091 | 42,538 |
| 65 + | 33.7 | 7118 | 9748 |
| | | 1,203,728 | 1,395,248 |
| | | <———> | |
| | | 15.9% | |

As seen in Table 4–4, the rate of growth in the nurse supply goes down sharply as the nurse population ages. The percentage of increase in the nurse supply between 1980 and 1985 was 49.6 percent. Between 1988 and 1993, the rate of increase is 12 percent, and between 1993 and 1998, it further slows to 8.7 percent. The expected work life of new graduates will continue to shorten, and the number of new graduates will have to increase substantially over the 1988 level of 70,561 to replace the nurses lost to the labor force because of aging. Although it is debatable whether a large growth in the nurse supply is desirable or not, it is clear that to maintain the growth in the nurse supply seen in the 1980 to 1985 period, approximately four times the number of nurses over and above the approximately 70,561 currently graduating each year would be needed. Thus, the replacement needs associated with the aging work force will continue to grow in future years.

Finally, the aged and employed nurses reported in Table 4–4 were distributed by the percentage in each category currently working in hospitals. As seen in Table 4–5, the rate of increase in the nurse supply available to work in hospitals is 15.9 percent, which compares with a 22.1 percent increase in the total registered nurse supply for the same time interval.

## Demand

Demand for registered nurses is more difficult to evaluate than the supply of nurses. To relate demand to shortage it may be helpful to think about demand as having two components: met and unmet. Met demand can be measured well in

**TABLE 4–6 Selected Indicators of Demand**

|  | 1977 | 1987 | % Change |
|---|---|---|---|
| Hospitals | 5881 | 5611 | −4.6 |
| Beds† | 969 | 958 | −1.1 |
| Admissions† | 34,373 | 31,601 | −7.8 |
| Census† | 715 | 622 | −13.0 |
| Length of stay | 7.6 | 7.5 | −5.6 |
| Inpatient days | 260,835 | 227,015 | −13.0 |
| Outpatient visits | 198,708 | 245,524 | +23.6 |

Source: American Hospital Association. (1988). *Hospital Statistics*. Chicago: American Hospital Association.
    † In thousands.

terms of the hours of nursing service purchased by employers; unmet demand is more problematic to measure in a reliable and valid manner. Unmet demand generally is expressed in terms of vacancy rates, and vacancy rates may be inflated in noncompetitive markets because employers report vacant positions but are unwilling to raise wages to attract the desired supply. Despite this limitation, relative vacancy rates may provide a useful picture of demand over time.

As described by Aiken (1982; Aiken & Mullinex, 1987) hospital vacancy rates were high in the 1960s when there were a reported 23 vacancies per 100 budgeted positions. In response, nursing salaries rose in comparison with salaries of comparable female workers, and the supply of nurses increased. During the 1970s, wage increases fell behind those of other groups and behind inflation itself, and by the end of the decade, vacancy rates of 13 percent were reported. The cycle repeated, with salaries increasing in the early 1980s and vacancy rates declining to approximately 8 percent. In 1983, when hospital reimbursement changed to a prospective payment system, which included cost-containment measures, demand for nursing services decreased. In the period 1983 through 1987, salary increases were low, under 5 percent, and vacancy rates have slowly increased to 13 percent in 1986.

Other indicators of demand for the most recent decade, 1977 to 1987, indicate a decline in all areas except outpatient services. Table 4–6, for example, illustrates that the total number of hospitals has decreased by 4.6 percent, and the number of hospitals that closed in 1986 and 1987 was double the average in the 5 previous years (American Hospital Association, 1989–90). Similarly, there have been declines in number of beds, admissions, census, length of stay, and number of inpatient days (American Hospital Association, 1989–90).

There are some counterbalancing forces to the overall indicators of decreased demand. For example, there are data to suggest that acuity of hospitalized patients has increased, and demographic trends indicate an aging patient population, which presumedly increases patients' needs for nursing care. Additionally, technologic advances have increased the complexity of services required by at least some patients, and as seen in Table 4–7, many more hospitals are offering an array of outpatient and home care services, at least some of which require significant nursing input.

**TABLE 4–7 Selected Changes in Percentage for Hospitals Offering Selected Services**

| Service | 1977 (%) | 1987 (%) |
|---|---|---|
| Home care | 7.1 | 35.1 |
| Outpatient chemical dependence | 7.1 | 18.8 |
| Outpatient rehabilitation | 12.7 | 41.0 |
| Outpatient general | 26.8 | 70.0 |

Source: American Hospital Association. (1988). *Hospital Statistics.* Chicago: American Hospital Association.

Although the data relevant to demand are mixed, the overall aggregate picture, as seen in Table 4–8, shows an increase in critical care (25,567) and a decrease in general medical-surgical and other beds (86,400), thus producing a net loss of 60,833 hospital beds.

The Commonwealth Fund report indicates that it takes four to six times as many nurses to staff an intensive care unit bed as it does to staff a general medical surgical bed (Roberts et al., 1989). Based on approximately 5 hours of care per day for a general medical-surgical bed, it can be assumed that a general medical-surgical bed requires approximately one nursing full-time equivalent (FTE). Under these conditions, the increase of 25,567 intensive care unit beds could account for between 41,435 and 92,569 nurses.*

Although it is not clear that the 60,833 lost beds were beds for which staff nurses were available, the shift to more nurse intensive care unit beds has at least partially been offset by the closure of beds and the shift toward ambulatory services, which historically have been less nurse-intensive than inpatient services.

**TABLE 4–8 Change in Distribution of Hospital Beds by Selected Services, 1979 to 1988**

| | 1988 | | 1979 | |
|---|---|---|---|---|
| | Number of Beds | % | Number of Beds | % |
| General medical-surgical | 651,045 | 66 | 765,448 | 72 |
| Intensive care unit | 87,540 | 9 | 61,973 | 6 |
| Other | 252,728† | 25 | 224,725‡ | 22 |
| Total | 991,313 | 100 | 1,052,146 | 100 |

Source: American Hospital Association. (1980, 1989–1990). *Hospital Statistics.* Chicago: American Hospital Association.

   † 1988 Other includes obstetrics, burns, neonatal, intermediate care, alcohol and chemical dependence, rehabilitation, long-term care, and other beds. Excluded are beds for psychiatric care and mental retardation.

   ‡ 1979 Other includes all bed categories in 1988 plus orthopedic, chronic disease, tuberculosis (TBC), and otolaryngologic.

---

\* $(4 \times 25{,}567) - 60{,}833 = 41{,}435$; $(6 \times 25{,}567) - 60{,}833 = 92{,}569$.

**TABLE 4–9 Staff Nurse Salaries**

| Year | % Change CPI | Average Starting Salary | % Change Starting Salary Adjusted for Inflation |
|------|------|------|------|
| 1989 | 4.6 | $23,488 | 0.2 |
| 1988 | 4.4 | $22,416 | 2.5 |
| 1987 | 4.4 | $20,964 | −1.3 |
| 1986 | 1.1 | $20,340 | 3.2 |
| 1985 | 3.6 | $19,500 | .6 |
| 1984 | 4.3 | $18,708 | −2.1 |
| 1983 | 3.2 | $18,312 | −0.2 |
| 1982 | 6.1 | $17,772 | 3.9 |
| 1981 | 10.4 | $16,116 | .6 |
| 1980 | 13.5 | $14,508 | −0.5 |
| 1979 | 11.3 | $12,816 | −4.7 |
| 1978 | 7.7 | $12,059 | −0.7 |

Source: University of Texas Medical Branch at Galveston. (1990, March). *National Survey of Hospital and Medical School Salaries 1978–1989.* (1978–1989 eds.). Galveston, TX: Bureau of Labor Statistics, Bulletin 2347, U.S. Department of Labor.

## Wages

Wages for registered nurses are shown in Table 4–9 for selected years. For the decade 1978 to 1988, there have been only 3 years when starting salaries of registered nurses were substantially higher than the rate of inflation. The salaries of registered nurses have been relatively low, and because they are better educated and more versatile than many other types of hospital workers, hospitals substitute registered nurses for other workers when economically possible (Aiken & Mullinex, 1987). In the period of 1981 to 1987, for example, hospitals increased registered nurse employment by 20.6 percent and simultaneously decreased employment of licensed practical nurses and ancillary personnel by 23.5 percent and 12.1 percent, respectively (Bureau of Health Professions, 1989). This substitution has been aided by the efforts of nurses to move toward all registered nurse staffs; however, it would not have occurred had the wages of licensed practical nurses been substantially

**TABLE 4–10 Wages for Selected Hospital Workers As a Percentage of Monthly Registered Nurse Wage**

| Job Catagory<br>Registered Nurse | 1983<br>$1507 | 1985<br>$1620 | 1987<br>$1747 | 1988<br>$1868 |
|------|------|------|------|------|
| Licensed practical nurse | 72.5% | 71.6% | 41.0% | 70.0% |
| Respiratory therapist | 90.0% | 92.2% | 87.0% | 88.0% |
| Physician's assistant | 117.0% | 117.5% | 113.0% | 111.0% |
| Medical technician | 96.5% | 97.0% | 95.0% | 93.0% |

Source: University of Texas Medical Branch at Galveston (1990, March). *National Survey of Hospital and Medical School Salaries 1978–1989.* (1978–1989 eds.). Galveston, TX: Bureau of Labor Statistics, Bulletin 2347, U.S. Department of Labor.

**TABLE 4–11 1986 Salary Progression in Various Occupations**

| Occupation | Average Starting Salary | Average Maximum Salary | % Salary Progression in Field |
|---|---|---|---|
| Attorneys | $31,014 | $101,169 | 226.2 |
| Chemists | $22,539 | $ 74,607 | 231.0 |
| Accountants | $21,024 | $ 61,546 | 192.7 |
| Engineers | $27,866 | $ 79,021 | 183.6 |
| Purchasing clerks | $13,994 | $ 29,834 | 110.0 |
| Computer programmers | $20,832 | $ 42,934 | 106.1 |
| Buyers | $21,242 | $ 41,304 | 94.4 |
| Personnel directors | $39,917 | $ 75,710 | 88.8 |
| General clerks | $10,478 | $ 19,744 | 84.5 |
| Accounting clerks | $12,517 | $ 21,872 | 74.7 |
| Secretaries | $16,326 | $ 28,051 | 71.8 |
| Personnel clerks | $14,193 | $ 23,702 | 67.0 |
| Staff registered nurses | $20,340 | $ 27,744 | 36.4 |

Source: Bureau of Labor Statistics. (1990, March). *White Collar Pay: Private Service-Producing Industries, March 1989.* Washington, DC: Department of Labor, Bulletin 2347, Government Printing Office.

lower than the wages of registered nurses. Table 4–10 illustrates the salary of selected hospital workers compared with wages of registered nurses. From 1980 to 1988, the salaries of licensed practical nurses ranged from a low of 69 percent to a high of 73 percent of the registered nurse salaries.

Finally, comparing nursing wages with those in selected occupations, Table 4–11 shows that salary compression has been a significant problem. The small difference between starting and maximum salaries in nursing indicates there has been little reward for the long-term employee. Now, however, this situation is beginning to change, as can be seen in Figure 4–1.

In 1989, wages at the top of the nursing salary scale increased by more than 10 percent to $35,442, which is double the rate of increase in base wages. Nationally, pay raises are running from 5 to 10 percent, and the range of staff nurse salaries is from $26,000 to $37,000 across the country (*American Journal of Nursing*, 1989b). Although the data relative to supply, demand, and wages are relatively straightforward, interpreting their meaning is not, and a number of factors need consideration.

## Interpretations of the Data

During the most recent round of the nursing shortage, the federal government named the Secretary's Commission on Nursing to study the problem and to make recommendations. As part of its activities, the Commission heard testimony from numerous sources, including the federal agency charged with responsibility for forecasting the nation's requirements for nursing personnel, The Division of Nursing, Bureau of Health Professions, Public Health Service. According to the Division of Nursing, the requirements of nurses and the available supply were in approximate balance (Division of Nursing, 1988). This view was not shared by many others deliv-

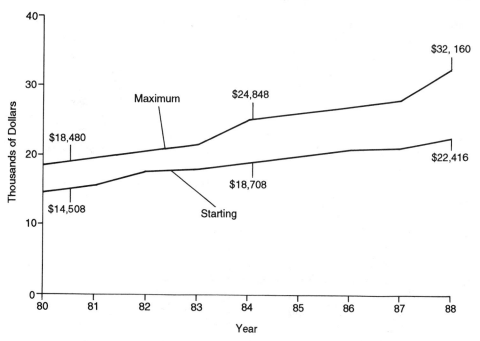

**FIGURE 4–1.** Maximum and starting salaries of staff nurses in hospitals.

Source: University of Texas Medical Branch at Galveston. *National Survey of Hospital and Medical School Salaries* (various years). Galveston, TX: Bureau of Labor Statistics, U.S. Department of Labor.

ering testimony, and questions were raised about how such a discrepancy could be explained. Several partial answers are suggested. First, there is little consensus regarding what level of vacancy constitutes a shortage. In 1980, for example, the American Hospital Association concluded that there was a severe and widespread nursing shortage (Mullner, Byre, & Whitehead, 1982). At that time, 67 percent of hospitals had either no vacancies or between one and nine vacant positions. Similarly, in 1987 the American Hospital Association reported that 59 percent of hospitals had less than 10 percent of their positions vacant, but the average vacancy rate of 13.6 percent was interpreted as indicative of a shortage (American Hospital Association, 1987). Clearly some (and in these two cases, the majority) hospitals had no or few vacancies, whereas others had more severe difficulties. As there is no benchmark indicator of what level of vacancy indicates a shortage, especially at the aggregate market level of analysis, it is difficult to tell if the claims of shortage at the time were the result of various parties advancing political agendas or of the loud voices of those individual institutions experiencing serious vacancy problems. In the past it has been to the advantage of hospitals for policy makers to declare a shortage, because that definition has led to federal efforts to increase the supply of nurses via subsidization of nursing education. This, in turn, has contributed to low wages and allowed hospitals to rely on solving their staffing problems with the influx of new graduates entering the work force each spring. If the federal response to a shortage had been different and had focused on stimulating wage competition among employers, hospitals might have been less enthusiastic about declaring a nursing shortage.

A second reason for disparate perceptions about a nursing shortage is related to methods used for examining the requirements for nursing personnel. At least some of the difference regarding the perception of shortage can be attributed to the method used to examine personnel requirements. For example, the Division of Nursing has used a professional needs model as the primary basis for its analysis of nursing requirements. This approach uses the expert opinion of clinicians to define what type and amount of services a given group of patients ideally should have. Need, as used by clinicians, is a normative concept that expresses professional goals unrestrained by the economics of health care. Clearly, need is a very different concept than demand, and statements of need generally advance in front of what, in fact, can exist. To the degree that professional goals are at considerable distance from the existing status quo, estimates of need can be judged to be unrealistic and unattainable.

Although there are a number of limitations to the professional needs model, the major weakness is that wages and other economic factors influencing employer demand are not included. Econometric models, on the other hand, are built on the assumption that labor supply and demand are equilibrated by wages and prices. These models are potentially more useful for examining labor shortage, but they, too, have been criticized because health personnel markets have not been well explained by economic factors alone. Other important considerations that impact on either supply or demand include technology, regulation and organization of service delivery, substitution among workers, and factors that influence productivity.

A third reason for discrepancies about whether the data are indicative of shortage or not relates to the time horizon of one's view of the nursing market. Markets are always fluctuating, and year to year changes in vacancy rates can be expected as markets seek a constantly changing equilibrium point. A long-term view, such as that provided by trend analysis across multiple years, is needed to identify significant disequilibrium in supply and demand.

Finally, discrepant views about a nursing shortage continue to exist because of data deficiencies. A recent review of the data needed at a national level to identify nursing shortage cited major data gaps and problems associated with wage and demand data in particular (Project Hope, 1989). In the past, data about the supply of nurses have come largely from the federal government based on sample surveys conducted at periodic intervals, most recently in 1977, 1984, and 1988. At this time the Division of Nursing is examining the feasibility of working with state boards that license nurses to create and maintain a current, accurate, and unduplicated master file of licensed nurses. Although this endeavor is very costly, in the long run it should be less costly than the previous approach to obtaining samples of nurses for the periodic sample surveys.

Data on employer demand and wages are more difficult to collect than is information about supply. In particular, it is difficult to impossible at this time to obtain reliable and valid data outside of the hospital sector. There is no organization, for example, representing all ambulatory care settings to parallel the data collection effort of the American Hospital Association. Since forecasts of shortage are only as good as the information on which they are based, rectifying data deficiencies is an important prerequisite to defining and solving shortage problems.

Despite discrepancies in views about what constitutes a nursing shortage and how to measure it with less than ideal data about supply, demand, and wages, it is relatively clear that the current situation in nursing in the United States is not indicative of a dynamic labor shortage. In view of the fact that the supply of nurses is at an all-time high, salaries have been relatively flat, and many indicators of demand suggest less rather than more need for nurses, how can the perceived shortage of nurses be explained?

## Explanations of Shortage

Part of the explanation has already been suggested, that is, (1) patients are sicker and older and require more care than in the past; (2) vacancy rates have been overstated owing to improperly functioning labor markets; (3) when the cost of nurses is inexpensive relative to other employees, substitution occurs; and (4) shortage can serve to advance political agendas by influencing policy makers to intervene in the labor market.

At least two additional explanations are advanced. First, nurses are not effectively used in hospitals because they are expected to perform the work of other departments, and second, because nursing practice is overly controlled and limited, nurses are not allowed to perform many patient care activities for which they are educated. Both of these situations result in too little professional nursing practice, one from the underutilization of nurses and the other from their utilization to do jobs that could and should be done by others (Diers, 1988; Prescott, 1989; Department of Health and Human Services, 1988).

The ineffective use of professional nurses is related to reductions in the numbers of licensed practical nurses, nurses' aides, orderlies, ward clerks, and unit managers and the absorption of their duties by registered nurses. In addition, nurses frequently perform the work of other hospital departments, such as pharmacy, transportation, housekeeping, laboratory, central supply, and dietary. This is especially true on evening and night shifts, weekends, and holidays, when many of these services are eliminated or severely curtailed. Taken together, the lack of support services and their performing the work of other departments contribute to nurses' spending a substantial amount of time in nonpatient care activities. In particular, nurses spend large amounts of time ensuring the smooth running of the patient care units. Historically, they have performed whatever activity was in danger of not being done, and their efforts have ranged from mopping the floor for housekeeping, enforcing hospital rules for administration, to performing lifesaving measures in the absence of physicians (Jacox, 1982). On a day-to-day basis, large amounts of registered nurse time are consumed by unit routines, such as checking narcotics and emergency carts, stocking supplies, ordering medications, transferring information from one form to another, and filling out reports. Many of these ritualistic tasks, if needed at all, could be performed by others.

On average, nurses spend large amounts of time in non–patient care activities, especially managing the patient care unit (*American Journal of Nursing*, 1989a). Making even relatively small changes in how nurses spend their time potentially could go a long way toward solving the shortage of nursing care experienced in hospitals today.

Factors that negatively influence the productivity of nurses have long been recognized in the literature as sources of job dissatisfaction. Until recently, however, they have not been emphasized as reasons for the perceived shortage of nurses. The recently completed final report of the Secretary's Commission on Nursing has recognized their importance (Department of Health and Human Services, 1988). Of the four general categories of recommendations that deal with nursing practice, two specifically address the problems identified above, that is, nurse decision-making authority and utilization of nursing time.

## Shortage Solutions: National Level

National labor force policy cannot be formulated until there are clear, agreed-upon, and consistent goals (Smith, Reinhardt, & Andreano, 1979). For example, concern has been expressed about cost, access, and quality of care, and personnel issues vary substantially, depending on which goal is emphasized. Further, rational labor force policy cannot be formulated based simply on extrapolation of historical trends, and meaningful labor force projections cannot be obtained and interpreted in isolation from the broader context of the economy in general, the health delivery system, and the interactions and substitutions among types of health care workers.

The shortage of nursing must be viewed within this complicated and continuous changing context. Not only are there multiple goals and multiple views of goals, problems, and solutions, there also are conflicting agendas whereby the solution for one group becomes a problem for another (Smith et al., 1979). Rather than focusing efforts at the national level on identifying the ideal number of nurses needed or demanded to solve the shortage problem, efforts might more profitably focus on a more multidimensional view of the problem, with particular emphasis on the kinds of interprofessional manpower mixes needed to deliver care at an acceptable level of access, cost, and quality. Solutions that are narrowly focused on nursing alone will fall short because of the interactional nature of the health care system.

At the federal level, policy makers need data and an approach to manpower forecasting that includes the analytic elements in Chart 4–1. Regardless of the occupation of specific interest, planners should pool resources and use common data and assumptions about demographic and population changes, economic growth in the economy, and growth in the health care sector of the economy; assumptions should be related to the organizational delivery, financing, and technology of health care, all of which significantly impact on work force requirements.

Of particular importance to a shortage of nursing personnel is the issue of substi-

**CHART 4–1 Analytic Components of a Model for Forecasting Imbalance in Supply and Demand for Health Care Personnel**

I. **Contextual Factors**
- Predictions about economic growth and its distribution across sectors of the economy
- Predictions about changes in the labor force and its distribution across economic sectors

II. **Technology, Delivery System, and Regulatory Factors**
- Labor-saving and labor-intensifying technologic changes
- Organizational and delivery system changes that significantly influence productivity
- Significant regulatory requirements that impact on staffing requirements

III. **Economic Factors**
- Prices and availability (quantities) of goods, services, and capital equipment
- Methods and levels of payment and associated economic incentives such as prospective payment
- Relative wages and wage elasticities for specific occupations and their relevant substitutes

IV. **Personnel Factors**
- Supply of target health care occupation
- Supply of relative substitutes
- Relative productivity of target occupation and substitutes

V. **Population Factors**
- Service utilization by various population subgroups
- Projected change in population by variables such as age, sex, race, income, health status

tution. Single discipline models do not have the potential for identifying this effect, which has been a significant factor in the current nursing shortage. Future efforts at analyzing the shortage should pay particular attention to the relationship among nurses, physicians, allied health workers, and selected other categories of hospital workers.

In the 1970s large amounts of federal resources were devoted to developing work force forecasting models. Budgets and accompanying personnel reductions have severely decreased the attention to health labor force issues, but the needs in this area are acute. Efforts to bring health care costs under control have not been successful, and concern over ever-rising costs of providing health care in this country are heard on a daily basis. Since labor costs account for more than one half of total hospital costs, it is time to devote more resources to a serious analysis of health personnel issues. Prerequisite to identifying optimal personnel mixes or solving shortages in specific target occupations is the need for national data bases that provide timely and accurate head counts by occupation and by employment sector within health care. Also needed are more data on wages and demand. Finally, much effort is needed to develop multioccupational models that contain the elements in Chart 4–1 and the ability to account for their interrelationships in interactional terms.

## Shortage Solutions: Individual Institutions

Shortage solutions at the level of individual employers are numerous and already well described in the literature (Aiken & Mullinex, 1987; Buerhaus, 1987; Diers, 1988; Fagin, 1989; Friss, 1989; Prescott, 1989; Roberts et al., 1989; Department of Health and Human Services, 1988).

The general tenor of these recommendations is that large supply increases are not likely to occur nor are they the primary solution to the problem. The one major exception to this statement refers to the part-time nursing labor force, which is substantial (26 percent in 1988). Even small increases in the number of hours worked by part-time nurses could substantially increase the nurse labor supply available to individual employers. Therefore, child care facilities, wage differentials, job sharing, and other flexible scheduling options are all possible solutions, which have already met with some success.

It is important to highlight the role of salaries and benefits in solving the shortage of nurses. Competitive relative wages are of critical importance at both the institutional level of individual employers and also at the aggregate market level. At the aggregate market level, increasing wages will serve to dampen employer demand and simultaneously will entice more labor in the form of new recruits into the field and/or into more hours of work from those already prepared as nurses. Freely rising nursing wages, relative to those in other fields now open to women, are the key to rectifying the chronic imbalance in the nurse labor market. As nurses become increasingly expensive relative to other types of workers, employers will substitute for them in favor of less expensive employees. The challenge for nursing will be to manage this decreased demand for registered nurse labor in such a fashion so as to not repeat the mistakes of the past.

In the past, use of nursing assistive personnel reduced the time professional nurses spent in the care of patients and changed their role to that of a care coordinator, as in the team mode of nursing delivery (Tappen, 1989). Team nursing decreased the hours of professional nursing care delivered to patients and produced a system of episodic and fragmented care that was not satisfying to nurses, patients, or physicians. It is important to realize that substitutes are not an effective solution to the shortage (Fagin, 1989). Instead employers need to identify solutions that enhance registered nurse time with patients. Use of complementary personnel rather than substitutes, changes that introduce labor-saving technologies such as computers for clinical management, decreased bureaucratic control over how nurses spend their time, better nurse-physician relationships, and more autonomous clinical practice of professional nurses are all partial solutions for the ineffective use of professional nurses (Christman & Jelinek, 1967; Koerner et al., 1986; Mowry & Korpman, 1987; Pellegrino, 1961; Prescott, 1989; Sovie, 1986; Zander, 1988).

Finally, wage increases cannot work to solve shortages at the level of individual employers, unless there are adequate differentials to draw nurses from one employer or employment setting to another. Hospitals have responded to this situation in a number of ways that may be thought of as short-term fixes as opposed to long-term solutions. For example, bounties have been offered to employees who find a new recruit, and money and prizes including trips and cars have been offered as sign-on bonuses. These rewards generally are available only when hospitals face an acute problem, and they are a one-time only pay that does not figure into base salaries. The same is true when hospitals use nurses from supplemental service agencies to augment their staff. Supplemental staff nurses are paid at a significantly higher rate than are hospital staff nurses. Although it is expensive, some hospitals have chosen this option because it avoids raising the wage rate of permanent staff and hence the overall marginal labor costs.

In general, competition among employers and competition across occupations are vital to assuring that adequate numbers of nurses will be attracted into nursing and then induced to work in it once their educations are completed. Because there is a positive relationship between wage and supply, anything that holds down wages will suppress the supply and increase the demand for labor. This does not mean that wages are the only factor of importance, and clearly the health care industry cannot afford unlimited wage increases for nurses or any other group.

Wages and benefits are an important component in any shortage reduction program. Overall solutions require a balanced and multidimensional approach that addresses both economic and professional considerations. Much progress could be made by shifting employers from reliance on recruitment to a focus on building serious programs of retention that recognize and reward professional nursing practice.

REFERENCES

Aiken, L.H. (1982). The nurse labor market. *Health Affairs, 1*(4), 30–40.
Aiken, L.H., & Blendon, R. (1981). The national nurse shortage. *National Journal, 13*(21), 948–953.
Aiken, L.H., & Mullinex, C. (1987). The nurse shortage: Myth or reality? *New England Journal of Medicine, 317*(10), 641–645.
American Academy of Nursing (1983). *Magnet hospitals: Attraction and retention of professional nurses.* Kansas City, MO: American Nurses Association.
American Hospital Association (1987). *The nursing shortage: Facts, figures and feelings.* Chicago: American Hospital Association.
American Hospital Association (1989–90). *Hospital Statistics,* Chicago: American Hospital Association.
*American Journal of Nursing* (1989a, September). Misuse of RNs spurs shortage, says new study: Only 26% of time is spent in professional care. *American Journal of Nursing, 89*(9), 1223.
*American Journal of Nursing* (1989b). Nurses gained new economic ground this year. *American Journal of Nursing, 89*(12), 1674–1684.
Bognanno, M., Hixson, J., & Jeffers, J. (1974). The short run supply of nurses' time. *Journal of Human Resources, 9*, 80–93.

Buerhaus, P. (1987). Not just another nursing shortage. *Nursing Economics, 5*(6), 267–279.

Bureau of Health Professions (1989). *Trends in hospital personnel 1981–1987: From the American Hospital Association Annual Surveys.* (Health Resources and Services Administration, Public Health Service, U.S. Department of Health and Human Services, ODANE Report No. 6-89). Washington, DC: U.S. Government Printing Office.

Burnstein, L. (1980). The analysis of multilevel data in educational research and evaluation. In D.C. Berliner (Ed.), *Review of research in education, 8* (pp. 158–233). Washington, DC: American Educational Research Association.

Christman, L., & Jelinek, R. (1967). *Modern Hospital, 108*(1), 78–81.

Department of Health and Human Services (1988). *Secretary's Commission on Nursing,* Final Report Vol. 1. Washington, DC: U.S. Government Printing Office.

Diers, D. (1988, February). *Nursing and shortage: Part of the problem or part of the solution?* Paper presented at the National Invitational Workshop on the Nursing Shortage Strategies for Nursing Practice and Education for the Division of Nursing, Department of Health and Human Services, Washington, DC.

Division of Nursing (1988). *Nursing: Sixth report to the President and Congress on the status of health personnel in the United States.* (U.S. Department of Health and Human Services, Accession No. HRP 0907204). Washington, DC: U.S. Government Printing Office.

Division of Nursing (1989). [1988 National sample survey of registered nurses.] Personal communication of unpublished data.

Edgren, J. (1976). The nursing shortage and the nurse training acts: Should the federal government be paying for the education of nurses? *Health Manpower Policy Discussion Series.* Ann Arbor: University of Michigan, School of Public Health.

Fagin, C. (1989). Why the quick fix won't fix today's nursing shortage. *Nursing Economics, 7*(1), 36–40.

Friss, L. (1989). Future prospects. *Strategic management of nurses; A policy oriented approach* (pp. 293–326). Owings Mills, MD: AUPHA Press, National Health Publishing.

Hannan, M.T. (1971). *Aggregation and disaggregation in sociology.* Lexington, MA: Lexington Books.

Herman, J.B., & Hulin, C.L. (1972). Studying organization attributes from the individual and organizational frame of reference. *Organization Behavior and Human Performance* (pp. 84–108).

Jacox, A.K. (1982). Role restructuring in hospital nursing. In L. Aiken (Ed.). *Nursing in the 1980's: Crisis, opportunities, challenges* (pp. 75–99). Philadelphia: J.B. Lippincott Co.

Koerner, B., Cohen, J., & Armstrong, D. (1986). Professional behavior in collaborative practice. *Journal of Nursing Administration, 16*(10), 39–43.

Mowry, M., & Korpman, R. (1987). Evaluating automated information systems. *Nursing Economics, 5,* 7–12.

Mullner, R., Byre, S., & Whitehead, S. (1982). Hospital vacancies. *American Journal of Nursing, 84,* 592–594.

National League for Nursing (1988). *Nursing Data Review.* New York: National League for Nursing, Publication No. 19-2290.

Nursing pay (1985, November). *Registered Nurse,* 33–39.

Pellegrino, E.D. (1961). The changing role of the professional nurse in the hospital. *Hospitals, 35*(24), 56–62.

Prescott, P.A. (1987). Another round of nurse shortage. *Image: Journal of Nursing Scholarship, 19*(4), 204–209.

Prescott, P.A. (1989). Shortage of professional nursing practice: A reframing of the shortage problem. *Heart and Lung, 18*(5), 436–443.

Prescott, P., & Bowen, S. (1987). Controlling nursing turnover. *Nursing Management, 18*(6), 60–66.

Prescott, P., Dennis, K.E., Cresia, J., & Bowen, S. (1985). Nursing shortage in transition. *Image: Journal of Nursing Scholarship, 17*(4), 127–133.

Project Hope (1989). *Assessment of gaps in available nurse data.* (Background paper 2, prepared for Health Resources and Services Administration under Basic Ordering Agreement #240-88-0057). Chevy Chase, MD: Project Hope.

Roberts, K.H., & Burnstein, L. (Eds.) (1980). *Issues in aggregation: New directions for methodology of social and behavioral science*, vol. 6. San Francisco: Jossey-Bass.

Roberts, M., Minnick, A., Ginsberg, E., & Curran, C. (1989). *A Commonwealth Fund report: What to do about the nursing shortage.* New York: Commonwealth Fund.

Rousseau, D. (1982). Technology in organizations: A constructive review of conceptual framework. In S.E. Seashore, E.E. Lawler, P.H. Miris, & C. Cammann (Eds.), *A field guide to organizational assessment.* New York: Wiley Intersciences.

Sloan, F. (1975). *The geographic distribution of nurses and public policy.* (Department of Health, Education, and Welfare Publication No. HRA 75-53). Washington, DC: U.S. Government Printing Office.

Sloan, F., & Richupan, S. (1975). Short run supply responses of professional nurses: A microanalysis. *The Journal of Human Resources, 10*(2), 241–257.

Smith, K., Reinhardt, U., & Andreano, R. (1979). Planning a national health manpower policy: A critique and strategy. In R. Scheffler (Ed.), *Research in health economics, a research annual.* Greenwich, CT: JAI Press, Inc.

Sovie, M. (1986). Nursing management considerations: Doing things differently and better. *Nursing Economics, 4*, 201–203.

Tappen, R. (1989). *Nursing leadership and management concepts and practice* (2nd ed.). Philadelphia: F.A. Davis Co.

U.S. Bureau of Census (1987). *Vital statistics of the United States*, Vol II, Part A. Washington, DC: U.S. Government Printing Office.

Yett, D. (1975). *An economic analysis of the nurse shortage.* Washington, DC: Lexington Books, Lexington, MA: Heath & Co.

Zander, K. (1988). Nursing case management: Strategic management of cost and quality outcomes. *Journal of Nursing Administration, 18*(5), 23–30.

## Chapter 5

# When Is Prevention Better Than Cure?

LOUISE B. RUSSELL

$P$REVENTION IS a recurrent theme in discussions of medical care policy. The argument is frequently put forth that the medical sector does not put enough emphasis on prevention, instead devoting too many of its resources to acute care aimed at treating disease once it has occurred. This allocation is thought to be a poor choice on two counts. First, it is argued that prevention is more effective than acute care as a way to improve health and extend life. Second, it is argued that prevention costs less than acute care, so that shifting more resources to prevention would actually reduce costs and help alleviate the problem of ever-escalating medical care expenditures.

Careful studies do not bear out the contention that prevention reduces medical expenditures. Instead, they show that the costs of preventive interventions usually outweigh any savings. In the following section, I discuss why expectation and reality on this issue are so far apart and cite evidence to show that prevention usually adds to medical expenditures.

The stress on prevention as a cost-saving measure is unfortunate because it has distorted the way preventive measures are discussed. Prevention often improves health and lengthens life in ways that acute care cannot. The real issue is not whether prevention is cheaper than treating disease but whether the additional health produced by prevention is worth the additional expense. Many preventive measures are worth undertaking because the gains in health are a good return for the expenditure. The second part of this chapter considers this point in more detail.

The last section discusses cost-effectiveness analysis as a way of evaluating prevention (and medical interventions generally). The methods of cost-effectiveness analysis make it possible to evaluate the benefits, risks, and costs of each intervention and to compare them with those of other interventions in a consistent framework. The discussion emphasizes how critically an evaluation depends on the medical evidence for an intervention's effectiveness.

## Prevention Usually Adds to Medical Expenditures*

At first glance, it seems obvious that prevention saves money. If people do not get sick, they do not have to go to physicians and hospitals. Since these are expensive services, much money is saved and it seems reasonable to believe that the savings will outweigh the costs of the preventive intervention. As a bonus, people are spared the pain and suffering of the disease.

The choice is often presented this way in radio and television advertisements, by physicians when talking with patients, and by speakers on the subjects of prevention and medical costs. One recent radio advertisement asks the listener to compare the cost of an annual blood pressure check with the expense of hospital care for the stroke or heart attack that might be caused by high blood pressure. The blood pressure test costs only a few dollars, whereas hospitalization costs thousands of dollars, with no guarantee that health can be fully restored.

But, a careful study of the costs of reducing high blood pressure found that savings offset only a small part of those costs (Weinstein & Stason, 1976). The study compared the costs of treating moderate and severe high blood pressures (a diastolic pressure of 105 mm Hg or higher) with the savings because disease is prevented. In addition, it estimated the gains in longer life and better health. The savings from fewer strokes and heart attacks amounted to only about one quarter of the costs of prevention. For mild hypertension, defined as a diastolic pressure between 90 and 105, the savings were even less.†

How can the study's conclusions differ so much from the simple comparison offered by the radio advertisement? The answer lies in two basic facts. The first is that the advertisement ignored most of the costs of preventing high blood pressure—the test is only the beginning. Second, it ignored the fact that not everyone who is tested has high blood pressure.

A brief consideration of the steps involved in screening and treating high blood pressure will make the issues clearer. The recommendation made by the Joint National Committee on High Blood Pressure—that adults should have their blood pressure checked at least every other year—means that millions of people must be tested repeatedly. Yet most of these people do not have and will not develop high blood pressure. Thus, the small cost of the test adds up as it is done over and over, particularly for many people who will never benefit from it. In addition, by itself, the test produces no improvements in health, and thus no savings. It merely identifies those who need further treatment, a major point overlooked in the simple comparison.

For those who do show elevated blood pressures, the test must be repeated.

---

\* Most of the discussion in this section and the next is based on Russell, L.B.: *Is Prevention Better Than Cure?* Washington, DC, Brookings Institution, 1986.

---

† The estimates included the cost of a single screening test. If the costs of regular rescreening for adults not identified as hypertensive by the initial test had been added, the savings would have been a still smaller percentage of total costs.

Elevated pressures are often transitory, and the best practice dictates that the patient be tested on at least two more occasions before a diagnosis of high blood pressure is definitely established. Once the diagnosis is established, additional tests are required to rule out the possibility that the hypertension is caused by undetected disease and to assess the extent of any damage that it may already have caused. Based on this information, the physician institutes treatment. For patients with moderate and severe high blood pressures, it is accepted practice to prescribe antihypertensive drugs. These cost anywhere from a few hundred to a thousand dollars a year, depending on the drug chosen. During the first year or so, extra visits to the physician are necessary to work out the best drug regimen and to evaluate and treat side effects. If the hypertension has been caught early, as it ideally should be, the drugs must be taken for many years. Chances are that no ill effects would occur during these years because it takes years of having high pressure before illness results. Thus the costs of prevention are high, immediate, and ongoing, whereas the savings do not occur until much later.

For the millions of people with mild hypertension, especially those with diastolic pressures in the range between 90 and 100 mm Hg, the physician may give nondrug alternatives a try—salt restriction, weight reduction, and exercise. All these have been shown to have some effect on blood pressure. If these do not work within a reasonable period of time, drugs may be prescribed. Again, the costs of extra visits to the physician and of drug prescriptions add up quickly.

When these costs are summed up to include the millions of adults who are tested and treated every year, the total reaches billions of dollars. The savings from prevented strokes and heart attacks—only in some people and usually not until years later—are much less. Although the original study, published in 1976, is rather old, experts who reviewed it in 1986 concluded that it is still accurate (Russell, 1987). Thus screening for and treating high blood pressure add to medical costs rather than reducing them. Prevention in this case does not save money.

At the same time, of course, screening and treating high blood pressure lead to better health and longer life for many people. The increase in life expectancy has been demonstrated in major clinical trials both for those with mild hypertension and those with moderate or severe hypertension. Thus screening and treating high blood pressure produce more good health, but at additional cost.

A small but growing number of careful studies show the same result for other important preventive measures: they add to medical expenditures at the same time that they improve health. In addition to screening and treatment for high blood pressure, these other measures include major cancer screening tests—the Papanicolaou smear, mammography, and tests for occult blood in the stool (American Cancer Society, 1980; Eddy, 1980, 1989); adult vaccines, such as the influenza and pneumococcal pneumonia vaccines (Office of Technology Assessment, 1979, 1981, 1984); childhood vaccines, such as the measles vaccine (Axnick, Shavell, & Witte, 1969); screening and treatment for lead poisoning in children (Berwick & Komaroff, 1982); screening and treatment for high cholesterol levels in children (Berwick, Cretin, & Keeler, 1980); and screening and treatment for high cholesterol levels in middle-aged men (Oster & Epstein, 1987; Taylor et al., 1990).

These studies look at the total costs of the preventive measure, no matter who pays them. Total costs, for a community or the nation, are the important number for public policy. Any change in medical practice shifts expenditures around, but this is cost shifting, not cost saving. It is important to be aware of this point when studies showing savings for a component of the total, such as a government program or a corporation, are cited as evidence that the nation will save money. The costs of all parties must be examined before that conclusion can be drawn. The studies cited here, which examine the costs of all parties, agree that prevention usually adds to medical expenditures rather than reducing them.

The statement is, however, an empirical observation, not a natural law. Although most preventive interventions add to medical expenditures, there are exceptions. For example, the Office of Technology Assessment (1979) estimated that, if pneumococcal vaccine were provided through a public program, the medical costs for people 45 years of age and older would be less than if the vaccine were not provided. If, however, the vaccine were provided through private physicians, as is currently the case, they estimated that medical costs would increase.

It is possible that prevention may save money in areas other than medical care, such as special education and custodial care, and that these savings may be enough to offset the additional medical costs. The studies of measles vaccine and lead screening for children both found substantial savings outside of medical care. Nevertheless, it is too soon to conclude that this is generally the case. Few good studies have looked at costs outside of medical care. Often the studies that do look at such costs estimate savings incorrectly and in such a way as to overestimate them. For example, if the preventive measure reduces the number of people requiring institutional care, the study may count the entire cost of institutionalization as a saving, without deducting the cost of living in the community for the same individuals.

At the same time, costs outside medical care are often ignored, especially if no one pays cash for them. Consider exercise, which has substantial health benefits. It uses a great many resources outside of medical care, including equipment, facilities, clothing, and perhaps most important, individuals' time. Even when no one pays for that time, it is a real resource, and one that can be used for many other purposes. People recognize this when they react to exercise as though it were expensive: "But, with my job/schoolwork/children/other activities, I can't find the time!" This example brings out the point that all resources used in providing an intervention must be counted, even those that fall outside the medical sector and those for which no money changes hands.

## Cost Saving Is Not the Issue

The idea that prevention does save money has led to the idea that it *must* save money to be worthwhile. Nothing could be further from the truth, and it is unfortunate that the cost-saving issue has created such confusion.

The truth is that good health is worth paying for. That may seem obvious when stated so baldly, but this basic fact has been lost in the argument over whether prevention saves money. It would be ideal, of course, to get better health at a saving. But even when prevention adds to medical expenditures, it is often a good investment. Making cost saving a requirement for prevention is wrong because it does not reflect our real values (we really do think better health is worth paying for) and because it makes prevention easy to shoot down by setting a standard that it cannot and should not have to meet. Thinking to make prevention more attractive, those of its supporters who stress the cost-saving argument have instead done it a disservice.

Indeed, most expenditures are made not to save money but to gain various other benefits. To draw a parallel from another area, people live in houses not because it is cheaper than living in tents but because it is better in many ways they think are worth the additional expense. They would not stop living in houses if someone pointed out that tents are cheaper. By the same token, we are not going to stop investing in prevention, but just as individuals must judge whether the benefits of a particular house are worth the cost, they also must judge whether the benefits of a particular preventive measure are worth the cost.

Many preventive measures are worth undertaking because the health gains are a good return for the expenditure. In its 1979 study, done at the request of Congress, the Office of Technology Assessment showed that pneumococcal vaccine added about $1000 in medical expenditures for each year of good health gained by people over 65. Even though the vaccine did not save money, Congress voted to provide coverage for it under Medicare because it brought better health at a reasonable cost. Pneumococcal vaccine thus became the first preventive measure explicitly covered by Medicare.*

To repeat the main point, prevention usually cannot be justified on the basis of cost saving, but it does not need to be. It is often worth doing because it produces better health, health that cannot be produced by alternative means, and better health is worth paying for. At the same time, the resources available to society, and the time and energy available to each clinician and patient, are limited. Each intervention must be evaluated on the basis of its health gains, risks, and costs to decide whether it is worth doing. Further, it is not possible to make blanket statements about preventive interventions in general (or, for that matter, about acute care in general). Each intervention must be evaluated individually.

## How to Evaluate Prevention

All the studies cited above use the methods of cost-effectiveness analysis. Although its application can be complicated, the basic idea behind cost-effectiveness analysis is simple. It is a formal process much like the informal one individuals go through when deciding to spend money or time. The individual thinks about what he or

---

* Some measures, such as treatment to reduce high blood pressure, are covered because, for insurance purposes, they are considered treatment rather than prevention.

she will gain, what the costs are, and how the gains compare with the costs. The cost-effectiveness studies cited above ask the same questions from a national, or societal, standpoint: What are the health gains from this intervention? What are the costs? How do the health gains compare with the costs?

In general, these studies estimate the costs and health benefits of a preventive measure according to the following formulas:

COSTS = medical costs of the preventive measure
          *minus* savings in medical expense because illness is prevented
          *plus* costs of treating side effects of the preventive measure

EFFECTS = lives or years of life saved by prevention
          *minus* lives or years lost to side effects*

These formulas are appropriate for interventions whose costs fall entirely in the medical sector, as they do for most of the interventions cited.

To show the balance between health effects (benefits) and costs, the analyst can present the results in several ways. Total health effects and costs are usually presented, along with subtotals for items of particular interest. For example, in the study of hypertension, health effects and costs were presented for men and women of different ages. In addition, it is usual to present cost-effectiveness ratios; these are the total costs for a group of people divided by the total health effects for the same group. When health effects are measured in years of life, a cost-effectiveness ratio shows the cost per year of life gained by the intervention. As an example, consider the Office of Technology Assessment's update of its 1979 report on pneumococcal vaccine (1984). That report estimated that the cost of vaccination for people 65 or older was between $300 and $6000 per year of healthy life in 1983 dollars. The range reflects different assumptions about the duration of immunity and about the percentage of all pneumonias that are pneumococcal and therefore susceptible to control by the vaccine.

Comparison is central to cost-effectiveness analysis. Its purpose is to array alternatives and compare them. The goal is to obtain as much health as possible from the resources available, and comparisons identify the alternatives that provide the most health in return for the resources used.

To clarify the importance of comparisons and the way cost-effectiveness results help to make them, consider a simplified example. Suppose a community has a choice of the three interventions described below, all of which have been proved effective by scientifically impeccable evidence:

---

\* Health effects may also be estimated using the method of the quality-adjusted life-year, also known as the well-year or the healthy year. This method assigns numerical values to different states of health so that changes in life expectancy and changes in health status can be combined into a single measure, the number of healthy years. See, for example, Kaplan et al., 1989.

| Intervention | Total Cost | Years of Life | Cost per Year | Intervention Might Be |
|---|---|---|---|---|
| A | $300,000 | 100 | $3000 | Childhood vaccination |
| B | $300,000 | 10 | $30,000 | Drug therapy for mild hypertension |
| C | $300,000 | 1 | $300,000 | Cholesterol level reduction for low-risk men |

The cost-effectiveness ratio, or cost per year of life, ranges from $3000 for intervention A to $300,000 for intervention C. The last column indicates actual interventions with cost-effectiveness ratios in this range.

If the community has $900,000 to spend, it will undertake all three interventions because they all contribute to better health. The total gain in health would be 111 years of life. If, however, the community has only $300,000 to spend, at least for now, it should choose to do A. That way, it will gain 100 years of life, the most possible with an expenditure of $300,000. If it invested in B, the next best alternative, it would gain only 10 years of life. The comparison shows that the cost of choosing B is having to give up A and C and the 101 years of healthy life they could produce. A is the better choice because only the 11 years produced by B and C are lost. Thus poor choices are a matter of concern because they mean that resources are not being used as productively as possible. The true cost is not measured in dollars but in health lost. To see that true cost requires information about what else the money could do.

To see some of these points in the context of a real intervention, consider a study of serum cholesterol level reduction for the prevention of heart disease in men (Taylor et al., 1990). This study was prepared for the United States Preventive Services Task Force, a group convened by the Department of Health and Human Services to develop recommendations for clinicians about the use of preventive interventions. To help encourage the use and understanding of cost-effectiveness analyses, the Task Force supported the preparation of a paper that applied cost-effectiveness analysis to several of the interventions it considered.

A particular strength of this study is the clarity with which it shows the importance to cost-effectiveness results of the evidence about medical effectiveness. The results of an analysis depend on costs, of course, but also, to a larger degree than is generally recognized, on evidence about whether the intervention is effective,* how effective, and for whom; these are the same issues that are debated when clinicians try to formulate recommendations on purely medical grounds.

The study of cholesterol reduction bases its estimates of the health effects on the Framingham model of coronary heart disease. This model relates risk factors, such as blood pressure, smoking habits, and cholesterol levels, to death from heart disease and is based on data from a longitudinal study of the population of Framingham, Massachusetts, which is an important source of much that is known about heart disease. The Framingham model uses a relationship of the multiple logistic form.

---

* If the intervention is not effective, there is no need to do a cost-effectiveness analysis, since the intervention should not be used.

**TABLE 5–1  Cost per Year of Life of a Dietary Program to Reduce Serum Cholesterol Levels in Men**

| Age | Cholesterol (mg/dl) | Cost per Year of Life Low-Risk Men† | High-Risk Men‡ |
|-----|---------------------|-------------------------------------|----------------|
| 40  | 180 | $360,000 | $42,000 |
|     | 240 | $180,000 | $21,000 |
|     | 300 | $ 94,000 | $11,000 |
| 60  | 180 | $540,000 | $43,000 |
|     | 240 | $280,000 | $23,000 |
|     | 300 | $160,000 | $13,000 |

Source: From Taylor, W.C., Pass, T.M., Shepard, D.S., Komaroff, A.L.: Cost-effectiveness of cholesterol reduction for the primary prevention of coronary heart disease in men. *In* Goldbloom, R.B., Lawrence, R.S. (Eds.): *Preventing Disease: Beyond the Rhetoric*, pp. 437–441. New York: Springer-Verlag (1990). Dietary program based on the Multiple Risk Factor Intervention Trial is expected to reduce serum cholesterol by 6.7 percent. Discount rate of 5 percent.

† Low risk is defined as no cigarette smoking; systolic blood pressure at the 10th percentile of the age- and sex-specific population distribution; and high-density lipoprotein cholesterol at the 90th percentile of the age- and sex-specific population distribution.

‡ High risk is defined as cigarette smoking; systolic blood pressure at the 90th percentile of the age- and sex-specific population distribution; and high-density lipoprotein cholesterol at the 10th percentile of the age- and sex-specific population distribution.

The important point about the multiple logistic form is that in it the risk factors act multiplicatively rather than additively, which means that a person with two or more risk factors has a much higher risk of death from heart disease than someone with only one risk factor. In turn, this means that the person with several risk factors will benefit much more from having one of them reduced than will the person with only one risk factor.

A few numbers may help make the point clearer. Suppose that men with no risk factors have a death rate of 1 per 1000. Men with a single risk factor, e.g., high cholesterol level, have a death rate of 3 per 1000, and those with smoking as their single risk factor have a death rate of 4 per 1000. According to the multiplicative Framingham model, someone with both risk factors, high cholesterol level and smoking, would then have a death rate of 12 (3 times 4), 12 times as high as the person with no risk factors. Reducing this person's cholesterol level would then reduce his death rate to that of the person with smoking as the only risk factor, a reduction of 8 per 1000 (12 minus 4). By contrast, the gain from reducing cholesterol level for a person whose only risk factor was a high level would be much less, only 2 (3 minus 1). Thus the health gain from reducing the cholesterol level of the person with two risk factors is much greater than the gain for the person whose only risk factor is a high cholesterol level.

This difference in health benefit drives the results of the cost-effectiveness analysis, as Table 5–1 demonstrates. The table shows the cost per year of life of an intervention modeled after the Multiple Risk Factor Intervention Trial. The intervention begins with a determination of serum cholesterol level that takes place at a physician visit made for some other reason, so that only the cost of the test is counted. Subsequent retests of cholesterol level and additional tests to rule out disease as a possible cause follow the recommendations of the Expert Panel on Detection, Evaluation, and Treatment of High Blood Cholesterol in Adults of the National Cholesterol Education Program. A program to change diet is then begun. In the first year it involves two extra visits to the physician and 10 visits to a dietitian, for a total first year cost of $557. Costs come to $150 for each subsequent year, for two serum cholesterol determinations, one physician's visit, and three visits to a dietitian. The intervention is ended after age 65, since the Framingham data indicate that cholesterol levels no longer have any impact on heart disease deaths after that age.

As the table shows, the cost per year of life gained from the intervention is much less for high-risk men (those with several risk factors) than for those with only one risk factor. This is true because although the yearly cost of the intervention is the same for all, the high-risk men gain much more in terms of improved life expectancy than the low-risk men. Thus the cost per year of life is much lower for the high-risk men. For example, the cost is $94,000 per year of life for a 40-year-old man with a cholesterol reading of 300 mg/dl and no other risk factors, compared with $11,000 for a man of the same age with the same cholesterol reading who also smokes and has high blood pressure and low high-density lipoproteins.* Thus, the results suggest that the intervention should focus first on high-risk men.

Taylor and his colleagues also estimated the cost of alternative approaches to reducing serum cholesterol, including a less expensive dietary program and two regimens in which two drugs, cholestyramine and lovastatin, were combined with a dietary program. Although the costs per year of life differed greatly among approaches, with approaches involving drugs being the most expensive, the contrast between low-risk and high-risk men held for all: it is always more cost-effective, that is, produces more health for the resources spent, to treat the high-risk men.

This study demonstrates especially clearly the importance of medical evidence for the results of cost-effectiveness analysis. Since the intervention is exactly the same for all men, the differences between the low- and high-risk men depend entirely on the effect the intervention is expected to have on their health.

## Conclusions

Careful studies of a wide range of important preventive measures show that prevention usually adds to medical expenditures at the same time that it improves health. This finding disappoints many of the supporters of prevention, who have argued that prevention deserves more resources in part because it will reduce expenditures. The focus on cost saving has unfortunately created confusion about how preventive measures should be evaluated. Good health is worth paying for, and prevention is often a worthwhile investment even when it adds to medical costs.

Since the nation's resources, which include the time and energy of clinicians and

---

* High-density lipoprotein cholesterol is a component of total cholesterol.

patients, are limited, however, decisions must be made about which preventive measures are worthwhile and for whom. The methods of cost-effectiveness analysis provide information crucial for these choices and have been briefly outlined. The results of cost-effectiveness studies depend as much on what is known about the medical effects of the intervention as on costs. A study of serum cholesterol level reduction in men demonstrated this point particularly well.

## REFERENCES

American Cancer Society (1980). *Guidelines for the cancer-related checkup: Recommendations and rationale.* American Cancer Society.

Axnick, N.W., Shavell, S.M., & Witte, J.J. (1969). Benefits due to immunization against measles. *Public Health Reports, 84,* 673–680.

Berwick, D.M., Cretin, S., & Keeler, E.B. (1980). *Cholesterol, children and heart disease: An analysis of alternatives.* New York: Oxford University Press.

Berwick, D.M., & Komaroff, A.L. (1982). Cost-effectiveness of lead screening. *New England Journal of Medicine, 306*(23), 1392–1398.

Eddy, D.M. (1980). *Screening for cancer: Theory, analysis, and design.* Englewood Cliffs, NJ: Prentice Hall, 1980.

Eddy, D.M. (1989). Screening for breast cancer. *Annals of Internal Medicine, 111*(5), 389–399.

Kaplan, R.M., Anderson, J.P., Wu, A.W., Mathews, W.C., Kozin, F., & Orenstein, D. (1989). The quality of well-being scale: Applications in AIDS, cystic fibrosis, and arthritis. *Medical Care, 27,* S27–S43.

Office of Technology Assessment, U.S. Congress (1979, September). *A review of selected federal vaccine and immunization policies: Based on case studies of pneumococcal vaccine* [technical memorandum]. Washington, DC: U.S. Government Printing Office, 1979.

Office of Technology Assessment, U.S. Congress (1981, December). *Cost effectiveness of influenza vaccination.* Washington, DC: U.S. Government Printing Office.

Office of Technology Assessment, U.S. Congress (1984, May). *Update of federal activities regarding the use of pneumococcal vaccine.* Washington, DC: U.S. Government Printing Office, 1984.

Oster, G., & Epstein, A.M. (1987). Cost-effectiveness of antihyperlipidemic therapy in the prevention of coronary heart disease: The case of cholestyramine. *Journal of the American Medical Association, 258,* 2381–2387.

Russell, L.B. (1986). *Is prevention better than cure?* Washington, DC: Brookings Institution.

Russell, L.B. (1987). *Evaluating preventive care: Report on a workshop.* Washington, DC: Brookings Institution.

Taylor, W.C., Pass, T.M., Shepard, D.S., & Komaroff, A.L. (1990). Cost-effectiveness of cholesterol reduction for the primary prevention of coronary heart disease in men. In R.B. Goldbloom, & R.S. Lawrence (Eds.), *Preventing disease: Beyond the rhetoric* (pp. 437–441). New York: Springer-Verlag, 1990.

Weinstein, M.C., & Stason, W.B. (1976). *Hypertension: A policy perspective.* Cambridge, MA: Harvard University Press.

## Chapter 6

# Health Care Technology and Its Assessment: Where Nursing Fits In

ADA JACOX

$S$IMPLY PUT, technology is the application of science. Where nursing fits in health care technology is a reflection of where nursing and nursing science fit in the health care arena generally. Questions such as what technology is used in patient care and who selects it, who does the research to determine if the technology is safe, efficacious, cost-effective, and has positive social benefits, who implements the technology, and who is reimbursed for its use are fundamental to a consideration of where nursing fits in health care technology and its assessment. This chapter describes health care technology, its regulation, the cross-disciplinary overlap in use of health care technologies, and nurses' involvement in its use and assessment.

### Health Care Technology: Definition and Cost

Whereas some people view technology narrowly as mechanical devices, the federal Office of Technology Assessment takes a broader view, defining health care technology as the drugs, devices, and procedures used in health care as well as the organizational and support systems within which such care is delivered (*Strategies for Medical Technology Assessment*, 1982). Thus, health care technology includes both prescription and over-the-counter drugs; devices such as fluidized air mattresses, pulse oximeters, and artificial hearts; procedures such as surgical operations and cardiopulmonary resuscitation techniques; and the personnel and organizational mechanisms that support the technology. Technology is pervasive throughout the health care system and is increasing in complexity and cost. Additionally, technology that formerly was found primarily in acute care settings increasingly is used in long-term care, ambulatory settings, and patients' homes.

The high cost of technology is widely acknowledged as a significant factor contributing to rapidly rising health care costs over the past two decades. Policy makers, health care professionals, third-party payers, and others increasingly are documenting the misuse and overuse of complex technology as contributing in unknown amounts to increased health care costs. Califano, for example, asserted that approximately 25 percent of health care expenditures are wasted, amounting to over 125 billion dollars in 1988 (*Medical Alert*, 1989, p. 31). Reportedly, 20 to 30 percent of work performed by physicians in hospitals is inappropriate, ineffective, or unnecessary, and 20 percent of diagnostic tests may be unnecessary (*Medical Alert*, 1989, p. 31). Perry, who was the first director of the National Center for Health Care Technology, established under the Carter administration, noted that inappropriate use of technology is "a serious factor in raising the cost of health care," with inappropriateness defined as "instances where the technology is used in ignorance, for a marginal benefit to the patient, in the absence of evidence of its value or in spite of the fact that conclusive studies have not been done" (*Medical Alert*, 1989, p. 32). It was estimated that "new technologies, new applications of existing technologies, or increased use of existing technologies in traditional ways are responsible for as much as 25 percent or more of the dramatic increases in health care costs over the past two decades" (*Medical Alert*, 1989, p. 31).

The cost of health care technology is difficult to determine precisely, given the broad definition used by the Office of Technology Assessment. Part of the difficulty in making accurate comparisons across categories of health care expenditures, including those related to technology, is that various agencies and researchers use different categories or categorize specific products and services differently. Nevertheless, all of the studies indicate substantial cost increases related to health care technology during the past 20 years, and it is possible to document the cost of components of health care technology, such as devices or drugs.

A medical device has been defined as "any item promoted for a medical purpose that does not rely on chemical action to achieve its intended effect" (Kessler, Pope, & Sundwall, 1987). The development and proliferation of devices have not received the same regulatory scrutiny that drugs have. The lack of clear regulatory authority and rigorous standards for development has given rise not only to misuse but also to enormous competition among manufacturers in developing and marketing various devices. In 1983, it was estimated that there were more than 1700 different types of medical devices, 50,000 separate products, and 7000 manufacturers of such devices (Kessler et al., 1987, pp. 357–358).

The development of devices has been profitable for manufacturers, and financial projections for the next few years indicate that such profitability will continue. *The Value Line Investment Survey*, a publication used by stock brokers and investors to evaluate the likelihood of earning profits in 98 different industries, projects that

> . . . the sales of medical supplies [including devices] will advance about 10% annually through 1992–94. Our nation's health care bill is expected to account for a greater proportion of GNP over the next few years, despite efforts to control costs. Underlying the greater demand will probably be new technology, and aging of the population, and perhaps a broader insurance coverage. . . . Profitability should be buoyed by new products, continued

efforts to limit manufacturing costs, and economy of scale. Overall, we look for earnings to grow 13–14 percent annually over the 3–5 year pull (*Medical Supplies Industries. The Value Line Investment Survey,* December 22, 1989).

The June 21, 1991 issue of *Value Line* ranked the medical supplies industry as fifth among the 98 industries in projected profitability over the next 12 months. Also on June 21, 1991, the drug industry was ranked first in projections of profitability. The cost of pharmacy and related expenditures for 1987 has been estimated at $34 billion (Letsch, Levit, & Waldo, 1988) or about 7 percent of total health care costs. *Value Line* noted that the 19 pharmaceutical companies followed by them showed a net profit margin of 16.1 percent in 1989. They projected that "In a year when corporate profits as a whole are likely to rise by 5% at best, drug manufacturers are on course to registering 1990 earnings gains on the order of 15%. The industry's profit rise is being fueled by healthy domestic sales of new drugs that command premium price tags, and by stringent cost controls" (*The Value Line Investment Survey,* May 11, 1990, p. 1258).

The medical services industry, which includes hospitals, nursing homes, and other health care agencies, was rated second in profitability by *Value Line* on June 21, 1991. One factor that *Value Line* identified as contributing to the health of the medical services industry is the major effort by both government and private agencies to improve the assessment of health care technology and its ability to produce cost-effective positive patient outcomes (*The Value Line,* November 10, 1989, p. 1277). Total costs for hospitals and nursing homes for 1987 were $235.3 billion (Levit & Freeland, 1988). The percentage attributable to carrying out health care procedures and to the support and administration of technology is unknown but is probably considerable given the pervasiveness and proliferation of technology. Berk and coworkers (1988) described the rapid growth during the 1960s of expensive technologies used in hospitals. The number of open heart surgical procedures performed increased from approximately 14,000 in 1967 to over 38,000 in 1971. In 1962, coronary care units were introduced, and by 1976 most hospitals with 300 beds or more had opened coronary care units, along with intensive care units used for patients with other conditions (Berk, Monheit, & Hagin, 1988, p. 53).

The recent response of hospitals to the expense of technology is reflected in a comment by Moxley (1988), president of a hospital chain, who noted that expenditures for both replacement and new technology must be markedly reduced. He referred to an announcement by the Hospital Corporation of America that they had reduced their capital expenditures by 50 percent, from 1.4 billion dollars in 1985 to 700 million dollars in 1986 (Moxley, 1988, p. 92). Moxley stated that "the pressures on hospitals at the present time are going to force them to be increasingly conservative purchasers of new and replacement technologies" (Moxley, 1988, p. 92).

## Regulation of Health Care Technology

Responsibility for the regulation of health care technology is far from clearly defined. In general, the only component of health care technology that has been closely regulated is drugs, which have been regulated by the Food and Drug Administration (FDA). Recent criticism has been directed at the long, complex, and expensive process required to gain approval to market new drugs, which is claimed to add to the costs of producing the drugs.

In contrast, there has been little regulation of devices. In 1976, the FDA was given authority for assuring that new devices were safe and effective before they were marketed (Kessler et al., 1987, p. 357). Kessler and colleagues observed that devices are regulated not only through federal statute by the FDA but also through federal reimbursement policy. They noted that "Medicare will cover an item or service that is generally accepted by the professional medical community as an effective treatment for particular conditions; payment will also be made if the safety and effectiveness of an item have been established, even if it is rarely used, novel, or relatively unknown" (Kessler et al., 1987, p. 361). Policies set by Blue Cross and Blue Shield and by the commercial insurance companies also determine which devices will qualify for reimbursement for their use; this constitutes additional regulation. Prior to the implementation of the Prospective Payment System in 1983, Medicare and other third-party payers reimbursed hospitals for the cost of devices on a cost-based pass-through system. The implementation of the Prospective Payment System and other forms of capitated payment means that now the cost of devices is included in the overall cost, and therefore use of devices within a particular diagnosis-related category (DRG) must be clearly justified as needed by patients in that particular group.

A current major concern is to try to ensure better review and regulation of devices. A "safe medical devices act," if considered by Congress, would necessitate more evaluation of devices after they have been marketed and implemented to identify problems. It also would require clinical trials for some products to demonstrate that the product is equivalent to an older model, since the 1976 amendments to the FDA law have permitted the entry of a number of products into the market that have not undergone extensive clinical trials (*The Value Line Investment Survey,* December 22, 1989).

The regulation of procedures is even more problematic. In the congressional hearing cited earlier, Perry estimated that 80 to 90 percent of all medical procedures have not been adequately assessed. "As a result, many new technologies have moved from research into the practice of medicine before their safety and effectiveness have been clearly defined. At the same time, Dr. Perry continued, many old, obsolete, and ineffective technologies continue to be used for years, even after new, more effective technologies have been introduced" (*Medical Alert,* 1989, p. 33).

Various approaches to assessment of procedures have been attempted, including randomized clinical trials, analysis of large data sets, and group judgment methods such as the National Institutes of Health "Consensus Conferences." In these conferences, expert panels analyze the results of available scientific evidence and develop guidelines for which procedures are most effective in particular situations. In general, however, many procedures used in health care have not received careful review of their effectiveness and agreement concerning appropriate use prior to implementation and widespread use.

A comparative perspective on the effects of regulation on the use of technologies across three different countries is given in a study of six technologies (open heart surgery, cardiac catheterization, organ transplantation, radiation therapy, extracorporeal shock wave lithotripsy, and magnetic resonance imaging) in the United States, Canada, and Germany, in which overall health care resources are comparable (Rublee, 1989). Canadian figures were for 1989, whereas German and United States figures were primarily for 1987. "Canada is an example of a country that has taken a tough stance on slowing the introduction of medical technologies; Germany is one that has taken a few small steps in that direction; the United States has done practically nothing" (Rublee, 1989, p. 179). There are wide variations across these countries in the use of cardiac catheterization; for example, it is being performed 1.5 per million persons in Canada, 2.64 per million persons in Germany, and 5.06 per million persons in the United States. "Given the differing approaches to constraining technological adoption, it is not surprising that there are significant differences between countries in the extent of technological availability. This is particularly the case in Canada, where some major technologies, for example, MRI [magnetic resonance imaging], are prohibited outside of hospitals" (Rublee, 1989, p. 181).

High variation illnesses are conditions that vary markedly from one locality to another in how they are treated because of the lack of medical consensus about the need for hospitalization. The lack of practice guidelines for health care technology has resulted in considerable geographic variation in the treatment and cost of treatment for various conditions. Wennberg (1988) began studying factors that influence variations in practice approximately 20 years ago. A resident of New Haven, Connecticut, for example, is twice as likely to have coronary bypass surgery as a Bostonian, but only half as likely to receive an endarterectomy (Tarlove et al., 1989). Bostonians are much more likely to have their hips and knees replaced, whereas New Haven residents have far more hysterectomies and back operations.

Noting the wide variation in practice styles and costs, Wennberg commented: "We remain ignorant of the consequences for patients of spending vastly different proportions of the gross national product (GNP) on health care. . . . Over the next decade or so, the issue of what is appropriate practice will dominate the health policy debate. The debate threatens to be increasingly acrimonious and devisive, pitting physician against physician, specialty group against specialty group, and the profession itself against the payer and the government, with the patient lost somewhere in the rhetoric" (Wennberg, 1988, pp. 100–101). Wennberg described the lack of evaluation of the outcomes of many treatments, including major surgery, invasive and risky diagnostic procedures, and the practice of treating many chronic and acute medical conditions in hospitals.

The recent recognition of wide variations in practice and cost has given rise to major research and evaluation efforts by private and public sector groups with the intent to assess the effectiveness of technology, with particular attention to patient outcomes. Such research is fundamental as a basis for appropriate and informed regulation. In the early 1980s the American College of Physicians established a program known as The Clinical Efficacy Assessment Program, which evaluates performance and cost-effectiveness of various technologies to determine when they can be used most effectively. The Rand Corporation is completing a major study of medical outcomes in which variations in patient health outcomes are related to factors such as clinicians' practice and the setting in which the care is given.

Various federal agencies also have undertaken major initiatives to study the effectiveness of various technologies. The Congressional Office of Technology Assessment, the United States General Accounting Office, the Health Care Financing Administration, the Food and Drug Administration, the National Institutes of Health (Office of Medical Applications), and the Prospective Payment Commission all have sponsored or conducted major studies related to technology assessment.

On December 19th, 1989, Congress established a new federal agency called the Agency for Health Care Policy and Research. Replacing the National Center for Health Services Research and Technology Assessment, the Agency for Health Care Policy and Research now serves as the federal government's focal point for health services research. Its goals are "(1) promoting improvements in clinical practice and patient outcomes for more appropriate and effective health care services; (2) promoting improvements in the financing, organization, and delivery of health care services; and (3) increasing access to quality care" (The Agency for Health Care Policy and Research, 1990, p. 1). The Agency is concerned with acquiring, developing, and transferring new knowledge through a program of research, demonstrations, evaluations, and information dissemination activities. The Agency sponsors individual and institutional national research service awards for academic training and research concerning health services research methods and problems. A major part of the Agency's activities is extramural research on the effectiveness of medical treatment on patient outcomes. This program is geared to improving the effectiveness and appropriateness of health care services and procedures. Another function of the new Agency is to arrange for the development, periodic review, and updating of clinically relevant practice guidelines. These guidelines are to be used by health care professionals, educators, and consumers to help determine how various health conditions can most effectively be prevented, diagnosed, treated, and managed. The initial guideline development by the Agency includes seven conditions (cataracts, benign hypertrophic prostate disease, clinical depression, sickle cell anemia, pain, urinary incontinence, and impaired skin integrity). At present nurses are chairing or cochairing three of these panels (those on pain, urinary incontinence, and impaired skin integrity).

One program in the Agency is specifically focused on technology assessment. This program "evaluates the safety and effectiveness of new or unestablished medical technologies being considered for Medicare coverage. The assessment process culminates in a report that is a detailed analysis of the safety, clinical effectiveness, and uses of new or unestablished medical technologies" (Agency for Health Care Policy and Research, AHCPR Program Note, *Publications in Print, 1989*, 1990, p. 9). Some of the areas in which the Agency has focused its health technology assessment are automated ambulatory blood pressure monitoring of hypertension, continuous positive airway pressure for the treatment of obstructive sleep apnea in adults, chemical aversion therapy for the treatment of alcoholism, cardiac rehabilitation services, and the role of speech-language pathologists in the treatment of dysphagia. Several nurses are employed in positions throughout the Agency, and four nurses were named as members of the advisory council to the Agency.

The increasing number of public and private organizations dealing with some aspect of technology assessment is reflected in the directory published by The Institute of Medicine (IOM) in 1988, which listed over 50 organizations concerned with technology in health care (*Medical Technology Assessment Directory*, 1988). An International Society of Technology Assessment in Health Care was formed in 1985. The technology assessment activities of other countries are documented in publications by the Society (1990), and the IOM's Council on Health Care Technology (Goodman & Baratz, 1990).

## *Technology Assessment: A Form of Policy Research*

Technology assessment provides guidelines for the systematic evaluation of new and established technologies to distinguish between those worthy of support and dissemination and those that should be restricted or discontinued (Pillar, Jacox, & Redman, 1990). The objective of technology assessment is to provide information for clinicians and policy makers. The information obtained is used by health care professionals to guide their practice, by legislators to formulate regulations and legislation for health care, by third-party payers to determine what services will be covered, by administrators to make purchasing decisions, by industry to develop products, and by consumers to make decisions regarding the care they will receive (Pillar et al., 1990).

Technology assessment includes four components: safety, efficacy/effectiveness, cost and benefit, and social impact. Although any single assessment of the technology usually does not incorporate all of these components, a comprehensive assessment of technology does. The primary concern is safety, which is evaluated in relation to risk. That is, the amount of risk accepted is related to the amount of benefit expected. Efficacy relates to the probability that persons in a defined population will receive benefit. Effectiveness relates to the benefits of a technology under average conditions of use in practice (*Assessing the Efficacy and Safety of Medical Technologies*, 1978).

The third major component considered in technology assessment is the cost of the technology, including the cost in relation to the benefits to be received. Cost benefit analysis measures costs and benefits in monetary terms, which is difficult to do and often involves arbitrary decisions in specifying the monetary value of outcomes such as reduced pain and improved quality of life. Cost-effectiveness analysis compares the effectiveness of one or more technologies in producing health-related outcomes such as greater functional ability, reduced complications, and increased quality of life.

Determining the social impact of a technology involves an analysis of the legal, ethical, and political effects of the technology on an individual, family, health care system, or on the society as a whole. The widely varying views of persons evaluating the social impact make this aspect of technology assessment one of the most complex, and it is often one of the components not or inadequately assessed.*

---

\* Interested readers are referred to the following article, which further details the components of technology assessment: Pillar et al. (1990).

The difficulty of evaluating the social impact of technology is apparent in considering ethical issues, such as who has access to care. Although many in this country have until recently espoused the notion that every citizen has a right to health care, the meaning of this assumption is increasingly being questioned. The fact that approximately 37 million Americans do not have any form of health coverage is in clear contradiction to the idea that everyone has a right to health care. Although it seems likely that some form of national health insurance eventually will be adopted to address this issue, it is equally clear that only certain health care services will be included in what are considered to be fundamental or basic services to which everyone should have access. Decisions will continue to be made by federal and state governments as well as by private insurers regarding what aspects of health care services will be covered by third-party payers. To the extent that consumers are unable to supplement third-party payers' reimbursement, those consumers will be limited in their access to health care, including particular health care technologies. The difficult issue of who should have access to what health care technologies is one that will increasingly be a major factor in the determination of health care policy.

There are many similarities between the process of technology assessment and the process of quality assurance. Brooks (1988), observing the integral links between the two fields, noted that both depend on a broad definition of health, both make evaluative judgments, and both must establish causal links between the process of care and patient outcomes. In spite of the similarities between the fields of quality assurance and technology assessment, there has been little overlap in the agencies and persons involved in those two fields. The Council on Health Care Technology of the Institute of Medicine sponsored a conference to consider the relationships between quality assurance and technology assessment (Lohr & Rettig, 1988). Conclusions drawn regarding the two fields were that both shared the common objective of existing to improve patient well-being and quality of care, both evolved in large part from public and private sector efforts to control the growth of health care expenditures, both have had major impact on the health care professions, and both fields use similar methods and data.

## Turfs and Overlapping Activities in Health Care Organizations

To understand where nursing fits in health care technology and its assessment and in health care generally, it is important to begin with the dominant position that physicians hold in the health care system. As Havighurst (1987, pp. 132, 134) noted, "Professional licensure laws have long made the provision of most personal health services the exclusive province of physicians. . . . Most state licensure laws proceed by creating an exclusive province for physicians and then carving out narrow enclaves within that province for various other licensed occupations. This legal recognition of the medical profession's sovereign sphere gives rise to serious jurisdictional struggles that state legislatures must referee."

The assumption by organized medicine that whatever is done in health care should be under the purview of the physician has had significant influence on the evolution of nursing as a profession. Nursing and other health occupations have continuously interacted with medicine and with each other in defining, defending, and expanding occupational boundaries. A recent study by the Institute of Medicine describing the rapid proliferation of allied health workers (*Institute of Medicine Allied Health Services: Avoiding Crises*, 1989) listed 79 instructional programs in allied health, which did not include medicine, nursing, dentistry, pharmacy, and other major health professions. The report noted wide variations in the extent to which the "turf" of various occupations is well marked and protected.

The proliferation of health care workers has been accompanied by considerable overlap in activities carried out by nursing and various other occupations. There is overlap in the technologies used by nurses and by physicians, dietitians, emergency medical technicians, respiratory therapists, psychologists, clinical pharmacists, and cardiovascular technologists, among others. This overlap makes it difficult to draw precise boundaries around nursing and nursing technologies, since these vary with time, place, and setting. The overlapping and changing boundaries also contribute to a lack of understanding by those outside of nursing concerning precisely what it is that nurses do.

## *Where Nursing Fits In*

In spite of the invisibility of much of what nurses do, the role of the nurse in health care technology and its assessment can be described in terms of use of the technology, nursing costs related to the technology, reimbursement for use of the technology, and the process of technology assessment.

Nurses' use of health care technology includes technology to carry out nursing functions, such as monitoring patients' vital signs with various electronic devices and using IVACS to monitor infusion of intravenous fluids. It also includes delivering technology-related care prescribed by a physician, such as maintaining patients on ventilators and administering intravenous chemotherapy. As noted above, defining precise boundaries regarding what is nursing technology and what is cross-disciplinary technology or technology used by several disciplines is not possible with the overlap among health care providers. However their use of health care technology is defined, nurses are heavily involved in implementing health care technology in acute and long-term care settings and in the home. Nurses' involvement in the use of technology varies depending on time, setting, and the presence of other types of health care providers who also use the technology.

The report of a conference sponsored by the Food and Drug Administration in 1988 (Smith & Murray, 1989) noted that nurses are the primary users of sophisticated health care technology and that attention needs to be given to the role of nursing education in the safe and effective use of medical devices. Recommendations made by conference attendees included the need for nurses to be employed as full-time consultants to product development task forces and other research and development groups and for nurses to be more involved in the development and assessment of technologic devices.

One way in which nurses are involved in decisions regarding use of technology is when they serve as case managers for a health care agency or third-party payer. As noted above, federal and private policies regarding reimbursement for health care technology are a major influence in the development, adoption, and diffusion of technologies. The widespread introduction of capitation plans throughout the health care system and the need to contain costs will have an effect on spending and reimbursement for health care technologies. One response to the need to slow the rate of cost increases has been the increased use of case management techniques in the health care system. Although case management has traditionally been viewed as a way for health care professionals to ensure that patients received needed health care services, it is increasingly used by payers of health care as a means of containing costs. Case managers are expected to monitor carefully the type and amount of care received to see that the most cost-effective methods are used and that various technologies are not used inappropriately or wastefully. In view of the general lack of knowledge regarding what kinds of drugs, devices, and procedures are most effective and least costly, case managers and those establishing the policy framework for their decisions clearly have some of the most difficult jobs in the health care system today.

In general, determining the cost of health care technology, including that used by nurses, is difficult because it has only been fairly recently that the health care system has been required to pay serious attention to costs. When the Prospective Payment System was introduced in 1983, for example, the payment algorithm was based on the assumption that approximately 80 percent of the operating costs of diagnosis-related categories were labor-related and 20 percent nonlabor-related. More recently, the assumption of 75 percent of labor-related costs has been used (Cromwell, 1989), reflecting improved knowledge of the various components of health care. One focus of study by the Health Care Financing Administration was labor–nonlabor costs related to medical devices costing over $300 (Prospective Payment Assessment Commission, 1986). The researchers identified 36 diagnosis-related categories in which the majority of expensive devices were used and recommended that several diagnosis-related categories should have their labor–nonlabor costs more precisely measured because hospitals in high wage rate areas received significantly higher payment relative to costs for those diagnosis-related categories with high nonlabor costs.

Another reason for not knowing the effect of use of health care technology on the cost of nursing care is that nursing care has begun to be separated out as part of overall hospital costs only recently. Even when the costs of the nursing department are separated, however, determining the costs of technology-related nursing care is difficult because of the tremendous overlap with other occupations in use of the technology.

In nursing, as in health care technology generally, there are significant gaps in the research literature regarding the most effective use of technology, including the aspect of cost-effectiveness. One study (Hutchinson, Milliken, & Larson, 1989) compared the costs of heparinized and normal saline flushes for peripheral intermittent intravenous devices (heparin locks). They found that the heparinized saline flushes required 120 to 160 seconds to perform versus 45 to 60 seconds for the normal saline flushes. Interestingly, although there were no significant differences in the incidence of clotting, phlebitis, or infiltration between the two types of flushes, significantly more locks flushed with heparinized saline (12.9 percent) had to be restarted because of leaking at the intravenous site than those flushed with normal saline only (7.5 percent). The authors estimated that savings for the total hospital in using normal saline flushes would be approximately $30,000 to $40,000 per year. This is the kind of research that will have to be done in the literally hundreds of technology-related aspects of nursing in order to determine how best to use the technology.

Also important to consider is the impact on nurses' work of how other professionals do their work. The variation in physician practice noted above is a case in point. Because many of the diagnostic, surgical, and other therapeutic procedures done on patients have a direct impact on the nursing care, nursing activities also are affected by the variation in medical practice to an unknown degree.

A second example of how decisions implemented by other professionals in the health care setting influence nursing activities and costs was reported in a study that compared the use of controlled versus noncontrolled analgesic agents (Kitz, McCartney, Kissick, & Townsend, 1989). The researchers reported on the amount and cost of nurses' time generated by the use of two different types of drugs, noting that recent studies have demonstrated that a noncontrolled oral analgesic (flurbiprofen) is as effective as some controlled analgesics (acetaminophen with codeine and morphine sulfate) for postsurgical analgesic therapy. Costs of nursing time in three nursing units were estimated as $34,000 per year more when the controlled analgesics were used. The increased costs were directly attributable to the nature and amount of nursing activities associated with the administration of each type of analgesic.

The extent to which nursing is reimbursed for the technology that nurses use is another important consideration. In general, reimbursement for organized nursing services is included in the costs of a hospital day, with a frequently unknown percentage representing nursing costs. Direct reimbursement to nurses for specific services carried out has been sought by some nursing organizations and nurses in private practice over the past several decades, with considerable resistance from organized medicine. The implications of the overlap across health care professionals for the reimbursement of nurses' work are seen in recent attempts to develop revised payment structures for physicians. The Physician Payment Review Commission, which is considering alternative payment methods for physicians, has used the current procedural terminology published by the American Medical Association to specify technologies used in various areas of medical practice. Activities listed as those for which physicians should be reimbursed include the following: nasotracheobronchial catheter aspiration, bladder irrigation, therapeutic injection of drugs, intermittent positive-pressure breathing treatment, training in activities of daily living, and educational services to a group of patients. Griffith (Griffith & Fonteyn, 1989) is surveying nurses in various specialty areas to determine how often they perform certain activities, the percentage of time they perform them compared with other providers such as physicians, and the percentage of time that they are directly supervised by a physician during the performance of a procedure. Griffith's work should serve both as a basis for documenting the extent of overlap in these activities and for reimbursement of nurses for the performance of these and similar activities.

Another area in which nurses carry out much of the work but are not in policy-making positions is in the assessment of health care technology. Various governmental and private agencies concerned with technology assessment commonly employ nurses as staff. This includes agencies such as the FDA and many commercial insurance companies that use nurses as case managers and in utilization review. Similarly, nurses frequently are employed in hospitals to carry out many of the quality assurance activities that relate not only to nursing but also to the activities of other health care professionals; however, they are conspicuously absent from the policy-making positions in many of these organizations.

## Summary and Recommendations

The intent of this chapter has been to describe the major efforts under way to assess health care technology in order to promote its appropriate and cost-effective use and to illustrate the pervasiveness of nursing in implementing and assessing health care technology but its near invisibility in policy-making bodies and reimbursement schemes. If nursing is truly to enter the mainstream of health care, health care technology, and technology assessment, there is a need for nurses to become involved in helping to steer the course and not simply providing the labor needed to implement health care policy made by others.

Toward this end, the following recommendations are offered:

- Organized nursing should undertake a coordinated effort to make nursing's role in health care technology and technology assessment more significant and more visible. This includes acknowledging nurses' responsibility for the use of technology and the need for nurses to have greater involvement in its assessment. Nursing should be concerned not only with nursing technologies but also with the assessment of technologies used across disciplines. Nursing should be well represented in organizations concerned with technology assessment, including the Congressional Office of Technology Assessment, the Health Care Financing Administration, the Food and Drug Administration, the Prospective Payment Assessment Commission, the Agency for Health Care Policy and Research, and the Institute of Medicine. Their involvement should include serving as members of policy-making groups and should not be limited to serving as staff.
- Several national centers should be established to address technology assessment in nursing. The centers could be part of national nursing organizations located in academic health centers or joint ventures undertaken between selected professional organizations and universities. A model for this is the Rand Corporation in Santa Monica, California, which plays a major role in the assessment of medical technology.
- Nurse researchers should work with nurse executives, economists, accountants, and others to add analyses of costs to their studies. Many clinical studies could be framed within a technology assessment approach, thus enhancing their usefulness in addressing policy questions.

- Nurse executives should broaden their focus on research and evaluation type activities to include technology assessment. The need for an empiric data base on which to base administrative decisions regarding the most appropriate and efficient use of resources has never been greater. The need has been acknowledged by many nurse executives who have established such departments in nursing services. The cost-cutting efforts of some administrators have been aimed at eliminating many personnel who do not provide hands-on nursing care. Eliminating personnel who carry out research and development activities that can serve as a basis for designing efficient nursing service delivery systems and for assignment of personnel may save dollars in the short run but is short-sighted in planning for the future.*

- Documentation of nurses' use of technology should serve as a basis for reimbursement policy both for organized nursing services and for individual practitioners. Reimbursement policy should acknowledge that it is nurses who use nursing and nursing-related technologies and who should be reimbursed for their use.

- Nursing should be more involved in the political debates regarding access to care and the appropriate use of health care services. This should include specification by nursing of what basic nursing care patients should expect to receive. Nursing technologies should be carefully scrutinized so that they are used appropriately and efficiently.

## REFERENCES

Agency for Health Care Policy and Research Program Note (1990, April). In *Publications in print, 1989* (p. 9). Rockville, MD: Agency for Health Care Policy and Research.

*Agency overview, current agenda, and planning activities* (1991). Prepared by Kathleen Hastings. Washington, DC: Agency for Health Care Policy and Research.

*Assessing the efficacy and safety of medical technologies* (1978, September). Washington, DC: Office of Technology Assessment.

Berk, M.L., Monheit, A.C., & Hagin, M.M. (1988, Fall). How the U.S. spent its health care dollar: 1929–1980. *Health Affairs, 7*(4), 46–60.

Brooks, R.H. (1988). Quality assessment and technology assessment: Critical linkages. In K.N. Lohr & R.A. Rettig (Eds.), *Quality of care and technology assessment: Report of a forum on the Council of Health Care Technology* (pp. 26–27). Washington, DC: Institute of Medicine: National Academy Press.

Cromwell, J. (1989, June). An analysis of the perspective payment systems labor-nonlabor share by diagnosis-related group. *Health Services Research, 24*(2), 214–236.

Goodman, C., & Baratz, S.R. (Eds.) (1990). *Improving consensus development for health*

---

* Suggestions for including technology assessment activities with other similar activities and programs in hospitals are given in an article by Jacox and Kerfoot on nursing "Technology assessment in hospitals," *Nursing Economics*, July/August, 1990.

*technology assessment: An international perspective.* Washington, DC: Institute of Medicine: National Academy Press.

Griffith, H.M., & Fonteyn, M.E. (1989, August). Let's set the payment record straight. *American Journal of Nursing, 89*(8), 1051–1058.

Havighurst, C.C. (1987). The changing locus of decision making in the health care sector. In L.D. Brown (Ed.), *Health policy in transition: A decade of health politics, policy, and law* (pp. 129–167). Durham, NC: Duke University Press.

Hutchinson, T.N., Milliken, E., & Larson, W. (1989). Comparison of normal vs. heparinized saline for flushing infusion devices. *Journal of Nursing Quality Assurance, 3*(4), 49–55.

*Institute of Medicine Allied Health Services: Avoiding crises* (1989) (p. 18). Washington, DC: National Academy Press.

International Society of Technology Assessment in Health Care (1990, May 20–23). *Abstracts.* 6th Annual Meeting, Houston, TX.

Kessler, D.A., Pape, S.M., & Sundwall, D.N. (1987). The federal regulation of medical devices. *New England Journal of Medicine, 317*(6), 357–366.

Kitz, D.S., McCartney, M., Kissick, J.F., & Townsend, R.J. (1989, January). Examining nursing personnel costs: Controlled versus noncontrolled oral analgesic agents [Financial Management Series]. *Journal of Nursing Administration, 19*(1), 10–14.

Letsch, S.W., Levit, K.R., & Waldo, D.R. (1988, Winter). National health expenditures, 1987. *Health Care Financing Review, 10,* 109–121.

Levit, K.R., & Freeland, M.S. (1988, Winter). [Data Watch]. National medical care spending. *Health Affairs, 7*(5), 124–136.

Lohr, K.N., & Rettig, R.A. (Eds.) (1988). *Quality of care and technology assessment: Report of a forum of the council on health care technology.* Washington, DC: Institute of Medicine: National Academy Press.

*Medical alert* (1989). *A staff report summarizing the hearings on "the future of health care in America"* (pp. 101–151). Subcommittee on Education and Health, Joint Economic Committee, Congress of the United States. Washington, DC: U.S. Government Printing Office, S.PRT.

*Medical Supplies Industries. The Value Line Investment Survey* (1989, December 22). Edition 1, p. 202.

*Medical technology assessment directory* (1988). Washington, DC: National Academy Press.

Moxley, J.H., III (1988). Technology assessment: View of a multi-hospital system. In K.N. Lohr & R.A. Rettig (Eds.), *Quality of care and technology assessment: Report of a forum on the council of health care technology* (p. 92). Washington, DC: Institute of Medicine: National Academy Press.

Pillar, B. (1991). The safety of medical devices and the role of the FDA. *Nursing Economics,* July–August (in press).

Pillar, B., Jacox, A., & Redman, B. (1990, January/February). Technology, its assessment, and nursing. *Nursing Outlook, 38*(1), 16–19.

Prospective Payment Assessment Commission (1986). PPS payments for expensive prosthetic and implantable devices and other medical supplies (pp. 87–89). *Technical appendices to the report and recommendations to the secretary.* U.S. Department of Health and Human Services. Washington, DC: Prospective Payment Assessment Commission.

Rublee, D.A. (1989, Fall). Medical technology in Canada, Germany, and the United States. *Health Affairs, 8*(3), 178–181.

Smith, R., & Murray, E.W. (1989, April). Nursing and technology: Moving into the 21st century—Conference Proceedings, May 16–18, 1988. Annapolis, MD: HHS Publication FDA 89-4231, 121 pages.

*Strategies for medical technology assessment* (1982, September). Washington, DC: Office of Technology Assessment.

Tarlov, A.R., Ware, J.E., Jr., Greensfield, S., Nelson, E.C., Perrin, E., & Zubkoff, M. (1989). The medical outcomes study: An application of methods for monitoring the results of medical care. *Journal of the American Medical Association, 262*(7), 925–928.

*The Value Line Investment Survey* (1990, May 11). Edition 8, Drug Industry, p. 1258.

*The Value Line Investment Survey* (1989, November 10). Edition 8, Medical Services Industry, p. 1277.

*The Value Line Investment Survey* (1989, December 22). Edition I, Medical Supplies Industry, p. 202.

*The Value Line Investment Survey* (1991, June 21). Part I, Summary and Index, p. 1.

Wennberg, J.E. (1988, Spring). Improving the medical decision-making process. *Health Affairs, 7*(1), 99–106.

# PART II

## Issues in Hospital Nursing Practice

## Chapter 7

# Fostering Professional Nursing Practice in Hospitals: The Experience of Boston's Beth Israel Hospital

JOYCE C. CLIFFORD

*I*N THE DECADE of the nineties, restructuring the work environment and redesigning the role of the registered nurse are common themes within acute care hospitals motivated by the threat of continuing nurse shortages. During the early and mid-1970s, the Beth Israel Hospital (BIH) in Boston undertook a major initiative to restructure the nurses' work environment and redesign their roles, stimulated by a desire to have the BIH become an attractive place to work for nurse professionals and a satisfying care system for patients and families. This change process resulted in the development of a professional practice system cited as a model for others (Fagin, 1990), and it transformed BIH from one of the most unsatisfying nursing practice systems, where nurses were "just little cogs in the wheel" (Kilroy quoted in Scherer, 1988) to "one of the best in the country" (Sunshine & Wright, 1987). In large measure, this change can be attributed to the implementation and refinement of primary nursing within the context of a managerial philosophy of decentralized decision making and an organizational structure that supports five dimensions of professional practice: caregiving, teaching, consulting, leadership, and research. This paper provides a brief summary of the major concepts underlying the professional practice model at BIH. A more detailed account can be found in Clifford and Horvath, 1990.

Caregiving remains the central focus of the professional practice model of BIH. The centrality of this dimension of professional practice relates to our firm belief in nursing as a practice discipline and our commitment to use management and scholarship as a means for strengthening and advancing that practice. The work of the clinical nurse, i.e., the care of patients, is in the long run the work of us all. Thus, an emphasis has been placed on developing roles, organizational structures, and overall systems that will facilitate and support the clinical or caregiving dimension of practice.

Between 1973 and 1978, BIH underwent tremendous change in the way nursing care was organized at the unit level to meet the expectations that the nursing staff and the hospital administration agreed were essential for good patient care. Motivating these changes was the dissatisfaction with patient care expressed by nearly all groups: nurses, physicians, administrators, and most significantly, by patients and families themselves. This dissatisfaction ranged from nurses' frustration over their inability to complete the "tasks" associated with care let alone patient care planning, to the frequent and sometimes serious complaints from patients, families, and physicians about the quality of the care. Fragmentation of patient care was the result of the task-focused, team nursing system in place for nursing care delivery. Abrasiveness too often characterized the nursing staff, who felt overworked, underpaid, and unrecognized. Nurses lacked the resources to do their jobs, and they had alienated the ancillary and support departments of the hospital because they were constantly found hoarding supplies in an effort to have enough on hand when a patient needed them. Such supplies included linen to use when a patient was incontinent, wheelchairs to transport a patient, specula for vaginal examinations, flashlights to use at night, and even medications to use after the pharmacy closed in the afternoon until the next morning.

This scenario, present at BIH in the middle 1970s, was not unlike the practice systems found in many hospitals in the United States at that time, or unfortunately still found in some hospitals even today. Although it is not the intent of this chapter to dwell on the problems of the past, they do become important in understanding what has shaped the nature of hospital nursing practice in this country and the frustration of nurse professionals who have worked in these systems. Such understanding is also critical in framing the argument that the nursing practice system of any hospital is as much a product of its *interaction* with the total hospital system as it is of anything else. Thus, any change process undertaken is one that must be integrated with the overall institution. The concept of timing also becomes an important element in effecting successful organizational change. It is linked to the need for the nursing administrative team to have a clear understanding of the nature of organizational development, especially their own, and to use this understanding in making decisions. The nurse executive of the hospital organization becomes an essential leader in ensuring that these two concepts, integration and timing, are understood by all members of the hospital team and are effectively carried out.

The professional-bureaucratic conflicts described by Etzioni (1964), Clifford (1981), and others have special meaning to the nurse executive as the quest for professional practice systems is undertaken. As a member of the institution's administrative team, the nurse executive has an obligation to develop a care delivery system that ensures, at a very basic and minimal level, the safety of patients. This often translates into assuring not only that the technical requirements of care are carried out effectively but also that other tasks, often related to ancillary and support services, are completed on behalf of the patient. Because there is a responsibility on the part of the nursing division to be sure that such work *is done*, much of this work has also come to be viewed as *the work of nursing*. The dilemma faced by nurses in attempting to reconcile the conflict is the basis for various attempts made in the past to sort out the responsibilities of registered nurses vis-à-vis others in the care process. Such clarification remains the focus of many of the current hospital restructuring processes.

The development of effective systems that support care is a necessary, fundamental step in designing a clinical practice system that removes the barriers between nurses and patients. Nurses need to have the appropriate support services to provide patient care, and the evolution of a professional practice system depends upon the concurrent development of these systems of support. Nurses, and especially nurse executives, have a responsibility to help others understand that these support systems are as critical to the work of the nurse as surgical instruments are to the surgeon or as the clinical laboratories are to the internist. These are the systems that provide nurses with the tools they must use to effectively and efficiently accomplish much of their technical work.

But the professional-bureaucratic dilemma of the nurse administrator goes beyond clarifying the respective responsibilities of the registered nurse and institutional support systems in the provision of care. The nurse executive must ensure not only that work will be accomplished in a safe and adequate manner but also that the professional services of the registered nurse will be available. Hence, it is not sufficient for the professional nurse to simply oversee and supervise the work of others; professionals also must be in a position of being able to utilize their knowledge and skill on behalf of patients. Clinical decision making and expert judgment are the components of the professional role that cannot be delegated to or substituted for by someone less well prepared. Substitution of the nurse professional as a direct care provider, therefore, runs the risk of removing from the care process the expert judgment and decision making that can only come from the professional nurse. Systems of care delivery that maximize the professional nature of the registered nurse's role, providing patients and families with the benefit of this health professional's knowledge and judgment, are indispensible if the cost-quality balance of health care is to be maintained.

## First Steps

Given the circumstances of clinical practice at BIH in the mid-1970s, the initial plans for redesigning the role of the registered nurse had to encompass some fundamental principles about the work environment as well as some basic understanding of the notions of responsibility, authority, and accountability. Even though nurses constantly stated they wanted "the authority to" or they wanted "to be autonomous" in practice, they were seldom able to connect these concepts with that of professional accountability. Among the first steps in developing a professional practice system is to develop a set of clear expectations for practice that incorporate a fundamental understanding of the rights *and* obligations of professionals in the work place. At Beth Israel, those expectations involved in the early change process attempted to avoid making this process cumbersome. The primary object was to describe the expectations of practice and outcomes for patients and, in doing so, to help others bring basic values to the surface. Attempts were made to always ask for simple clarification, to be clear about what was acceptable and what was unacceptable, and to frequently ask questions such as "How does this relate to your professional responsibility to the patient and family?" and "What options were/are available to you?" Constant vigilance for the basic concept of accountability has been important to the members of the BIH nursing staff. Helping nurse professionals move from a task-oriented work model to a model of professional accountability is a prerequisite for eventually developing most other systems considered part of a professional model.

These tactics provide an opportunity to accomplish many things but most of all to be sure that everyone involved is operating from the same set of expectations in terms of the values and principles to be operationalized.

Having a clear set of values that can be articulated and understood throughout the organization is extremely critical in the development of an effective professional practice model. Values set the direction and provide the foundation as well. They become the stability of the organization's culture, and they become the measuring stick when there is a tendency to stray off course. Taking detours is really never the problem in organizational change—the important thing is knowing whether or not this particular detour will still bring you to the same outcome. Changing course may be necessary, for example, in a restricted labor force market. But understanding the consequences of the decisions made is the essential element and must be factored into the overall strategic plan. For example, because the need to give basic technical care is so demanding in hospitals, it is often the rationale used in a restricted economy or labor market for not developing a professional practice environment. There is an overwhelming sense of responsibility in hospital nursing practice to ensure that the technical aspects of care are carried out. Consequently, it is often easy to get caught up in the tasks to be accomplished or the work that must be done, inadvertently neglecting to lay the groundwork for the development of a professional model of care delivery that in the long run will have more significant outcomes for everyone involved.

## The Foundation: Primary Nursing

*Accountability* of practice and *continuity* of care are the two central concepts in a professional nursing model, and both are integral to primary nursing, the professional nursing model implemented at Beth Israel. Primary nursing remains central to the professional model of care at BIH today and is expected to remain as the delivery system throughout any foreseeable changes the hospital and the nursing division undertake.

The principles used in establishing primary nursing at BIH provide for its continued expansion and evolution. These principles remain as relevant for the future as they have been for the past. For example, as case management emerges as a nursing delivery system, the need to strengthen rather than delete or substitute for the primary nursing role surfaces. Since the implementation of primary nursing at BIH now nearly two decades ago, the role of the clinical (staff) nurse has, in concept as well as in practice, included a responsibility for the coordination of all aspects of the patient's care plan, including those that are provided by other clinical disciplines. The emphasis given to this coordinating role has varied according to patient population and other resources available at any given time. The need to develop the clinical competency and judgment of clinical nurses was critical to the success of primary nursing in the early years of implementation. Because *coordination* could, at that time, be easily misunderstood as an invasion of another discipline's practice area, this practice expectation did not always receive the priority the health care system now requires for it.

For BIH nurses, the concept of case management includes designating the primary nurse as *the accountable professional* for the development of an ongoing plan of care. This includes the coordination of all components, including those determined necessary by other disciplines or traditionally provided by other health professionals. In order to fulfill this responsibility, the nurse must be designated as the professional with the *authority to coordinate* all aspects of care. This designation of authority and accountability is in keeping with the previously defined role of the primary nurse as the coordinator of clinical services for the patient and family. For some patient populations, nurse professionals have assumed responsibility for managing elements of patient care across inpatient and ambulatory settings. The restructuring of the Beth Israel nursing practice model for the future includes broadening the concept of acute care, hospital-based nursing practice to incorporate caring for patients across the spectrum of illness. This will require a restructuring of clinical practice across the traditional settings of inpatient, ambulatory, and home care.

Integrating case management functions more fully within the primary nurse role is in keeping with the principles of the professional model previously established at BIH. Effective patient care management depends upon very close collaboration with other disciplines, especially medicine and hospital administration. Collaboration with both of these groups was an early focus of the development of our practice system and continues to be a major focus of current redesign efforts. The complexity of patient care calls for joint planning and goal setting, not just cooperation and good communication between disciplines. To this end, a collaborative care unit was established in 1988 at BIH in an effort to more fully investigate and understand all the complexities of these collaborative relationships. Collaborative relationships remain highly valued in our system.

An examination of our current practice system has led us to an even greater understanding of, and respect for, primary nursing. Primary nursing, as implemented at BIH, is more than simply a system of personalized care, an outcome we highly value; it is a system that represents a way for nurses to balance the needs of hospitalized patients for expert technical competence *and* humanistic care. Maintaining stability in the delivery system of primary nursing is of paramount importance for us in the achievement of ongoing hospital and professional goals. The fundamentals of this system, which allow for the continuous care of patients by an identifiable clinical nurse, provide a stable relationship that remains a critical element in assuring the balance of efficiency and effectiveness sought in today's health care environment.

Continuity in caregiving is a distinguishing element of primary nursing. Dissatisfaction of the patient, family, nurses, and other health care providers with the fragmented and interrupted care planning that occurs with the more conventional systems of team and functional nursing led us to incorporate continuity of care and accountability for that care by an identifiable professional into all aspects of our practice model. Some of the early organizational elements needed to operationalize these components included the stabilization of staff, scheduling, and assignments.

Continuity cannot be achieved if clinical staff members are reassigned from their primary unit on any regular basis. Stabilizing staff so they become home based and able to maintain a stable assignment of patients from admission through discharge becomes a first-level challenge in the development of a professional model. Placing trust in the judgment of the unit-based nurse manager and clinical staff to determine their staffing needs and to accept responsibility for their own coverage when needed became an early focal point in their socialization to the concept of what it means to be an accountable professional. Floating staff and using temporary agencies to supplement staff are practices that were rejected by us, beginning with the early redesign of the nursing practice system. Because of the existence of such a strong nurse-patient relationship, nurses at the unit level have been willing to extend themselves individually and as a work group to meet the staffing requirements for safe patient care. Today, the concepts of self-managed work groups are more frequently used, and patient care units are considered very self-sufficient with respect to these components.

At the Beth Israel, we have used patient classification systems to provide management information about the dependency or acuity of patients for overall planning purposes and quality assurance activities. We have rejected the use of these systems as decision-making tools to guide daily staffing needs on the unit. As institutions advance in the area of automation for nursing documentation and patient care activity, information regarding the acuity of patients should be created automatically as a byproduct of other pertinent clinical information. This eliminates the need for nurses to separately classify patients. Such information should be more reliable and more useful to hospitals in understanding the costs of caring for the multiple "case types" represented by the patient population of the institution.

Although changes in staffing have occurred since the implementation of primary nursing and the development of a professional model at BIH, the initial change to primary nursing was accomplished within the same budgeted guidelines approved for the more traditional delivery system. But as roles changed and nurses became patient-focused, not task-focused, the number of nurses *available for direct care* increased without an increase in budgeted full-time equivalent (FTE) positions. This was possible as the need for charge nurses, medication nurses, assistant head nurses, and clinical supervisors was eliminated. These roles were returned to the unit as direct care provider roles. The management and supervision of nurse professionals are quite different when each individual accepts accountability for her own actions and clinical support systems are in place through the role of the clinical nurse manager and other expert clinicians. Mentoring, precepting, and peer review processes are all elements firmly in place and considered indispensible in further developing the professional role of the clinical nurse.

## Decentralization and Leadership

As the rights, obligations, and roles of professionals were examined and clarified and systems redesigned to facilitate and support the nurse professional's role in patient care delivery, one of the most frequently asked questions became, "who has the right to make this decision?" For us, decentralization relates predominantly to decision making. Our interest was to place decision making as close to the point of delivery of service as possible. Thus, many conventional practices found in hospitals were challenged and replaced with practices that allowed for decentralized decision making. Flattening the organizational structure was one of the first steps, as was clarifying the roles of staff nurse, head nurse, and nursing supervisor. Clarification of roles includes identification of the authority and accountability points for decision making within the organization, not simply the rewriting of job descriptions. Role clarification within the context of authority and accountability relationships must first occur.

The fostering of a professional practice model requires the development of many systems that facilitate decentralized decision making. For a professional nursing department, the development of a strong committee structure is as important to the successful implementation of decentralization as flattening the hierarchical organizational structures. Coordination of efforts, standard development, and monitoring practice against those standards are all essential elements to have in place to ensure nursing's willingness to be accountable for its own practice. The committee structure of BIH serves as an alternative to shared governance models. We prefer to think of this level of participation as one of the necessary systems for integration of clinical and administrative practice and overall integration of nursing within the larger institutional policy and decision-making system. Nurses at BIH are not only actively involved in the many nursing committees and task forces in place—they are also active participants on hospital-wide committees and medical executive subcommittees. The vice-president for nursing/nurse-in-chief participates with other hospital executives at Board of Trustee meetings and committees and also with other clinical chiefs at their meetings. Decentralization is implemented throughout the hospital, and nurses are considered important contributors to the policies and practices that evolve from these committee efforts.

Of great significance in the successful development of a professional practice model is the development of the unit-based leadership role, traditionally titled head nurse and now more frequently called clinical nurse manager. The development of this managerial role has proved critical for the successful implementation of decentralized decision making. Professional practice systems change the communication patterns that have existed within the hospital. For the most part, the nurse manager has served as the central resource for all other members of the health team, including other members of the nursing department. Changing this pattern often requires a number of hospital-wide policy changes, including such basics as allowing phone calls to come directly to the primary nurse, providing the primary nurse with the authority to call the physician's office directly, developing an integrated patient care record, or, just as simply, people needing to learn the names of many nurses and not just a few! In the mid-1970s these practice changes seemed revolutionary to some, but to most clinical nurses they seemed logical and long overdue.

Clarification of the head nurse's decision-making authority did not simply mean determining what he or she must give up doing in order for primary nurses to assume their rightful authority and accountability in the decision-making process. Nurse managers needed to learn how to disengage from the specifics of individual patient care management and yet still involve themselves freely in patient care activities in order to assist primary nurses to develop as professionals. A consistent part of clinical management practice must be how to place accountability for patient care on staff and how to hold them accountable for this care.

This expectation of the nurse manager requires a management style that is open and honest in its communication, nonjudgmental and yet comfortable in expressing ideas, and quick to praise and compliment others. A willingness to continue their own learning and development is essential in order for nurse managers to continue to value the learning and developmental needs of clinical staff. Nurse managers at BIH take their dual role of a hospital manager and clinical leader very seriously. They are as intent on managing their own cost center resources as they are on putting the educational needs of patients and staff as a top priority and serving as mentors for clinical nursing staff.

## Professional Salary Model

Salary and benefits are often cited as being among the most significant issues to be addressed if the health care industry and the nursing profession seriously expect to change the career decisions of nurses or decrease the amount of movement that occurs within and among health care institutions (Aiken & Mullinix, 1987; Prescott, 1987; Sovie, 1989).

Because ideas are continuously evolving, BIH regularly evaluates its clinical practice model for its effectiveness in meeting the needs of nurses as well as patients. One area of continuous evaluation is that of salary and benefits. Even though local labor market competition is a strong motivator in establishing annual compensation programs for nurses, the Beth Israel has attempted to design its compensation program for nurse professionals within an overall framework of a professional rather than a labor model.

In keeping with the underlying values that support the concept of professionalism in the practice setting, the compensation program for registered nurses is designed to provide a salaried approach to wage administration rather than the traditional, hourly labor approach used by most hospitals. Although the salary range is within the market range of other Boston teaching hospitals, there are other economic considerations to this compensation approach for registered nurses. Increments for clinical advancement and merit review are established within a salary model that takes into account the total compensation package of salary and benefits.

As hospitals begin to incorporate a salaried approach for professional nursing staff, there is a need to evaluate the economic impact of this method of compensation over the traditional hourly wage approach. Salary practices should be closely monitored to ensure its fairness to nurses, who by the nature of their work are often unable to control the reasons for frequently working beyond the scheduled work hours. In addition, nurses often must adjust to rotation to undesirable work hours, a factor that many salaried professionals do not face. Exploitation of nurses has been part of nursing's history (Reverby, 1987), and the move away from the hourly payment system should not promote such exploitation in any way. There is the additional need to evaluate the effectiveness of this method of compensation in changing the self-image of the nurse sufficiently to influence his or her career decisions. Clearly, this is a desired outcome motivating the change to a salaried approach at BIH.


## Education and Scholarship

As primary nursing developed at the Beth Israel, so did the level of preparation of registered nurses employed. This delivery system places nurses in the very center of relationships, communication, and coordination with patients and families, physicians, other nurses and health professionals, and hospital administration. The skills, knowledge, and overall know-how required to communicate, collaborate, confront, coordinate, and provide continuity of care in a complex academic medical center led first to the demand from nursing staff for more hospital-sponsored continuing education programs and then more opportunity to return for more formal education. It was the latter phenomenon, the return to formal education by staff nurses, that led nurse managers and senior nursing leadership to adopt the practice of employment of the baccalaureate degree–prepared nurse. Beth Israel has distinguished itself as a hospital that has utilized the bachelor of science, nursing–prepared nurse well. In 1990, 93 percent of the nursing staff were prepared at the bachelor of science (nursing) or master of science (nursing) level of education, a fact considered by us to signify tremendous success considering that in 1974 the hospital found it difficult to attract bachelor of science (nursing)–prepared nurses even for leadership positions. From our viewpoint, we have found this level of educational preparation to be the most effective in accomplishing the goals of quality patient care, even in a financially constrained health care environment.

We now have a large cadre of well-prepared nurses on staff. As a consequence, many activities are extremely decentralized in our practice model, providing us with the opportunity as a hospital to avoid the expense of a cumbersome organizational structure to support a variety of activities. Activities range from staff orientation to nursing research. Nurses at the unit level participate actively in the development as well as the implementation of many programs, including educational initiatives, quality assurance, continuing care, nursing research, and other professionally satisfying yet organizationally required activities. We have been able to blend and integrate these responsibilities so nurses feel involved in standard setting and decision making without feeling exploited. Enhancement of the opportunities for professional growth for clinical nursing staff is an ongoing goal of the nursing division. The need to restructure the work setting to maintain the expertise of very experienced and well prepared nurses at the bedside who are delivering direct patient care services is considered essential in our practice model.

Work redesign, task analysis, and clarity of decision making once again become the focus of the BIH's nursing department's next step into the future. Benner's (1984) conceptualization of the domains of nursing and advancing from novice to expert practice have become fundamental concepts in the continuing evolution of the Professional Advancement and Recognition Program of BIH. Developing an organizational structure that appropriately utilizes and recognizes the differentiation of nurse professionals by competencies has become an essential component for the next generation of professional practice at Beth Israel. An examination of the role of nursing in a teaching hospital has raised a number of interesting questions about our responsibilities for career development of nurse professionals and development of supporting structures to operationalize these responsibilities. Experience has shown that the first work experience of the new graduate becomes all important in fostering professional behaviors and commitment to patient care. Yet, the nursing profession has not established standards directed at the programmatic development for a careerist in nursing. Once they graduate from the basic educational program, the career trajectory of nurses becomes their own responsibility, since few generic professional criteria are required. Formal career development programs are conspicuously absent in nursing. The need for professional practice models in teaching hospitals to accept some responsibility for developing such standards is an area the BIH in Boston expects to investigate in the decade of the nineties.

## Summary

The key to understanding the professional practice model of the BIH is to concentrate on the underlying, basic values and principles used to establish the beginning practice system. These continue to be used to test, refine, and further develop the professionalism of nurses and the delivery of quality patient care. At the heart of this model is the clarity of the components described earlier—accountability for practice, continuity of care, and mutual respect—the tasks or work that need to be accomplished on behalf of patients and the capacity of nurse professionals to have a significant effect on the well-being of patients and families when given the opportunity to maximize and use their knowledge and skill.

Although they are well integrated at the BIH, clarity of mission, role, and responsibility, authority, and autonomy are all considered basic elements of the professional practice system and essential first steps in fostering professional practice and improving patient care. Clinical and administrative role responsibilities are articulated as complementary and not in competition with each other. Decentralized decision making is considered as essential for the clinician as it is for the nurse manager. Hospital-wide systems are in place to support these values, and the contributions of nurses are considered by all to be indispensible to meeting the hospital's mission.

Although clinical practice is the central focus of Beth Israel's practice model, the professional development of nurses is considered vital to assuring our patient population that well-prepared care providers are in place and ready to accept accountability for the outcomes of patient care. To that end, scholarly endeavors are pursued by clinical staff and supported by the hospital. Research and publication have become standard practices for many experienced and expert nurses. At all times, their interest in pursuing these activities can be traced to their primary concern—quality patient care.

## REFERENCES

Aiken, L., Mullinix, C. (1987). Special report: The nurse shortage—myth or reality? *New England Journal of Medicine, 316*(10), 641–646.

Benner, P. (1984). *From novice to expert.* Menlo Park, CA: Addison-Wesley.

Clifford, J.C. (1981). Managerial control versus professional autonomy: A paradox. *The Journal of Nursing Administration, 11*(9), 19–21.

Clifford, J.C., & Horvath, K.J. (Eds.) (1990). *Advancing professional nursing practice: Innovations at Boston's Beth Israel Hospital.* New York: Springer Publishing Company.

Etzioni, A. (1964). *Modern organizations.* Foundation of Modern Sociology Series. Englewood Cliffs, NJ: Prentice Hall.

Fagin, C. (1990). Foreword. In J.C. Clifford & K.H. Horvath, (Eds.), *Advancing professional nursing practice: Innovations at Boston's Beth Israel Hospital* (pp. xi–xii). New York: Springer Publishing Company.

Prescott, P. (1987). Another round of nurse shortages. *Image: Journal of Nursing Scholarship, 19*(4), 204–209.

Reverby, S.M. (1987). *Ordered to care: The dilemma of American nursing, 1850–1945.* New York: Cambridge University Press.

Scherer, P. (1988). Hospitals that attract (and keep) nurses. *American Journal of Nursing, 88*(1), 34–40.

Sovie, M. (1989). Clinical nursing practices and patient outcomes. *Nursing Economics, 7*(2), 79–85.

Sunshine, L., & Wright, J.W. (1987). The hospitals: Beth Israel Hospital, Boston, Massachusetts. In L. Sunshine & J.W. Wright (Eds.), *The best hospitals in America* (pp. 131–135). New York: Henry Holt and Company.

## Chapter 8

# Initiatives to Restructure Hospital Nursing Services*

PAULINE M. SEITZ
BARBARA A. DONAHO
MARY KAY KOHLES

*T*HE RESTRUCTURING of hospital nursing services is not a new idea. From the Goldmark Report published in 1923 through the 1988 Final Report of Secretary Bowen's Commission on Nursing, expert panels and chartered commissions as well as the professional nursing literature have stressed the need to create institutional environments that promote optimal use of nursing resources, improve patient care in a cost-effective, efficient manner, and provide satisfying service designs for patients as well as nurses and other staff. The 1980s began and ended with nursing shortages and recommendations to restructure hospital nursing services (American Nurses Association, 1983; U.S. Department of Health and Human Services, 1988; Roberts et al., 1989; United Hospital Fund Paper, 1989).

Despite repeated exhortations for professional restructuring of hospital nursing services, efforts to convert the theory of reorganizing the work of patient care into practical models have often been limited to essentially marginal attempts to reassign tasks. In response to cyclical shortages of nursing supply and an ever climbing demand curve for nursing services, multiple variations on task substitution models were initiated, redefined, and resubmitted starting in the 1940s through to the 1970s. If registered nurses were in short supply, aides, orderlies, and technicians were assigned their work until economic constraints shifted the balance and nurses once again were able to replace professional, ancillary, and support personnel.

In past supply and demand imbalances, short-term solutions centered on increasing the nurse supply through educational sudsidies and increasing entry-level salaries for new graduates. Efforts by hospitals to address the more difficult challenges of the demand side of the equation were not forthcoming (Aiken & Mullinix, 1987).

The challenges that hospital management must address in the 1990s reflect changes that are occurring within our society. Health care is the third largest of the

---

* The views expressed in this chapter are solely those of the authors; official endorsement by The Robert Wood Johnson Foundation is not intended and should not be inferred.

service industries, employing over eight million people. The low birth rate of the 1970s has now led to a reduction in the number of people in the health care work force. Because of technologic advances, the health care industry has demonstrated an ever increasing need for knowledgeable workers, particularly in view of the challenge to deal with cost and quality. There are increasing concerns about the characteristics of the work force because of the gap identified between the basic skills of the young worker and the skills required by the employer. The skill gap will have a direct impact on the alternatives management can select to deal with productivity as is mandated by the consumer, the government, or the industry itself.

As a result of the declining number of young people entering the labor market, recruiting practices will become more aggressive. Management practices will have to address new strategies to retain key performers if they are to be successful in managing cost and quality and improving productivity (Johnson & Packer, 1989). This will require reviewing and revising the work of the health care institution and changing how care is delivered by the multiple professional and service departments.

The management leadership as well as the leaders of the various professions must recognize that the projected shortage of workers mandates that the demand side of the equation be addressed, that the productivity of the existing work force be increased, and that unnecessary demands on workers be eliminated. Although this is not a startling new concept, the health care industry has focused predominantly only on the human resources supply part of the equation and not on restructuring the work required. This cannot continue if the shortage of human resources is to be effectively addressed. The work involved in reassessing systems of patient care in the context of changing social norms, cost constraints, burgeoning technology, and an increasingly regulated environment has been deferred or avoided by most American hospitals.

## Strengthening Hospital Nursing: A Program to Improve Patient Care

Recognizing the long-standing need to address the serious challenge of restructuring the role of hospital nursing in an increasingly complex patient care environment, in August, 1988, The Robert Wood Johnson Foundation and the Pew Charitable Trusts announced a jointly developed grants initiative—"Strengthening Hospital Nursing: A Program to Improve Patient Care." The program seeks to improve patient care by addressing the problems that deter nurses from providing optimal nursing services. It recognizes that only through institution-wide restructuring is it possible to develop enduring models that address issues such as:

- the organization of patient care systems
- communication between nursing and medical staff
- the coordination of service units such as housekeeping, dietary, pharmacy, and central supply with nursing care systems
- compensation and benefits

- nursing's role in hospital governance and executive management
- evaluation of the productivity and cost of nursing services
- institutional commitment to change, specifically the degree of support from hospital trustees, medical staff, and administration

In the first phase of the program, 80 planning grants of $50,000 each were awarded. During the planning grant year, the grantees participated in workshops on organizational change attended by each hospital's chief executive officer, the chief nursing officer, the chief medical officer, and a trustee. At the end of the planning grant year, 20 of the most promising designs for national models were awarded 5-year implementation grants of up to $1 million. The Strengthening Hospital Nursing Grants Program was structured with four times as many planning grants in order to stimulate institutional interest in work redesign. The Foundation and Trusts anticipate that the interest and commitment to the models developed in the planning phase of the program may carry the work forward even if the specific institution was not among the 20 selected for implementation grants.

The response to the program's call for proposals indicates the interest and willingness of hospitals to engage in work redesign efforts. A total of 608 completed applications for the program were received, 448 from individual hospitals of over 300 beds and 150 applications from consortia of all sizes. The consortia ranged in size from 2 to 23 institutions. One sixth of the country's hospitals applied to the program. The completed applications came from 48 states and involved a total of 1118 of the 5003 hospitals eligible for the program. At each hospital, the chief executive officer, chief nursing officer, medical staff director, and trustee chairman signed the proposal and provided letters of support. The 80 hospitals and consortia selected for planning grants represent the full spectrum of acute care settings, from small isolated rural institutions that are best described as frontier to large inner-city academic health science centers. Over 200 hospitals in 41 states participated in planning grants. They were selected because they demonstrated a clear recognition of the internal and external barriers that impeded their ability to provide optimal nursing services, a strategic plan for developing solutions for the identified problems, and a conceptually sound change process that was institution-wide in its approach.

It is too soon to identify the specifics of the work redesign the participating hospitals are incorporating into their models, but the barriers identified in their applications and interim progress reports on the processes being used in model development suggest a number of the approaches that will be used in restructuring hospital nursing services. The interventions being developed address the external and internal barriers described by the applicant pool and reflect the socioeconomic and organizational challenges that will confront the nation's health care system throughout the 1990s. Although there was variability in the priority and emphasis placed on specific external and internal barriers to provision of patient care in applicant institutions, the themes were consistent. Problems in supply and demand imbalances, reimbursement and regulatory policies, demographic patterns and allocation of nursing resources, and departmental support services were generic issues described in both the total pool of 608 applications to the program and the subset of the 80 proposals selected for planning grants.

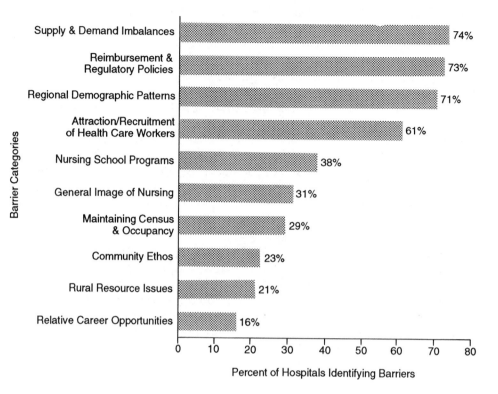

FIGURE 8–1. External barriers identified: All proposals (overall n = 80).

*Source:* Health Systems Management Center, Case Western Reserve University.

## Barriers to Patient Care

A detailed content analysis of the 80 planning grant applications selected for funding was done by the program's evaluation team at the Health Systems Management Center, Case Western Reserve University's Weatherhead School of Management. The sample size of 211 is based on the total number of hospitals involved in the 80 planning grants funded by the Foundation and Trusts as either single institutions or consortia (Taft, 1990). The evaluation team found that the most common external barriers described were supply and demand imbalances such as understaffed nursing units, decreased nursing school enrollments, and increased demand for nursing services (Fig. 8–1). These were reported by 74 percent of the applicants. Reimbursement and regulatory practices were identified in 73 percent of the proposals and included problems with diagnosis-related groups and payment modalities, length of stay, declining revenue bases, cost containment, federal and state regulations, and Joint Commission on Accreditation of Healthcare Organizations (JCAHO) requirements.

In 71 percent of the applications, regional factors such as age, patient acuity, acquired immunodeficiency syndrome, drug abuse, the local economy, poverty, and uncompensated care were cited as barriers to patient care. Inadequate attraction and recruitment of health care workers resulting in limited human resource pools were noted overall by 61 percent of the applicants; with 100 percent of the rural and 53 percent of the urban hospitals reporting problems in this area. Other external barriers to the provision of optimal nursing services described in the applications included community expectations of the institution and the image and social valuing of nursing. A perceived separation between nursing education and nursing service was expressed in terms of difficulties in the readiness of new graduates for practice resulting in "reality shock" and time- and resource-consuming orientations. Providing continuing education and advanced academic experience was a special issue for many of the rural areas. Finally, the existence of multiple entry levels into the profession of nursing was noted as a barrier in terms of obtaining a heterogeneously prepared work force that had to meld into essentially homogeneous roles in the hospital work environment (Taft, 1990).

Among the internal barriers described by the hospitals, nursing resource issues such as staffing, turnover, recruitment, retention, use of foreign and agency nurses, differing levels of education and experience, and unit leadership were discussed in 85 percent of the applications (Fig. 8–2). At 76 percent of the hospitals, problems related to nursing practice were reported. Examples cited were nursing's control over nursing practice and patient care, quality of care, role definition, and role confusion. The category of nursing practice also encompassed autonomy, professionalism, and unions. Additionally, problems regarding professional communications among nurses and with other hospital departments were detailed, and practice models such as primary care, case management, self-governance, and differentiated practice were discussed.

Departmental support services for patient care were described as a barrier by 76 percent of the grantees. Characterized under this rubric are professional turf issues; nonnursing functions performed by nurses; relationships with dietary, pharmacy, transport, and other hospital departments; and human resource allocations. Compensation and benefits were identified as issues at 63 percent of the applicant hospitals, with rural hospitals (75 percent) indicating more problems than urban ones (59 percent). The concerns specified in this area included wage compression, child care, and weak relationships between incentives and work performance. Nursing and medical staff relations were considered a barrier by all types of hospitals, with 60 percent describing problems in this area; rural hospitals (81 percent) indicated more concern with this area than urban hospitals (55 percent). The issues described were working relationships, rotating house staff, traditional roles, historical tensions between nursing and medicine, and the desire for collaborative practice models (Taft, 1990).

Job satisfaction for staff nurses, which encompassed morale and stress issues such as burnout, workload, organizational culture, and environment and unit working relationships, was discussed by 54 percent of the funded hospitals. The role of nurses in hospital decisions and the concomitant areas of strategic planning, financial allocations, policy, and work structuring was identified as a barrier by 59 percent. The issues grouped within this category included nurse participation in governance,

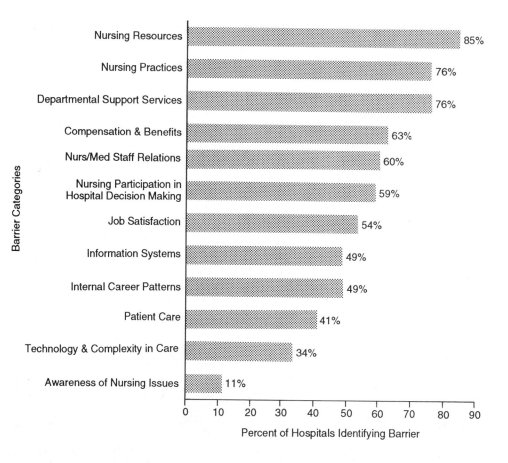

**FIGURE 8–2.** Internal barriers identified: All proposals (overall n = 80).

*Source:* Health Systems Management Center, Case Western Reserve University.

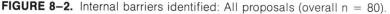

planning and management, work design and distribution, revenue and cost centers, organizational structure, and communications.

Additional internal barriers identified in the content analysis of the applications for planning grants were the impact of technologic advances in patient care, computer and information systems, and internal career opportunities for nursing staff (Taft, 1990).

Many factors described in the external barriers area are beyond the domain of the Strengthening Hospital Nursing Program and in any case are not readily amenable to change. Reimbursement and regulatory policies will be enduring problems throughout the 1990s, and it is safe to predict that their influence on the health care system will be felt throughout the decade. Utilization review, quality assurance, and risk management committees are examples of reimbursement regulatory mandates that intrude into hospital organizational structure. Successful models will identify and assess the weight that present and potential exogenous issues such as the local economy and population projections bear on individual institutions. Flexible systems are needed that can respond to the specific external stresses that are indigenous to each area, whether it is the geographic isolation and declining population base in remote rural areas or a high density of acquired immunodeficiency syndrome patients or the medically indigent in urban areas.

The internal barriers identified by the applicants reflect more immediate although difficult issues that hospitals can directly address to develop more productive and satisfying work environments. Changing the culture and leadership style of their institution's patient care system and/or nursing service has been a long-standing desire of many hospitals. However, the transition from authoritarian to participatory models of governance, from hierarchical to matrix organizational designs, and from centralized to decentralized management systems requires an institutional will and resources that extend beyond the realm of nursing. The challenge for many hospitals is not in identifying the components of successful models they would like to initiate, such as primary nursing, case management, collaborative practice, or self-governance, but in overcoming the institution-specific internal barriers, such as territoriality, limited fiscal and human resources, and resistance to change.

## *Model Development**

Bearing in mind that the context of the restructuring and work redesign for nursing services in the 1990s is a health care system in the midst of seismic changes in its financing, technology, and patient and provider demographics, it is not likely that template solutions to the problems being encountered by most American hospitals will have much success. A "silver bullet" or single model that could be readily adopted by most hospitals to quickly alleviate their pain is not likely. In restructuring efforts, a strong emphasis on process is more important than dissemination of a specific model because of the high probability that most template models will be outdated before they can be fully implemented.

Despite common themes, the proposals received for the Strengthening Hospital Nursing Program and the interim reports from the planning teams at the funded hospitals indicate great variation in institutional environments. The content analysis confirmed the initial impressions of reviewers and the program office that differing emphasis is placed on identified barriers by different kinds of hospitals, i.e., urban, rural, teaching, and community hospitals. Consequently, the interventions and strategies that address the needs of an urban community hospital may differ considerably from those of a neighboring academic teaching center or a suburban community hospital.

Human nature is far more consistent than the economics of health care, and resistance to change is a constant across institutional and regional settings. The

---

* Most of the discussion in this section is based on Ackoff et al. (1984). *A guide to controlling your corporation's future.* New York: John Wiley & Sons; and Walton, M. (1986). *The Deming management method.* New York: Dodd, Mead & Company, Inc.

grantees in the Strengthening Hospital Nursing Program were encouraged to place considerable effort into developing institution-wide communication networks that could endure beyond the planning and implementation process. By involving the hospital's major stakeholders—nurses, physicians, administration, trustees, and supportive services—systems can be developed to detect and respond to environmental changes as an ongoing process rather than as a crisis.

Incorporation of organizational management techniques into the planning process provides a vital component in nursing services model development. If there is no "buy-in" by key stakeholders in patient care systems, the best designs will lie fallow. Grantees in the Strengthening Hospital Nursing Program were provided with a series of educational opportunities on organizational change. The purpose of the educational seminars was to assist the institution's leadership, specifically the hospital administrator, the chief nurse executive, the chief of the medical staff, and a trustee representative in identifying planning processes and change models that could be adapted to meet their institution's needs. In the selection of a conceptual framework for work redesign and acceptance of change, models based on a systems approach that utilizes multidisciplinary, multilevel group techniques offer the best opportunities for institution-wide acceptance and support.

In the Strengthening Hospital Nursing Program, the initial emphasis on organizational change and a planning process that relied on collaboration and consensus building horizontally as well as vertically within the institution made the hospitals less reliant on external consultants than had originally been anticipated. Many of the hospitals used their funding resources for staff time to participate in nominal groups and delphi type discussions of the ideal patient care model, the barriers to attaining it, and the solutions to overcoming the barriers and implementing the model. The reliance on internal resources represented a shift from original plans to seek outside consultation from nationally known accounting and management firms or experts in a particular nursing model such as case management, or primary nursing, or dyads linking a registered nurse with a licensed practical nurse or nurse's aide. Organizational and management consultants were used to facilitate the planning groups' ability to envision models that incorporated features from multiple designs rather than one specific model.

The multidisciplinary nature of the planning groups, with participation from nurses, physicians, pharmacists, radiology technicians, dietitians, transport workers, and other ancillary and support services, provided an opportunity to look at the roles of all the participants in patient care and the positive or negative impact that any proposed changes would have on their work. Professional territoriality or "turf issues" are endemic in most planning processes. The use of an interactive process focused on the different provider's relationship to the patient rather than the relationships between the providers, e.g., nursing and pharmacy or nursing and dietary, thus expanding the interest in and commitment to the work redesign project from the leadership team to all levels of hospital personnel. Cross-training of professional staff in low population census rural hospitals and of ancillary staff in high volume urban hospitals is more likely to be an acceptable alternative when it emerges from a bottom-up process instead of being enforced from the top down.

Cross-training was a staffing trend that was evident in many of the applications to the program. In the rural areas, low population census and remote location, combined with a declining population base, created a need for hospital nurses with enough versatility to cover all the services in the hospital, including pharmacy, radiology, and supplies. In more populated areas, economics more than demographics created an interest in ancillary and support staff able to integrate roles such as transport, dietary and housekeeping tasks, or clerical and supply. The impact of such reorganization moves beyond the institutions involved to local unions and state regulations. A harbinger of the changes to come could be seen in job titles, which were more functionally descriptive than task-oriented. For example, the title environmental management technician replaced housekeeper, an indication of an emergent trend toward clear delineation of "hotel services" as distinct from nursing services that a patient may need.

Unbundling hotel services from patient care services opens several avenues of discussion for future care models. Allowing patients to select from a continuum of services may be possible and desirable in some circumstances, i.e., opting to eat in the cafeteria or having family bring in meals instead of having room service. However, for patients with limited family or financial resources, problematic issues of equity and equality of care are raised. Multidisciplinary planning is needed to determine the cost benefits of such services in terms of quality of care, accounting and billing procedures, reimbursement, and liability.

The institution-wide impact of new practice models was evident in interim reports from hospitals exploring options to expand professional development opportunities for the nursing staff. Differentiated practice models with clear delineations of registered nurse role expectations based on education as the sole criteria were rarely proposed. The criteria for multiple levels of nursing practice entailed a combination based on performance, experience, and education linked to a tiered system of wage and benefit packages. Development of the new compensation scales led to discussion not only of how the wage and benefit increases would be financed but also of how they would affect the expectations of other hospital personnel.

Professional practice models were of interest to many of the applicants. Their enthusiasm about case management or primary nursing was tempered, however, by assessments of the regional nurse supply and limited fiscal resources for rapidly increasing salaries for registered nurses. Many applicants planned institutional adaptations of primary or managed care with use of ancillary or support staff pairings with specific registered nurses or as part of patient care teams that could free registered nurse staff from identified nonnursing tasks.

During the planning process, attention to the details of implementing a strategy such as increased autonomy in patient care or self-governance of individual nursing units brought into focus the interconnectedness of various model components. For example, in self-governance models, nurses assume responsibility for the staffing of the unit (including hiring and termination) set performance standards, and negotiate their compensation and benefits. When the self-governance model is combined with a cross-training model for unit-based ancillary staff, multiple constituencies are affected. The reporting relationships, disciplinary protocols, and compensation packages of non-nursing staff must be acceptable to labor unions and management groups that have a vested interest in the planned change. During the planning period, a tolerance for ambiguity was identified as a learned skill by many grantees. The freedom to generate ideas and be creative instead of concrete facilitated development of a common language necessary for negotiating the details of implementation. Despite a turnover in administrative leadership at many of the grantee hospitals, the multilevel planning process continued uninterrupted.

## Conclusion

The outcome of planning for organizational change can only be speculative, but the Strengthening Hospital Nursing grantees have generated not only interest but also excitement within the nursing community as well as the industry at large. To date, the program has resulted in the key stakeholders acknowledging their interdependence and beginning a planned process to analyze the work of patient care, its efficiencies and inefficiencies, the duplication effort among the caregivers, and the rationale used to determine how, why, and when the work is done. This has been energizing for all and more important is resulting in a very comprehensive analysis and resultant acknowledgment that the hospital system and structure of work must change. Acceptance of this premise is the first critical step and has the potential to produce a change process that will equip the employees within a health care institution with the tools to appropriately adjust a system that must respond to both the continuing changing technology and a rapidly changing work force. The result should be more appropriate and effective utilization of the professional nurse.

## REFERENCES

Ackoff, R., Gharajedaghi, J., & Vergara, F.E. (1984). *A guide to controlling your corporation's future.* New York: John Wiley & Sons.

Aiken, L., & Mullinix, C. (1987). Special report: The nurse shortage—myth or reality? *New England Journal of Medicine, 317*(10), 641–646.

American Nurses Association (1983). *Magnet hospitals: Attraction and retention of professional nurses.* Task Force in Nursing Practice in Hospitals. Kansas City, MO: American Academy of Nursing.

Johnston, W., & Packer, A. (1989, July). *Workforce 2000. Work and workers for the 21st century.* Washington, DC: Hudson Institute, Inc., Corporate Press Inc.

Roberts, M., Minnick, A., Ginsberg, E., & Curran, C. (1989). What to do about the nursing shortage (pp. 17–20). New York: Commonwealth Fund.

Taft, S. (1990). *Strengthening hospital nursing program: Report of the phase I proposal content analysis.* Unpublished manuscript, Cleveland: Health System Management Center, Case Western Reserve University.

The nursing shortage: New approaches to an old problem (1989, October). United Hospital Fund Paper, Series 12, p. 29. New York: United Hospital Fund.

U.S. Department of Health and Human Services (1988, December). *Secretary's Commission on Nursing, final report,* volume 1 (pp. 17–20). Washington, DC: U.S. Government Printing Office.

Walton, M. (1986). *The Deming management method.* New York: Dodd, Mead & Company, Inc.

## Chapter 9

# Advanced Nursing Practice: Future of Clinical Nurse Specialists

### LUTHER CHRISTMAN

$C$LINICAL SPECIALIZATION at the graduate level of nursing education did not develop until about 30 years ago. It has gathered much momentum, but there is still much that can be done to strengthen the clinical posture of the nursing profession. At least 25 percent of nurses, instead of the approximately 6 percent currently at this level of preparation, are needed to enable nurses to become viable contributors to the multidisciplinary health care teams of the future. This may understate the prevailing view in the profession that graduate education should be the entry level requirement for nursing positions. This is a long way from the early specialization of nurses which, for many years, was labeled postgraduate education but primarily was a form of on-the-job experience in a clinical area. The duration of this practical experience was from 6 months to a year. Very little, if any, formal preparation was included, and nurses were expected to acquire advanced competence by some form of "living" in a specialty milieu.

Consistently and over a long period of time nurses have been comparing and contrasting nurses with nurses. This preoccupation appears to have led to more rancor than accord. This lack of unity and constructive proactive change may be an indication of the constant inward orientation of the profession and the slowness of accommodation to the major developments in other professions. This intense examination of self appears to have fostered analyses from without as well. Beginning with the Goldmark Study (Goldmark, 1923), the nursing profession probably has had more national studies and commission reports than any other profession. Rather than deliberate planned change and growth to new professional heights as an outcome of all these data, only changes that came with the natural drift of society seem to have occurred.

Is this apparent inertia within the profession a structural problem that is a strong residual of the beginnings of modern nursing and the fateful placement of nursing education as a product of hospital activity instead of a component of higher education? It is interesting to note that two other clinical professions, physical therapy and dietetics, which were spun off from the nursing profession, moved into higher education completely. There appears to have been no inquiry into why the offspring were more avid for a richer and more independent education than the parent profession. The end result of this educational lag leaves about 30 percent of nurses holding only baccalaureate degrees. This is a narrow base for the preparation of clinical specialists who are capable of providing desirable leadership in the clinical management of patients. These observations are made to emphasize the fullness and extent of the problem in preparing for the future.

## Scientific Factors That Influence the Future

The massive results of scientific research overwhelm every profession and discipline. Clinicians, scientists, and scholars alike are inundated with increasingly large amounts of new data that are being disseminated at an almost overwhelming rate. As far back as 1961, an educator (Nyquist, 1961) asserted that because of the rapid obsolescence of knowledge, faculty members probably were teaching errors much of the time. If this intellectually exciting statement had significance then, the current situation is even more serious. The vertical and horizontal expansions of knowledge are outstripping even the expectations that persons held just 10 years ago. Horizontal expansion is a term used to indicate the refinement of present knowledge into more and more precise elements. Vertical expansion is a term applied to the creation of entirely new knowledge. This approach tends to predict an exponential expansion of knowledge. If, for example, knowledge is expanding exponentially every 2 years, in 10 more years there will be 32 times as much scientific knowledge in the world as there is today. A state of instant obsolescence is a likely end result—that is, new knowledge will be created faster than it can be absorbed and utilized. Thus the proliferation of knowledge, when synchronized with a similar growth in technology, constitutes part of the milieu in which nurse specialization must be projected in order to have even a suggestion of validity.

Clinical science is applied science—that is, the transforming of the theory and content of all the various sciences into a social good called clinical care. There is nothing theoretical about this approach. It is the exquisite use of the methods of science around the problems of care for each individual patient. It implies a prevailing investigative attitude when caring for patients. Each care plan is treated as if it were a miniresearch endeavor in order to ensure that all data needed are collected and analyzed and the decisions implemented. This calls for rigorous scientific training and appropriate content.

The knowledge needed for specialty practice will have a large role overlap among clinicians in various disciplines but in the same specialty area. Clinical psychologists, psychiatrists, social workers, and nurses working in adult psychiatry (if all are at the doctoral level) will have more common than different knowledge. Psychiatric nurses and psychiatrists share more similar knowledge bases, as do oncology nurses and oncologists, than either psychiatric and oncology nurses or psychiatrists and oncologists. The same can be said about all the specialty areas. Thus it is far wiser to examine nurse specialization vis-à-vis the clinical specialists in the other groups that constitute the health care team than to contrast nurses with nurses. In the specialty model the landmarks are fairly well in place and the acquisition of the needed expertise can be readily delineated. In the nurse-nurse model only the comparison with other nurses is present. The increase in knowledge base may make a difference between nurses but might be insufficient to give nurses equal social power on the health care team.

We are constantly informed by the media about the growth of knowledge. The industrialized world has, in some respects, become a gigantic research laboratory. With the decline in enmity and hostility among nations and a growing desire for cooperation and harmony, the scientific enterprise should flourish more than ever. The reduction of barriers to travel, the availability of computerized translations, the natural affinity of scientists around their common interests, the omnipresent media, and the general elevation in education among people of the world all augur well for the rapid dissemination of new knowledge. Because good health is an important cultural variable in every country of the world, it is a natural target for a high degree of cooperative research and development endeavor. Nurses around the world, unfortunately, are poorly positioned to become major contributors in the early stages of this operation because the majority of nurses worldwide have been educated in hospital schools of nursing with very weak basic and clinical preparation. Inroads are being made in many countries to improve these conditions; therefore, the door is opening to change. As yet, however, Iceland is the only country that has mandated baccalaureate education as the only basic form of nurse preparation. Several countries are moving in this direction. As specialization becomes an accomplished fact, other countries may follow the example set by Iceland so that rational planning for specialization may occur. The development of such expertise will be a means of facilitating the health goals of all nations.

Overlapping knowledge among clinicians will foster joint educational programs in the various sciences that are heavily used in their respective specialties. Common education will present the opportunity for developing a common scientific language for communication across disciplines, for developing multidisciplinary research, for gaining insight into the most pressing areas for research, and for mutual respect. Furthermore, such coeducation will facilitate the understanding of complementary and supplementary roles to ensure a stronger clinical umbrella for each patient who needs care. Instead of splendid isolation, the health care team can become welded together by the desire to utilize science to decrease human suffering.

## Role Formation*

The full professional role for any of the clinical professions encompasses the activities listed under the concepts of practice, education, research, management, and consul-

---

* Ever since the behavioral scientists have researched, analyzed, and discussed the concepts of role, role formation, role change, and similar issues, there has been a growing interest in the phenomena of role by others. The nursing literature, as an example, is replete with articles about role. However, nurses and many other professional and occupational types often do not have the depth of understanding of role construction of occasional behavior. Thus role development can often be more superficial, less complete, and more ineffective than its title would indicate.

tation. Nurses generally adopt only one of these subroles and insist on forcing that particular subrole into a full role activity, causing a diminution in quality of role performance. The predilection to enact the role in this manner seems more akin to a "business" model than to the clinical model exhibited in other clinical disciplines. Additionally, when large numbers of nurses make this kind of decision, the profession becomes atomized. The growing edge of each part is narrowed and lacks regular stimulation. This same growing edge has a far different quality when the full professional role is achieved. It compares favorably with the progress identifiable in the other major clinical professions such as medicine, dentistry, and psychology. The preference of nursing for a business type of model may be a primary structural barrier to obtaining the goal of clinical competence.

Over a long period of time and even up to the present, there has existed an intense concentration on functional role development instead of clinical expertness. This seems almost a contradiction of identity that does not have an analogue in the other major clinical professions. For many years nurses received their advanced preparation under such rubrics as education, management, or supervision. This advanced preparation usually was devoid of clinical content, and, therefore, the scientific content necessary to bring about change and advance the quality of the profession occurred more by means of a trickle-down effect of what was happening in health care than by the dynamics of professional content. It also meant that nurses had to teach or manage without enriched clinical content. This kept nursing growth at the practical and ordinary levels. This may be one of the reasons that nurse specialists threaten nurse managers, who do not have extensive clinical training, and why they are downplayed or underemployed by these administrators. It may be that nurses became out of step with other types of clinicians by being first accepted for college education by teachers' colleges at the time when this concept of role was rife among educators. This educational motif persisted even into doctoral education for nurses, where many programs focus primarily on research methods content and do not provide enrichment of clinical content. The essence of research is asking the proper questions, and for clinicians, this knowledge comes from highly developed insight into the clinical phenomena gained through sophisticated care. Very few, if any, of the PhD programs in nursing have a clinical program as potent as that found in clinical psychology or in the boards of dentistry and medicine, or a program as rich in content as that for scientists at the doctoral level of preparation. It is not difficult to speculate what the state of health care in our society would be if all the clinical professions had concentrated on functional rather than clinical content for full role development.

The concentration on subrole performance has helped to inhibit the development of clinical nursing competence. That persistent attention to and concentration on limited role enactment fits more nearly into a businesslike approach can be seen in the draining off of many nurses into functional graduate education instead of clinical preparation; the stronger attachment of economic rewards to functional role activity; the tight and specific job descriptions that leave little or no discretionary flexibility; and the institutionalizing of ward routines and procedure books. This limited role enactment and these ramifications stem from the concept of scientific management as developed by Taylor and others in the early part of this century. This approach assumes that management is all-knowing and that workers are unimaginative and need direction. All power is vested in the top of the organization, and complete powerlessness is characteristic of the lower levels. Practically all communication is downward. The many years of functional nursing, team nursing, and care through others are a direct product of the industrial model. The persistence of a multilevel entry system fits this model because the emphasis is placed on routine technical tasks rather than the skillful application of the theory and content of the various sciences in an inventive way with patients. The wide gulf—almost deliberate separation—between education and service stems from subrole specialization. The resulting weak clinical base of most nurses (70 percent without a college education) adds to the impediments hampering full professional role development. The evolution of the clinical specialist's role traveled an arduous route, considering that nurses purport to be clinicians. It is clear that structural barriers were a major contributor to the sluggish pace of clinical development.

The recognition of this deficit in role strength first occurred among psychiatric nurses: A small group banded together and was instrumental in obtaining a federal grant to alter the direction of graduate education (National League for Nursing, 1958). From this small beginning, graduate programs in this specialty slowly began to emerge, and the notion of clinical specialization spread to other majors. The nurse practitioner had similar beginnings. Both psychiatric patients, who were then concentrated mostly in rural state hospitals, and children in rural areas were not being adequately managed clinically because of a shortage of physicians and other clinicians in these underserved areas. The field was ripe for opportunistic change that would fill the void. A small critical mass of nurses moved into these areas of clinical endeavor and established, for the first time, behavioral models of clinical practice, offering an alternative to functional role preparation. The clinical doctorate in nursing took considerable time to evolve and was first conceived and implemented at Boston University. This transition also occurred first in psychiatric nursing.

The nurse practitioner evolved some several years later and seemed to have more acceptance. The disparity in acceptance between the clinical specialist and the nurse practitioner may be explained by the acute physician shortage that existed at the time. Nurse practitioners were viewed as a means of easing the physician shortage by being extenders of physician services. The physician assistant programs won acceptance for the same reason and emerged about the same time. These extender roles could erode if a physician surplus develops. In countries such as Italy and Germany where physician surpluses are the norm, nurses tend to have minor roles. In breaking new ground at the graduate level, the nurse specialist was perceived as a threat to the status quo because she took as her model the full professional role in its broadest sense. This had threatening implications for those who wanted to cling tenaciously to traditional ways. Not only did this role create uneasiness in staff nurses with weak clinical preparation but it also posed problems for nurses in administrative positions. Nurse specialists knew much more about clinical care and how to be innovative by using new research findings and thus stimulating steady ripples of change that might be beyond the understanding of their administrative superiors. It is not easy to gain acceptance under these circumstances. Furthermore, some specialists avoided line responsibility and were often seen as expensive appendages instead of valuable assets. Because of the business-oriented attitudes of many directors of nursing and practically all hospital administrators, the immediacy of the daily tasks usually took precedence over the long-range development of quality. Because of the dearth of clinical leadership, the deficit of numbers during nurse shortages may be more marked than necessary because many leaders are incapable of giving strong clinical direction. Clinical innovation in nursing care will lag behind until clinical competence becomes the criterion for appointing nurse administrators. Hence resources are not as wisely used as they might have been if clinical specialists had been available. A quality shortage is more prevalent than a real number shortage. The business analogue can be observed in American business in general. When we find ourselves in competition with Germany, Japan, and other countries that have long-range quality as their goal, because of the here and now of the American business orientation, there is growing difficulty in competing effectively. In Germany and Japan, the use of those with a Master's in Business Administration is downplayed, and industry is run by engineers and scientists who know and understand the goals of the future. Full role content, which utilizes the methods of science, appears to be more effective than functional role outcomes.

## The Economic Factors Attached to Clinical Practice

The economics of health care are looming larger than ever, and all indicators point to an even greater influence in the near future. Health care is losing much of its aura as a humanitarian mission and taking on some of the characteristics of a public utility needing regulation. The split organizational structure (Rosengren, 1980; Denton, 1978; Jules, 1954) of hospitals may be one of the reasons nurses appear to be caught in an economic bind. The polarization of hospitals into two major and differing structures has been given the label of the "pine tree-oak tree" relationship. The pine tree element is the highly structured, multidepartment, tight job description portion in which there is very limited discretionary deviance from role allocation. The oak tree element is relatively flat and one in which roles are fluid enough to coalesce quickly around the exigencies of care. Nurses are embedded in both organizational elements. In addition, they usually are the only ones in both prongs who are available continually and consistently; thus they are expected to react to every gap, major or minor, in the work flow of each element. The bureaucratic pressures to fill the needs of the nonclinical departments are ever present. Thus nurses spend an enormous amount of time in trying to make an inefficient system efficient (Christman & Jelenick, 1967). Much of the nursing shortage may stem from this structural arrangement (Aiken, 1988). Almost all the studies of nurses have ignored this structural variable. The federal government and private foundations that are funding projects to assist in easing the nurse shortages have not focused intensely on eliminating the large amounts of nonclinical activities encountered in the daily work of nurses. The calls for funding of nurse extenders may become a form of entrapment of nurses, especially if the prerequisite for funding mandates, overtly or covertly, that they report to nurses. This approach is another indication that nurses are being locked into a business administration model rather than one stressing clinical growth. It will be difficult to enforce accountability in the other departments if it continues to be customary for nurses to pick up all the slack. Writers have called for structural change (Christman, 1967), but there does not seem to have been much interest in restructuring the hospital to alleviate the artificial shortage that is a direct outcome of nurses being involved in a large amount of nonclinical activities. At present a project funded by the Illinois Hospital Association is under way, with ten participating hospitals, representing a cross-section of the state, to approach restructuring so as to diminish (or eliminate) the participation of nurses in nonclinical activities. The ability to concentrate on clinical practice and the concomitant specialization may become feasible if the duress of shortage is eliminated. For example, if nurses are distracted 30 percent of their time from clinical activities, it is easy to project that a nurse surplus would occur as a result of structural rearrangement.

A controlled field experiment to test the effectiveness of clinical nurse specialists in a hospital found that the lowest cost and the highest quality per unit of care were outcomes of using master's–prepared nurse specialists in line positions (Georgopoulos & Christman, 1990). In addition, registered nurse turnover decreased on these units as contrasted with conventional units. During this study, a nurse specialist was unattached and made available to nurses on both the experimental and control units for clinical consultation. Her services were unused. The reasons given were varied, but apparently when nurses concentrate on role types instead of direct care, all kinds of tacit turf barriers result. The findings of this study suggest that wide use of nurse specialists in line positions might aid in achieving two goals—cost effectiveness and quality care—at one and the same time. Although it is readily conceded that each person does not always use the knowledge she or he has, it also is axiomatic that no one can use knowledge she or he does not have. The use of expert knowledge, as demonstrated in this experiment, can bring about constructive change. The practice differences were documented and costs and quality were one to one with education. The next lowest costs and the next highest quality stemmed from the nurses at the baccalaureate level, and the highest cost and lowest quality from nurses without college preparation. It should be clearly and carefully stated that this was not deliberate behavior but the outcome of these nurses having substantially less knowledge than that possessed by nurse specialists.

## The Effects of Nursing Education

Unlike other disciplines and professions, nursing is limited in obtaining candidates for advanced preparation because only 30 percent of nurses have a college education and a fair number of these graduates do not meet the criteria for further education. Furthermore, many university schools of nursing have insisted on one or more years of practice at the baccalaureate level before admission. The extent of this inhibition of enrollment does not seem to have been studied very carefully. The other clinical professions and scientific disciplines do not impose this requirement but instead encourage immediate enrollment. The widespread pattern of separating service and education also may be another inhibitor. Students do not have their faculty members as behavioral models of practice but must emulate nurses with lesser preparation, since these are the only nurses they usually can observe. In the controlled field experiment mentioned above (Georgopoulos & Christman, 1990), education and service were separated. Students were interviewed individually, but the majority had the same perception. They asserted that they were caught in covert guerrilla warfare between service persons and faculty members, and that all they were learning were survival skills to graduate so that they could learn nursing practice at that time. When asked whether they planned to go on to graduate school, most stated that they enjoyed working with patients, and if they went to graduate school they probably would be the same as their teachers and would never care for patients. The subtleties of the role induction process apparently were at work. Although this area needs much more exploration, the above clues may be part of the reason why there is such a small percentage of nurses with graduate degrees, especially at the doctoral level. The figures might be substantially different if nursing students could be induced to go on to doctoral programs immediately upon graduation at the baccalaureate degree level. They would then be in their middle twenties when they finished their education, with the promise of a fruitful professional life.

## Ethical Considerations

Professions are a public trust and as such are more subject to ethical scrutiny than other forms of livelihood. In return for a public monopoly, there are expectations of a higher order of service to the public. An ethical question can be raised in this fashion: Can nurses maintain their ethical commitment to patients if they do not keep pace with the burgeoning output of science and technology? Can nurses, as a collectivity, continue to withhold the application of knowledge to patient care by maintaining programs at less than the baccalaureate level? Can nurses continue to have a very low percentage of their membership at the graduate level and yet continue to assert that they are patient advocates? Can it be expected ethically that nurses will be as strong in their specialty training as are other professionals? Can nurses maintain strong ethical standards without a high level of expert practice as a base? Others may raise even more searching questions. High-level ethical practice is more than doing no harm. It is the deliberate moral effort to embrace the golden rule in principle and practice. In "people processing" organizations (Georgopoulos & Mann, 1972), this is an obligation rather than a privilege.

## The Future

Currently there is a plethora of information in the media and the scientific and professional journals about the forthcoming decade and the impact that will come from the merging of science, technology, economics, and political influences on the quality of life in a global way. All this information states a view of the past and present from which the future not only must be projected but is the base from which all change must spring.

It is not unreasonable to assume that a completely automated health care system will come into being in this decade and be more sophisticated in the next. Such a development will call for radical changes in the structure, preparation, and licensure of all health care personnel. The establishment of a national system of research and clinical knowledge as a basic foundation for the management of health is a very strong possibility. All medical centers and research facilities will be in a computerized network into which new information will be constantly fed so that all clinical information will be of the latest order. Nurses will be able to seek consultation from other nurses, even though they may be many miles away. Each person's health history will be on a chip that can be inserted into the system and analyzed (Lesse, 1981). The main requirement for using all this knowledge correctly will be the ability to ask the right questions when dealing with all the issues surrounding each patient.

The clinical preparation of nurse specialists will be at the doctoral level. The appropriate scientific and clinical content will be the major component of graduate education. Research methods courses will be another but lesser component to enable nurses to acquire investigative abilities and to sharpen their clinical approaches by fostering an investigative attitude. The major investigators into clinical practice will prepare themselves through the DNSc-PhD route. Scientific training will be rooted in the sciences most closely related to nurses' respective clinical practice. This form of preparation is not novel and has been used by veterinarians, dentists, and physicians to enable them to become effective investigators.

The future can be scrutinized more easily by conceiving of all care in the clinical model, with each of the health care professions as a subset. Instead of a nursing model or medical model and similar appellations that divide the health care team, it seems best to have an all-encompassing clinical model, with each profession drawing upon its basic content. Physiology (or any other science) is the same in theory and content whether a physiologist, a nurse, a physician, or a dentist is using it. It is the role expression of knowledge that is different. The way the conglomerate of role functions is a composite of scientific depth of training, legal restrictions, organizational patterns, and tradition. The proliferation of science will impact heavily on role expression, and those with the most content will be able to be most expressive and creative. Nurses, because of their restrictive time and space binding with patients, will have a different form of role expression than physicians. However, the merging of the competencies of the two at the level being suggested could have a profound effect on the good of patients.

The greatly increased mass of scientific theory and content of all types will practically mandate that very astute clinicians give direction to nursing services, because most innovation and change start at the top. The line of command will continue this linkage system so that excellence will be a continuous theme. As outcomes become a chief means of assessing care, the demand for a direct line of nurse specialists from top to bottom will be obvious. Nurses will be in a perfect accountability pattern, that is, each error of omission or commission will be traced unerringly to the person committing the error. Each act of competence and innovation will be ascertained in a similar fashion. The computerized system will have this capability. Eventually, the computer system will be used to evaluate all practitioners, and scores will be printed out at stated intervals. Those who practice at or above the norm will have their licenses and privileges renewed, and those who do not will have theirs suspended. With this technologic capability, the bureaucratic structure will be very flat, and hence most specialists will be direct caregivers. In order to achieve efficiency of effort, the training of nurse practitioners and nurse specialists will be merged into the broader perspective to better ensure competence.

The role induction of students will become more stimulating and be of a higher order. In the interest of both economy of effort and cost-effectiveness, service and education will be unified. Students will have as behavioral models the expert practitioners on the faculty. Observing skilled performance will stimulate students to aspire to similar capabilities. Mentoring in action can be more readily understood than word portraits.

As a consequence of concerted world action of governments, combined with an emphasis on illness prevention and health maintenance, nurse specialists will be working in three main areas. One will be in prevention activities, where each person will be regularly monitored for health; the second will be in intensive care, where all the complexities of technology will be employed. The third, and very large segment, will be in out-of-hospital care arrangements. The miniaturization of technology, remote monitoring, two-way visual contact by dedicated television lines, the availability of voice-activated computers, the development of fuzzy logic (computers reacting to words rather than the digital system), genome mapping, and the availability of health knowledge systems to patients through their own personal computers as well as to clinicians will constitute an arena in which sharp, clinical judgments, often within a complex set of circumstances, will have to be made continuously. This kind of care can be handled best by specialists. It is not difficult to forecast that nurses from different specialty areas will be collaborating on these problem areas. All health care formats will be clinically arrayed. The historical use of those with a Master's in Business Administration as managers will erode, and the leadership will be given to clinicians who know the product as well as the challenges of the future.

## A Policy Agenda

A policy agenda for the enhancement and preservation of nurse specialization at the sophisticated level needed to keep pace with the other professions will grow out of the exigencies of future health care needs. A more rapid movement toward graduate clinical preparation will enable nurses to move more comfortably into the impending, scientifically dramatic changes during this decade. As the complete cybernetic system* eventually falls into place, it will become obvious that nurses with limited preparation will not be able to cope with this means of sophisticated care.

It can be predicated that a cybernetic health care system will create a reduction in the numbers of physicians, nurses, and other clinical personnel needed to staff the system. Concomitantly, the competence of those utilized will have to be at the highest level.

The survival of the nursing profession depends on producing and implementing a policy agenda. It is hoped that a proactive stance will be taken by university educators, who will take the lead in steering this agenda. An entire reorganization of the health care delivery system must be envisioned. The new organizational structures should remove encumbrances from nurses by filling the gaps left by others in the clinical-nonclinical portions of the system. In the close time and space binding of nurses with patients, there is an important and enormous possibility for an effective and needed means of reducing suffering and stress in the health care of patients. Cooperation in framing a strong agenda should be sought from the American Nurses Association and the National League for Nursing. History has shown that it is very difficult to obtain a high degree of agreement within the profession. The unwillingness to cooperate stems from the various levels of entry into the profession. An overriding concern, however, is the welfare of patients. The ethics of deliberately withholding the benefits of science from patients by less adequate preparation than the other clinical professions is an underlying theme in nursing that eventually will demand clarification and action. It is far better to be proactive and set an agenda that empowers nurses to be effective and highly valued than to constantly and perhaps inappropriately react to change when it is inevitable. The nursing profession has enough fertile minds and capable people to bring this about, but it will take a leadership group that understands the full implications of the task to create the momentum needed to achieve the goals of thorough preparation and excellent service.

In forming the agenda, nurses could take a cue from Warren Kingston (Kingston, 1983). He stated:

> In a general hospital, the patient's needs are manifested primarily on the ward. The organizational problem in promoting patient-focused care may

---

* In a cybernetic system, health care will be very highly automated. The miniaturization of technology will have a profound effect. Much of the present work of physicians, nurses, and other types of clinicians will be done by technologic devices. Computer diagnoses will be more accurate than those of humans. The monitoring of vital signs will be done more accurately and efficiently by technology than by clinicians. Alerting devices, furthermore, will be built into these mechanisms to warn health care team members about impending changes, so that proper resources and clinical talent can be mobilized to manage these crises. Sensors will monitor therapeutic drug levels and automatically adjust them to the designated level without clinician interface. Anxiety levels will be monitored in a similar manner. Teaching machines will be available for patients to learn about their disease processes and to enable them to be more active participants in their care. Automation will be extensive. The clinical plans of physicians, nurses, and others will be more congruent because of the interface with the computer. Clinical information will constantly be updated in the computer memory and be available instantly by asking the right questions. The system will be increasingly more sophisticated, complex, and accurate.

be then restated as how to ensure that the ward is run to meet the patient's needs, which includes enabling doctors and other professionals involved to provide their services and have prescribed tests and treatments carried out. This immediately suggests that the nursing profession might be the key group which ought to carry overall responsibility for seeing that the patient's needs, medical and otherwise, are met. Poorly designed or filled nursing structures and inappropriate definitions of nursing work and its relation to other work might therefore be expected to play a large part in reducing the quality of care available to patients.

Although Kingston makes his statement from a position of hospital care, his concepts can be extended to apply to the entire gamut of care. If nurses flex their intellectual muscles and are able to view the future from a position of greatly enlarged clinical strength, they will have an enormous impact on the health care system. Imagine, for a moment, the amount of impact 250,000 nurses, prepared at the doctoral level to be clinicians, would have on patient care. This number is only about 25 percent of all nurses in the country. It is, however, a critical mass that could be a catalyst for change. It is a modest figure and, therefore, it is achievable. Even the same number of nurse specialists at the master's level would enhance the power of the nursing profession and raise the level of care. No more effort is needed to think big than to think small. Those who think big do big things, and those who think small must settle for much less. The clinical model (Christman, 1971, 1987) has within its parameters the sense of direction, the basic content, and the professional growth potential to enable nurses to far surpass the dreams of those who started the clinical specialist movement. The growing richness of science, the strong effects of economics, and the desire for greater professional recognition can be welded together to help nurses reach the potential that is inherent in the concept of nursing care. Are nurses visionary enough to become the extremely beneficial and powerful clinicians they have the potential to be? The power of knowledge is a wonder to behold.

## REFERENCES

Aiken, L.H. (1988). Assuring the delivery of quality patient care. *Proceedings of the State-of-the-Science Invitational Conference: Nursing Resources and the Delivery of Patient Care* (p. 8). Bethesda, MD: U.S. Department of Health and Human Services, U.S. Public Health Service, National Institutes of Health.

Christman, L. (1967, February 4). As an example see "Would a Stewardess Help?" *Saturday Review*, 65–67.

Christman, L. (1971). The nurse specialist as a professional activist. *Nursing Clinics of North America, 6*(2), 231–235.

Christman, L. (1987, Winter). The future of the nursing profession. *Nursing Administration Quarterly, 11*(2), 1–8.

Christman, L., & Jelenick, R. (1967). Old patterns waste half the nursing hours. *Modern Hospitals, 108*, 78–81.

Denton, J.A. (1978). *1978 Medical sociology*. Boston: Houghton Mifflin.

Georgopoulos, B., & Christman, L. (1990, March). *The effects of clinical nursing specialization: A controlled organizational experiment*. (Studies in Health and Human Services, vol. 14) Lewiston, NY: The Edwin Mellen Press.

Georgopoulos, B.S., & Mann, Floyd D. (1972). The hospital as an organization. In E. Gartly Jaco (Ed.), *Patients, physicians and illness*, 2nd ed. New York: The Free Press.

Goldmark, J. (1923). *Committee for the study of nursing education, nursing and nursing education in the United States*. New York: The Macmillan Co.

Jules, H. (1954). The formal structure of a psychiatric hospital. *Psychiatry, 17,* 139–151.

Kingston, W. (1983). Hospital organization and structure and its effect on inter-professional behavior and the delivery of care. *Social Science and Medicine, 17*(16), 1159–1170.

Lesse, S. (1981). *The future of the health sciences, anticipating tomorrow*. New York: Irvington Publishers.

National League for Nursing (1958). *The education of the clinical specialist in psychiatric nursing*. New York: National League for Nursing.

Nyquist, E.B. (1961). *The wisest man who had not the gift of foresight*. Unpublished paper presented at the Annual Conference of Directors and Faculty Members of Nurse Preparing Programs in New York State, Buffalo.

Rosengren, W.R. (1980). *Sociology of medicine: Diversity, conflict and change*. New York: Harper & Row.

## Chapter 10

# Medicare Prospective Payment and the Changing Health Care Environment

EILEEN V.T. LAKE

*D*URING ITS FIRST two decades, the Medicare program paid all the "reasonable costs" incurred by hospitals for care of the nation's elderly. In 1983, Medicare began to pay hospitals a fixed rate, set in advance, for the entire hospital stay of an elderly person (Iglehart, 1983). Since its legislation, this new, prospective payment system has been the subject of intense scrutiny, debate, and criticism. This controversy, over what may seem to be a bureaucratic technicality, reflects both the radical nature of this policy change and its potential to affect a considerable segment of health care interests in the United States: federal dollars, elderly Americans, and hospitals. In 1989, Medicare expenditures for inpatient hospital services reached $49 billion (Health Care Financing Administration, 1989). Medicare enrollment now includes 33 million beneficiaries (Health Care Financing Administration, 1989). About 5600 hospitals, or 84 percent of all American hospitals, care for Medicare beneficiaries (Health Care Financing Administration, 1989). Medicare payments account for about 40 percent of inpatient hospital revenues, on average (Prospective Payment Assessment Commission, 1989). Beyond the direct impact on the Medicare program, its patients and providers, major Medicare policy changes affect nearly all institutions and individuals that provide, consume, or pay for health care.

This chapter reviews the history, implementation, and consequences of the Medicare prospective payment system (PPS). The enactment of the Medicare program is described and the developments that led to prospective payment are described. The purpose, goals, and design of the PPS are then described. The system was implemented in October, 1983. The seven years since its implementation have seen profound changes in the delivery of hospital services, with repercussions evident throughout the American health care system. These changes and the repercussions are detailed. The question of whether and how the PPS met its stated goals is explored. The likely future of Medicare hospital payment policy is considered. The chapter closes with an assessment of the influence of the PPS on our national health policy priorities and trends.*

---

* For readers who would like more detail on prospective payment, a recent book by Louise Russell provides a very readable, comprehensive treatment of this subject (Russell, 1989).

121

## *The Medicare Program and Health Care Cost Escalation*

With the rise of the welfare economy following World War II, the government began to subsidize health care through broader tax exclusions for employer-paid health insurance (Durenberger, 1985). The health care needs of the elderly, disabled, and poor, however, were not addressed by these measures. With nearly 30 percent of elderly Americans living below the poverty level in the early 1960s (Health Care Financing Administration, 1989), national attention turned to whether the elderly could afford or had access to needed health services.

In 1965, the Medicare program was enacted to provide health insurance for the elderly. Through Medicare, the government insures the elderly against the expense of acute hospital and nursing home services (called Part A insurance). Part A insurance is free to the elderly and is funded by mandatory Medicare payroll taxes on America's labor force. Realizing that the elderly have expenses for more than just acute services, a supplementary insurance for other medical services (Part B) was devised for which beneficiaries pay 25 percent of the premium.

Upon its implementation in 1966, the Medicare program had 19 million elderly enrollees (Health Care Financing Administration, 1989). In 1973, the program expanded to cover blind and disabled Americans, since they could not obtain employer-sponsored health insurance. At present, the blind and disabled account for fewer than 1 in 10 enrollees (Health Care Financing Administration, 1989).

The method the government chose to pay the providers of health services to the elderly was based on costs. The government paid whatever "reasonable" costs a provider incurred in the course of caring for a Medicare patient.

The first two decades of the Medicare program saw tremendous growth in health care spending. National health expenditures rose from $41.9 billion (1965) to $419.0 billion (1985) (Health Care Financing Administration, 1989). This tenfold increase outpaced the growth of the United States economy. That is, the share of gross national product accounted for by health care spending grew from 5.9 percent (1965) to 10.4 percent (1985). The growth in Medicare spending paralleled that of national spending for health care: from $7.1 billion (1970) to $69.3 billion (1985) (Health Care Financing Administration, 1989). By 1980, Medicare expenditures accounted for about 15 percent of national spending on health care (Health Care Financing Administration, 1989, computed from tables on pp. 24 and 30). The majority (67 percent) of Medicare spending was for hospital services (Prospective Payment Assessment Commission, 1989, computed from p. 145).

Alarming as these trends may seem, growth in health care spending is not intrinsically harmful. It may reflect a change in society's values, with an increased priority on health. Note that between 1965 and 1980, per capita spending on health care grew from $200 to $1000 per year (Health Care Financing Administration, 1989). This may indicate desired improvements in social welfare. Nevertheless, growth of this magnitude requires explanation and consideration of the prudence of these expenditures and the availability of resources to support them.

The increase in health care spending over this period has been attributed to a mix of demographic, economic, and policy factors.

- The "graying of America," i.e., the increasing number of elderly persons as a percentage of the United States population, has increased the demand for health care. Whereas in 1960 9.3 percent of our population was over age 65, by 1980 this proportion had increased by 21.5 percent to 11.3 percent (Prospective Payment Assessment Commission, 1989).*
- The expansion of both public and private health insurance over this period increased the use of, and expense for, health services. Medicare and Medicaid were the fastest growing government programs in the 1970s. (Medicaid, the federal/state health insurance for the poor, also was enacted in 1965.) The growth in private health insurance is reflected in total claims paid, which in 1980 were eight times the payments in 1965 ("Source book of health insurance data 1989," 1989).
- The growth in medical care prices between 1967 and 1980 exceeded the price inflation of goods and services overall, and of food, housing, and transportation in particular ("Source book of health insurance data 1989," 1989). The development and diffusion of quality-enhancing but cost-increasing technologies contributed to the rise in medical care prices.
- Medicare's cost-based method of payment itself contributed to cost escalation. All covered services were reimbursed, regardless of their cost. Thus, there was no incentive for hospitals to provide services efficiently or to consider the balance between the cost of additional care and expected improvements in health status. Annual inflation in hospital room prices was in the double digits for most of this period ("Source book of health insurance data 1989," 1989).

## Health Care Spending in the Political Context

Beginning in the early 1970s, the federal government began to face unprecedented budget deficits (U.S. Bureau of the Census, 1987). By 1980 the deficit reached a historical high of $73.8 billion. In the early 1980s, President Reagan's plan to substantially reduce taxes and increase defense spending placed great budgetary pressure on Congress. At that time, the annual increase in Medicare hospital expenditures was 19 percent. By 1980, it was projected that the Medicare program would be bankrupt before the end of the decade.

## Responses to Increased Health Care Spending: Cost Containment Efforts

In the face of looming deficits and dramatic health care inflation, the federal government initiated a variety of measures to contain health care costs. Most initia-

---

* It is important to note that the graying of America simultaneously affects Medicare spending and revenue. The employment base to support the Medicare benefit is eroding as the demand for it is increasing. Currently, the ratio is four workers to each Medicare beneficiary. By the middle of the 21st century, there will be only two workers per beneficiary.

tives promoted Reagan's agenda to encourage competition in the health sector. Medicare and Medicaid health maintenance organizations (HMOs) were started. Coverage expanded to include benefits such as ambulatory surgery and hospices, to enable the delivery of services in lower cost settings and thereby purchase services more prudently.

Parallel efforts to increase efficiency in the delivery of health care were pursued in the private sector. Business and labor became active in controlling health care costs by redesigning health benefits, offering HMOs, and starting programs such as surgical second opinion.

Government policy makers had recognized early on that Medicare's cost-based reimbursement method did not sufficiently encourage efficiency. Legislation in 1967 and 1972 directed Medicare to experiment with alternatives. Over the 1970s, seven states began alternate payment systems. Debate intensified in the late 1970s, with consensus that the system needed to be replaced.

## The Introduction of the Prospective Payment System

Prospective payment emerged in the political context of Reagan's agenda to encourage competition in the health sector. The financial realities of staggering Medicare expense and pending bankruptcy and soaring federal budget deficits required action. The principal goal of the PPS was to curtail Medicare costs by providing the incentive for hospitals to deliver services more efficiently. Under prospective payment, Medicare pays a flat rate to a hospital for a patient's stay. The hospital is allowed to keep the profits if its costs fall below this rate, but it must absorb the losses if costs are above this rate. By placing the hospital at financial risk for medical actions, this method introduced an economic incentive dramatically different from that of cost-based reimbursement. Each hospital became responsible for making prudent choices for itself, and in the larger context, for the Medicare program.

Despite the great potential for the PPS to control Medicare expenses, there were concerns about the impact of the system on hospitals and beneficiaries. An independent advisory body, the Prospective Payment Assessment Commission (Pro-PAC), was created to advise the secretary of health and human services and the Congress on maintaining and updating the system.

### The Diagnosis-Related Groups Classification System

A critical step in the development of a prospective system was how to recognize and classify a hospital's patient mix for payment purposes. Since hospitals treat different mixes of patients, it would be unfair to pay the same rate for the care of all patients. The method that was selected assumes that patients with similar conditions will need similar amounts of hospital resources. It classifies patients into groups of related diagnoses; thus the term "diagnosis-related groups" (DRGs). Other criteria, including patient age and other diagnoses, and whether the patient has had surgery, also affect DRG classification. The DRGs were developed by researchers, including nurse John Thompson, at Yale University. There are about 475 DRGs.

Each DRG has a relative cost weight, which reflects the average cost across all hospitals of treating patients in that DRG, compared with the average cost for all DRGs (Prospective Payment Assessment Commission, 1985). The average weight is 1.0000. In 1989, the DRG weights ranged from .1242 for DRG 382 (false labor) to 14.7080 for DRG 103 (heart transplant) (Prospective Payment Assessment Commission, 1990). Thus, on average, a Medicare heart transplant hospitalization costs 118 times that of a hospital stay for false labor. The DRG definitions and weights are revised annually to account for changing practice patterns and costs.

The actual hospital payment is the product of the cost weight of the DRG and a standard payment amount, which is based on historical hospital costs. In 1989, this standard payment amount was about $3100 (Health Care Financing Administration, 1988, computed from p. 38545). To support payment equity across hospitals, payment is adjusted for other factors that affect a hospital's service costs. These include differences in hospital location (urban versus rural), cost of labor, service to the poor, and teaching commitment.

Thus, the hospital receives an average payment, with the expectation that, although some patients' illnesses will be more costly than this average, others will be less costly, and overall the hospital will be paid fairly. A safety valve was included in the PPS to provide extra payments for unusually costly or lengthy hospital stays.

The PPS applies to inpatient hospital care only. Capital expenses, outpatient services, and the direct costs of medical education are excluded. The exclusion of capital expenses from PPS is noteworthy, since Medicare payment policy may considerably influence hospitals' choices to build or invest in new equipment, which in turn can have an enormous impact on health care costs. Although capital expenses were to be incorporated into the prospective rate in 1986, the hospital industry resisted this plan. The compromise has been reimbursement for capital expenses at a reduced rate. Initially reduced to 96.5 percent of costs in 1987, this rate had declined to 85 percent by 1989. The inclusion of capital expenses into the PPS is now planned for 1992 (Prospective Payment Assessment Commission, 1990).

## PPS Policy Design and Implementation

The change to a prospective system was expected to have substantial financial and administrative impact on hospitals. To cushion the negative consequences on hospitals with higher than average costs, the shift to prospective rates was planned to be phased in over a 3-year period, by gradually shifting from each hospital's own costs to national payment rates. Ultimately, hospitals successfully lobbied to stop the transition at the level of regional payment rates. The result is distinct rates in 18 specified geographic or urban/rural locations, developed from each hospital's average costs (Prospective Payment Assessment Commission, 1985).

Policy makers were aware of the potential for undesirable hospital responses to these new incentives. Two major concerns were that hospitals would increase admissions in order to increase total payments or compromise the quality of care in order to contain costs.

Although the PPS's fixed payment per stay was designed to encourage hospital cost efficiency within a patient stay, hospitals could skirt this incentive by increasing the total number of stays. For example, hospitals could admit a patient for diagnostic tests and then readmit the patient for the indicated treatment. This possibility had negative implications for both total costs and quality of care.

From the outset of the implementation of the PPS, the potential for a decline in quality of care given to hospitalized elderly patients was recognized (Berenson & Pawlson, 1984). Access to hospital care could be compromised if hospitals sought to identify and avoid admitting very costly patients (Stern & Epstein, 1985). The quality of inpatient care could suffer if hospitals failed to provide essential services in an effort to contain the costs of a patient's stay (McPhee, Myers, Lo, & Charles, 1984). For example, a hospital could discharge a patient too early. Since every day of a hospital stay has a cost associated with it, a simple way to cut costs would be to cut days.

To guard against these possibilities, a monitoring system was set up in which physicians review the medical record of the hospital stay to evaluate the hospital care. This watchdog mechanism is called the Medicare Utilization and Quality Peer Review Organization (PRO). Utilization review focuses on whether a hospital admission was necessary and whether diagnostic information is valid. Quality review focuses on whether care was complete and adequate. A small sample of all hospital stays plus a larger proportion of specific types of hospitalizations is reviewed.

In the early years of the PPS, PRO review was oriented toward limiting admissions to those that were medically necessary and preventing financially motivated record coding (Cislowski, 1987). The last several years have seen increasing emphasis on the role of PROs in measuring and assuring quality of care. Quality review areas include patient stability at discharge, unscheduled returns to surgery, and patient injury or complications.

## After Six Years of PPS, Did Medicare Costs Decline?

The most obvious question after 6 years of this complex and controversial system is whether it has been successful in slowing Medicare hospital expenditures. The simple answer is yes. Health economist Louise Russell (& Manning, 1989), in her estimate of the savings of the PPS to Medicare, found that the PPS had reduced Medicare's hospital costs substantially. Projected expenses were $12 billion less (adjusted for inflation) in 1990 than would have been expected compared with the pre-PPS trend. Further, this 20 percent savings has not been offset by an increase in nonhospital expenditures.

As with expenditure growth, it is important to understand why and how expenditures slowed. Russell's analysis indicated that about one third of the Medicare savings was the result of fewer hospital admissions, and another segment was due to restricted payment rates.

### Change in the Use of Hospital Services

The most dramatic and unexpected response to the PPS was a decline in the rate and number of hospital admissions, that is, even as Medicare enrollment was increasing, total Medicare hospital admissions were declining. Before the PPS, the rate of Medicare admissions had been increasing slightly each year (Guterman & Dobson, 1986). This rate peaked in 1983 and thereafter declined 15.6 percent through 1987, when it stabilized (Health Care Financing Administration, 1989). In the aggregate, this amounted to one million fewer hospital admissions in 1987 than in 1983, an 8.5 percent absolute decline.

This surprising change has been attributed to the early emphasis of PRO review on inappropriate hospital use (Russell & Manning, 1989). Medicare would not pay the hospital if PRO review found the stay to be "unnecessary." An example of a procedure that was targeted for PRO utilization review is cataract extraction with intraocular lens implantation. Hospital admissions for this procedure declined 59 percent in both 1985 and 1986 (Prospective Payment Assessment Commission, 1989). A study of Medicare hospitalizations in late 1984 estimated the potential for a shift of some hospital admissions to outpatient care ("National DRG validation study: Unnecessary admissions . . .," 1988). About 10 percent of hospital admissions were found that could have been treated on an outpatient basis. It has been difficult to assess comprehensively, however, whether and how much of the actual 8.5 percent decline represents an appropriate shift to other sites of care or the denial of needed access to hospital care.

The PPS also initially accelerated the existing downward trend in hospital length of stay (Guterman & Dobson, 1986). Length of stay had been declining since the late 1970s. In 1978, the average Medicare length of stay was 10.6 days, and by 1983, it had fallen about a day to 9.7. Since the PPS was implemented, length of stay has fallen further to just less than 9 days and remained stable.

## Restricted Payment Rates

The standard PPS payment amount had to be updated over time to account for changes in hospital costs. The PPS legislation directed the secretary of health and human services to update this amount annually. The Prospective Payment Assessment Commission was required to recommend an update to the secretary, giving consideration to changes in hospital inflation and other factors affecting hospital costs, e.g., technology advances, hospital productivity, and quality of care (Prospective Payment Assessment Commission, 1985). The quality and skill levels of professional nursing were explicitly noted in relation to maintaining quality care.

Setting the cost update has involved a protracted struggle each year among hospitals, the Congress, and the administration. Congress overruled the secretary's update for the first several years. In 1986, Congress assumed the authority to set the update. This unusual expansion of the legislative role into technical program decisions reveals the use of the PPS update as a budgetary tool and reflects the enormous budget pressure on the Congress.

Each year, the legislated update has been substantially less than actual hospital inflation. Many factors have been debated in determining the update, from hospital financial welfare to errors in the original cost estimates. The precise impact of these restricted updates has been difficult to measure. Simultaneous, substantial increases in hospitals' DRG case mix have resulted in per case payment increases nearly double those resulting from the updates and other policy decisions (Prospective

Payment Assessment Commission, 1989). The change in case mix is discussed further below.

### Expense for Nonhospital Services

Medicare's nonhospital expenses have increased, both absolutely and proportionately, since the advent of the PPS. The share of total Medicare spending accounted for by physician, nursing home, home health, and outpatient hospital services increased from 35.4 percent (1984) to 42.9 percent (1988) (Prospective Payment Assessment Commission, 1989, computed from Table 6–2, p. 145).

### Medicare Costs Outlook

Evidently, the ability to constrain Medicare spending by addressing inpatient care only is limited. Furthermore, the observed declines in utilization that have the greatest effect on costs (i.e., admissions and length of stay) have leveled off more recently. Perhaps the lower limits of these utilization patterns have been reached, yielding a one time although substantial savings that cannot persist as a trend.

## The Impact of the PPS on Patients and Hospitals

### Beneficiaries

Much attention has been given to the impact of the PPS on beneficiary welfare, particularly whether beneficiary access or quality of care has declined. The fact that little conclusive evidence has been produced after 6 years remains one of the more troubling aspects of the PPS. Evaluative efforts have been hampered by the early stage of quality of care measurement and by data limitations. Attempts to do before and after PPS quality comparisons have been undermined by the lack of systematic study prior to the start of the PPS.

These limitations aside, most of the evidence suggests that neither quality of care nor access to care has changed substantially since the PPS. There were early anecdotal reports that patients were being discharged from the hospital "quicker and sicker." A pre- and post-PPS analysis of 500 hospitals revealed that the rate of discharges to subacute facilities had increased since the start of PPS, whereas the lengths of stay before transfer to such facilities had declined (Morrisey, Sloan, & Valvona, 1988). A study by the Office of Inspector General ("National DRG validation study: Special report . . .," 1988) found that 1 percent of patients had been discharged prematurely from hospitals in 1984. Another study found that 7 percent of patients received poor quality hospital care, which involved mostly errors of omission ("National DRG validation study: Quality of patient care . . .," 1988).

Studies on quality have been either wide or deep in scope but rarely both. For example, studies of all hospitals nationally have indicated that patient deaths related to hospitalization have remained stable since the advent of the PPS (Prospective Payment Assessment Commission, 1989). Mortality, however serious an outcome, is limited as an indicator of quality of care. Alternatively, studies of two Indiana hospitals have raised concerns that some hip fracture patients may be less likely to regain ambulation since the advent of PPS (Fitzgerald et al., 1987; Fitzgerald et al., 1988). However, the extent to which the PPS itself can be implicated remains debatable (Vladeck, 1988). The same study in a third Indiana hospital found no difference in several patient outcomes, including ambulation status at discharge or 6 months after discharge (Palmer et al., 1989). A large study of the PPS and quality of care by the RAND Corporation is addressing these study weaknesses and should shed needed light on these quality of care questions (Eggers, 1987).

Patient access to new technologies or procedures may be affected by the adequacy of DRG assignment and payment. The Prospective Payment Assessment Commission concluded in 1989 that hospital acquisition and use of many major new technologies have continued to grow since the advent of the PPS. Examples include cardiac catheterization, magnetic resonance imaging, and thrombolytic agents. A recent case study, however, indicates that persistent PPS underpayments have restrained the use of and thus patient access to cochlear implants, which are devices that may improve hearing (Kane & Manoukian, 1989).

Beyond the narrow question of hospital quality is the ongoing concern over whether patients who are not admitted or no longer need acute hospital services receive the support or services they need in place of a hospital stay or upon hospital discharge. In a 1986 survey, hospital discharge planners reported increased difficulty placing patients in skilled nursing facilities since the start of the PPS ("Posthospital care . . . ," 1987). The rights and welfare of the elderly have been promoted by increasingly effective special interest groups, such as the American Association of Retired Persons.

## Hospital Financial Condition Under PPS

Prospective payment has been feast and famine for hospitals. In the early years, Medicare payments greatly exceeded costs, and hospitals' Medicare profit margins reached historically high levels of over 14 percent. This pattern reversed in 1985, however, and by 1989 the PPS profit margin was projected to approach zero (Prospective Payment Assessment Commission, 1989).

This financial roller coaster reflects both the transition to the PPS and the impact of the decline in hospital admissions. Expectations of tight revenue constraints under the PPS may have led hospitals to control their costs initially. Initial payments were high, however, because the payment rates were phased in. Hospitals' experience of unprecedented profits may have blunted their incentive to control costs. Thereafter, increasing hospital costs have outpaced payment updates. Declines in admissions have in turn decreased hospital occupancy and precipitated hospital bed closures. These changes fuel hospital cost per admission by decreasing the base over which to spread fixed costs.

Some hospitals in severe financial straits have been forced to close. Between 1980 and 1987, 343 community hospitals (nearly 6 percent) closed (Prospective Payment Assessment Commission, 1989). In contrast, the number of hospitals had increased slightly (less than 1 percent) in the late 1970s. The hospitals that have closed have been disproportionately smaller, nonteaching, nonaccredited facilities with poor financial status or in a competitive environment.

Although the 1980s began with the recognition that the hospital industry had excess capacity and that the PPS had the potential to weed out the excess, concern remains over whether the hospitals that have closed were efficient hospitals or whether they served patients who had no alternative sites of care.

### Hospital Payment Equity: DRG Case Mix and Severity of Illness

A hospital's DRG payments and Medicare's outlays are highly dependent on the distribution of patients across DRGs, or the DRG case mix. Higher-weighted DRGs generate higher payments, and vice versa. Each 2 percent change in DRG case mix translates into one billion Medicare dollars (Carter, Newhouse, & Relles, 1989).

Since the DRG system was first implemented, the patient distribution overall has shifted considerably toward the higher weighted DRGs. This reason for this shift and its impact on payments have been one of the ongoing controversies of the PPS. Case mix increase may be attributable to several factors, including increasing complexity of hospitalized patients, changing treatment patterns, and changing hospital documentation or coding practices.

Increases in DRG case mix have resulted in dramatic increases in PPS payments per case. Patient shifts to higher weighted DRGs should generate higher payments if they reflect a real increase in resource needs, but they should not if they are only due to coding improvements or "upcoding." It is complex indeed, however, to separate case mix increase into real change versus upcoding. A recent analysis indicates that about two thirds of the increase in the years 1986 to 1987 was real, thus justifying most of the additional payments to hospitals for this period (Carter et al., 1989).

A related and controversial issue is the inability of the DRGs to capture differences in patient "severity of illness" (Horn et al., 1985). That is, although one hospital may consistently care for more severely ill patients within a given DRG than another hospital, both hospitals receive the same payment. Efforts to incorporate more precise measures of severity of illness into the DRGs have been undermined by data limitations, although major refinements are now being explored.

### Hospitals' Responses to the PPS

Hospitals have initiated a variety of marketing, service, and administrative responses to prospective payment and other cost containment initiatives.

One concern was whether hospitals would begin to curtail unprofitable services and as a consequence restrict patient access. In fact, hospitals have instead sought to increase the volume of profitable services by increasing their patient base or by shifting their payer mix to cost-based services (Prospective Payment Assessment Commission, 1989). To achieve these objectives, hospitals have diversified their service mix, specialized in selected services, increased advertising, recruited physicians, and contracted with HMOs and PPOs. Hospital revenues also have been enhanced by an increasing volume of outpatient services. The share of hospital revenue from outpatient services increased from 12.5 percent in 1980 to 20 percent in 1988. Since the PPS was initiated, the number of hospital-based home health agencies has increased by 100 percent (Prospective Payment Assessment Commission, 1989). Other cost containment strategies hospitals have used include integrating with other hospitals to spread costs over a larger base, and contracting for services.

Within hospitals, departments have been created that scrutinize all phases of hospitalization. These departments' goals are to ensure and maximize hospital payment and to minimize hospital expense. They achieve these goals by evaluating whether admissions are "medically necessary," by monitoring the volume and type of hospital services used, and by expediting patient discharge.

Under prospective payment, the patient's medical record has attained an elevated status and medical records departments have grown in importance as well. The record is the basis for the discharge abstract, which determines DRG assignment and thus hospital payment. The record is also the object of PRO review. This level of attention has spawned new administrative roles in hospitals, complemented by a new computer software industry, to ensure maximum DRG payment and favorable PRO judgment through thorough record documentation and "optimal" DRG coding (Hines, 1988).

Hospitals' employment strategies have changed as well. In the first 4 years of the PPS, hospitals downsized their inpatient staff an average of 2 percent each year (Prospective Payment Assessment Commission, 1989). This contrasts with staffing increases in the years prior to the PPS. Hospitals have also increased the skill mix of their inpatient staff. This trend is most evident for nursing personnel. Registered nurses constituted 65 percent of nursing personnel in 1987 compared with 49 percent in 1980 (Prospective Payment Assessment Commission, 1989). This pattern of downsizing while upgrading staff in the context of the low relative wage of the staff nurse is considered a prominent factor in the current hospital nurse shortage (Aiken & Mullinix, 1987; Project HOPE Health Policy Research Center, 1988).

## The Impact of the PPS on Other Segments of the Health Care System

Although the institutions principally affected by the PPS have been hospitals, other providers have been affected by the changing patterns of hospital patient mix and service use.

### Nonhospital Institutions

A spillover effect of the PPS has been the increased complexity of patients needing posthospital care. Professionals in rehabilitation hospitals report a higher incidence of acute illness since the introduction of the PPS (Heinemann, Billeter, & Betts, 1988). The number of rehabilitation hospitals has increased by 100 percent since the PPS began (Prospective Payment Assessment Commission, 1989). Nursing home and home health care since the start of the PPS have required substantially more intensive medical and nursing care (Gamroth, 1988; Harron & Schaffer, 1986; Shaughnessy & Kramer, 1990; Tresch et al., 1988). Also, the proportion of patients dying in nursing homes rather than in hospitals has increased (Sager, Easterling, Kindig, & Anderson, 1989). Whether nursing homes and home health agencies have had the resources to manage this trend is unclear.

Alternative sites of care, such as ambulatory surgery and diagnostic centers, have flourished in recent years. Between 1984 and 1987, the number of surgery centers increased 40 percent annually (Prospective Payment Assessment Commission, 1989). Ambulatory care centers, diagnostic imaging centers, and freestanding cancer, cardiac, and dialysis centers also have increased over this period.

## Nurses and Nursing*

The demand for and the nature of nursing care within and beyond hospitals have changed over the 1980s.

A more intense nursing environment has been reported in rehabilitation, home health care, and nursing homes as well as hospitals (Harron & Schaffer, 1986; Jaffe, 1989; Mitty, 1988; Phillips, et al., 1989). For example, the use of nutritional support in home care accelerated following the beginning of the PPS (Orr, 1989). In nursing homes, demand for registered nurse skills has increased because of the use of high-technology procedures, e.g., telemetry, infusion pumps, and blood transfusions (Mitty, 1988). This increased clinical intensity across service settings, in the context of widespread nurse vacancies, probably compounds the current nurse shortage by contributing to nurse stress and burnout.

Increasing attention has been given to the quality, allocation, productivity, and cost of nursing care, particularly in hospitals (Jacox, 1987; Pointer & Pointer, 1989; Shaffer & Preziosi, 1988). The development of nursing classification tools for allocating and costing nursing resources is described in Chapter 11.

With earlier hospital discharges and later admissions, continuity of care across service settings has grown in importance. Nurses have demonstrated successfully the cost-effectiveness of a nursing transitional care model (Brooten et al., 1986; Pappas & VanScoy-Mosher, 1988). Another promising development has been the evolution of nursing case management (Zander, 1988a; Zander, 1988b).

The changing role of nurses in health care delivery has significant implications for nursing education and research (Brooten, 1988; Shaffer, 1988; Van Ort et al., 1989). Although curricula have incorporated health policy and ethics, content relevant to patient acuity across settings, particularly clinical experiences, needs to be addressed. Researchers have begun to explore the nurse's role in cost-effectiveness and quality across the continuum of care (e.g., discharge planning, transitional care, home care, and case management).

---

* Karen K. Knibbe, R.N., M.S.N., contributed to this section.

## *Physicians and Medicine*

Physicians perceive the PPS as government interference in medical practice with potentially negative consequences for quality of care. The PPS also complicates relations between medicine and administration in hospitals.

In a survey of 650 internists, two thirds believed that the PPS system has hurt quality of care ("The impact of prospective payment . . .," 1988). Their greatest concerns were pressure to discharge patients sooner than medically appropriate (63 percent of respondents) and to delay admission until the patient was sick enough to meet admission criteria (55 percent).

Physician practice and the incentives of the PPS conflict in several ways. Physician services continue to be paid on a fee-for-service basis. Physicians' oath of beneficence, particularly in the context of medical liability, encourages them to do all they can for patients. Hospital administrators and the shadow of peer review, however, exert pressure on physicians to modify their behavior.

Nevertheless, physicians remain integral to hospital admissions policies. Administrators must balance efforts to contain costs against attempts to satisfy physician requests for new equipment, specialty staff, or other resources.

## *Other Payers*

Historically, hospitals have attempted to shift the costs of public and uncompensated care (from low or zero payment levels) to private payers, e.g., Blue Cross and commercial insurers. There were concerns that the PPS would exacerbate such cost shifting (Iglehart, 1982). In fact, other payers have responded to and benefited from the example set by the PPS (Prospective Payment Assessment Commission, 1989). They have set up cost containment programs such as preadmission review, second surgical opinion, managed care, and limiting the patient's selection of providers ("Questions and answers . . .," 1987).

## The Role of Non-PPS Developments

It is important to recognize that other developments have contributed to the dramatic changes in health care observed in the 1980s. The positive and negative changes attributed to the PPS may be due to other factors or the combination of the PPS with other factors. The acquired immunodeficiency syndrome crisis, the boom in health care technology, cost containment efforts by all parties including employers, increasing consumer acceptance of alternative sites of care, and sociodemographic changes all have contributed to these changes. For example, technology advances have permitted technology use in less-tertiary settings.

## PPS for Medicare Hospital Payment: Assessment and Outlook

### *Assessment*

The PPS was designed to curb Medicare expense through more efficient use of hospital services. The PPS not only has generated sizable savings but has precipitated substantial changes in health care delivery. Inpatient care has intensified, with corresponding impact on ambulatory and long-term care. Whether Medicare's savings under the PPS reflect prudent choices and efficiency gains is uncertain. Hospital costs rise relentlessly. The shift of services to nonhospital settings may provide a generally safer, more comfortable, and less costly environment. Nevertheless, coverage for and availability of nonhospital services may be problematic.

Although the concept of prospective payment is simple, the structure of the PPS is necessarily complex. Implementing and adapting to PPS have been difficult for both the Medicare program and hospitals. The transition to the PPS meant different payment structures for each hospital for each year. Nearly annual revisions to DRG classification and payment adjustments have contributed continuing complexity. Because such revisions alter PPS incentives and impact, they generate an ongoing dynamic between Medicare revisions and hospital responses.

The PPS amply demonstrates the potential for a payment system to become a political instrument. The efforts of Congress and interest groups to manipulate this system underscore the dominant role of federal and hospital budgets in policy decisions.

## Outlook

It is unlikely that Medicare payments to hospitals will see a dramatic overhaul in the near future. Other health care concerns, in particular the 37 million uninsured Americans and the elderly's long-term care needs, demand national attention. In this context, the relative success of prospective payment and the incremental nature of policy change will inhibit any dramatic change. In fact, Medicare's prospective payment frontier is extending to other settings. Ambulatory surgery centers are now paid prospective fixed rates, and prospective payment for outpatient services is under development.

The progress to date notwithstanding, inpatient prospective payment deserves continuing attention and technical refinement. Major areas of potential improvement include the DRG measurement of hospital case mix and patient severity of illness, the efficacy and efficiency of peer review, and payment equity among hospitals.

## The PPS and Our Health Care Priorities

The lessons of the PPS have helped to shape our national health care priorities in both obvious and subtle ways.

Realizing the limits of inpatient savings, federal attention has turned to payment reform for outpatient services, particularly physician services. One of the last legislative achievements of the 1980s was the enactment of a new Medicare payment method for physician services. The method, which is detailed in another chapter, rivals the PPS as the most radical health policy development of the 1980s.

A significant contribution of the PPS to health care delivery has been in the measurement of quality of care. The potential for the compromise of quality under the PPS demanded that Medicare systematically monitor hospital care quality. The PPS thus catalyzed the advancement of quality of care research. A major development in quality assessment over the 1980s has been the shift in orientation from measures of hospital care structure and process to measures of outcomes of hospital care.

In a concurrent development, health services researchers recognized and began to tap the wealth of data in our federal health care systems. Extensive Medicare data are now available for public use.

As health care has become more oriented to business and less toward social good, the patient's role has evolved as well. Patients are becoming informed consumers of health care rather than passive recipients. The changing patterns of health care delivery depend in part on patient acceptance of alternative delivery styles. Patient expectations influence physician behavior, especially in our contentious malpractice environment. Thus, patient education has become vital to the wise use of our health resources.

As changes in health care delivery blur the boundaries between levels of care, the focus of health policy must shift from acute hospital care to an episode of illness. The policy questions become: Who coordinates the services and guides the consumer across a continuum of care? How can financing be integrated to ensure that needed services are provided across settings? Nurse practitioners are well qualified to manage patient care across settings. Financing for this nurse role, however, remains unresolved.

Spiraling costs and an aging population, the major impetuses for the enactment of the PPS, continue to overwhelm our health care system. Our national strategy continues to focus on encouraging more efficient health care spending rather than deliberate rationing of health services. The merits of a refined and more broadly applied PPS and newer efficiency initiatives will unfold over this new decade.

## REFERENCES

Aiken, L.H., & Mullinix, C.F. (1987). The nurse shortage: Myth or reality? *New England Journal of Medicine, 317*(10), 641–646.

Berenson, R.A., & Pawlson, L.G. (1984). The Medicare prospective payment system and the care of the frail elderly. *Law and Public Policy, 32*, 843–848.

Brooten, D. (1988). Effect of DRGs on research. *Nursing Clinics of North America, 23*(3), 587–597.

Brooten, D., Kumar, S., Brown, L.P., Butts, P., Finkler, S.A., Bakewell-Sachs, S., Gibbons, A., & Delivoria-Papadopoulos, M. (1986). A randomized clinical trial of early hospital discharge and home follow-up of very-low-birth-weight infants. *New England Journal of Medicine, 315*(15), 934–939.

Carter, G.M., Newhouse, J.P., & Relles, D.A. (1990, April). *How much change in the case mix index is DRG creep?* Santa Monica, CA: The RAND Corporation.

Cislowski, J.A. (1987). *The peer review organization program* (CRS Rep. No. 87-860 EPW). Washington, DC: Congressional Research Service.

Durenberger, D. (1985). Twenty years of Medicare and Medicaid [commentary]. *Health Care Financing Review, 7* (Suppl.), 75–79.

Eggers, P.W. (1987). Prospective payment system and quality: Early results and research strategy. *Health Care Financing Review* (Ann. Suppl.), 29–37.

Fitzgerald, J.F., Fagan, L.F., Tierney, W.M., & Dittus, R.S. (1987). Changing patterns of hip fracture care before and after implementation of the prospective payment system. *Journal of the American Medical Association, 258*(2), 218–221.

Fitzgerald, J.F., Moore, P.S., & Dittus, R.S. (1988). The care of elderly patients with hip fracture: Changes since implementation of the prospective payment system. *New England Journal of Medicine, 319*(2), 1392–1397.

Gamroth, L. (1988). Long-term care resource requirements before and after the prospective payment system. *Image: Journal of Nursing Scholarship, 20*(1), 7–11.

Guterman, S., & Dobson, A. (1986). Impact of the Medicare prospective payment system for hospitals. *Health Care Financing Review, 7*(3), 97–114.

Harron, J., & Schaffer, J. (1986). DRGs and the intensity of skilled nursing. *Geriatric Nursing, 7*(1), 31–33.

Health Care Financing Administration (1988). Medicare program; changes to the inpatient hospital prospective payment system and fiscal year 1989 rates; final rule. *Federal Register, 53*(190), 38476–38640.

Health Care Financing Administration (1989). *1989 HCFA statistics* (HCFA Publication No. 03294). Baltimore: Health Care Financing Administration.

Heinemann, A.W., Billeter, J., & Betts, H.B. (1988). Prospective payment for acute care: Impact on rehabilitation hospitals. *Archives of Physical Medicine and Rehabilitation, 69*(8), 614–618.

Hines, G.L. (1988). DRGs: Nursing documentation contributes to the bottom line. *Nursing Clinics of North America, 23*(3), 579–587.

Horn, S.C., Bulkley, G., Sharkey, P.D., Chambers, A.F., Horn, R.A., & Schramm, C.J. (1985). Interhospital differences in severity of illness: Problems for prospective payment based on diagnosis-related groups (DRGs). *New England Journal of Medicine, 313*(3), 20–24.

Iglehart, J.K. (1982). Health policy report: The new era of prospective payment for hospitals. *New England Journal of Medicine, 307*(20), 1288–1292.

Iglehart, J.K. (1983). Medicare begins prospective payment of hospitals. *New England Journal of Medicine, 308*(23), 1428–1432.

Jacox, A. (1987). Determining the cost and value of nursing. *Nursing Administration Quarterly, 12*(1), 7–12.

Jaffe, K. (1989). Home health care and rehabilitation nursing. *Nursing Clinics of North America, 24*(1), 171–178.

Kane, N.M., & Manoukian, P.D. (1989). The effect of the Medicare prospective payment system on the adoption of new technology: The case of cochlear implants. *New England Journal of Medicine, 321*(20), 1378–1383.

McPhee, S.J., Myers, L.P., Lo, B., & Charles, G. (1984). Cost containment confronts physicians. *Annals of Internal Medicine, 100*(4), 604–606.

Mitty, E. (1988). Resource utilization groups: DRGs move to long-term care. *Nursing Clinics of North America, 23*(3), 539–557.

*National DRG validation study: Quality of patient care in hospitals.* (1988). Washington, DC: Office of Inspector General, Department of Health and Human Services.

*National DRG validation study: Special report on premature discharges* (Report No. OAI-05-88-00740). (1988). Washington, DC: Office of Inspector General, Department of Health and Human Services.

*National DRG validation study: Unnecessary admissions to hospitals* (Report No. OAI-09-88-00880). (1988). Washington, DC: Office of Inspector General, Department of Health and Human Services.

Orr, M.E. (1989). Nutritional support in home care. *Nursing Clinics of North America, 24*(2), 437–445.

Palmer, R.M., Saywell, R.M., Jr., Zollinger, T.W., Erner, B.K., LaBov, A.D., Freund, D.A., Garber, J.E., Misamore, G.W., & Throop, F.B. (1989). The impact of the prospective payment system on the treatment of hip fractures in the elderly. *Archives of Internal Medicine, 149*(10), 2237–2241.

Pappas, C.A., & VanScoy-Mosher, C. (1988). Establishing a profitable outpatient community nursing center. *Journal of Nursing Administration, 18*(5), 31–33.

Phillips, E.K., Fisher, M.E., MacMillan-Scattergood, D., & Baglioni, A.J., Jr. (1989). DRG ripple and the shifting burden of care to home health. *Nursing & Health Care, 10*(6), 324–327.

Pointer, D.D., & Pointer, T.K. (1989). Case-based prospective price reimbursement. *Nursing Management, 20*(4), 30–34.

*Posthospital care: Discharge planners report increasing difficulty in placing Medicare patients* (Rep. No. PEMD-87-5BR). (1987). Washington, DC: General Accounting Offfice.

Project HOPE Health Policy Research Center (1988). An examination of the relationship between Medicare prospective payment and the nursing shortage. *Nursing Economics, 6*(6), 317–318.

Prospective Payment Assessment Commission (1985). *Report and recommendations to the Secretary, U.S. Department of Health and Human Services April 1, 1985.* Washington, DC: U.S. Government Printing Office.

Prospective Payment Assessment Commission (1989). *Medicare prospective payment and the American Health Care System: Report to the Congress. June 1989.* Washington, DC: U.S. Government Printing Office.

Prospective Payment Assessment Commission (1990). *Report and recommendations to the Secretary, U.S. Department of Health and Human Services, March 1, 1990.* Washington, DC: U.S. Government Printing Office.

*Questions and answers about the Blue Cross and Blue Shield organization.* (1987). Chicago: Blue Cross and Blue Shield Association.

Russell, L.B. (1989). *Medicare's new hospital payment system: Is it working?* Washington, DC: The Brookings Institution.

Russell, L.B., & Manning, C.L. (1989). The effect of prospective payment on Medicare expenditures. *New England Journal of Medicine, 320*(7), 439–444.

Sager, M.A., Easterling, D.V., Kindig, D.A., & Anderson, O.W. (1989). Changes in the location of death after passage of Medicare's prospective payment system: A national study. *New England Journal of Medicine, 320*(7), 433–439.

Shaffer, F.A. (1988). DRGs: A new era for health care. *Nursing Clinics of North America, 23*(3), 453–463.

Shaffer, F.A., & Preziosi, P. (1988). Nursing: The hospital's competitive edge. *Nursing Clinics of North America, 23*(3), 597–613.

Shaughnessy, P.W., & Kramer, A.M. (1990). The increased needs of patients in nursing homes and patients receiving home health care. *New England Journal of Medicine, 322*(1), 21–27.

*Source book of health insurance data 1989.* (1989). Washington, DC: Health Insurance Association of America.

*The impact of prospective payment on patient care: A survey of internists' experiences under DRGs.* (1988), Washington, DC: American Society of Internal Medicine.

Stern, R.S., & Epstein, A.M. (1985). Institutional responses to prospective payment based on diagnosis-related groups: Implications for cost quality and access. *New England Journal of Medicine, 312*(10), 621–627.

Tresch, D.D., Duthie, E.H., Newton, M., & Bodin, B. (1988). Coping with diagnosis related groups: The changing role of the nursing home. *Archives of Internal Medicine, 148*(6), 1393–1396.

U.S. Bureau of the Census (1987). *Statistical Abstract of the United States: 1988* (108th ed.). Washington, DC: U.S. Government Printing Office.

Van Ort, S., Woodtli, A., & Williams, M. (1989). Prospective payment and baccalaureate nursing education: Projections for the future. *Journal of Professional Nursing, 5*(1), 25–30.

Vladeck, B.C. (1988). Hospital prospective payment and the quality of care [editorial]. *New England Journal of Medicine, 319*(21), 1411–1413.

Zander, K. (1988a). Nursing case management: Strategic management of cost and quality outcomes. *Journal of Nursing Administration, 18*(5), 23–30.

Zander, K. (1988b). Nursing case management: Resolving the DRG paradox. *Nursing Clinics of North America, 23*(3), 503–520.

## Chapter 11

# Diagnosis-Related Groups and the Measurement of Nursing

DONNA DIERS

$D$IAGNOSIS-RELATED GROUPS (DRGs) were developed to define the mix of cases treated in hospitals so that comparisons for cost and quality could be made among institutions or services. Without such definition, it is not possible to compare the productivity of institutions or to *manage* clinically the efficient and effective use of resources. As it turns out, the federal government was also interested in management—management of the Medicare program to limit unrestrained growth and make the government a "prudent purchaser" of hospital services on behalf of Medicare enrollees. DRGs provided a way to pay for care that was defined by what patients *need* rather than what was done to or for them.

The payment system itself is described in Chapter 10 and is lucidly summarized in Louise Russell's book (1989). Although it is not possible to discuss DRGs without reference to money, the focus of this chapter is on the clinical and nursing management implications of DRGs as case mix definitions and the possibilities of using DRGs and measures of nursing to improve the quality and quantity of hospital services.

### Background

Hospital administrators will argue that the reason their costs are high is because their patients are "sicker." Actually, there are three possible reasons for the documented vast differences across institutions in hospital costs: hospitals are treating different kinds of patients (case mix); the patients are the same but the treatment protocol is different; or the patients and the treatment are the same but some hospitals do it more efficiently. It is not possible to detect efficiency differences or quality (treatment) differences, however, unless the patients themselves can be defined. We cannot manage what we cannot measure. Thus DRGs were devised to provide a measure of case mix, allowing comparisons of cost or quality within relatively homogeneous groups of cases.

The most obvious way to define patient condition is by diagnosis, or in the case of those having surgery, by surgical procedure. Diagnoses are coded in the International Classification of Diseases (ICD), now in its tenth revision, and surgical procedures are also named and labeled in this classification. But there are thousands of ICD codes for diagnoses and only a slightly smaller number for surgical procedures, and there are sometimes very small distinctions among the codes. To define case types by relatively like conditions requires collapsing the diagnoses and procedures into groups of relatively similar conditions.

The principles that guided DRG construction were that there should be a manageable number of classes (under 500); that the classes should be clinically coherent; that the classes should be defined using commonly available variables (no new data need be collected); and that the classes produced should be statistically stable, that is, persons in the class should have similar expected measures of resources used in their care (Fetter, Shin, Freeman, Averill, & Thompson, 1980). Inevitably, in grouping diagnoses or surgical procedures, some precision is lost. It is very important to understand what is inside any given DRG, because the labels attached were invented. Thus DRG 127, Heart Failure and Shock (one of the highest volume Medicare DRGs), has ten diagnostic codes; eight are variations on heart failure and two are "shock," but only cardiogenic shock. DRG 370, Cesarean Section with Complications/Comorbidities, lists more than 500 codes that would classify a woman in the "complicated" DRG. Some of them are quite minor—abnormal vulva; varicose vein in leg—but most are major—e.g., grand multiparity; primary uterine inertia; locked twins; rupture of the uterus (*DRG's—Diagnosis Related Groups Definition Manual*, 1985 and annually). To use DRGs for clinical management or research requires knowing what is inside of each one.

DRGs are *discharge* classifications, using the "principal diagnosis"—the condition determined after discharge and *after study* to have been responsible for the hospitalization. DRGs are usually assigned by the medical records department, from the physician's written or dictated discharge summary, using a computer "grouper" program that has built-in error detection routines. For example, such programs would flag a record in which a hysterectomy code had been assigned to a male patient. There are only certain comorbidities and complications that qualify as secondary diagnoses and put the patient into a more resource-intense class. Patients admitted with one condition (e.g., a myocardial infarction) who subsequently have another (e.g., a stroke) will be coded according to the principal diagnosis, which may not have been the admitting diagnosis. Patients with a pre-existing condition (comorbidity), for example, chronic obstructive pulmonary disease, whose present hospitalization is for something else, perhaps a broken ankle, will be coded by the reason for the present inpatient hospitalization, with the chronic obstructive pulmonary disease as a comorbidity (for those DRGs that use complications/comorbidities for definition). Patients are assigned to one and only one DRG, and the data used for assignment are only the data contained in the Uniform Hospital Discharge Data Summary, a format prescribed for hospital use by the National Center for Health Statistics. Uniform Hospital Discharge Data Summary variables are diagnoses and surgical procedures, gender, age, length of stay, discharge disposition (to home, nursing home, etc.), and patient and physician identifiers. These data were the only set uniformly available when DRGs were being formed (and this is still the case), which explains why the DRG definitions developed the way they did.

Diagnosis-related groups (fifth revision) explain about 15 to 23 percent of the variance in length of stay, depending on what percentage of outliers are included (McGuire, 1990). As medical record coding has improved, the explained variance has risen. The psychiatric DRGs have been a problem from the beginning because length of stay depends more on treatment philosophy than on patient diagnosis. Hospital stays for rehabilitation also do not fit the model well, nor does long-term care for persons with cancer. Thus special cancer hospitals, rehabilitation units, psychiatric units, and children's hospitals have been exempt from the DRG-based payment system. There are few children in the Medicare program.

Under Medicare's Prospective Payment System, DRGs are examined annually and changes are made according to new data. For example, as the quality of coding of the medical record began to improve, the use of the advanced age (>70) definition no longer improved the predictability of resource use, and therefore this age criterion has been dropped from DRG definitions. New DRGs or new combinations have been put into place as technical advances dictated. Transluminal angioplasty was not being performed in 1980; now it is included. Acquired immunodeficiency syndrome was not identified in 1980; a New York State version of DRGs now includes human immunodeficiency virus–related conditions as separate categories. Version 8 has separate DRGs for conditions or treatments that do not fall within any one Major Diagnostic Category such as liver transplant, multiple trauma, bone marrow transplant, and temporary tracheostomy. The last was identified as a signal of high resource use in the most recent DRG refinement project (Health Systems Management Group, 1989). The neonatal DRGs have been refined to take birth weight and ventilator support into account (National Association of Children's Hospitals and Related Institutions, 1985). (These latter changes have not been adopted by Medicare, since little neonatal care is paid for under that program. They have, however, been used in states in which all third-party payers use DRGs as the basis for payment rates.)

When DRGs were formed, length of stay was used as the basis for putting relatively similar diagnoses or surgical procedures into the same group. Thus an average "price" for each case type can be calculated. The actual method for assigning prices to DRGs is beyond the scope of this chapter (Schweiker, 1982). For now, it should be known that the price set is an average for an average length of stay, which means that any given case may actually come in below or above the price that will be paid. Thus, there is an incentive to deliver services more efficiently because if the final costs are lower than the assigned price, the hospital can keep the difference between what the hospitalization "actually" costs and the price paid. Of course, if final costs are higher than the assigned price, the hospital cannot charge more for Medicare patients. Special payments are made for very long-stay patients— "outliers." Over a long enough period of time, about as many patients will be discharged earlier than the average as will be discharged later. However, since hospitals and clinicians tend to think of "my patient, now" and do not have information about how the previous 100 patients in the same DRG fared, the "average" has been used as the standard target; as a result, hospital administrators' worries about exceeding the limit roll down on nurses, who are told that the patient has reached his or her "DRG days." There is no such number, except in the sense that the Professional Review Organizations use the average length of stay as a point at which to check on whether the Medicare patient needs continued hospitalization. However, there is a continuing fantasy, fueled by the media, that DRGs themselves set the limit for how long anyone can stay in the hospital. No hospital, of course, congratulates any professional for discharging patients before the "limit."

Knowing what the price will be for each DRG, knowing the volume in the past year by DRG, and taking into account local changes in technology or patient mix, hospital managers can predict their budgets, at least for Medicare patients, within fairly tight limits. Third-party payers or health maintenance organizations, who use DRGs to define their own case types of enrollees, may also better predict their outlays of funds. DRG information can also be used in short- and long-range planning as population-based data. And information produced by DRG-based information systems may be used for quality assessment and utilization review, as was originally intended.

Some 17 countries are experimenting with the use of DRGs for dispersing global budgets to regions, districts, hospitals or general practitioners, which is the way health care is funded in countries with nationalized health care systems. Portugal, for example, began to pay hospitals according to case mix by DRGs in 1990, and it is possible that when the next Australian government contracts with States are negotiated in 1993, hospital budgets will be determined by DRG case mix. These experiments suggest that even if the United States were to evolve "per head" population-based capitated payment structures, a case mix measure would still be used in calculating budgets or prices.

Since the only payment program over which the United States federal government has complete control is Medicare, only under Medicare is prospective payment (which is really prospective rate setting—hospitals are not actually *paid* in advance of service delivery) mandated. Some states have passed legislation to require all third-party payers to use DRGs and to prospectively set rates, and other states have amended their Medicaid programs to include DRG-based rates (Thorpe, 1987). Whether states have taken such steps or not, the fact that so much of hospital business is paid by Medicare has meant that the data systems based on DRGs are nearly uniformly in place.

Before being adopted by the federal government, DRGs were tested as a basis for rate setting in New Jersey. The New Jersey Nurses Association negotiated to have special funding for a study to weight DRGs by a measure of nursing resources (Joel, 1984). It was argued that medical diagnosis, which is used to form DRGs, is not a precise indicator of the requirements for (and costs of) nursing care. This deal carried with it the promise that when a reliable method was invented and tested, it would become part of the payment mechanism. A study was conducted (Caterinicchio, 1983; Caterinicchio & Davies, 1983; Grimaldi & Micheletti, 1982; Trofino, 1985), but it was sufficiently flawed and controversial that the nursing weighting method—RIMS (Resource Intensity Measure)—was never implemented in the payment structure. Nursing woke up abruptly to two problems: (1) hospital payment was going to be based on a measure that allegedly did not include nursing's concerns (the "medical model"); and (2) nursing, as clinical work or resource, was not visible within the DRG/Prospective Payment System payments or the information systems. Thus organized nursing's response in public testimony was essentially conceptual distress with the medical model, petulance at somehow being excluded from DRG construction, and anxiety about the effect on nursing jobs (Cole, 1982; Curtis, 1983). But nursing data, which had been collected for years, were simply not available to be used for DRG definition.

The remainder of this chapter deals with these issues and with the opportunities the DRG/Prospective Payment System has provided for understanding nursing resources, defining nursing's contribution, and even grasping more fully what nursing in hospitals is all about.

## Diagnosis-Related Groups and Nursing Data

Apart from the individual patient record with its pages of nurses' notes, nursing information comes in two categories: nursing as resource (nursing patient classification plus nursing time), and nursing diagnosis. Both can be measures of nursing.

### Nursing Patient Classification

Modern nursing patient classification rose out of industrial management studies of hospitals in the early 1960s. Charles Flagle at Johns Hopkins is usually credited with the first effort to establish measures of patient requirements for nursing care (Flagle, 1962). The early research was an attempt to make requirements for nursing *staffing* more predictable and flexible, so that staffing would vary with what patients needed. The literature on nursing patient classification has been collected and annotated by Aydelotte (1973), analyzed by Giovannetti (a student of Flagle) (1978), extended to the United Kingdom by Hearn (1972), and distilled by Thompson and Diers (1990).

Giovannetti distinguishes among three types of patient classification systems: patient profiles, nursing task documents, and critical indicator systems (Giovannetti & Mayer, 1984). Patient profiles are descriptive narratives of the "prototype" patient, and although they were used in the early days of classification, they have nearly died out now. Actual patients were matched to the prototype and assigned to a category or class of care requirements, to which a time frame could be assigned. It is possible that nursing diagnoses could be gathered together to form a contemporary version of the prototype system (Halloran, 1988a).

In nursing task documents, the majority if not all of the direct nursing care tasks or activities are listed and checked off for each patient. Each task or activity is associated with a standard time value, and values are accumulated into categories or levels of care.

The most common type of classification is based on critical indicators for care rather than tasks. The critical indicator systems all contain, at a minimum, the basic activities of daily living or "dependence," such as the ability to feed oneself or move about out of bed. Each indicator is given a unique numerical weight, usually developed by consensus of the nurses involved. The weight is a relative value for nursing effort. For example, "Admission/Transfer in" might have a value of 3, "Specimen collecting/testing" a value of 2, "Major physiologic instability" a value of 8, and "Tube care" a value of 6. The weights are points that are summed, and the total assigns the patient to a level of care that has been assigned standard times for care by the service or unit. In general, hospitals have adopted their own definitions of the cutoffs that define levels of care using their own frequency distributions.

The possibilities for listing either nursing tasks or patient characteristics are nearly endless, and all existing systems must reduce these points to a manageable number. The San Joaquin system, perhaps the most widely used of the nonproprietary systems, reduces nursing tasks to nine from an original 200 (San Joaquin General Hospital, 1976). The Rush-Medicus system has about 40 patient characteristics (Jelinek, Haussman, Hegyvary, & Newman, 1974). Contemporary efforts attempt to include more of the cognitive dimension of nursing practice alleged to be missing from the task and patient characteristic documents (Prescott & Phillips, 1988). Giovannetti notes that there are more similarities than differences among the patient classification systems and that little increase in validity is to be gained by adding more than the basic activities of daily living/medication/monitoring items (Giovannetti & Mayer, 1984). There are a large number of patient classification systems increasingly available on computer software. One system has been designed specifically for intensive or critical care (Cullen et al., 1974; Keene & Cullen, 1983).

In using both task documents and critical indicators, standard time values are associated with each task or indicator, based either on consensus of the nurses or on time-motion studies. The times are based on an accepted standard of quality of care. Constants or other weights are added to reflect indirect nursing activity. When the times are totaled over all the patients on a given unit, they can be converted to hours; divided by eight, they produce full-time equivalents that become the staffing target. Or at least that was the initial reasoning. The Joint Commission on the Accreditation of Health Care Organizations in the United States and the Canadian equivalent organization now mandate that each hospital have a way of assigning nursing staff that takes patient classification into account.

This way of approaching nursing as task, indicator, or time has been criticized as an outmoded way of thinking that does not match the professional models of care. Indeed, enlightened institutions are no longer using their patient classification system for assigning staff but are increasingly employing the information to track patient acuity, to monitor equity of workload among nursing staff, and to discern changing patterns of nursing work or patient requirements. Nurses are also using the information to argue for increased staff or to plan for new services such as the step-down units now springing up like weeds. None of this was possible before there were computers to store the vast amount of data such systems produce.

The issue concerning patient classification systems is not which one is perfect and exactly captures patient needs and requirements in adequate detail, but which one the nurses will *use*. If nurses punch the buttons or fill out the forms every shift and nothing happens with the information—no more staff is produced or no information is fed back to the staff—the system is useless.

Researchers and manpower policy analysts are sometimes frustrated by the proliferation of nursing patient classification approaches in the United States. It has been thought that the fact that each hospital makes its own decision about which instrument to invest in precludes the possibility of interinstitutional comparisons, to say nothing of establishing a reimbursement policy that would recognize nursing's contribution. In a nationalized health system, the government can simply prescribe the use of a particular system, as has been the case in France, which has adopted Quebec's PRN system (Chagon, Audette, Lebrun, & Tilquin, 1978). In the United States' private health care system, government would approach such prescription very gingerly. But since all such systems eventually can be converted to a standard measurement—time (and thence to dollars)—they can be made equivalent when comparisons are of interest.

Nursing patient classification information is increasingly being used for yet another purpose: variable billing. Some hosptials are now billing differentially for nursing, depending on the level of care required by the patient.* First, they use the patient classification system with its standard times to attach a cost to nursing that reflects both direct care given to individual patients and nursing activities that cannot be assigned to individuals but are spread equally across all patients on the unit. A charge is then calculated that takes into account the nursing salaries and fringe benefits as well as the allocated costs of nursing administration. The charge appears as a line item on the bill: "Nursing Level II—$60." This breaks nursing out of the room and board charge and allows nursing care to be separately identified as a legitimate charge. When the income thus tagged and generated is accounted back to the nursing service department, nursing turns from a cost center to a revenue center, with all the policy, political, and managerial connotations of any income-producing service (Sovie & Smith, 1986).

The link of nursing care to the patient's bill has other ramifications. Since bills are rendered for individual patients by DRG, even when the third-party payer is not Medicare, it becomes possible to relate patient acuity and nursing intensity to the larger data sets. Nursing information enters the budget system, and even when

---

* Information on hospitals using variable billing is collected and updated by Van Slyck & Associates ([Ann Van Slyck] 4033 East Mission Lane, Phoenix, Arizona 85028-9955). As of June, 1990, 22 hospitals that use variable billing have agreed to share their information through contact persons listed with Van Slyck.

hospitals decentralize budgets to the service or unit level, it is possible to predict nursing resources by knowing past volume by DRG and projecting to the next budget year. Such information would also be useful when hospitals enter into capitation contracts with health maintenance organizations and when global budgets need to be assigned to individual services or units. The costs of nursing vary considerably by DRG, by service, and even by unit (Sovie et al., 1984; Thompson & Diers, 1988).

Finally, if enough nursing intensity information were gathered and linked to DRGs, it would be possible to "weight" DRGs by a measure of nursing time and thus to reflect nursing resources more accurately in payment policy, as was intended in the Resource Intensity Measure study.

## Nursing Diagnosis and Diagnosis-Related Groups

> Nursing must be able to name itself and to describe what it does in order to function effectively in a world where computerized information is used to establish everything from diagnosis-related groups (DRGs) to cardiac output. Until nurses can name what they do and assign a computer code to that name, we may be neither reimbursed nor recognized as a profession with unique skills and knowledge (*Classification Systems for Describing Nursing Practice—Working Papers*, 1989, p. 3).

It is argued that patient classification, as discussed above, might fulfill the agenda of hospital administrators or payers but that it does not meet nursing's agenda—to name and label the "phenomena of interest" and thus to establish nursing as a definable, separate profession. Thus one thrust of the nursing diagnosis movement has been to work toward including nursing data within federally mandated data systems such as the Uniform Hospital Discharge Data Summary.

One proposal is essentially to add five new variables to the Uniform Hospital Discharge Data Summary: nursing diagnosis; nursing intervention; nursing outcome; intensity of nursing care; and a unique number for the principal registered nurse provider (Werley et al., 1986; Werley & Lang, 1988; Werley & Zorn, 1989). If such data were to be collected nationally, comparisons between institutions or providers could be made, research on effectiveness of care could be done, and nursing would understand more about the scope and variety of patient services. Eventually, nursing diagnoses would be included in future versions of ICD codes.

The proposal assumes that, from the point of view of Uniform Hospital Discharge Data Summary-type data systems, nursing diagnosis is parallel to medical diagnosis, and nursing intervention is parallel to procedure codes. (There is no Uniform Hospital Discharge Data Summary equivalent to "nursing outcome.") Apart from the problem of obtaining significant agreement on either nursing diagnosis or intervention classification, there are conceptual and empirical differences that have implications for data set definition and use. Nursing diagnoses occur in multiple forms and combinations over a patient's stay. Medical diagnostic nomenclature and procedure definitions are issued once and then they stick; a patient who has appendicitis and has an appendectomy has each just once, and neither is eliminated in the data definition. The problem of entering these nursing variables into the present data system is very complicated. At present, there is considerable resistance to the notion of weighting nursing diagnoses, which would be the only way to reduce them to a single item. But surely there are some that are more difficult, time-consuming, or important than others, and some nursing diagnoses are more important in the context of the patient's medical diagnosis than others. For example, "knowledge deficit" might be critical in a person newly diagnosed with diabetes but not so troubling in a person facing herniorrohaphy.

The idea of weighting nursing diagnoses, or otherwise converting them into a quantitative measure, even by adding up how many there are, runs counter to describing patient needs and nursing intervention qualitatively. In a resource-based information system, nursing diagnoses must be converted to fit. Would one count *all* of the nursing diagnoses ever issued, and if so, what would one do about repeated ones? Would all nursing diagnoses be weighted the same? Remember that the Uniform Hospital Discharge Data Summary is a *discharge* summary and cannot possibly include everything that ever went on with a patient—it is a *minimum* data set. The discharge summary is a way to enter or access the whole patient record, if daily changes are of interest (Thompson, 1988). In the absence of a way of collapsing nursing diagnoses into the discharge summary, DRGs will remain the easiest way to access the medical record.

The importance of the nursing diagnosis work is that it points up the possibility that there are patient conditions in addition to medical diagnosis or surgical procedure that play a part in resource consumption as cost. Halloran is one of the few researchers to attempt to link nursing diagnosis to resources. He has shown that nursing diagnosis *in combination* with DRGs explains a greater proportion of the variance in length of stay than DRGs alone, and nursing diagnoses predict nursing time better than DRGs (Halloran, 1985; Halloran & Kiley, 1987). To do this, however, he had to use only one day's nursing diagnoses—the day of admission for medical patients, and day 3 after surgery for surgical patients. It is of interest that in early versions of Halloran's patient classification form, which is composed of nursing diagnoses, medical diagnosis is almost treated as a "weight" to nursing, an interesting idea that has not been pursued further (Halloran & Halloran, 1985).

## Uses of Diagnosis Related Groups–Based Nursing Information

Interprofessional politics in the United States—the dread of being a captive of the "medical model," the qualitative/quantitative debate about the development of nursing science (Gortner, 1990), and the push toward nursing models of organizing service and delivering care—have perhaps militated against using DRGs as information and nursing patient classification as data for anything other than the very most beginning inquiries. In countries with nationalized health care systems where DRGs are increasingly being used to define budgetary priorities, nurses are making use of the information to match nursing work to cost and case mix (*Nursing and Casemix,* 1990).

## *The Severity Issue*

A vast literature on the extent to which DRGs adequately capture relative "severity" within the groups exists, and the problem was identified in the American Nurses' Association testimony to Congress referred to earlier. The issues (Smits et al., 1984; Jencks & Dobson, 1987) are summarized here.

It is argued that there is no common definition of severity. To physicians, it may mean involvement of more than one body system; to hospital administrators, it means "my patients are sicker and we ought to get paid more"; to nurses, it may mean complicating family or personal circumstances, handicaps, or depression, which make care more difficult; to a pathologist, it may mean the size of the infarct or tumor. Numerous attempts have been made to add variables to DRG definition in order to capture this severity, but implementing any of the proposals would require collecting new data, which is expensive, or they involve variables that might create perverse incentives in the payment system. For example, it would be possible to count laboratory tests or procedures and reason that the more there are, the more severely ill the patient is, but that would create an incentive to perform more. Or, it would be possible to take some measure of the use of intensive or critical care as an index of severity, but that also adds a perverse incentive in situations in which admission to critical care is, in some sense, discretionary (Wagner, Kraus, Draper, & Zimmerman, 1983). The most recent proposal is to link *specific* complications and comorbidities to DRG definitions. This method requires no new data, just a new grouping program, and it increases the amount of variation explained in length of stay and hospital charges by some 45 percent (Health Systems Management Group, 1989).

The within-DRG variation in resources is less of a problem in surgical DRGs than in medical ones because the surgical treatments are more standardized and their effects better known, including to nurses. One small study (Fosbinder, 1986) found very large variances in nursing time in two specific DRGs—Esophagitis and Heart Failure/Shock—in one San Diego hospital. Another study grouped patients within selected DRGs into three length of stay groups. This exercise produced nonoverlapping patterns of nursing resource use for medical DRGs, especially for stroke and angina. In both cases, nursing resource use was lower for the shorter stay patients, suggesting that there are at least some DRGs that could be better specified if nursing time were added to the DRG definitions (Thompson & Diers, 1990). Sovie and Smith (1986) propose that "severity" may really mean "nursing intensity," but it will remain for future researchers to pin down what, within the variables used in nursing patient classification, makes nursing work more intense. One hypothesis not yet tested is whether there is an inverse relationship between nursing resource consumption and charges for ancillary services (e.g., laboratory tests, x-rays, certain procedures, and drugs). Another fruitful line of inquiry would involve tracking nursing resources occasioned by new technologic interventions. There are some that are relatively inexpensive as technology but that make patients very sick before recovery and the care of which requires a great deal of nursing time to manage. Radiation and chemotherapy are two such possible targets for this research.

## Case Mix Analysis

Diagnosis-related groups provide a way to compare hospitals by the kinds of patients they treat. While this information has been particularly interesting for third-party payers, including government, and for analysis of relative hospital mortality, it might be of interest to nurses as well.

Smaller and rural hospitals tend to have higher case mix indexes than do larger, tertiary teaching hospitals, which has implications for recruitment, staffing, and organizing nursing care. Larger hospitals can coast on their obstetric services, where a large number of inexpensive normal deliveries offset more expensive cases. Smaller, rural hospitals have to serve a wide variety of community needs (especially if they have emergency rooms, which most do).

Publicly funded hospitals have a case mix that is typical of the problems of poverty, with more patients with psychiatric disorders, cirrhosis, gastrointestinal disorders, and drug-related problems. The requirements for nursing care are likely to be different in such institutions. Analysis of nursing intensity within DRGs across public and private institutions might provide more ammunition to argue for different staffing where nursing variables matter the most. In one small analysis comparing five hospitals, there was considerable difference in the DRGs ranked highest in nursing intensity (Thompson & Diers, 1990). In one hospital, the most nursing-intense DRG was Poisoning and Toxic Effects of Drugs < 17 (age under 17), which ranked only 103rd in another. The first hospital is in an inner city environment in one of the seven poorest cities in the United States. When the mix of patients within that DRG was examined, it turned out that there were two distinct groups: children under 5 who probably ingested poisonous substances accidentally, and adolescents 15 and over whose hospitalization was probably for overdoses of street drugs (Bailey, 1989). In another analysis, DRG 112, Vascular Procedures, was the fourth highest in nursing intensity in small community hospitals, although it never ranked higher than 25th in other, larger institutions. The speculation was that vascular procedures probably represent "high tech" in small hospitals, with the requirement for considerable nursing resources, whereas vein ligation and stripping are considered much less complex by medical center nurses. One hospital had apparently specialized in cardiovascular procedures, and the volume of coronary artery bypass grafts performed was very high. Not coincidentally, nursing intensity for that DRG was the lowest of the five institutions, because nurses become adept at doing the work.

Some case mix comparisons have been done with international data, and it is interesting to guess at what these differences mean in standards of nursing time and requirements for nursing across countries. The highest volume nonmaternity DRG in the Netherlands, for example, is T and A (tonsillectomy and adenoidectomy); in France, it is cirrhosis. Skin cancer is a very high-volume DRG in Australia (remember that DRGs are hospital discharge assignments, so this must be very serious skin cancer). In general, international comparisons show much longer lengths of stay in the hospital than do American data. For example, the average length of stay for cesarean section without complications is 5.4 days in the United States, 12.1 days in selected French hospitals, 9 days in selected Portuguese hospitals, 7.9 days in Stockholm, 10 days in Victoria, 9.5 days in New South Wales, and 9.8 days in South Australia (Palmer, Freeman, & Rodrigues, 1990). These data and other comparisons suggest that the health care systems in other countries are very different from those in the United States, although some nursing issues such as shortages of staff are the same (Aiken, 1990). Case mix information may be useful in explaining how vastly different nurse-to-bed ratios still produce shortages.

Very simple case mix analyses can also be instructive. For example, Sovie found that on one cardiology unit, only nine DRGs accounted for some three quarters of the patients. This suggested to her that generic nursing care plans could be developed by the primary nurse, with a consequent saving of nursing time estimated to be one full-time equivalent nurse. This time could then be reassigned to quality assurance, staff education, or any other identified priority (Sovie, Tarcinale, Van Puttee, & Stunden, 1984).

As third-party payers, including the government, increasingly examine the cost-effectiveness of various hospitals, and as Preferred Provider Organizations multiply, it will be very important for nurses to understand their own institutions and how they might differ in mix of services, quality, and cost. Further, the possibility of using DRG-based national and international comparisons to better understand what nursing is and does will greatly expand our ability to participate in policy direction and decisions.

### Costs of Nursing

Nurse managers will sometimes argue that of course they know how much nursing costs—just take the nursing budget, divide by the number of patient days in the past year, and you have nursing cost per patient day. That assumes, of course, that all patients get the same amount of nursing care every day, which is not true. Furthermore, this kind of calculation leaves the nurse manager in the position of managing only the total nursing budget, not the clinical variability.

Sovie reported eightfold differences in the costs of caring for the same kinds of patients between Strong Memorial Hospital and Rochester General Hospital (Sovie et al., 1985). Fosbinder (1986) compared a San Diego hospital, a northern California hospital, a Los Angeles hospital, and Strong Memorial Hospital on both length of stay and nursing costs. She found that length of stay and cost for patients in DRG 209, Major Joint Procedures, was 75 percent lower in San Diego than in northern California (Stanford), which she attributes to a special orthopedic nurse practitioner effort in San Diego with early discharge planning and patient education. Strong Memorial Hospital was always lower in cost than the San Diego hospital in three compared DRGs. Fosbinder notes that the Strong Memorial Hospital costs do not include management above the head nurse, which San Diego costs do, and she emphasizes the need to establish precise causes of excess cost and to standardize this kind of reporting. Sovie's review of the research on variable costs of nursing care in hospitals emphasizes the problems of interhospital comparison as well as the advantages of patient-specific (DRG-based) nursing intensity information as the basis for nursing management as well as for comparative studies (Sovie, 1988).

## Clinical Management by Diagnosis-Related Groups

When nursing patient classification information can be linked to DRGs, patterns of daily nursing resource requirement can be identified by DRG. Elective surgery patients have a pattern of predictable nursing care requirements that begins at a moderate level, peaks the day after surgery, and then declines. Trauma patients have a pattern that begins very high, then gradually declines but never gets as close to the baseline as the pattern of elective surgical patients. Terminally ill patients have a pattern that begins at a moderate level and increases until death, at least in institutions with special oncology units so patients are not transferred to intensive care as death approaches.

Knowing such patterns, and knowing how many of each type of patient is present on a given unit could allow primary nurses or nurse managers to predict nursing workload and arrange for it to be provided when needed. Or more adventurously, if it is known that the surgical patient requirements not only peak predictably but do so on Tuesdays and Wednesdays, the nurse manager might either argue for more staff on those days or argue to change the surgical schedule to even out the work week.

Halloran (1988b) has done some interesting work in relating nursing diagnoses to discharge disposition, on the theory that discharge to a nursing home is less desirable than discharge to one's own home. He found that the variable that best predicted nursing home placement within DRGs was incontinence (surely something that could be attended to by nurses).

There are information systems that will assign a "working DRG" to a patient on hospital admission, to which various kinds of standards for monitoring resource use can be programmed (McMahon, Creighton, Bernard, Pittinger, & Kelley, 1989). Such standards are developed out of the hospital's own data and could include, for example, expected hours of nursing care by day of stay along with other expected needed resources such as laboratory tests, x-ray studies, or procedures. Then patients whose resources do not follow an expected pattern (are either higher or lower than a set standard deviation from the mean for the DRG for the day) can be examined to see if the patient is clinically unique, if there is a potential quality problem, or if discharge planning is needed. These systems have not included nursing resources to date, but they could.

Data on DRGs can also be used to study the effects of institutional changes or problems. For example, if primary nursing or some other system change is instituted, it is possible to examine resources (or quality assurance [Q/A] indicators) by DRG before and after the innovation is in place. Flood's study of the effects of short staffing used DRGs to define groups of patients cared for under different staffing conditions (Flood & Diers, 1988). She found that within the same DRG, patients on the inadequately staffed unit had longer lengths of stay and more complications than patients on the adequately staffed unit. The effect of the presence of clinical nurse specialists, the effect of changes in protocols for admission to the intensive care unit, new quality assurance efforts, discharge planning—any topic of clinical management interest—can profit from the methodologic control offered by DRGs and the data systems spawned by them.

## Toward Quality and Standards

Finally, DRGs can be used as they were originally intended—for analyses of quality of care. Fosbinder (1986) found that fully one third of the patients discharged from her hospital who were classified in DRG 127, Heart Failure and Shock, were outliers, patients whose length of stay exceeded 1.95 times the standard deviation for the DRG. There has been essentially no published analysis of outliers. One small study examined 32 patients identified as "nursing intensity outliers"—people whose length of stay and nursing requirements were both significantly higher for the DRG (Talerico & Diers, 1988). Many of the patients were clinically unique and had unusual nursing requirements because of depression, handicap, or conditions related to poverty or alcoholism. But infection was the most common secondary diagnosis, and only half the patients with infections had them on admission. There were also five cases of patients falling out of bed.

Two small studies of critical care have produced hints at quality issues. In one, older patients in certain DRGs were more often admitted to intensive care units after surgery than were younger patients in the same DRG. Yet their requirements for nursing in the intensive care unit were *lower* than those of younger patients (Kiesel, 1988). Intensive care is not especially good for older people, and yet it appears that in this institution, age is being used as a criterion for intensive care unit admission. In another study, patients were discharged from a cardiac surgical intensive care unit at the highest levels of nursing requirement, whereas other patients remained in the unit who had relatively low levels of nursing care requirements (Corcoran & Diers, 1989). Again, the absence of protocols for intensive care unit use, which nurses surely may participate in developing, appears to be at issue, and the implications for nursing workload both inside and outside the intensive care unit are obvious. Since the reason for admission to the hospital is the need for nursing, nurses might also determine when patients should be moved from special care to another service or discharged altogether. The fact that patients are being discharged "quicker and sicker" is hardly arguable any more, but whether they are too sick to be discharged and whether there are consequences for quality of care are still unanswered questions. One attempt at an answer would be an analysis of requirements for nursing on the last day of the hospital stay, with particular attention to those items of patient classification that require skilled care.

Standards for the *utilization* of nursing services have never been developed. It would now be possible to test at least three such standards. The first would be the percentage of patients within each DRG who received any care in a special care unit. It is suspected that intensive care is used differently in different hospitals and under different conditions of staffing shortage. A related standard would be percentage of total days in special care and nursing care requirements in the unit. Finally, outliers and nursing intensity outliers, as described above, may be selected for study (Thompson & Diers, 1990).

## Conclusions

Diagnosis-related groups are certainly not perfect, nor is the payment system that uses them. By themselves, DRGs are simply a measure of case mix, no more and no less, but they are better than nothing at all. Whatever criticisms the DRG-based payment system deserves, the critique must distinguish between the categories per se and the uses to which they have been put.

The notion of describing cases by relatively homogeneous groups of patient variables is likely to be around for a long time, no matter what happens with the payment systems. In fact, extension of a DRG-like patient classification to outpatient surgery is already mandated for inclusion for hospital payment in 1992. Classification systems resembling DRGs for outpatient care and long-term care have already been tested and are being examined by the federal government for implementation in paying for these services (Schneider et al., 1988; Fries & Cooney, 1985; Hsiao et al., 1988). Some beginning work has identified variables that determine nursing requirements in home care (Pasquale, 1987, 1988).

When DRGs and the Prospective Payment System began, nurses worried, with some reason, that the consequences would entail cutting nursing positions from budgets. In fact, the increased acuity of patients in shorter hospital stays contributed to the well-documented nursing shortage, with the just as well documented benefits to nursing in terms of salary gains, publicity, and public concern. It is likely that the same thing will happen when payment for outpatient, long-term care, and home care services come to be based even more than DRGs on nursing care requirements. It is hoped that nursing will recognize early the opportunities in this form of measurement and use it not only as a fulcrum for policy participation but also for its own interests in developing nursing practice, the knowledge on which it is based, and the visibility of nursing's contribution.

REFERENCES

Aiken, L.H. (1990). Charting the future of hospital nursing. *Image: Journal of Nursing Scholarship 22*(2), 72–78.

Aydelotte, M.K. (1973). Nurse staffing methodology: A review and critique of selected literature. Department of Health, Education, and Welfare Publication No. 73-433. Washington, DC: U.S. Government Printing Office.

Bailey, C.P. (1989). Nursing resource variation among children and adults across DRGs. Unpublished master's thesis, New Haven: Yale University School of Nursing.

Caterinicchio, R.P. (1983). A debate: RIMs and the cost of nursing care. *Nursing Management, 14*(5), 36–39.

Caterinicchio, R.P., & Davies, R.H. (1983). Developing a client-focused allocation statistic of inpatient nursing resource use: An alternative to the patient day. *Social Science in Medicine, 17*(5), 259–272.

Chagnon, M., Audette, L., Lebrun, L., & Tilquin, C. (1978). A patient classification system by level of nursing care requirements. *Nursing Research, 27*(2), 107–113.

*Classification systems for describing nursing practice—working papers* (1989). Kansas City: American Nurses' Association.

Cole, E. (1982, November 22). *Testimony before the House Subcommittee on Health and Environment of the Committee on Energy and Commerce.* Washington, DC: GPO (Serial 97–183).

Corcoran, L., & Diers, D. (1989). Nursing intensity in cardiac surgical care. *Nursing Management, 20*(2), 80I–80P.

Cullen, D.J., Civetta, J.M., Briggs, B.A., & Ferrara, L.C. (1974). TISS: A method for quantitative comparison of patient care. *Critical Care Medicine, 2*, 57–60.

Curtis, B. (1983, February 14). *Testimony before the Subcommittee on Health of the House Ways and Means Committee.* Washington, DC: GPO (Serial 98–6).

*DRGs—diagnosis related groups definition manual* (1985 and annually). New Haven: Health Systems International (HSI).

Fetter, R.B., Shin, Y., Freeman, J.L., Averill, R.F., & Thompson, J.D. (1980). Case mix definition by diagnosis related groups. *Medical Care, 18*(2) (Suppl.), 1–53.

Flagle, C.D. (1962). Operations research in health services. *Operations Research, 10*(6), 591–596.

Flood, S.D., & Diers, D. (1988). Nurse staffing, patient outcome and cost. *Nursing Management, 19*(5), 34–36.

Fosbinder, D. (1986). Nursing costs/DRG: A patient classification system and comparative study. *Journal of Nursing Administration, 16*(11), 18–23.

Fries, B.E., & Cooney, L.M. (1985). Resource utilization groups: A patient classification system for long-term care. *Medical Care, 23*(2), 110–122.

Giovannetti, P. (1978). *Patient classification systems in nursing: A description and analysis.* Department of Health, Education, and Welfare Publication No. HRA 78–22. Hyattsville, MD: U.S. Government Printing Office.

Giovannetti, P., & Mayer, G. (1984). Building confidence in patient classification systems. *Nursing Management, 15*(8), 31–34.

Gortner, S. (1990). Nursing values and science: Toward a science philosophy. *Image: Journal of Nursing Scholarship, 22*(2), 101–105.

Grimaldi, P.L., & Micheletti, J.A. (1982). RIMs and the cost of nursing care. *Nursing Management, 13*(12), 12–23.

Halloran, E.J. (1985). Nursing workload, medical diagnosis related groups and nursing diagnoses. *Research in Nursing and Health, 8*(4), 421–433.

Halloran, E.J. (1988a). Conceptual considerations, decision criteria and guidelines for development of the Nursing Minimum Data Set from an administrative perspective. In H.H. Werley & N.M. Lang (Eds.), *Identification of the Nursing Minimum Data Set* (pp. 48–66). New York: Springer Publishing Company.

Halloran, E.J. (1988b, June 10). *Incidence and outcomes of urinary incontinence among hospitalized patients.* Paper presented at the Yale University Hospital Administration Alumni Association, New Haven.

Halloran, E.J., & Halloran, D.C. (1985). Exploring the DRG/nursing equation. *American Journal of Nursing, 85*(10), 1093–1095.

Halloran, E.J., & Kiley, M. (1987). Nursing dependency, diagnosis-related groups and length of hospital stay. *Health Care Financing Review, 8*(3), 27–36.

Health Systems Management Group (1989, February). *DRG refinement with diagnostic specific comorbidities and complications*. R.B. Fetter, Principal Investigator. Final Progress Report to the Health Care Financing Administration, Cooperative Agreements 15-C-98930/1-01 and 17-C-98930/1-0251. New Haven: Yale University School of Organization and Management.

Hearn, E.R. (1972). How many high care patients? *Nursing Times*, Part I, *68*, 472–478; Part II, *68*, 65–68.

Hsaio, W.C., Braun, P., Yntema, D., & Becker, E.R. (1988). Estimating physicians work for a resource-based relative-value scale. *New England Journal of Medicine, 319*(13), 835–840.

Jelinek, R.C., Haussman, R.K.D., Hegyvary, S.T., & Newman, T.F. (1974). *A methodology for monitoring quality of nursing care*. U.S. Department of Health, Education, and Welfare Publication No. HRA 74-25. Washington, DC: U.S. Government Printing Office.

Jencks, S.F., & Dobson, A. (1987). Refining case mix adjustment: The research evidence. *New England Journal of Medicine, 317*(11), 679–686.

Joel, L.A. (1984). DRGs and RIMs: Implications for nursing. *Nursing Outlook, 32*(1), 42–49.

Keene, A.R., & Cullen, D.J. (1983). Therapeutic intervention scoring system: Update 1983. *Critical Care Medicine, 11*, 1–3.

Kiesel, A. (1988). Nursing intensity in the surgical ICU. Unpublished master's thesis, New Haven: Yale University School of Nursing.

McGuire, T.E. (1990, April). *DRGs: The state of the art 1990*. New Haven: Health Systems International—₃m^tm.

McMahon, L.F., Creighton, F.A., Bernard, A.M., Pittinger, W.B., & Kelley, W.N. (1989). The integrated inpatient management model—a new approach to clinical practice. *Annals of Internal Medicine, 111*(4), 318–326.

National Association of Children's Hospitals and Related Institutions (1985). *Children's hospitals' casemix classification project. Phases I and II*. Alexandria, VA: National Association of Children's Hospitals and Related Institutions.

Nursing and casemix (1990, May). *Proceedings of the Conference*. Melbourne, Australia: Australian Nursing Federation.

Palmer, G.R., Freeman, J.L., & Rodrigues, J.M. (1990). Development and application of DRGs in other countries. In R.B. Fetter (Ed.), *DRGs—design, development and application*. Ann Arbor: Health Administration Press.

Pasquale, D. (1987). A basis for prospective payment for home care. *Image: Journal of Nursing Scholarship, 19*(4), 186–191.

Pasquale, D. (1988). Characteristics of Medicare-eligible home care clients. *Public Health Nursing, 5*(3), 129–134.

Prescott, P.A., & Phillips, C.Y. (1988). Gauging nursing intensity to bring costs to light. *Nursing and Health Care, 9*(1), 17–22.

Russell, L. (1989). *Medicare's new hospital payment system: Is it working?* Washington, DC: The Brookings Institution.

San Joaquin General Hospital (1976). *San Joaquin Classification*. Stockton, CA: San Joaquin General Hospital.

Schneider, K.C., Lichtenstein, J.L., Freeman, J.L., Newbold, R.C., Fetter, R.B., Gottlieb, L., Leaf, P.H., & Portlock, C.S. (1988). The AVG system for ambulatory care. *Journal of Ambulatory Care Management, 11*(2), 1–12.

Schweiker, R. (1982). *Hospital prospective payment for Medicare: Report to the Congress*. Washington, DC: Department of Health and Human Services.

Smits, H.L., Fetter, R.B., & McMahon, L.F. (1984). Variation in resource use within DRGs: The severity issue. *Health Care Financing Review* (Ann. Suppl.) 6(2), 71–77.

Sovie, M.D. (1988). Variable costs of nursing care in hospitals. *Annual Review of Nursing Research, 6*, 131–150.

Sovie, M.D., & Smith, T. (1986). Pricing the nursing product: Charging for nursing care. *Nursing Economics, 4*(5), 216–226.

Sovie, M.D., Tarcinale, M., van Puttee, A., & Stunden, A. (1984, November). *A correlation study of nursing patient classification, DRGs, other significant patient variables and costs of patient care.* Rochester, NY: Strong Memorial Hospital.

Sovie, M.D., Tarcinale, M., van Puttee, A., & Stunden, A. (1985). Amalgam of nursing acuity, DRGs and costs. *Nursing Management, 16*(3), 22–42.

Talerico, L., & Diers, D. (1988, Spring). Nursing intensity outliers. *Nursing Management, 19*(6), 27–35.

Thompson, J.D. (1988). The minimum data set for nursing and effectiveness of nursing care. In H.H. Werley & N.M. Lang (Eds.), *Identification of the nursing minimum data set.* New York: Springer Publishing Company.

Thompson, J.D., & Diers, D. (1988, Spring). Management of nursing intensity. *Nursing Clinics of North America, 23*(3), 473–492.

Thompson, J.D., & Diers, D. (1990). Nursing resources. In R.B. Fetter (Ed.), *DRGs—design, development and applications.* Ann Arbor: Health Administration Press.

Thorpe, K.E. (1987). Does all-payer rate setting work? The case of the New York prospective hospital reimbursement methodology. *Journal of Health Politics, Policy and Law, 12*(3), 391–408.

Trofino, J. (1985). RIMs: Skirting the edge of disaster. *Nursing Management, 16*(7), 48–51.

Wagner, D.P., Knaus, W.A., Draper, E., & Zimmerman, J.E. (1983). Identification of low risk monitor patients within a medical-surgical intensive care unit. *Medical Care, 21*(3), 425–434.

Werley, H.H., & Lang, N.M. (Eds.) (1988). *Identification of the nursing minimum data set.* New York: Springer Publishing Company.

Werley, H.H., Lang, N.M., & Westlake, S.K. (1986). The Nursing Minimum Data Set Conference: Executive summary. *Journal of Professional Nursing, 2*, 117–124.

Werley, H.H., & Zorn, C.R. (1989). The nursing minimum data set and its relationship to classifications for nursing practice. In *Classification systems for describing nursing practice—working papers.* Kansas City: American Nurses' Association.

# PART III

## Challenges and Opportunities Across Practice Settings

## Chapter 12

# Nurse-Midwives and Nurse Anesthetists: The Cutting Edge in Specialist Practice

DONNA DIERS*

*M*IDWIFERY IS THE oldest role for women healers. Nurse anesthesia is the oldest specialty *within* the nursing profession. Midwifery was in existence before obstetrics, and although surgeons created anesthesia, nurse anesthetists existed before anesthesiologists. The history and development of nurse-midwifery and nurse anesthesia provide the screen upon which to project current and future issues common to both professional groups: are nurse-midwives and nurse anesthetists nurses or not? complement or substitute? money and power. The same issues confront newer nursing specialties, and there are lessons to be learned from these pioneers.

## Brief History

In the beginning, there were midwives:

> And it came to pass, when she was in hard labour, that the midwife said unto her, Fear not . . . (Genesis 35:17).

The king of Egypt tried to compel Hebrew midwives to kill all male children, but they did not obey. When called to task, the midwives dissembled: "And the

* The author is extremely grateful to Ira P. Gunn, R.N., C.R.N.A., F.A.A.N., Consultant, Nurse Anesthesia Affairs, and Helen Varney Burst, R.N., C.N.M., M.S.N., Professor, Yale University School of Nursing, the acknowledged experts in their respective fields, who gave generously of their time and insight to provide information and interpretation. Sarah D. Cohn, R.N., C.N.M., J.D., Counsel, Medico-Legal Affairs, Yale New Haven Hospital, pointed out references in the legal literature, and her unique insights as a nurse-midwife and attorney were very helpful. The Reverend Rowan E. Greer, III, Walter H. Gray Professor of Anglican Studies, Yale Divinity School, donated an important piece of biblical scholarship. Susan Molde, R.N., M.S.N., made valuable editorial suggestions.

midwives said unto Pharoah, 'the Hebrew women are not as the Eygptian women, for they are lively and are delivered ere the midwives come unto them' " (Exodus 1:19). Their actions pleased God, who "dealt well with the midwives . . . " and "made them houses" (Exodus 1:21–22), although one interpreter wrote, "their disobedience herein was lawful, but their dissembling evil" (*Geneva Bible*, 1560, p. 244). One of the male children saved was Moses.

In ancient Greece, some women were designated midwives (obstetrice), but many women assisted each other in birthing without official designation. The practice of medicine and surgery was restricted to men; if the work could be done equally well by women, the status of males and hence their fees would be reduced (Donnison, 1988). One Athenian woman, Agnodice, passed herself off as a male and was trained in surgery. She became such a popular birth attendant that physicians accused her of seducing her patients. To counter the charge, she revealed her true gender and was condemned to death for practicing medicine without a license. But Athens' principal matrons, many of whom she had assisted in childbirth, rallied around her, and the law was amended to allow women to practice medicine and surgery (Donnison, 1988).

International midwifery does not require training as a nurse, and contemporary efforts to move midwifery into nursing in the United Kingdom are controversial (Clay, 1987). Midwives first came to the United States with the slave trade in 1619, bringing the histories, traditions, art, and folklore from the mother country and handing them down to their daughters (Robinson, 1984). Midwives also came to this country later with the waves of European immigration. Bridget Lee Fuller traveled on the *Mayflower* and probably aided in three births on the voyage (Litoff, 1982). Anne Hutchinson, a rebellious colonist midwife, held meetings with women to discuss, among other things, opposition to the established church. She was tried as a witch and banished from Massachusetts to be massacred in what later became New York (Williams, 1981). The Hutchinson River Parkway is named for her. Until the 17th century, the personal experience of childbirth was considered an essential prerequisite for practicing midwifery (Donegan, 1978).

Midwifery gave a little-known gift to early scientific medicine. Ignatz Semmelweiss is justly credited with making parturition safer by insisting that medical students and faculty wash their hands between cases. What is not often discussed is how he got this idea. There were two services in the Allegemeinne Krankenhaus in Vienna, one in which midwives gave care to the poor and the other the teaching service for the school of medicine. Semmelweiss noticed that the incidence of puerperal fever in women who were delivered in the midwifery service was a great deal lower than the incidence in the medical school ward. Midwives did not perform autopsies, and it was the germs from autopsy material that were being carried back to the wards by the physicians' hands.

By the early 1900s, the appalling rate of infant mortality (124 out of 1000 births) was attributed in part to the fact that half the births were attended by traditional midwives. After World War I, "the government began insuring itself for future wars by ploughing money into public health. For the first time children were recognized as future members of the military . . . " (Tom, 1982, p. 7), and women were producers of future fighting men. The Sheppard-Towner Act of 1921 supported public health nurses to train midwives, state laws requiring registration of births and licensing of midwives were passed, and very soon, statistics began to document lowered maternal and infant mortality rates and eradication of neonatal ophthalmia at quite low cost. Organized medicine withdrew its support of the federal legislation, however, because the programs were not under physician direction or control, and the legislation was allowed to lapse.

Nurse-midwifery began with the Frontier Nursing Service in Kentucky, under Mary Breckinridge, a nurse and British-trained midwife, in 1925. In 1931, the Lobenstine School of Midwifery, affiliated with the Maternity Center Association in New York City, began its formal training program for nurses. Formal preparation of nurse-midwives was thought by some to be a stopgap between traditional midwives and total control of birthing by obstetricians. In 1932, there were 3 million births and only 600 obstetricians, which made the American Medical Association's intended plan to eliminate nurse-midwives "impractical" (Hemschemeyer, 1943).

As of 1990, there were 26 nurse-midwifery programs, most of which are located within or affiliated with schools of nursing; 16 provided the master's degree and 10 are certificate programs. About 4000 nurse-midwives have been certified by the American College of Nurse-Midwives in the United States (Adams, 1989) since it began offering certification in 1971. In recent years, there has been a resurgence of lay midwives ("direct-entry midwives," "traditional midwives"), who are recognized by law in ten states and prohibited by law in ten others (Butter & Kay, 1988).

Before Crawford Long, M.D., removed two tumors from James Venable's neck under the influence of inhaled ether in 1842, whatever assistance people were given to control the pain of surgery or injury came from alcohol, sometimes champagne. In the wild days of the expanding American frontier, snake oil salesmen entertained mining camp audiences with demonstrations of nitrous oxide gas, and ether-sniffing was recreational. Long knew Venable liked to sniff ether (Long did too) and suggested this application in surgery. Long himself both administered the anesthesia and performed the surgery (Thatcher, 1953).

Lister's discovery of asepsis, published in 1867, and the later discovery of antisepsis made it possible for surgeons to cure something, but not without pain (and also not without the attendance of Florence Nightingale's trained nurses, who kept the environment clean and healthy, but that is another story). Long's use of ether as anesthesia, Horace Wells' and William T.G. Morton's experiments with nitrous oxide for dental extractions, and Morton's public demonstration of ether anesthesia at Massachusetts General Hospital in 1846 (Thatcher, 1953) made it possible for surgeons to invade the body cavity. Surgeons began to need help.

"Anesthizers" were surgeons in training, often more interested in observing the surgery and learning technique than in monitoring the anesthesia. As students, anesthizers were not paid; "the surgeon took whatever fee was paid, considering that the privilege of assisting him and seeing how he did his work was ample reward . . . " (Galloway, 1899, p. 1173 in Bankert, 1989). If the anesthizer was paid at all, it was a trivial portion of the surgeon's fee, perhaps $5 for a $200 operation—an early example of fee-splitting. There was no incentive for new physicians to take on anesthesia as a full-time job, since it was neither lucrative nor visible.

But surgeons needed help, and so they turned to nurses and trained them. In the beginning, they were religious sisters, who also did not have to be paid. The first identifiable nurse anesthetist was Sister Mary Bernard at St. Vincent's Hospital in Erie, Pennsylvania in 1877 (Bankert, 1989). The Sisters of the Third Order of St. Francis established a community and hospitals throughout the midwest and contracted with the Missouri Pacific Railroad to manage hospitals for railroad employees. One of the hospitals was St. Mary's in Rochester, Minnesota. The Sisters' explicit condition was that Dr. William Worrell Mayo take charge of it (Bankert, 1989). The Mayo Clinic had no interns in the beginning; therefore anesthesia was administered by nurses. "And when the interns came, the brothers [Mayo] decided that a nurse was better suited to the task because she was more likely to keep her mind strictly on it . . . " (Bankert, 1989, p. 30).

One of the first two nurse anesthetists married Dr. Charles Mayo, and her place was taken by the "mother of anesthesia," the amazing Alice Magaw. She collected and reported her work in a series of papers beginning in 1899, which were published privately by the Mayo Clinic, since nurses could not be published in the medical literature. By 1906, she had participated in over 14,000 cases without a single death directly attributable to the anesthesia (Thatcher, 1953, p. 59).

The need for nurses to administer anesthesia was so widespread that Isabel Hampton Robb devoted a chapter to it in her first textbook (1893). Alice Magaw and early nurse anesthetists used both ether and chloroform, although Magaw preferred ether. The popularity of chloroform was greatly enhanced when Queen Victoria used it in delivering two of her children (Thatcher, 1953, p. 17).

The first formal course in anesthesia was organized at one of the Sisters' hospitals in 1912; it admitted secular nurses in 1924. By the beginning of World War I, there were five postgraduate schools of anesthesia, the most important of which was at Lakeside Hospital in Cleveland. There, George Crile, a surgeon, recruited Agatha Hodgins to become a nurse anesthetist, and they experimented together on animals with nitrous oxide gas and oxygen. They were also apparently the first to use morphine and scopolamine as adjuncts to anesthesia (Crile, 1947). The Lakeside program trained both physicians and nurses.

Hospital-sponsored units such as the Lakeside Unit, which were not part of the military, made anesthesia available near World War I battlefields, thereby greatly decreasing mortality. The enthusiasm for nurse anesthetists during and after the war did not escape the attention of physician anesthetists, and a long campaign began "to legislate her [sic] out of existence" (Thatcher, 1953, p. 108). World War II also helped to establish nurse anesthesia, since the military clarified the standing of nurse anesthetists in the service. Immediately after that war, the American Association of Nurse Anesthetists began to offer certification (1945). Men were admitted to membership in the association in 1947, and special programs for men nurse anesthetists (who could double as stretcher bearers) began. During the Vietnam War, a special draft of male professional nurses was issued; nurses who were women were specifically excluded (Redman, 1986). Of the ten nurses killed in Vietnam, two were male nurse anesthetists.

As of 1989, there were about 23,000 certified registered nurse anesthetists, 40 percent of whom were men. However, there were also 22,100 physician anesthesiologists. Nurse anesthetists administer over 65 percent of the anesthesia given in this country (American Association of Nurse Anesthetists, 1989) and 70 percent or more in rural areas (Bankert, 1989, p. 175).

## Nurses or Something Else

Nurse-midwives describe themselves as being educated in two disciplines—nursing and midwifery.

> The *nurse* part of the term . . . acknowledges that being a registered nurse is prerequisite to being a certified nurse-midwife. It also emphasizes the primary focus of the professional nurse on the . . . individual patient as well as on patient education, counseling and supportive care (Varney, 1987, p. 3).

Midwifery, however, is a profession in its own right, which in other countries does not require nursing as a base. Three legal cases in the United States have dealt with the practice of registered nurses whose preparation for midwifery was not obtained in a nurse-midwifery program (*Leggett v. Tennessee Board of Nursing*, 1980; *Leigh v. Board of Registration in Nursing*, 1984; *Smith v. State of Indiana ex rel. Medical Licensing Board of Indiana*, 1984). In all three, but for different reasons, the courts have held essentially that the nurse has to make a choice: if she holds herself as practicing midwifery, she is not practicing nursing; if she holds herself as practicing nursing, that is not midwifery and certainly not nurse-midwifery if she is not certified. The wording of state practice acts is crucial to these interpretations. Nurse-midwifery is the only advanced nursing specialty that is regulated in some states outside the nurse practice act, sometimes even by the board of medicine (Kelly, 1987). There has never been a case of nurse-midwives being sued for practicing medicine without a license. Such a case would be difficult to prosecute because midwifery existed before medical obstetrics and because it is often specifically excluded from definitions of the practice of medicine (*Leggett v. Tennessee Board of Nursing*, 1980; Harlow, 1988).

Anesthesia was a natural role for nurses to perform as they assisted the surgeon. Nurses were recruited into a field shunned by physicians after it was determined that interns lacked the "deftness and tender touch which patients required for a successful anesthetic" (Olsen, 1940, p. 4). The nurse's gender was important too: " . . . just as soon as the patient lies down to take his ether, if he is a man he gives up to the nurse, but if a man is going to administer that ether the feeling of resistance and fight is in him . . . " (Truesdale, 1913, p. 283).

Ira Gunn is perhaps the most articulate spokesperson for nursing within nurse anesthesia. "By rendering the patient incapable of providing care for himself, the anesthetist must become the care provider—and this care is basically nursing" (Gunn, 1975, p. 136). She argues that the practice of anesthesia does not fit medicine's defined turf—to diagnose, treat, prescribe, or operate in order to cure—since it is rarely administered as a diagnostic or therapeutic regimen. Rather, anesthesia "facilitates" cure just as nursing and dietetics do (Gunn, Nicosia, & Tobin, 1987, p. 97). Anesthesia is a comfort measure, in this view, and thus within the sphere of nursing.

Agatha Hodgins at Lakeside Hospital became a leader in nurse anesthesia practice and education, and she was the founder and first president of what became the American Association of Nurse Anesthetists. She was committed to the notion that the anesthesia service (which at this time was *only* nurse anesthetists) should be separate from the nursing service in hospitals (Thatcher, 1953, p. 132; Bankert, 1989, p. 68) because it was a special field requiring special education and recognition not possible if it were contained within the nursing department.

Both professional groups have danced around the relationship with organized nursing (and medicine; see later on) with a certain amount of dissembling. For both, the official relationship with the American Nurses' Association (ANA) was definitive for how they evolved as professional organizations.

At their very first meeting in 1931, the nurse anesthetists' new association decided "to affiliate with the American Nurses' Association" (Thatcher, 1953, pp. 184–185). (Note: They did not "seek" affiliation.) A long period of correspondence and negotiation ensued. At first, the ANA's issue was that the *International* Association, as they then called themselves, could not be accommodated because ANA's membership was only "American." The nurse anesthetists then changed the name to the *National* Association. Agatha Hodgins wrote: "In regard to being a section, as the work is not nursing . . . ," she proposed an affiliate relationship with ANA, not quite in, not quite out (Hodgins to Marie Louis, February 15, 1932, cited in Bankert, 1989, p. 70). According to Thatcher, there were several reasons why the ANA refused to accept the application for affiliation. The ANA argued that individual membership was already open to anesthetists as nurses.

> It was considered that, since in some states the administration of an anesthetic was regarded as a medical activity, the question could arise of nurse anesthetists' practicing medicine. Furthermore, if the [nurse anesthetists] were to be accepted as an affiliated group, it might bring upon the ANA some legal responsibility for them (Thatcher, 1953, p. 196).

The nurse-midwives' dealings with the ANA started in the 1950s, when the three nursing organizations were sorting themselves out. The nurse-midwives (not yet an official organization) asked, as did the nurse anesthetists, for a special interest group. Nurse-midwives had had a section in the National Organization of Public Health Nursing and published the first descriptive data about nurse-midwives (Hemschemeyer, 1947). But when it merged with what became the National League for Nursing, that section fell out. The ANA simply invited the nurse-midwives to be part of a study of maternal-child health. The new National League for Nursing assigned midwives to the Interdivisional Council, which encompassed pediatrics, orthopedics, crippled children, and school health, too broad a constituency to serve nurse-midwifery's interests (Varney, 1987, p. 8). Therefore the nurse-midwives organized their own association, incorporated in 1955. By then, the nurse anesthetists had an organization that was over 20 years old. Some leaders of the American Association of Nurse Anesthetists still wistfully wished to come under the ANA umbrella, but the ANA was not disposed to consider special interests.

Rebuffed by the ANA, and not wanting to affiliate with the anesthesiologists' organization (even had they been welcomed), the nurse anesthetists accepted the offer of the American Hospital Association to provide space, money, and moral support. Since anesthesia services were a hospital service, this affiliation made some sense.

Things came full circle in 1973 with the formation of the National Federation of Nursing Specialty Organizations and the ANA, when the ANA belatedly tried and failed to generate enthusiasm for a specialist forum under its own umbrella. The ANA and the American Association of Nurse Anesthetists, among others, were founding members of the Federation, and the American College of Nurse-Midwives also joined. Perhaps as payment for ANA support of the efforts of the American Association of Nurse Anesthetists to become the accrediting arm for nurse anesthesia educational programs, the American Association of Nurse Anesthetists supported the ANA's credentialing study and subsequent activities; the American College of Nurse-Midwives declined membership on the committee, although it sent observers (Fullerton, 1982). Nurse anesthetists took the leadership in 1989 by creating the Specialty Nursing Forum, Inc. It publishes a newsletter edited by Ira Gunn, which reports on specialist practice, legal or legislative issues such as prescriptive authority, and National Federation of Nursing Specialty Organizations news.*

Nurse-midwives seized the opportunity to build their new organization and the profession of nurse-midwifery and essentially backed away from organized nursing. Although the American College of Nurse-Midwives requires licensure as a registered nurse for initial certification by the association, it does not require continuing licensure (individual states may, however); continuing competency assessment is required every 5 years. By 1984, all states, as well as the District of Columbia, Guam, Puerto Rico, and the Virgin Islands, had recognized nurse-midwifery by name in law or regulation (Varney, 1987). The American College of Nurse-Midwives began to establish criteria for the approval of nurse-midwifery education programs in 1962, and its Division of Accreditation is recognized as the accrediting body for nurse-midwifery programs by the Office of Education. Not satisfied with being contained within the nursing literature, the official journal of the American College of Nurse-Midwives, the *Journal of Nurse-Midwifery*, fought for 15 years to be included in *Index Medicus*.

Just prior to World War II, the nurse anesthetists challenged the military nurse corps on whether nurse anesthetists would be considered nurses with the same pay and privileges but also with the obligation to perform staff nursing if no surgery was scheduled. At first the military waffled, but when war was declared and nurse anesthetists became necessary, they came to have a special place in military nursing—a clinical nursing specialty (Bankert, 1989).

---

* *Specialty Nursing Forum,* published by Specialty Nursing Forum, Inc., 216 Higgins Road, Park Ridge, Illinois 60068-5790; (708) 692–7050.

The American College of Nurse-Midwives testified in favor of the American Association of Nurse Anesthetists' becoming the accrediting body for nurse anesthesia education in 1975 (Bankert, 1989, p. 158), but other than this activity, there has apparently been little communication between the two groups. Both have evolved independently of each other and of organized nursing.

## Complement or Substitute?

The relationship between professions is not only a political question but is also an economic one (Griffith, 1984). However, challenges to the practice of nurse-midwives and nurse anesthetists from organized medicine are more often phrased as matters of safety and control, thus concealing their economic basis.

In production economics, complements are either jointly used in the production process or consumed with each other as a good or service. Thus bread and butter are consumed together. An increase in the demand for one will cause an increase in the demand for the other. A decrease in the price of one (bread) will cause an increase both in the demand for it and for its complement (butter). But if the two are total substitutes for one another, an increase in the price of one (butter) will cause an increase in demand for the other (margarine).

Nurse-midwifery never grew up as a complement to medical obstetrics; nurse-midwives were not there to help out, except in the most remote sense of an increased demand for obstetric care that exceeded the supply of hands. But nurse anesthesia was a complement to surgery, necessary to its performance. Nurse-midwifery is a complete substitute for medical obstetrics in the care of the "essentially normal" patient, in family planning, and in well-woman gynecology. Nurse anesthesia is a complete substitute for anesthesiology, to the limits of its scope of practice. The political battles center on substitutability.

The legal authority to practice is a property right—a way to make a living—and thus interference with it is subject to litigation. This was the basis for early physician challenges to the legality of nurse anesthesia: nurses were stealing their property right.

The series of incursions against nurse anesthesia began in 1911, when the New York State Medical Society took it upon itself to declare that the administration of anesthetic by a nurse was a violation of state law (Thatcher, 1953, p. 108). This went nowhere. The following year the Ohio State Medical Board passed a resolution that no one other than a registered physician could administer an anesthetic (Thatcher, 1953, p. 110). This provoked nothing more serious than some editorials. But in 1916, the Ohio Medical Board was asked to take action against the Lakeside program as the "chief source of the nurse-anesthetist abuse" ("Use of nurses as anesthetists," 1916). A "spirited" hearing before the Board took place, and the upshot was that the edict against Lakeside was withdrawn (Thatcher, 1953, p. 113). After the complaint was withdrawn, Crile got an amendment to the Medical Practice Act passed to prevent the Act from applying to or prohibiting the administration of anesthetic by a registered nurse "under the direction of and in the immediate presence of the licensed physician" and also provided that the nurse had taken a prescribed course in anesthesia (Thatcher, 1953, pp. 116–117). He was taking no more chances in Ohio.* But next door in Kentucky, upon the request of the Louisville Society of Anesthetists, the attorney general delivered an opinion to the effect that the administration of an anesthetic is "unquestionably the practice of one of the branches of medicine and surgery" (Thatcher, 1953, p. 117). The Kentucky State Medical Association passed a similar resolution.

With what was to become a pattern of assertiveness, a Louisville surgeon, Louis Frank, and Margaret Hatfield, his nurse anesthetist, insisted on a court test; they sued the State Board of Health. The trial court ruled in favor of the defendants, but the case was appealed and reversed in 1917. In an opinion so strongly worded and memorable it is still quoted among nurse anesthetists, the judge wrote:

> . . . [These] laws have not been enacted for the peculiar benefit of the members of . . . professions, further, than they are members of the general community, but they have been enacted for the benefit of the people (*Frank et al.* v. *South et al.*, 1917).

Miss Hatfield was "not engaged in the practice of medicine."

The increasingly hostile climate for nurse anesthetists in California set another stage. To shorten a long and interesting story, Dagmar Nelson had been recruited from the Mayo Clinic to work as a nurse anesthetist for Dr. Verne Hunt in Los Angeles, at St. Vincent's hospital. The Anesthesia Section of the Los Angeles County Medical Association asked the Superior Court to permanently enjoin Nelson from giving anesthesia. Hunt hired lawyers, who argued that the Medical Association had no standing to sue. The politics got really dirty after the court sustained this argument. The Medical Society's *Bulletin* incorrectly reported that an injunction had indeed been granted. A furious blast from Hunt's lawyers made the *Bulletin* print a retraction with a curious introduction: " . . . the information . . . which appeared in the *Bulletin* was sent to the Editor's Desk from what appears to be an authentic source . . . " (Thatcher, 1953, p. 144).

Since the Medical Society could not sue, one physician, William Chalmers-Frances, took up the cudgels on their behalf. He argued that because the surgeon was separated from the anesthetist by a screen, he could not supervise the actual administration of anesthesia; that an anesthetic was a drug and the anesthetist was using medical judgment in deciding the amount and thus was treating the patient; and that the anesthetist was observing the physical signs of patients and acting on them, thus diagnosing and practicing medicine (*Chalmers-Frances v. Nelson*, 1936). Hunt's lawyers presented expert testimony and other evidence to the effect that

---

* Ohio is relevant here. The fight against nurse anesthetists was led by Francis Hoeffer McMechan, M.D., of Cincinnati, just across the river from Louisville. McMechan took on this cause as a personal vendetta apparently, explicitly protecting the property right, and pursued it for years, often using his position as editor of the annual *Anesthesia Supplement* to the surgery journal as a personal platform. He had personal reasons apart from the public political ones. After he died, his wife continued to support this losing cause. His odd role is colorfully discussed in both Thatcher (1953) and Bankert (1989).

giving drugs upon direct or *understood* instruction of a physician was a recognized practice within the definition of nursing and that supervision by a physician could be direct or *understood* (Thatcher, 1953, p. 146, emphasis in Thatcher). The trial took 12 days; 3 days later, the judge ruled that since Miss Nelson was under the direction and supervision of surgeons, her work did not constitute practicing medicine or surgery.

The ruling was appealed at the instigation of the Anesthesia Section, and the newly formed National Association of Nurse Anesthetists filed an amicus brief. Two years later, the Supreme Court of California stated: ". . . it is the legally established rule that they [nurse anesthetists] are but carrying out the orders of the physicians to whose authority they are subject . . . " (Thatcher, 1953, p. 148); the original judgment was upheld. The Anesthesia Section could not let it die, and they asked the county Medical Association to help pay the lawyers' fees ($2500). The Association declined.

*Frank et al. v. South et al.* (1917) and *Chalmers-Frances v. Nelson* (1936) provide the legal basis for nurse anesthesia practice as nursing and are still cited if the need arises. Although the right of certified registered nurse anesthetists to practice anesthesia has apparently been sealed by these two decisions, further attempts have been made to hack off portions of their anesthesia practice. The American Society of Anesthesiologists has issued proclamations stating that regional anesthesia (e.g., spinal blocks, epidurals and caudals) should be administered only by physicians and intra-arterial lines should be placed only by physicians (Bankert, 1989). Physician-owned malpractice insurance companies have taken these resolutions to heart and have written into the malpractice insurance policy for nurse anesthetists that they would not be covered for administering regional anesthesia (Blumenreich & Wolf, 1986). As the malpractice insurance crisis has heated up, some surgeons have attempted to distance themselves from "supervision" of anesthesia and have editorialized that somehow surgeons are more liable if anesthesia is administered by a certified registered nurse anesthetist than if it is administered by an anesthesiologist. Actually, courts have determined that the surgeon's supervision does not mean control, and therefore the liability is not automatically the surgeon's (Blumenreich, 1989).

A landmark case, *Oltz v. St. Peter's Hospital* (1986), established nurse anesthetists' standing to sue for anticompetitive strategies when anesthesiologists conspire to restrict or revoke their practice privileges. Another case has established their capacity to be awarded damages for illegal economic discrimination through exclusive contracts (*Bhan v. NME Hospitals, Inc. et al.*, 1985). The issue of exclusive contracts is a difficult one for nurse anesthetists because they may well profit from being part of a practice group with anesthesiologists who have such a contract. One case has gone all the way to the Supreme Court on this issue (*Jefferson Parish Hospital v. Hyde*, 1984). In a split vote, the Court ruled that exclusive contracts are not illegal on their face ("per se"). Justice Sandra Day O'Connor suggested a more subtle standard of "adverse economic effects and potential economic benefits" (Blumenreich, 1984).

Antitrust and restraint of trade are extraordinarily difficult and time-consuming cases to mount and prove, depending, as the federal law does, on evidence of conspiracy. The full case of two nurse-midwives in Tennessee who could not obtain hospital practice privileges and whose collaborating obstetrician's malpractice coverage was cancelled has yet to be heard in court nearly 10 years after the incident in question. In the one part of the case that has been heard, the court ruled against the physician owners of the insurance company, reasoning that their activity was not "the business of insurance" but was actually anticompetitive (*Nurse-Midwifery Associates v. Hibbert*, 1983). The Federal Trade Commission also ruled against the insurance company, which filed a consent decree to terminate the practice of denying coverage to physicians who were in practice with nurse-midwives.

The Federal Trade Commission also obtained a consent order against the medical staff of Memorial Medical Center in Savannah, Georgia, where the obstetricians argued that a nurse-midwife, Rebecca Almand, should not be granted hospital privileges because "there was no shortage of obstetricians in the Savannah area" (*In Re Medical Staff of Memorial Medical Center*, 1988). The Federal Trade Commission order explicitly states, "Because nurse-midwifery services can substitute for certain kinds of obstetrical services . . ." nurse-midwives offer "a greater range of choices for consumers and increase competition in the provision of obstetrical care" (*In Re. Medical Staff of Memorial Medical Center*, 1988). Time-consuming as the process of appealing to the Federal Trade Commission and obtaining a consent decree is (Almand's case took 5 years), the appellant does not have to pay for lawyers—the Federal Trade Commission's lawyers bring the case to the Commission.

Nurse-midwives have generally faced challenges to their practice in legislative hearings or local forums rather than in the courts. Organized physician groups have tried to prevent legal authorization of nurse-midwifery, prescriptive authority, licensure of out-of-hospital birthing centers, and third-party reimbursement. Nurse-midwives have also encountered attempts to restrict their practices by specifying that they may not conduct deliveries anywhere but in a hospital or that there must be a physician present at all deliveries. In the unfortunate situation at Boston City Hospital, the physicians unilaterally ruled that women with previous cesarean sections who desired a vaginal birth and women with minor chronic medical problems were too "high risk" for nurse-midwifery care. In addition, women with any meconium staining were to be delivered in the delivery room in stirrups, and a nothing-by-mouth policy was established for all women on the labor and delivery unit, even if they were in early labor or just there for a nonstress test. Finally, certified nurse-midwives were deemed unqualified to carry out initial prenatal history taking and physical examinations. These and other more blatant attacks on the nurse-midwifery service, which at its zenith in Boston had eleven nurse-midwives and seven physicians delivering services in two hospital-based clinics and nine neighborhood health centers, compromised the nurse-midwifery service in favor of residents and attending staff (Breece, Israel, & Friedman, 1989).

Nurse-midwives were at the center of the malpractice insurance issue, caught up in the same tort liability crisis that hit circuses, restaurants, and the Boy Scouts. The company that had covered nurse-midwives through the American College of Nurse-Midwives abruptly withdrew that coverage. The American Nurses' Association negotiated with their own insurance carrier to cover nurse-midwives, but that carrier withdrew support and in addition called into question its coverage of nurse practitioners and others in expanded roles. Eventually the American College of Nurse-Midwives was able to put together a consortium of insurance carriers to issue coverage, but it is a great deal more expensive than the previous coverage, and the policy stipulates that nurse-midwives must be "employees," which confuses practice quality issues with employment relationships.

The malpractice insurance situation has also affected obstetricians. In 1986, there were approximately 31,400 obstetricians; 35 percent of the 35,000 family practice physicians included obstetrics in their practices and an unknown number of general practitioners did so as well (Scholle & Klerman, 1988). One estimate indicated that 12.4 percent of obstetricians gave up obstetric practice (but continued their gyneco-logic practice), with considerable variation from state to state (8.3 percent in New York, 25.1 percent in Florida). Nearly half of general-family practice physicians have given up obstetrics (Scholle & Klerman, 1988). What effect this will have on nurse-midwife practices is not yet known.

In an exhaustive review of the legislation, Hadley argues that prescriptive author-ity makes nurses in expanded roles less complementary and more substitutable (Hadley, 1989). The economic analysis helps explain the resistance of organized medicine (and organized pharmacy too, to the extent that they wish to move beyond "dispensing" to "prescribing") to granting prescribing privileges to nurses. In gen-eral, prescriptive authority has been less of an issue for nurse-midwives than for nurse anesthetists, partly because the need of the former for access to pharmaceuti-cals is relatively limited. Nurse-midwives function under mutually agreed-upon medically approved standing orders that specify particular drugs for particular symp-toms or conditions. Nurse-midwives, however, have had an interest in the authority to prescribe birth control devices (e.g., intrauterine devices) and to order laboratory tests and procedures (ultrasonography, for instance), which may be covered in the same laws or local policies.

Nurse anesthetists' issues regarding prescriptive authority have had to do with how the range of medications is limited by law or regulation; they need access to controlled drugs in all of the five Schedules of the Federal Controlled Substance Act (1981). Many of the 26 states that at present have some form of prescribing authority for nurses in advanced practice limit it to formularies or only Schedule II drugs.

Nurse anesthesia has formulated a unique argument about prescriptive authority. Gene Blumenreich, General Counsel of the American Association of Nurse Anesthe-tists, opines that since most surgery cannot be performed without anesthesia, sched-uling a patient for surgery, which only a physician can do, is "generally equivalent to the prescription for anesthesia" (Blumenreich, 1988, p. 91). Thus, the physician prescribes "anesthesia" and leaves it up to the nurse anesthetist to determine the specifics (*Kamalyan v. Henderson*, 1954). A nurse anesthetist is obliged, as is any other nurse, to carry out the physician's order unless it is unlawful, the wrong medication, the wrong dose, or the wrong time, or if the nurse is not qualified to carry out the order or manage the potential (more immediate) complications and other providers are not sufficiently close to help (Ira Gunn, personal communication, April 11, 1990).

Both nurse-midwives and nurse anesthetists have used published statements about their practice to advantage, but quite differently. The American College of Nurse-Midwives, the American College of Obstetricians and Gynecologists, and the Nurses' Association of the American College of Obstetricians and Gynecologists issued their first joint statement in 1971, recognizing and supporting the development and utilization of nurse-midwives in teams "directed by a physician." A later supplementary statement made it clear that neither physical presence nor employment by physicians was intended. The most recent joint statement (American College of Nurse-Midwives, 1983) still stands. Nurse-midwives have been able to wave these statements in the faces of physicians or legislators who might question the working relationship and to hold obstetricians to the published words of their association. Negotiating such statements obviously requires that the participants communicate. The American Society of Anesthesiologists will not even meet to negotiate contemporary troubling issues with the American Association of Nurse Anesthetists. Thus, the American Association of Nurse Anesthetists has issued its own statements.

The anesthesia standards of the Joint Commission on the Accreditation of Health Care Organizations specify that an independent licensed practitioner is responsible for the determination of the patient's physical status and capacity to undergo anesthesia even though she or he need not perform these functions directly. To establish firmly that the certified registered nurse anesthetist is the *independent* licensed practitioner and perhaps to head off future battles, the American Association of Nurse Anesthetists has issued a position statement on "Relationships Between Health Care Professionals," which states that as independent licensed practitioners, certified registered nurse anesthetists function with the *consent* of another licensed provider who "supervises" but does not "control" the practice (American Association of Nurse Anesthetists, 1987). The statement has been distributed widely to hospitals, departments of anesthesiology, and government agencies. The American Association of Nurse Anesthetists and the American Society of Anesthesiologists have accepted editors' invitations to argue in publication, since they cannot talk in private, on who should train and supervise nurse anesthetists (Ditzler, 1979; Gunn, 1979) and in response to a policy analysis of anesthesia payment (Beutler, 1988; Weiss, 1988).

Linguists might find amusing research opportunities in tracing the changing language in the interprofessional statements, court cases, and legal arguments: from "direction" or "medically directed team" to "supervision" to "understood supervision" to "consent" and whatever comes next. The choice of the word "direction" (even when modified in nurse-midwifery to provide for "consultation, collaboration, and referral") in position statements contrasts with the efforts of other nursing groups to get out from under such terminology when nurse practice acts are revised. The landmark case, *Sermchief v. Gonzales* (1983), turned in part on just such a change in legislative language (Wolff, 1984). But in the political context in which both groups evolved, that terminology probably helped, and as the practices have matured, the "direction" has become more and more pro forma.

Whether there is truly a shortage or a surplus of physicians, a point that is hotly debated (Schwartz et al., 1988, 1989; Ginsberg, 1989), the American Medical Association has made its agenda all too clear. In 1985, the American Medical Association's House of Delegates passed a resolution "to combat legislation authorizing medical acts by unlicensed individuals" (American Medical Association, 1985). It commits state medical societies to fight off all attempts to expand the practice of "unlicensed" individuals (the license to practice *medicine* as the property right is the only one that counts). The American Medical Association will provide funds, speakers, position papers, and reviews of state legislation to any medical society facing a challenge [sic], as well as contributing financially to the political campaigns of sympathetic legislators.

The rhetoric of the American Medical Association emphasizes safety and physician authority, but the issue is really something else: money.

## Money

Nurse-midwives and nurse anesthetists pursued third-party reimbursement in the same period, and eventually with the same success, but apparently without joining forces. Nurse-midwifery was written into third-party reimbursement legislation first in the Civilian Health and Medical Program of the Uniformed Services for military dependents who receive care outside military hospitals, and in 1980, in Medicaid, with the support of Senator Daniel K. Inouye (D-Hawaii), who is proud to announce that he was delivered by a midwife. The American College of Nurse-Midwives was able to effectively use the considerable literature on the success of nurse-midwifery with poor and underserved people (Diers & Burst, 1983). The Medicaid provision said that reimbursement for nurse-midwifery services was mandated in all jurisdictions with "legal authorization" for nurse-midwifery. In states without clear authorization in law or regulation, nurse-midwives worked to make sure language appeared using the Medicaid carrot to political advantage. Senator Inouye also got nurse-midwifery included in Medicare coverage where certified nurse-midwife services are available to handicapped women; certified nurse-midwives are also moving into the area of postmenopausal gynecology. Reimbursement for nurse-midwifery is also available under the Federal Employees Health Plan. These programs require only one act of one central government, which is a great deal easier than going through every state's insurance laws. Senator Inouye, alerted by the American College of Nurse-Midwives that some states were dragging their feet, asked the General Accounting Office to find out how many states had complied with the Medicaid provisions (Medicaid, 1987). By then, 44 states had amended their Medicaid programs and the General Accounting Office report signaled the Health Care Financing Administration to get after the others, who had lame excuses. As a mandated benefit under these federal plans, the government had the possibility of exercising punishment—withdrawal of all of the Medicaid funds for noncompliance.

The first (unsuccessful) efforts of the American Association of Nurse Anesthetists to obtain direct reimbursement targeted Medicare in 1976–1977, when Congress first expressed concern about the growing Part B Medicare payments for anesthesia, pathology, and radiology (Ira Gunn, personal communication, April 11, 1990). In 1982, under the Tax Equity and Fiscal Responsibility Act (TEFRA), which set the stage for diagnosis-related group (DRG)-based prospective payment, certain constraints were placed on billing of anesthesiologists. The Prospective Payment System threw a wrench in the works for certified registered nurse anesthetists, creating major reimbursement disincentives for hospitals to use them.

First, all nonphysician services provided within the hospital were considered to be covered by the DRG-based payment under Medicare Part A. Given an adequate number of anesthesia providers in the area, it was not in a hospital's interest to employ certified registered nurse anesthetists and bundle their services in the DRG-based Part A payment, when anesthesiologists could be paid under Part B, outside the hospital billing system. The law prohibited unbundling services previously provided as a package. Further, the DRG-based payment was a composite of costs reported by hospitals, some of which employed certified registered nurse anesthetists and some of which did not. If hospitals had not employed certified registered nurse anesthetists, their zero contribution to this composite had the effect of lowering the base for the rate calculation (the American Association of Nurse Anesthetists estimated that 17 percent or more of hospitals fell into this category, enough to make a difference [Garde, 1988]).

The American Association of Nurse Anesthetists developed a comprehensive strategy with two explicit agendas: to constrain costs and to create a level playing field in any competitive market (no inherent incentives or disincentives to use particular providers, and with all providers being paid out of the same pot—Part A or Part B—under the same constraints but not necessarily on the same payment rate). They sought and obtained a temporary 3-year cost pass-through for hospital-employed certified registered nurse anesthetist services. Then, in a rare show of support, some groups within the American Society of Anesthesiologists joined the successful proposal of the American Association of Nurse Anesthetists for a single exception from the unbundling provision for certified registered nurse anesthetists employed by anesthesiologists. Finally, the American Association of Nurse Anesthetists sought direct reimbursement for certified registered nurse anesthetists under Medicare, crafting the proposal to be budget neutral and guaranteeing acceptance of the assignment (to take the Medicare payment as full payment). Trying to move anesthesiologists into Medicare Part A proved too politically troublesome for Congress; therefore, nurse anesthetists were moved into Part B in legislation implemented in January, 1989.

The payment method for anesthesia services amounts to a pork barrel for anesthesiologists. In brief, there are pre-established "base units" that reflect the difficulty of a particular case. Then one time unit is added for every 15 minutes the patient is under anesthesia. The rationale here is that the length of the case is not under the control of the anesthesia provider. The sum of these units is multiplied by an allowable conversion factor in order to arrive at a payment rate. Those anesthesiologists who "medically direct" certified registered nurse anesthetists bill for the medical direction under two schedules: if they employ the certified registered nurse anesthetist, they bill for 15-minute time units; if they "direct" hospital-employed certified registered nurse anesthetists, they may only bill for 30-minute time units (assuming they are physically in the hospital), whereas the hospital bills for the certified registered nurse anesthetists' services. Anesthesiologists are the only physicians allowed under Medicare to bill a medical direction fee. The President's FY 1990 budget called for reductions in anesthesia Medicare fees of 25 percent, paying certified registered nurse anesthetists and anesthesiologists the same amount. Only one fee would be permissible. For the hospital-employed certified registered nurse anesthetist where the anesthesiologist "medically directs" the service, the hospital and anesthesiologists would have to negotiate who gets what portion of the fee. It has occurred to nurse anesthetists, as it has to nurse-midwives, that the sensible thing to do would be to hire physician anesthesiologists or obstetricians as consultants, paying them out of fees billed in the certified registered nurse anesthetist's or certified nurse-midwife's name.

In a Health Care Financing Administration contracted policy analysis, Cromwell and Rosenbach (1988) analyzed anesthesia payments. The report ends with an unusually forthright statement:

> Any maldistribution of anesthesiologists should not be solved by raising the reimbursement bridge in rural areas, but rather by lowering the reimbursement river in overdoctored cities. With an annual net income in excess of $140,000 . . . it seems extravagant for society to be offering extra bonuses to anesthesiologists . . . [U]nless some real reform is initiated soon, the opportunity to achieve an efficient anesthesiologist/CRNA mix could be lost, program outlays will remain unnecessarily high, and another occupation providing valuable care at low cost will be put on the endangered list (p. 17).

Insurance coverage in the private sector varies from state to state. Some states mandate reimbursement for nurse anesthetists if they are not practicing as another reimbursable health provider's employee or as a contractor. All states permit direct reimbursement to certified registered nurse anesthetists, but some Blue Cross/Blue Shield plans do and some do not. In 1982, Haire surveyed third-party payers and found that the vast majority of private insurance companies covered nurse-midwifery services directly even when the written policy did not mention nurse-midwifery. But the rate of coverage under Blue Cross/Blue Shield was much lower, reflecting the fact that the policy boards of many of these organizations are heavily weighted with physicians (Haire, 1982). Nurse-midwives have made considerable headway in health maintenance organizations, which are, after all, insurers as well as providers. Health maintenance organizations have found certified nurse-midwives to be cost-effective and highly marketable. Since health maintenance organizations do not employ anesthesia providers, this has not been an option for certified registered nurse anesthetists, although there is no particular reason why such groups could not contract to deliver anesthesia to a health maintenance organization's patients. Medicaid permits certified registered nurse anesthetists to be directly reimbursed, but allows states to make the decision; they are reimbursed under Medicaid in 22 states. Certified registered nurse anesthetists are eligible to seek direct reimbursement from the Civilian Health and Medical Program of the Uniformed Services.

The confusion of the employment relationship with professional supervision calls into question the notions of "supervision," "direction," and "control" of practice, which are holdovers from history. Nurse-midwifery has been more successful in separating the employment and economic issues. Nurse-midwifery has also made more coin out of data on the effectiveness of nurse-midwifery for underprivileged clientele, in effect painting a political picture of willingness to go where others will not. Nurse anesthetists have more often used the cost-effectiveness argument and have played upon politicians' and bureaucrats' charge to promote equity (the "level playing field").

Value—societal or otherwise—is money. Nurse-midwives have successfully argued their place as caregivers having different values and practices, relieving the high technology, pregnancy-as-a-disease orientation of physicians. Nurse anesthetists do not have as many opportunities to argue for the specialness of nursing, although an outsider reading their literature and the anesthesiology literature might detect a clear difference that parallels the difference between nurse-midwifery and obstetrics. Nurse anesthesia's rhetoric emphasizes care, comfort, use of distraction and other low technology interventions, communication and nurse-patient relationships, easy induction, and natural levels of sleep consistent with the surgical procedures. Anesthesiology's rhetoric conceptualizes anesthesia as a technical service necessary to keep the body's functions in balance while surgery is performed. More could be made of these parallels.

While nurse anesthetists may enjoy unconventional employment relationships, nurse-midwives also have moved into nontraditional or alternative settings for practice, such as out-of-hospital birthing centers. There is no equivalent opportunity for nurse anesthetists, who must practice where surgeons, dentists, or obstetricians do.

A large national study (N = 11,814) of out-of-hospital birth centers (Rooks et al., 1989) showed that the patient outcomes—complications, transfer rates, mortality—were in the same range as outcomes from earlier studies of low-risk women delivering in hospitals. An editorial that accompanies the report of the birth center study generally agrees with the conclusion that birth centers offer lower cost, greater availability of service, a high degree of patient satisfaction, and comparable safety; however, it still proposes that proximity to a hospital is the factor most to be adhered to in the future (Lieberman & Ryan, 1989). How close is close (in miles, attitudes, collaboration) is central to considering the relative independence of practice of nurse-midwives in these or traditional settings. The same issue is explicit in anesthesiology, phrased as the extent to which nurse anesthetists are a "close substitute" (Weiss, 1988). Here, the reference is to scope of practice, safety, and money. Is physician presence always required? If knowing the limits of one's ability or training is the "hallmark of the professional," as Michael Wolff argued in *Sermchief v. Gonzales* (Wolff, 1984), would it not seem that the appropriate practice relationship for both nurse-midwives and nurse anesthetists would be consultative, with the nurse specialists determining when consultation should occur? That, of course, makes the nurses gatekeepers . . . (Diers & Molde, 1983).

## Conclusions

As specialist practice has matured through experience, education, regulation, accreditation, licensure, and economic independence, nurse specialists have drifted away from the tight relationship with medicine and traditional practice sites, and this is exactly what physicians worry about.

In spite of early resistance to primary care by nurses (Ford, 1982), the climate for nurse specialization has changed considerably since nurse-midwives and nurse anesthetists had their disappointing negotiations with the American Nurses' Association. However, other nursing specialties, notably oncology nurses and emergency department nurses, have also created their own organizations and literature, in the first instance deliberately outside the structure of the American Nurses' Association and in the second instance because they, too, were put off by the professional organization (Kelleher, 1990). Although psychiatric nurses have stayed within the American Nurses' Association, the fact that they have been swept up into a generic "therapist" title in many settings suggests an ambivalence about nursing, similar to nurse-midwives, and nurse anesthetists. Primary care nurse practitioners have created new organizations and journals outside the professional organization. Nurse-midwives, nurse anesthetists, psychiatric nurses, and nurse practitioners are the substitutable roles. The more complementary roles of the medical-surgical subspecialties and community health nursing may find a more sympathetic home within the professional organization.

Complementarity and substitutability are perhaps not as distinct as once was thought. And the different, sometimes overlapping, roles should surely not create the newest divisiveness within the profession. Nurse anesthesia might provide an interesting model for how a specialist practice can evolve wearing two hats. Practices do not have to be substitutable to be autonomous or powerful.

Nurse anesthesia profited from having friends in high places. Surely the early work of nurse anesthetists in the Mayo Clinic and Lakeside Hospital brought the specialty both influence and power and a high profile. Nurse-midwifery also had distinguished connections (Diers & Burst, 1983), and Mary Breckinridge herself was the daughter of an ambassador. Nurses in other kinds of expanded roles have found highly placed colleagues, and this is a helpful strategy to remember.

Nurse anesthesia has more often fought its battles through the courts than through legislation, and nurse anesthetist practice is most often contained within Nurse Practice Acts. The American Association of Nurse Anesthetists hires lawyers. Nurse-midwifery has more often turned to public forums such as the legislature and has sought legal authorization outside Nursing Practice Acts. The American College of Nurse-Midwives hires lobbyists. Nurse-midwifery has been able to generate consumer enthusiasm and rely on attention to mothers and babies for public exposure and pressure. Nurse-midwives' natural political constituency is families. Nurse anesthetists hardly have such a satisfied customer relationship, since their clients, even if they know their anesthesia was administered by a nurse, are asleep. Outpatient surgery may provide nurse anesthetists with more patient contact and more public presence because the surgery is shorter and the patients more often are awake, at least for part of the time. Careful analysis of natural constituencies for other nursing specialists is clearly in order. The hospice and oncology nurses have made good use of their poignant patient stories; the emergency nurses have natural allies in physicians, patients, and possibly the police.

Nurse anesthetists and nurse-midwives have leap-frogged over organizational, legislative, and legal issues—a success here for certified nurse-midwives, a success there for certified registered nurse anesthetists—yet there is scant evidence that they have studied one another's roles and activities. Their successes are remarkably consistent, requiring heroic effort. Perhaps nursing is now mature enough to learn from the lessons of those who have gone off in new directions so that we no longer have to reinvent the wheel.

It would be naive to think that competition with organized medicine is over for nurse-midwives, nurse anesthetists, or any other nurse specialists. The fact that there are now so many definable nursing specialties is a strength rather than a weakness for nursing. The shared experience suggests that the natural constituency for nursing is nursing itself.

Despite the American Medical Association's declaration of war on advanced practice nursing, there are signs of some easing of tensions between medicine and nursing as the Association's membership declines and ages and newer physicians have learned to respect nursing's contributions. If the United States health care system ever moves to making access to health care universal, the need for nurses in all specialties will far exceed the available supply. A recently released federal report projects the need for 40 percent more nurse anesthetists by 2010, despite the growing number of anesthesiologists (Health Economics Research, 1990). We should be prepared to take advantage of this new desirability to help us, among other things, understand interprofessional relationships.

Substitutable practices are alternatives. The more fully substitutable the practice, including prescribing authority and payment for service, the more real is the choice for patients, hiring institutions, and third-party payers. Alternatives must not only prove themselves but also of necessity must *improve* to remain viable. Nurse-midwifery and nurse anesthesia have made enviable progress on quality control through accreditation and competency assessment, which might be a lesson for other specialties.

The final implication of this analysis is the critical power of data. Both specialty groups began early to record the results of their practices, long before data were needed politically. In effect, the data established the legitimacy of the practices, which were then embedded in legislation or court decisions. As nurse-midwifery and nurse anesthesia have no longer needed data for defense of quality or right to practice, their information has become increasingly sophisticated and tuned to policy issues. This direction should be a more general agenda for nursing. If nursing practices can be demonstrated to produce quality outcomes and to preserve natural and normal processes as much as possible, at a competitive cost, their future is assured.

REFERENCES

Adams, C.J. (1989). Nurse-midwifery practice in the United States, 1982–1987. *American Journal of Public Health, 79*(8), 1038–1039.
American Association of Nurse Anesthetists (1987). *Guidelines for nurse anesthesia practice.* Park Ridge, IL: American Association of Nurse Anesthetists.

American College of Nurse-Midwives, American College of Obstetricians and Gynecologists (1983). *Joint Statement on Maternity Care*. Washington, DC: The College.

American Medical Association (1985). *Resolution: To combat legislation authorizing medical acts by unlicensed individuals*. Chicago: The Association.

Bankert, M. (1989). *Watchful Care—A history of America's nurse anesthetists*. New York: Continuum.

Beutler, J.M. (1988). Perspectives: A nurse anesthetist. *Health Affairs*, 7(3), 26–31.

*Bhan v. NME Hospitals, Inc. et al.* (1985). 772 F. 2nd 1467 (9th Cir.).

Blumenreich, G.A. (1984). Jefferson Parish Hospital v. Hyde—The last chapter. *Journal of the American Association of Nurse Anesthetists*, 52(4), 462–463.

Blumenreich, G.A. (1988). Nurse anesthetists and prescriptive authority. *Journal of the American Association of Nurse Anesthetists*, 56(2), 91–93.

Blumenreich, G.A. (1989). Surgeons' responsibility for CRNAs. *Journal of the American Association of Nurse Anesthetists*, 57(1), 6–8.

Blumenreich, R.A., & Wolfe, B.L. (1986). Restrictions on CRNAs imposed by physician-controlled insurance companies. *Journal of the American Association of Nurse Anesthetists*, 54(6), 538–539.

Breece, C., Israel, E., & Friedman, L. (1989). Closing of the nurse-midwifery service at Boston City Hospital—What were the issues involved? *Journal of Nurse-Midwifery*, 34(1), 41–48.

Butter, I.H., & Kay, B.Y. (1988). State laws and the practice of lay midwifery. *American Journal of Public Health*, 78(9), 1161–1169.

*Chalmers-Frances v. Nelson* (1936). 6 Ca. 2nd 402.

Clay, T. (1987). *Nurses—power and politics*. London: William Heinemann Medical Books.

Crile, G.W. (1947). *George Crile: An autobiography*. Philadelphia: Lippincott.

Cromwell, J., & Rosenbach, M.L. (1988). Reforming anesthesia payment under Medicare. *Health Affairs*, 7(3), 6–18.

Diers, D., & Burst, H.V. (1983). The effectiveness of policy related research: Nurse-midwifery as case study. *Image Journal of Nursing Scholarship*, 15(3), 68–74.

Diers, D., & Molde, S. (1983). Nurses in primary care. The new gatekeepers? *American Journal of Nursing*, 83, 742–745.

Ditzler, J.W. (1979). Nurse anesthetists should be trained and supervised by anesthesiologists. In J.E. Eckenhoff (Ed.), *Controversy in anesthesiology* (pp. 205–210). Philadelphia: W.B. Saunders.

Donegan, J.B. (1978). *Women & men midwives: Medicine, morality and misogyny in early America*. Westport, CT: Greenwood Press.

Donnison, J. (1988). *Midwives and medical men—A history of the struggle for the control of childbirth* (2nd ed.). London: Historical Publications Ltd.

Federal Controlled Substance Act of 1981. 21 U.S.C.A. at 801–971 (West 1981 and Suppl. 1989).

Ford, L. (1982). Nurse practitioners: History of a new idea and predictions for the future. In L.H. Aiken (Ed.), *Nursing in the '80's* (pp. 231–248). Philadelphia: J.B. Lippincott.

*Frank et al. v. South et al.* (1917). *Kentucky Reporter* 175:416–428.

Fullerton, J.D.T. (1982). The ACNM and the NCHCA: The significance of membership . . . the evolution of the health credentialing agency, the National Commission for Health Certifying Agencies. *Journal of Nurse-Midwifery*, 27(3), 27–30.

Galloway, D.H. (1899, May 27). The anesthetizer as a specialist. *The Philadelphia Medical Journal*, 1173.

Garde, J.F. (1988). A case study involving prospective payment legislation, DRGs, and certified registered nurse anesthetists. *Nursing Clinics of North America*, 23(3), 521–530.

*Geneva Bible: A facsimile of the 1560 edition* (1969). Madison, Milwaukee, and London: University of Wisconsin Press.

Ginzberg, E. (1989). Physician supply in the year 2000. *Health Affairs, 8*(2), 84–90.

Griffith, H. (1984). Nursing practice: Substitute or complement according to economic theory . . . working relationships between physicians and nurses. *Nursing Economics, 2*(2), 105–110.

Gunn, I.P. (1975). Nurse anesthetist-anesthesiologist relationships: Past, present and implications for the future. *Journal of the American Association of Nurse Anesthetists, 43*(2), 129–139.

Gunn, I.P. (1979). Nurse anesthetists should control the teaching and practice of their profession. In J.E. Eckenhoff (Ed.), *Controversy in anesthesiology* (pp. 211–220). Philadelphia: W.B. Saunders.

Gunn, I.P., Nicosia, J., & Tobin, M. (1987). Anesthesia: A practice of nursing [editorial]. *Journal of the American Association of Nurse Anesthetists, 55*(2), 97–100.

Hadley, E. (1989). Nurses and prescriptive authority: A legal and economic analysis. *American Journal of Law and Medicine, 15*(2–3), 245–300.

Haire, D. (1982). Health insurance coverage for nurse-midwifery services: Results of a national survey. *Journal of Nurse-Midwifery, 27*(6), 35–36.

Harlow, M.O. (1988). Midwifery: State regulation. 59 *ALR* 4th 929–948.

Health Economics Research (1990). *Nurse anesthetists: Supply and demand.* Report to the National Center for Nursing Research and the Division of Nursing, U.S. Public Health Service. Washington, DC: U.S. Government Printing Office.

Hemschemeyer, H. (1943). The nurse-midwife is here to stay. *American Journal of Nursing, 43*(10), 916.

Hemschemeyer, H. (1947). Obstetrical nursing today and tomorrow. *Public Health Nursing, 39*(2), 35–39.

*In Re Medical Staff of Memorial Medical Center* (1988, June 1). Federal Trade Commission Docket No. C-3231, Decision and Order.

*Jefferson Parish Hospital v. Hyde,* (1984). U.S. Supreme Court, March 26.

*Kamalyan v. Henderson* (1954). 277 P. 2nd 372.

Kelleher, J.C. (1990). When dreams come true [editorial]. *Journal of Emergency Nursing, 16*(1), 1–2.

Kelly, M.E. (1987). Control of the practice of nurse practitioners, nurse-midwives, nurse anesthetists and clinical nurse specialists. In C. Northrup, & M.E. Kelly (Eds.), *Legal issues in nursing* (pp. 469–486). St. Louis: C.V. Mosby.

*Leggett v. Tennessee Board of Nursing* (1980). 612 South Western Reporter, 2nd, 476.

*Leigh v. Board of Registration in Nursing* (1984). 481 N.E. 2nd 401 (Ind. App.).

Lieberman, E., & Ryan, K.H. (1989). Birth-day choices. *New England Journal of Medicine, 321*(26), 1824–1825.

Litoff, J.B. (1982). The midwife throughout history. *Journal of Nurse-Midwifery, 27*(6), 3–11.

*Medicaid: Use of certified nurse-midwives* (1987, November). Report to the Honorable Daniel K. Inouye, U.S. Senate. U.S. General Accounting Office (GAO/HRD-88-25). Washington, DC: Government Printing Office.

*Nurse Midwifery Associates v. Hibbert* (1983). 577 F. Supp. 1273.

Olsen, G.W. (1940). The nurse anesthetists: Past, present and future. *Bulletin of the American Association of Nurse Anesthetists, 8*(4), 298.

*Oltz v. St. Peter's Community Hospital* (1986, November). CV 81–271–H–Res, Montana District Court.

Redman, R. (1986). The nurse and the draft in the Vietnam War. *Bulletin of the American Association for the History of Nursing, 10*(2), 2–3.

Robb, I.H. (1893). *Nursing: Its principles and practice for hospital and private use.* New York: E.C. Koechert.

Robinson, S.A. (1984). A historical development of midwifery in the black community: 1600–1940. *Journal of Nurse-Midwifery, 29*(4), 247–250.

Rooks, J.P., Weatherby, N.L., Ernst, E.K.M., Stapleton, S., Rosen, D., & Rosenfield, A. (1989). Outcomes of care in birth centers—the National Birth Center Study. *New England Journal of Medicine, 321*(26), 1804–1811.

Scholle, S.H., & Klerman, L.V. (1988, August). *The actual and potential impact of medical liability issues on access to maternity care.* Paper prepared for the Committee on the Effects of Medical Liability on the Delivery of Maternal and Child Health Care. Washington, DC: Institute of Medicine, National Academy of Sciences.

Schwartz, W.B., Sloan, F.A., & Mendelson, D.N. (1988). Why there will be little or no physician surplus between now and the year 2000. *New England Journal of Medicine, 318*(14), 892–897.

Schwartz, W.B., Sloan, F.A., & Mendelson, D.N. (1989). Debating physician supply: The authors respond. *Health Affairs, 8*(2), 91–95.

*Sermschief v. Gonzales* (1983). 660 SW. 2nd 683.

*Smith v. State of Indiana ex rel. Medical Licensing Board of Indiana* (1984). 459 NE. 2nd 401 (In. App. 2 Dist).

Thatcher, V. (1953/1984). *History of anesthesia with emphasis on the nurse specialist.* Philadelphia: J.B. Lippincott.

Tom, S.A. (1982). The evolution of nurse-midwifery: 1900–1960. *Journal of Nurse-Midwifery, 27*(4), 4–13.

Truesdale, P.E. (1913). *Transactions of the American Hospital Association, 15,* 283.

"Use of nurses as anesthetists in Ohio hospitals in violation of State law is charged; Medical Board acts." (1916). *Ohio State Medical Journal, 12*(12), 679.

Varney, H. (1987). *Nurse-midwifery* (2nd ed.). Boston: Blackwell Scientific.

Weiss, J.B. (1988, Fall). Perspectives: An anesthesiologist. *Health Affairs, 7*(3), 20–25.

Williams, S.R. (1981). *Divine Rebel—The life of Anne Marbury Hutchinson.* New York: Holt, Rinehart & Winston.

Wolff, M.A. (1984, February). Court upholds expanded practice roles for nurses. *Law, Medicine & Health Care,* 26–29.

## Chapter 13

# The Organization and Financing of Long-Term Care

CHARLENE HARRINGTON

$L$ONG-TERM SERVICES include those health, social services, housing, transportation, income security, and other supportive services needed by those with chronic illnesses or disabilities. Such services may be intermittent or continuous and may be given after hospitalization or for chronic illnesses and disabilities unrelated to hospitalization (Kane & Kane, 1982). The current private and public financing programs generally create an arbitrary distinction between short- and long-term services by placing time limits on short-term covered services and excluding long-term services (Estes et al., 1983; Harrington et al., 1985). The need for long-term care arises out of physical, mental, or cognitive limitations in a person's ability to perform tasks that are essential to living independently. The need and demand for long-term care services are increasing with the aging of the population.

The United States has a complex and often overlapping array of financing and service programs for those with chronic illnesses and disabilities. The financing system for long-term care services is a combination of public and private financing, which places the financial burden most heavily on those who are disabled and do not have private insurance and do not qualify for public programs (InterStudy 1988a). It works by making individuals and their families spend down their personal funds until they qualify for public assistance under one of the special categorical funding programs available. In most instances, the net effect of this approach is that individuals must virtually impoverish themselves before they become eligible for public program assistance (U.S. General Accounting Office, 1988).

Faced with growing long-term care expenditures and increasing numbers of individuals who need help, public policy makers are considering a wide range of new strategies for meeting the need for long-term care. Congress has introduced a number of serious legislative proposals that are incremental and would expand the eligibility and/or benefits for the current Medicare and/or Medicaid programs (Rovner, 1988). The current limitations on federal revenues and spending, the budgetary deficit, and the limited amount of federal discretionary funds, however, are all factors that discourage public policy reform. Offsetting these concerns is the growing public priority on long-term care financial protection (Wiener, Hanley, Spence, & Murray, 1989).

This paper examines the problems with the current financing and delivery system for long-term services and the public policy options. Any financing system has options in establishing services, eligibility, the delivery system, utilization, and cost controls. Beyond these components, options exist for a private, public, or combination financing system. A public insurance model is recommended by many experts to provide universal coverage for the public, so that those in need of services would receive services without becoming impoverished. A mandatory public insurance model that uses financial risk pooling through progressive taxing mechanisms is discussed. This model would provide protection at a far lower cost than having each family bear the cost. Tax options for financing a long-term care system are also discussed. And finally, the implications for nursing are discussed.

## Current Financing of Long-Term Care

The nation's total expenditures for long-term care are difficult to estimate, but in 1990 these included $54.5 billion for nursing home services, $14.1 billion for equipment and appliances, and $10.6 billion for home health and other professional services (U.S. Department of Commerce, 1990). Some proportion of the nation's expenditures for drugs and medical sundries was for those individuals needing long-term care services. In addition, about 10 percent ($25 billion) of the total hospital costs were spent on psychiatric and long-term hospital services (American Hospital Association, 1986; U.S. Department of Commerce, 1990). Most estimates of long-term care expenditures have focused on the elderly; therefore accurate data for the population as a whole have not been developed.

Public programs finance half of the total formal long-term care, primarily through the Medicaid program. The United States Congressional Budget Office (1987) estimated that 48 percent of nursing home expenditures were paid for by Medicaid, 2 percent by Medicare, and 3 percent by other public payers. Private insurance pays for less than 2 percent, and consumers pay 45 percent of total costs directly out of pocket (U.S. Congressional Budget Office, 1987; U.S. Department of Health and Human Services, 1988; Division of National Cost Estimates, 1987; Levit & Freeland, 1988). For home health agency services and other services in the home, the United States Congressional Budget Office (1987) estimated that 40 percent is paid directly by consumers. Thus, the role of Medicare in paying for long-term care remains limited.

Some 80 federal programs provide direct or indirect services to individuals with long-term care problems. In addition to Medicare, Medicaid, and the Veterans Administration programs, the Older Americans Act and Title XX Social Services Funds are important funding sources (U.S. Senate, 1989). Other public programs that provide long-term care include those for the developmentally disabled and the mentally disabled and state disability insurance programs.

United States cost estimates do not include informal or unpaid long-term services. Data from the 1982 National Long-Term Care Survey showed that of the 4.6

million disabled elderly, more than 70 percent (3.2 million) relied exclusively on unpaid sources of care (Liu, Manton, & Liu, 1985). Almost 22 percent relied on a combination of both formal and informal care, and 5 percent used formal care exclusively (Liu et al., 1985; Stone, 1986; Stone et al., 1987; U.S. Senate, 1989).

The average $29,000 per year for nursing home care in 1987 is beyond the level many individuals can afford (Rivlin & Wiener, 1988), so that formal service users rapidly spend their savings and become eligible for Medicaid and other public programs. A recent study showed that the average individual exhausts his or her resources (spends down his or her resources to become eligible for Medicaid) within 13 weeks after admission to a nursing home for the single older person (age 75 and over) (Branch et al., 1988; U.S. House Committee on Ways and Means, 1987). Although Spence and Wiener (1989) argue that the percentage who become impoverished by nursing home care is less (only 10 percent of private patients), they also show the high probabilities of impoverishment for those who are older, single, and in lower income groups as lengths of nursing home stay increase. Since only 15 percent of the elderly had incomes above $25,000 in 1984, many elderly are unable to finance their long-term care costs beyond a few months (U.S. Social Security Administration, 1984). For those with incomes below $25,000 and in need of long-term care, the risk of impoverishment is significant.

## Services

Currently, each public and private insurance program has different benefits, making it difficult for consumers to understand the system. Most Medicare beneficiaries incorrectly believe they are covered for long-term care services (R.L. Associates, 1987). Unfortunately, Medicare limits nursing home care to 100 days of care per spell of illness with 3 days of prior hospitalization required, and it limits home health visits to those who are homebound and who require skilled nursing or therapy up to 5 days a week for 2 to 3 weeks (Commerce Clearing House Inc., 1989). Private insurance plans generally do not include long-term service benefits beyond those covered by Medicare, unless the policy is specifically for long-term care services. Furthermore, most long-term program benefits are biased toward acute and institutional programs rather than community and socially oriented services, even though state Medicaid programs have been adding more community services (U.S. Senate, 1989). The fragmentation of the estimated 80 public long-term care programs, state disability programs, and the private insurance programs create complex benefit rules with many gaps in coverage.

One policy option to lessen the fragmentation is to create a uniform benefit package for all public programs that is comprehensive in nature, which would include medically and socially oriented services as well as institutional services, community-based services, and expanded services such as drugs. The advantages of comprehensive benefits are that they ensure the availability of the most appropriate services; may prevent high-cost hospitalizations or other institutional services; and respond to consumer demand. Most individuals want to remain in their own homes and be as independent as possible. The elderly overwhelmingly support programs that provide community-based care, even if such benefits increase costs (R.L. Associates, 1987; Rivlin & Wiener, 1988).

Many policy makers argue for a limited or restricted benefit package for long-term care, primarily on the grounds of controlling costs. Other policy makers argue that long-term care proposals should include a broad array of benefits but place limits or restrictions on benefit use, as is currently the case with Medicare. Neither approach is appropriate (Firman, Weissert, & Wilson, 1988). Cost containment can be achieved by means other than limiting benefits, including prior authorization and utilization review procedures. More important, limited benefits have proved costly to the Medicare and other programs by encouraging the use of high-cost institutional services. As long as public and private long-term care benefits continue to be limited, access to appropriate long-term care delivered by nurses and other professionals will be hampered.

## Eligibility

Currently, each public and private financing program for long-term care has its own eligibility criteria, including age, disability, and income. Medicare covered 32.4 million individuals who are elderly (65 years and over) and/or disabled and their dependents in 1988 (Gornick et al., 1985; U.S. Senate, 1989). Even though an individual is eligible for a general program, specific rules apply to long-term care service eligibility. For example, Medicare long-term care services are specifically limited to a spell of illness and not for those with long-term chronic illnesses. In 1988, Medicaid covered an estimated 24.2 million individuals, including 6.9 million aged, blind, and disabled people who were poor enough to be eligible for the federal Supplemental Security Income program or who had spent down to become eligible for the program (Congressional Research Service, 1988). The Older Americans Act programs have an age requirement of 60 and older but are not tied to disability. Social service, mental disability, and development disability programs are primarily targeted to the poor and have their own eligibility criteria. This complex array of public and private eligibility policies creates serious difficulties for nurses and other caregivers who provide long-term care services because frequently individuals in need do not meet the eligibility requirements for coverage and many are unable to pay for such services directly out of pocket.

One of the basic issues in designing a long-term care financing program is determining who should be eligible for the program. All of the current federal legislative proposals for long-term care financial coverage would restrict eligibility to those who are age 65 and over. The argument for focusing on older individuals is that they have significantly greater utilization and expenditures rates for long-term care services than the under age 65 groups (Rice & Feldman, 1983). The advantages of age restrictions are that they are easy to administer and determine eligibility for; they make administration less costly and complex than some other eligibility criteria;

they limit the overall program costs; and they are easily understood and accepted by the public.

The disadvantages are that they would exclude the large number of those individuals under the age of 65 who commonly need long-term care services because they have permanent or progressive symptoms from a variety of complex illnesses such as Alzheimer's disease, acquired immunodeficiency syndrome, stroke, brain tumors, accidents, infections, and many other diseases. Many children have severe disabilities (they constitute 5 percent of the disabled) and are not eligible for coverage under existing public programs (Schoenborn & Marano, 1988). Seventy-eight percent of the disabled who receive Social Security or Supplemental Security Income/SSP nationally and 14 percent of those currently in nursing homes are under 65 years of age (Hing, Sekscenski, & Strahan, 1987). Thirty-four percent (11 million) of the noninstitutionalized population who have limitations in activity owing to chronic conditions are under 65 (Schoenborn & Marano, 1988). Thus, the disabled population under 65 is an important group that needs coverage.

A national long-term care program could be limited to those who are poor or almost poor or could cover all income groups. A limited program could use the Medicaid model by restricting services to those with low incomes and assets (i.e., a "means test" of an individual's income at a specified level is used). This approach to eligibility targets scarce public resources to those with the greatest economic need and reduces the total program costs to government. "Means testing" for program eligibility is opposed by many for several reasons. It is difficult to determine income and costly to administer, it creates a stigma against those who are eligible, and it is not necessarily cost saving for the public because individuals may postpone treatment and then have higher costs in the long run (Blumenthal, Schlesinger, & Drumbeller, 1988). Income tests could undermine the political support for the program.

Universal eligibility for everyone judged to need services based upon pre-established criteria and using an entitlement or social insurance program is the most ideal. This type of approach is used for Medicare, in which individuals are required to pay into the program and eligibility is unrelated to financial status. Such a program could eliminate inequities based upon income. The primary argument against universal eligibility is one of program costs. To address this issue, long-term care services could be limited to those that have an established need for service based on a specified level of disability. Many different definitions of disability are currently being used by public programs and therefore one uniform set of eligibility criteria that would be used for all long-term care is needed.

## Delivery System

The current delivery system is highly fragmented among many acute, ambulatory, and long-term care providers. Long-term care providers are frequently situated in small, freestanding organizations. The fragmentation of long-term care services creates unnecessary duplication of administrative services and potentially higher costs and fails to achieve economies of scale in organizations with few clients (Zawadski,

1983). The irrational system makes it difficult to monitor quality of care and utilization of services.

A serious consequence of delivery fragmentation is the confusion and frustration experienced by individuals and families when seeking help. Without a single point of entry for coordinated long-term care beyond the primary physician, patients and families must search through information and referral services for compartmentalized services. It is not uncommon for individuals seeking help to be "assessed" again and again, pay fees for each encounter, and repeatedly have to request medical records from physicians. Few physicians and other health providers, including those primarily serving the elderly, are informed about services in the community and still fewer have staff to assist patients seeking help.

Ideally, the health care system should be coordinated, consolidated, efficient, accessible, and innovative. Two approaches encourage the coordination and delivery of long-term care services: the brokered system model (which does not change the organizations that provide services in a community but rather attempts to systematically coordinate services among organizations); and the consolidated delivery model (in which all services are provided by a single organization). Prepaid health plans and health maintenance organizations (HMOs) are the principal organizations that currently deliver health care through a consolidated model, but most offer only limited long-term care services to members. An example of the brokered system model was the national channeling demonstration project in which case management services were added to long-term care programs to coordinate and facilitate the delivery of services. Most of these types of demonstration projects have increased long-term care costs (Kemper, Applebaum, & Harrigan, 1987).

Two long-term care demonstrations have used consolidated program models: the social health maintenance organizations and the On Lok Senior Health Service demonstration in San Francisco. In both models, the organization provides a full range of acute, ambulatory, and long-term care services. On Lok targets only the frail elderly population but provides a full range of health services under a capitated payment system. Social health maintenance organizations are capitated programs similar to HMOs, except that they provide additional long-term care benefits beyond those covered by Medicare for those who are chronically ill. There are four social health maintenance organization demonstration sites in the country that enroll a cross-section of the elderly Medicare beneficiaries. They use case management and resource coordinators to coordinate the services and manage resources (Harrington et al., 1989; Newcomer & Harrington, 1988).

Consolidated models may be more cost-effective than brokered models. On the other hand, brokered models may be more practical because they require less restructuring of provider organizations and relationships than do consolidated models. Brokered or consolidated models probably have greater capacity for improved service delivery and cost containment than traditional fee-for-service provider arrangements and should be encouraged through financial and other public policy incentives.

Both brokered and consolidated systems for long-term care rely heavily on case management services by nurses and social workers. By using skilled professionals, assistance can be provided to individuals and their families and caregivers in planning, coordinating, and monitoring long-term care services but also in ensuring high quality of care. Case managers for those who are frail and disabled and need assistance are critical components of a long-term care system and should be mandated and paid for by any newly created system. The services of nurses are essential where clients have physical and psychological problems, whereas the services of social workers are valuable for social and financial management issues. These two types of professionals may work together, in combination with multidisciplinary team members (e.g., physicians, homemakers, home health aides, and therapists) because of the complexity of long-term care problems that face many individuals and their families and caregivers.

The delivery system should integrate, or at least coordinate, acute and ambulatory services with long-term care services, since they are "inextricably linked and mutually dependent" (Kane & Kane, 1987). Some believe that acute and ambulatory care utilization can be substantially reduced, allowing for potential shifts in acute care to less expensive community-based long-term care services (Kane & Kane, 1987). The pattern of health expenditures among the elderly shows that 66 percent is spent on hospital and physician services compared with 21 percent for nursing home care and 13 percent for other care (Waldo & Lazenby, 1984). Since long-term care is closely tied to acute and ambulatory care services, it is difficult if not illogical to separate them. Failure to integrate and coordinate services may lead to adverse outcomes in terms of access, quality, and costs for those who need long-term care.

## Utilization Controls

One major concern about expanding the financial coverage for long-term care services is that more individuals will demand formal long-term care services than currently use them. Rivlin and Wiener (1988) estimate that long-term care insurance coverage could result in a 20 percent increase in nursing home utilization and a 50 percent increase in community and home health care use. Increases in utilization resulting from expanding financial coverage may be expected to level off after the initial period, as reportedly occurred in Canada after about 3 years of long-term care coverage (Kane & Kane, 1985).

Even though some increases in utilization may be expected, the key to any financing system is to install utilization controls that can be used to prevent overuse or inappropriate utilization. Traditionally, utilization for nursing homes has been limited under Medicare and Medicaid by 3-day prior hospitalization requirements and by specific level of care requirements. The 3-day requirements can actually increase the hospital and overall costs and have not been examined for overall cost-effectiveness. Under the new 1990 proposed Medicaid rules for nursing homes, physician certification and recertification, which were used as gatekeeping methods, are abolished (Federal Register, 1990). Physician authorization of home care services has also traditionally been used as a gatekeeping approach. The regulation is frequently inappropriate and hinders nurses from making professional decisions regarding home care services. Prior authorization procedures for services, generally conducted by nurses or social workers, have also been used, as have preadmission screening programs in which individual physical and mental assessments are made by professionals to determine need. Again, these types of programs introduce gate-keeping barriers to care but do not guarantee that the most appropriate, cost-effective services are provided.

Utilization controls alone, without the provision of information, referral, and coordination of services, can limit access and create serious problems for those in need of services. Many states have combined gatekeeping programs with case management and community services and have demonstrated that such programs can be effective in preventing unnecessary institutionalization and ensuring the use of appropriate services (InterStudy, 1988b; Justice, 1988). Thus, utilization controls are necessary but must be combined with information and referral, case management, care coordination, and other such services where appropriate.

Case management by nurses and social workers appears to be an effective method for controlling utilization by providing assessment, planning, authorization, coordination, and monitoring of long-term care services. This approach can ensure that individuals have a need for services based on standardized criteria before services are authorized, while at the same time providing professional assistance in planning and coordination of appropriate services (Mechanic, 1987; Ruchlin, 1982; Kemper et al., 1987). At the same time, professional judgment is needed to ensure that utilization controls are sensitive and flexible, to ensure access to those with special needs, and to take into account informal caregiver resources and individual prefer-ences for services. By placing the utilization control responsibilities in the hands of professional nurses, cost controls can be monitored at the same time that access is guaranteed to those with the greatest needs and appropriate case management ser-vices are provided.

## Costs

Like other health care expenditures, the costs of long-term care have been increasing rapidly. Fee-for-service payment systems, where each provider is paid for a unit of service delivered, have been considered inflationary. Public and traditional private insurance plans, which pay for services to providers on a fee-for-service basis, have given incentives to providers to increase the number and complexity of services and their subsequent costs. These types of traditional plans are steadily disappearing from the general health market and are expected to constitute no more than 5 to 10 percent of the market in the near future. They are being replaced by managed care programs, such as HMOs, Preferred Provider Organizations (PPOs) and self-insured purchasers (Hale & Hunter, 1988).

Cost controls are essential to ensuring the affordability of a long-term care financ-ing system for the government. Managed care, transferring financial risk to providers (within limits), regulation of payments, and financial disclosure of income, costs, and earnings are ways to control costs. Managed care programs that are financially at risk have built-in incentives to control costs. These organizations may encourage more appropriate utilization of services because providers have no incentives to use services unnecessarily and may encourage efficiency through the use of low cost and low technology services.

More important, the regulation of provider rates is needed to control costs, equalize reimbursement rates across all public and private payers, and ensure cost-effective systems (Harrington et al., 1985). The current system allows public and private payers to use different reimbursement methods and rates with wide rate variations. In some instances, nursing homes and other long-term care providers have not met the minimum staffing and other requirements in order to keep costs low (Hawes & Phillips, 1986). All-payer rate regulation or annual global budgeting for facilities and services (as is done in Canada) can be established to ensure adequate levels of payment for direct service costs and to equalize rates across payers. The costs of care for public programs would probably increase, but this balance could be phased in over time. Public rate setting could ensure that rates are reasonable to provide appropriate levels of professional and other staffing while preventing arbitrary price inflation by providers. Uniform and rational rate setting for institutional or home care providers would not necessarily affect nurses or other caregivers negatively; wage increases could be passed through with inflation while controlling growth in profits and unnecessary administrative costs.

Issues of profit making are particularly problematic in long-term care, an area in which 75 percent of the nursing homes and a growing percentage of home care agencies are proprietary (National Center for Health Statistics, 1987). A wide variation exists in profitability among nursing home providers, and providers are also allowed to increase their private pay rates to offset costs for public payers. Providers also have minimal audits and thus have little accountability to the public for public or private revenues. The great variability in rates, fees, standards of payment, and conditions of provider participation in public programs adds significantly to the administrative costs of paying for care for both purchasers and providers and does not reflect wide differences in patient need. Unfortunately, none of the current legislative proposals addresses the issues of profit taking and the effects of profit making on health care.

## Financing Options

There are four public policy financing options for long-term care. One approach is to make no changes in public policies and hope that voluntary private insurance will gradually expand to cover long-term care services without public policy intervention. A second option is to adopt public policy interventions to provide public funds to expand or subsidize private long-term care insurance. The third approach is to expand public financing of long-term care incrementally and/or to combine some public financing with private dollars. The fourth approach is to develop public financing for all of long-term care.

Recent attention has been focused on the viability of expanding private sector financing for long-term care services, particularly private insurance (Meiners, 1983; Anlyan & Lipscomb, 1985). Private insurance plans have been growing rapidly, but still only about 1 million policies were sold in 1988 (U.S. Department of Health and Human Services, 1987; U.S. General Accounting Office, 1989; U.S. Senate, 1989). Generally speaking, these private insurance policies favor nursing home care over home care and offer only limited indemnity coverage (flat rates of payment per day) (Consumer Reports, 1988; U.S. General Accounting Office, 1987; U.S. Senate, 1989). Premiums vary by the duration, coverage, and deductible period but are generally expensive, and costs increase dramatically with the individual's age when the policy is initially purchased (U.S. General Accounting Office, 1987; Rivlin & Wiener, 1988; Firman et al., 1988). Because of the benefit restrictions, the chances for not collecting any benefits are high (Firman et al., 1988). To respond to criticisms, private insurance carriers and other advocates have formulated alternative strategies for reducing their risk and improving their products.

Brookings-ICF (Rivlin & Wiener, 1988) have recently published an extensive analysis of the demand and public costs likely to result from enrollment in private long-term care insurance. They conclude that only one third of the elderly would be able to afford a moderately comprehensive policy in the period from 2016 to 2020. Since the market would be composed primarily of upper and upper-middle income individuals, the Brookings-ICF study concluded that private insurance will have little effect on reducing future public long-term care costs.

## Public Financing Model

Many experts have recommended expanded public financing of long-term care (Rivlin & Wiener, 1988; Blumenthal et al., 1988; InterStudy, 1988a; Villers Foundation, 1987; Lewin & Associates, 1987; Kane & Kane, 1985). Most other proposals recommend an expansion of the current Medicare program and focus primarily on the aged. An alternative proposal would develop a comprehensive national health program for long-term care, similar to the Canadian model (Kane & Kane, 1985). In Canada, long-term care services are basic entitlements for everyone (regardless of age or income) and are another component of a basic health care plan. Canada has been able to provide broad nursing home and community-based services without runaway inflation by using a case management system to determine need for services and to authorize such services. And finally, the Canadian system for long-term care is administered at the provincial and local levels so that models vary somewhat across the different provinces (Kane & Kane, 1985).

Public insurance models have a number of advantages over private financing models. One is that overall program efficiencies could be engendered. By consolidating existing public programs, administrative efficiencies should be achievable. By establishing similar rules for benefits, eligibility, utilization controls, reimbursement, and other program components, cost savings over the current administrative structure may be possible. Duplicated administrative costs across the public and private programs could be eliminated.

Another major advantage of public insurance models would be to lower the overall program administrative costs below those that currently exist in the private market. Overall, state and federal program administration costs have been estimated to be about 5 percent of total program costs for the Medicaid program nationally, with a payout ratio of 95 percent for services (Rivlin & Wiener, 1988). In contrast, Blue Cross/Blue Shield had a payout ratio on its premiums of 92 percent; self-insured plans had an average ratio of 91.7 percent; prepaid plans had a ratio of 88.3 percent; and private insurance had a ratio of 81.1 percent in 1986 (Division of National Cost Estimates, 1987). Those dollars not paid on benefits are used for administration, profits, and other program costs. Some Medicare supplemental plans have a payout ratio of only 60 percent or less (U.S. General Accounting Office, 1986). Thus, it is expected that a public program would have lower overhead costs for marketing, administration, and profits.

Other potential advantages of a public program are that uniform benefits and eligibility would be easier to achieve; benefits received could be proportionate to premiums invested; financial risk could be spread across the working age population as well as the elderly; lower overall provider rates could be achieved by concentrating purchasing power; and discrepancies in quality and access between private and public payers could be eliminated. Cost savings should result in administrative savings that could be used to expand long-term care services.

Finally, public opinion surprisingly supports a public program model. A 1987 public opinion survey by the American Association of Retired Persons and Villers Foundation found that the majority of Americans believe that a public rather than a private program would best safeguard the elderly's long-term care needs of the elderly. Public programs administered by the federal government were preferred over private insurance programs by a margin of 3 to 2 (R.L. Associates, 1987). This poll found by a 2 to 1 margin that the public believed that private insurance companies would undermine quality of care because of profits. Although the respondents wanted a federally financed program, they supported the administration of such a program at the state level (R.L. Associates, 1987).

The disadvantages of a public financing program are that direct public expenditures would be increased; consumers may not support increases in taxes for such a program; costs are difficult to estimate and control and could be higher than expected; more individuals would be entitled to services and therefore utilization and costs could increase; and reductions in out-of-pocket costs could lead to increased service use. In spite of the disadvantages, a publicly financed system appears to be the most viable approach for ensuring access to needed services by the population and controlling costs.

Another issue is whether or not participation in financing long-term care should be voluntary or mandatory or a mix of both provisions. Because voluntary participation gives individuals choices between public and/or private programs, many have advocated this approach (Davis & Rowland, 1986; Blumenthal et al., 1988). Problems can occur with voluntary models because many older persons are unaware of the need for coverage. The Brookings analysis (Rivlin & Wiener, 1988) showed that if a voluntary private insurance model were the primary approach to funding long-term care, many individuals would not join the system. Many of those with the greatest need and who are at risk for long-term care are likely to be low-income persons who cannot afford the premiums. Mandatory participation requires all individuals to be enrolled regardless of their health status or perceived health status. This approach eliminates the problems of what is termed "adverse selection," where the sicker individuals are left to be covered by public programs and the private programs are able to enroll healthier individuals (favorable selection) (Lewin & Associates Inc., 1987). A mandatory public program could reduce the costs of the program per participant by spreading the financial risks, reduce adverse selection by eliminating those who are disabled or ill, and reduce the need for a public safety-net program.

Public and private funds could be combined or pooled into a single public insurance program for the population. Such a mandatory public insurance approach could be administered by a new or existing public program (Himmelstein & Woolhandler, 1989). A single public administrative system, as used in Canada and many Western European countries, allows a concentrated public purchasing power. If used in the United States, it would mean pooling all funds used to purchase long-term care services in an existing state government agency or in one created especially for the purpose. This approach would allow for consolidation of each state's multiple programs. Blumenthal and coworkers (1988) argue that a single administrator has many advantages in terms of administrative simplification. The single administrator reduces administrative costs by eliminating duplication of administration, marketing cost, quality monitoring, and related activities; vests enormous purchasing power in a public entity, resulting in great leverage when negotiating prices and quality standards with providers; and simplifies eligibility and benefit design and related budgeting. On the other hand, some providers may fear concentration of power in the hands of the government (Enthoven & Kronick, 1989), and others object to greater vulnerability to political influences unrelated to health needs (e.g., disputes over abortion can affect budgeting and services development). Although these objections may cause political problems in gaining acceptance of the plan, the advantages of a single administration outweigh the political objections by special interest groups.

## Financing Sources

The key question is who should pay for long-term care: federal, state, and/or local government, private health insurance, patients, families or relatives, employers, or others. Most financing systems in the United States have been based on combinations of payers and include a premium base. Premiums are generally fixed flat-rate payments that the insured must pay to be eligible for service coverage. Under Medicare, for example, the monthly premium for Part B coverage is $28.80 and will gradually increase with the new Medicare catastrophic legislation (Commerce Clearing House Inc., 1989). Premiums offer the advantage of being fixed and predictable and spread the risk among all beneficiaries, not just service users. On the other hand, flat premiums are regressive in placing the highest burden on lower income groups (Blumenthal et al., 1988). If premiums are too high and not adjusted by income, they undermine access to services for poor persons. For these reasons, the use of premiums should not be supported.

A variety of public revenue sources can be used to finance a long-term care system. These include income taxes, payroll taxes, estate taxes, sin taxes (on cigarettes and alcohol), tax credits, or deductions for long-term care expenses, home equity conversions, tax deductions for medical IRAs, lottery funds, or other sources. These options fall into two broad categories: (1) taxes levied on the general population (e.g., payroll taxes, general revenues, income taxes, estate taxes, sin taxes, value added taxes, and selected excise taxes), and (2) taxes levied on the elderly and the disabled (e.g., insurance premiums, income tax surcharges and credits, home equity conversions, tax deductions for medical IRAs, supplementary health insurance taxes, and liens on estates) (Long & Smeeding, 1984). The latter types of tax proposals are regressive in their financial impact on those with lower incomes and place an undue burden on those who are unfortunate enough to become disabled.

The financing of long-term care should ideally use public financing through a progressive taxation system. Thus, the most desirable system would be the income tax system as one of the most progressive tax methods. Currently about 20 percent of the total Medicare program costs (Blumenthal et al., 1988) and all of the Medicaid and other public programs are financed through general revenues. An increasing portion of long-term care could be financed by expanded general taxes. Expanding the current Social Security payroll taxes now established for Medicare would build upon the existing tax system and ensure a broad tax base without unduly burdening individual workers. Blumenthal and associates (1988) have recommended increasing the earned income tax credit for lower income workers to lower their payroll tax burden. The current ceiling on Social Security payroll taxes could be removed to make the system more progressive and to increase revenues without having a negative impact on lower income groups (Blumenthal et al., 1988). Estate taxes are another logical source of funds for long-term care and would have less negative impact on low income groups.

## Conclusions

In summary, a publicly financed system could be developed using the Canadian model. Although a public program model could be developed by expanding or allowing voluntary buy-in to the existing Medicaid program or could be an expansion of the existing Medicare program for the aged, we do not recommend an incremental approach. The most comprehensive public insurance model could be adopted as a single mandatory plan for the population that would combine new public revenues with existing public program dollars. This approach would ensure universal access, comprehensive benefits, improved service delivery, greater cost control, and potentially improved quality of care. Most important, the financial costs can be spread across the entire population and financed through a progressive taxing approach from a combination of sources.

The nursing profession, as one of the primary providers of long-term care services, and the public have a direct and immediate interest in reforming the current financing and delivery system for long-term care. The current inadequately financed system is the greatest barrier to the professional practice of nursing in long-term care. Although there is growing public policy concern about long-term care services, most of the current federal legislative proposals are narrowly focused on limited expansion of benefits to the elderly under Medicare or Medicaid and the encouragement of expansion of private long-term care insurance. The expansion of benefits under public programs is essential, because private sector solutions do not appear viable.

Nursing as a profession should support a major reform of the financing and delivery of long-term care, under a mandatory publicly financed system modeled after the Canadian system, with broad benefits, universal coverage, delivery system reform, controls on reimbursement rates, and utilization controls. Local, state, and national nursing organizations should become familiar with the problems of long-term care and give full support to candidates and policies that will bring about a major reform, not simply small incremental changes in the financing and delivery of long-term care services.

## REFERENCES

American Hospital Association (1986). *Hospital statistics: 1986 edition.* Chicago: American Hospital Association.

Anlyan, W.G., & Lipscomb, J. (1985). The National Health Care Trust Plan: A blueprint for market and long-term care reform. *Health Affairs, 4*(3), 5–31.

Blumenthal, D., Schlesinger, M., & Drumbeller, P.B. (1988). *Renewing the promise: Medicare and its reform.* New York: Oxford University Press.

Branch, L.G., Friedman, D.J., Cohen, M.A., Smith, N., & Socholitzky, E. (1988). Impoverishing the elderly: A case study of the financial risk of spend-down among Massachusetts elderly people. *The Gerontologist, 28*(5), 648–652.

Commerce Clearing House, Inc. (1989, December 8). Medicare Catastrophic Coverage Repeal Act of 1989, HR 3608. *Medicare and Medicaid guide.* CCH #603. Chicago: Commerce Clearing House.

Congressional Research Service, Subcommittee on Health and the Environment, Committee on Energy and Commerce (1988, November). *Medicaid source book: Background data and analysis.* Washington, DC: U.S. Government Printing Office.

*Consumer Reports* (1988, May). "Who can afford a nursing home?" *Consumer Reports, 53*(5), 300–311.

Davis, K., & Rowland, D. (1986). *Medicare policy: New directions for health and long-term care.* Baltimore: Johns Hopkins University Press.

Division of National Cost Estimates, Office of the Actuary, Health Care Financing Administration (1987). National health expenditures, 1986–2000. *Health Care Financing Review, 8*(4), 1–36.

Enthoven, A., & Kronick, R. (1989, January 12). A consumer-choice health plan for the 1990s. *New England Journal of Medicine, 320*(2), 94–101.

Estes, C.L., Newcomer, R.J., and Associates. (1983). *Fiscal austerity and aging.* Beverly Hills, CA: Sage Publications.

Federal Register, Department of Health and Human Services (1990, March 23). 42 CFR Part 405, Medicare and Medicaid programs; Nurse aide training and competency evaluation programs and preadmission screening and annual resident review; proposed rules. *Federal Register,* 10938–10981.

Firman, J., Weissert, W., Wilson, C.E. (1988). *Private long term care insurance: How well is it meeting consumer needs and public policy concerns?* Washington, DC: United Seniors Health Cooperative.

Gornick, M., Greenberg, J.N., Eggers, P.W., & Dobson, A. (1985). Twenty years of Medicare and Medicaid: Covered populations, use of benefits, and program expenditures. *Health Care Financing Review,* Ann. Suppl., 13–59.

Hale, J.A., & Hunter, M.M., at InterStudy (1988, June). *From HMO movement to managed care industry: The future of HMOs in a volatile healthcare market.* Excelsior, MN: InterStudy.

Harrington, C., Newcomer, R.J., & Friedlob, A. (1989, September). Medicare beneficiary enrollment in S/HMO (Chapter 4). In R.J. Newcomer, C. Harrington, & A. Friedlob, *Social health maintenance organization demonstration evaluation: Report on the first thirty months.* Prepared for Health Care Financing Administration, Contract No. HCFA 85-034/CP.

Harrington, C., Newcomer, R.J., Estes, C.L., and Associates. (1985). *Long term care of the elderly: Public policy issues.* Beverly Hills, CA: Sage Publications.

Hawes, C., & Phillips, C.D. (1986). The changing structure of the nursing home industry and the impact of ownership on quality, cost, and access. In B.H. Gray (Ed.), Institute of Medicine, *For-profit enterprise in health care.* Washington, DC: Academy Press.

Himmelstein, D.U., Woolhandler. (1989). A national health program for the United States: A physician's proposal. *New England Journal of Medicine, 320*(2), 102–108.

InterStudy (1988a, September). *InterStudy's long-term care expansion program: A proposal for reform.* Volume I. Excelsior, MN: InterStudy.

InterStudy (1988b, September). *InterStudy's long-term care expansion program: Issue papers.* Volume II. Excelsior, MN: InterStudy.

Justice, D. (1988). *State long term care reform: Development of community care systems in six states.* Washington, DC: National Governor's Association.

Kane, R.A., & Kane, R.L. (1982). *Values and long-term care.* Lexington, MA: Lexington Books.

Kane, R.A., & Kane, R.L. (1987). Long-term care: Principles, programs, and policies. New York: Springer Publishing Company.

Kane, R.L., & Kane, R.A. (1985). *A will and a way: What the United States can learn from Canada about care of the elderly.* New York: Columbia University Press.

Kemper, P., Applebaum, R., & Harrigan, M. (1987). Community Care demonstrations: What have we learned? *Health Care Financing Review, 8*(4), 87–100. HCFA Pub. No. 03239. Office of Research and Demonstrations, Health Care Financing Administration, Washington, DC: U.S. Government Printing Office.

Levit, K.R., & Freeland, M.S. (1988). National medical care spending. *Health Affairs, 7*(5), 124–136.

Lewin and Associates, Inc. (1987). Draft proposal long term care social Insurance Program Initiative. Prepared for Advisory Committee. Sponsored by the American Association of Retired Persons, Older Women's League and the Villers Foundation. Washington, DC: Lewin and Associates Inc.

Liu, K., Manton, K.G., & Liu, B.M. (1985). Home care expenses for the disabled elderly. *Health Care Financing Review, 7*(2), 51–57.

Mechanic, D. (1987). Challenges in health and long-term care policy. *Health Affairs, 6*(2), 22–34.

Meiners, M. (1983). The case for long-term care insurance. *Health Affairs, 2*(2), 55–79.

National Center for Health Statistics, Hing, E., Sekscenski, E., & Strahan, G. (1987). The

National Nursing Home Survey; 1985 summary for the United States. *Vital and Health Statistics*, Series 13, No. 97. Department of Health and Human Services Publication No. (PHS) 89-1758. Public Health Service. Washington, DC: U.S. Government Printing Office.

National Center for Health Statistics, Schoenborn, C.A., & Marano, M. (1988). Current estimates from the National Health Interview Survey: United States, 1987. *Vital and Health Statistics*, Series 10, No. 166. Department of Health and Human Services Publication No. (PHS) 88-1594. Public Health Service. Washington, DC: U.S. Government Printing Office.

Newcomer, R.J., & Harrington, C. (1988). Social health maintenance organizations (S/HMOs): Assessing their potential role in health and long-term care service delivery. In California Health and Welfare Agency, *A study of California's publicly funded long-term care programs 1988* (pp. 169–216). Sacramento, CA: California Health and Welfare Agency.

R.L. Associates (1987, October). *The American public views long term care: A survey conducted for the American Association of Retired Persons and the Villers Foundation*. Princeton, NJ: R.L. Associates.

Rivlin, A.M., & Weiner, J.M. (1988). *Caring for the disabled elderly: Who will pay?* Washington, DC: The Brookings Institution.

Rovner, J. (1988, April 9). Lawmakers taking hard look at problem of long-term care. *Congressional Quarterly, 46*(15): 939–940.

Ruchlin, H.S. (1982, January 14). Management and financing of long-term-care services. *New England Journal of Medicine, 306*(2), 101–106.

Spence, D.A., & Wiener, J.M. (1989, March). Medicaid spend-down in nursing homes: Estimates from the 1985 National Nursing Home Survey. Unpublished paper prepared for the Brookings Institution, Economic Studies Program.

Stone, R. (1986, September 30). Aging in the eighties, age 65 years and over–Use of community services: Preliminary data from the supplement on aging to the National Health Interview Survey: United States January–June 1985. *NCHS Advance Data, 124*, 1–8.

Stone, R., Cafferata, G.L., & Sangl, J. (1987, October). Caregivers of the frail elderly: A national profile. *The Gerontologist, 27*(5), 616–626.

U.S. Congressional Budget Office (CBO). (1987, October 1). Statement of Nancy Gordon, Assistant Director for Human Resources and Community Department, CBO, before the Health Task Force Committee on the Budget, U.S. House of Representatives, Washington, DC.

U.S. Department of Commerce (1990). International Trade Administration. Health and Medical Services. *U.S. Industrial Outlook 1990*. Washington, DC: U.S. Department of Commerce.

U.S. Department of Health and Human Services (1987). Task Force on Long-Term Care Policies. *Report to Congress and the Secretary: Long-term health care policies*. Washington, DC: U.S. Government Printing Office.

U.S. Department of Health and Human Services (1988, November 18). National health expenditures 1987. *HHS News*. Washington, DC: Department of Health and Human Services.

U.S. General Accounting Office (1986, October). Report to the Subcommittee on Health, Committee on Ways and Means, House of Representatives. *Medigap insurance law has increased protection against substandard and overpriced policies*. Washington, DC: U.S. General Accounting Office.

U.S. General Accounting Office (1987, May). Report to the Subcommittee on Health, Committee on Ways and Means, House of Representatives. *Long-term care insurance varies widely in a developing market.* Washington, DC: U.S. General Accounting Office.

U.S. General Accounting Office (1988, November). Report to the Subcommittee on Health, Committee on Ways and Means, House of Representatives. *Long-term care for the elderly: Issues of need, access and cost.* Washington, DC: U.S. General Accounting Office, HRD-89-4.

U.S. General Accounting Office (1989, April). Report to the Subcommittee on Health, Committee on Ways and Means, House of Representatives. *Long-term care insurance: State regulatory requirements provide inconsistent consumer protection.* Washington, DC: U.S. General Accounting Office.

U.S. House, Committee on Ways and Means (1987, April 23). *Medicare Quality Protection Act of 1986.* Hearing. Serial No. 99-75. Washington, DC: U.S. House of Representatives.

U.S. Senate (1989, January 28). *Developments in aging: 1988, Vol. 1, Vol. 2, Vol. 3.* A report of the Special Committee on Aging, United States Senate. Washington, DC: U.S. Government Printing Office.

U.S. Social Security Administration (1984). Department of Health and Human Services. *Income and resources of the population 65 and over.* Washington, DC: U.S. Government Printing Office, Social Security Administration Publication No. 13-11727, p. 11.

Villers Foundation (1987). *Long term care conference.* Washington, DC: Villers Foundation.

Waldo, D., & Lazenby, H.C. (1984, Fall). Demographic characteristics and health care use and expenditures by the aged in the United States: 1977–1984. *Health Care Financing Review, 6*(1), 1–31.

Wiener, J.M., Hanley, R.J., Spence, D.A., & Murray, S.E. (1989). We can run but we can't hide: Toward reforming long-term care. *Journal of Aging & Social Policy, 1*(1/2), 87–102.

Zawadski, R.T. (1983, Fall/Winter). The long term care demonstration projects: What they are and why they came into being. *Home Health Care Services Quarterly, 4*(3/4), 3–19.

## Chapter 14

# Nursing Homes: Residents' Needs; Nursing's Response

MATHY MEZEY

*A* NURSING HOME STAY is now a common event for the elderly population in America. Although only 5 percent of the elderly reside in nursing homes at any point in time, the lifetime risk of entering a nursing home is approximately 20 percent. One out of every five individuals living past the age of 65 and one out of three aged 85 or older will spend some time in a nursing home.

As a result of the "aging" of society and changes in hospital practices, the character of nursing homes has changed dramatically in the past 10 years. Gone are the relatively small institutions that provided a permanent home for the elderly who, for the most part, were in good physical health but lacked the capacity to live independently in the community. Nursing homes are now complex institutions caring for people who because of severe incapacities need both subacute and chronic care.

Despite the increasing acuity of residents, the need to improve the overall quality of care in nursing homes remains largely unaddressed. Where quality care is delivered, professional nursing is pivotal in achieving high standards. But the majority of homes continue to be hampered by minimal standards, limited expectations, and restrictive reimbursement. Despite intermittent concern regarding inadequate care ("Neglect at Nursing Home," 1990; Institute of Medicine, 1986), many nursing homes continue to function without an on-site professional provider. A registered nurse may be "in charge" but not necessarily present. And the professional nurse-to-patient ratio provides on average no more than 12 minutes of registered nurse time per resident per day. Recent legislative and regulatory recognition of substandard care has led to some reforms, for example, enhanced requirements for resident assessment and nurse's aide training. However, the need for a professional nursing presence in nursing homes has yet to be fully recognized.

The purpose of this chapter is to provide an in-depth description of elderly nursing home residents and their caregivers, and, based on recent findings from several demonstration projects, to propose a specific strategy—the use of nurse specialists—as a proven mechanism for improving overall quality of care.

198

## Nursing Homes: An Overview

Nursing homes provide around-the-clock services in an institutional setting to residents who have physical and/or mental disabilities that do not allow them to live in the community (Spector, Kapp, & Eichan, 1988). Encouraged by the Medicaid and Medicare programs, beginning in 1965 there was a rapid growth in nursing home beds, with bed capacity increasing an additional 38 percent between 1973–1974 and 1985 (National Center for Health Statistics, 1987b) (Table 14–1).

In contrast to hospitals and, until recently home care agencies, the for-profit nature of nursing homes has greatly influenced society's response to the "legitimacy" of nursing homes as responsible providers of health care. Proprietary (for profit) homes account for 75 percent of all nursing homes and 69 percent of beds (National Center for Health Statistics, 1987b). Today, the nursing home industry is a multibillion dollar business, with one of the highest growth rates in expenditures among all health services (Harrington, Swan, & Grant, 1988). There are more nursing homes than acute care beds. Chain nursing homes, those that are members of a group of facilities operating under one general authority or general ownership, make up 41 percent of total homes and 49 percent of total beds (National Center for Health Statistics, 1987b).

In 1989, the nation spent over $35 billion on nursing home services, representing 9 percent of the total personal health care dollars spent in the United States that year (Health Care Financing Administration, 1989). Once patients are admitted to nursing homes, approximately 50 percent of funding comes from out-of-pocket payments, 41 percent from Medicaid, and 5 percent from Medicare (National Center for Health Statistics, 1987b).

## Case Mix in Nursing Homes

A typical nursing home resident is a very old, white female, with no surviving spouse or children, who is admitted to the home directly from a hospital with multiple diagnoses, including some evidence of impaired mental function. The median age of nursing home residents is now 81 years. Seventy-five percent of elderly residents are female and 93 percent are white (National Center for Health Statistics, 1987a). Over 60 percent of these patients evidence impaired mental capacity in addition to severe functional and physical disabilities.

This composite picture, however, masks the complexity and heterogeneity of nursing home residents and services. The flow of patients in and out of nursing homes is more fluid than was previously thought (Lewis et al., 1987; Shaughnessy & Kramer, 1990). Nationally, nursing home use is approximately evenly divided between those persons having stays of less than 90 days (short stayers) and those with stays over 90 days (long-stay residents). Short-stay residents almost always enter a nursing home for recuperative services following a hospital stay, for example, following a stroke or hip fracture, or for quasi-"hospice" type services in the period

**TABLE 14–1 Percent Distribution of Nursing Homes, Beds, and Beds per Nursing Home by Selected Nursing Home Characteristics: 1985\*†**

| | Nursing Homes N = 19,100 % | Nursing Home Beds N = 1.6 million % | Beds per Nursing Home |
|---|---|---|---|
| *Ownership* | | | |
| Proprietary | 75 | 69 | 78 |
| Voluntary nonprofit | 20 | 23 | 98 |
| Government | 5 | 8 | 132 |
| *Certified Facilities* | 76 | 89 | 99 |
| *Bed Size* | | | |
| < 50 beds | 33 | 9 | 24 |
| 50–99 beds | 32 | 28 | 72 |
| 100–199 beds | 28 | 43 | 130 |
| 200 beds or more | 6 | 20 | 272 |
| *Affiliation* | | | |
| Chain | 41 | 49 | 102 |
| Independent | 52 | 42 | 68 |
| Government | 5 | 8 | 132 |
| Unknown | 0.5 | 0.7 | 116 |

\* Note: Figures may not add up to totals due to rounding.

† Adapted from the National Center for Health Statistics. Strahan, G. *Nursing Home Characteristics Preliminary Data from the 1985 National Nursing Home Survey. National Center for Health Statistics Advance Data,* 131, 1987, p. 3.

prior to death. Long-stay residents, on the other hand, are generally older, more physically and mentally disabled, and have fewer family and social network ties than short-stay residents.

Irrespective of whether a nursing home stay is for the short or long term, nursing home residents are sicker than in the past and are more disabled than persons utilizing home health services. Thus nursing homes now provide unique services that do not duplicate hospital or home care.

## The Health Status of Nursing Home Residents

There is no question that people now admitted to nursing homes are sicker than was the case even 5 years ago. The disability and acuity of nursing home residents, expressed as a nursing home's case mix, have increased substantially. The dominant concerns of a few years ago regarding inappropriate placement of people in nursing homes (Vladeck, 1980) have been replaced by debate over whether the nation has enough facilities to care for those very debilitated elderly who truly need nursing home services.

Acuity in nursing homes is assessed through case mix classification systems that group nursing home residents according to common characteristics. The basis for almost all case mix classification systems in nursing homes is functional ability, as reflected in performance of activities of daily living. Activities of daily living (e.g.,

**TABLE 14–2 Percentage of Nursing Home Residents 65 Years of Age and Over by Type of Dependency in Activities of Daily Living\***

| | Total | |
|---|---|---|
| Dependency Status | 1977 | 1985 |
| Requires assistance in bathing | 88.6 | 91.2 |
| Requires assistance in dressing | 77.7 | 77.7 |
| Requires assistance in using toilet room | 54.8 | 63.3 |
| Requires assistance in transferring | | 62.7 |
| Continence—difficulty with bowel and/or bladder control | 47.3 | 54.5 |
| Requires assistance in eating | 33.6 | 40.4 |

\* Data from the National Center for Health Statistics. E. Hing. *Use of Nursing Homes by the Elderly: Preliminary Data from the National Nursing Home Survey.* Advance Data from *Vital and Health Statistics*, No. 135, Department of Health and Human Services Publication No. (Public Health Service) 87-1250. Public Health Service, Hyattsville, MD: May 14, 1987.

bathing, dressing, toileting, transferring, and feeding) are thought to provide an indirect measure of "vitality" (Spector et al., 1988) and to be more sensitive than disease or severity of illness as indicators of health. Age of resident and other indicators of disability may also be considered when classifying nursing home residents.

One has only to examine the decline in average functional levels of residents in nursing homes between 1977 and 1985 to appreciate the enormity of case mix changes (National Center for Health Statistics, 1987a; Spector et al., 1988) (Table 14–2). Of 4000 new admissions to nursing homes in 1985, 51 percent were dependent in five activities of daily living (Spector et al., 1988). In addition to a very high level of functional disability, nursing home residents experience frequent exacerbations of chronic illnesses as well as new episodes of acute illness. One in four residents is hospitalized annually, and one in three requires a hospital emergency room (Aiken, Mezey, Lynaugh, & Buck, 1985).

Four factors—the aging of the population; the Prospective Payment System (PPS); restriction of bed supply; and case mix reimbursement—have each substantially contributed to the increase in acuity of nursing home residents.

*The Aging of the Population.* Of 1.6 million nursing home residents, those aged 85 and over constitute the largest age group (45 percent) and account for 76 percent of the 17 percent overall increase in nursing home utilization between 1977 and 1985 (National Center for Health Statistics, 1987b).

Residents in nursing homes who have long stays are more likely to be older and functionally and mentally impaired at the outset of their nursing home stay, and as this cohort of residents "ages in place" in the facility, they are at ever-increasing risk of greater morbidity (Spector et al., 1988). Nationally, the average number of dependencies in activities of daily living is 3.8 for residents aged 75 to 84 in contrast to 4.2 for those 85 and over (National Center for Health Statistics, 1987b).

*Prospective Payment for Hospital Care.* Since the introduction of the Medicare PPS for hospital care, a stay in a nursing home substitutes for time previously spent in a hospital (Lyles, 1987; Morrisey et al., 1988). Moreover, there is disturbing evidence that admission to a nursing home after a hospital stay, other things being equal, reduces the probability of the resident's ever returning to the community.

The greatest proportion of residents (39 percent) are admitted to nursing homes directly from general or short-stay hospitals (National Center for Health Statistics, 1987b). Since PPS was first introduced, although hospital length of stay for Medicare beneficiaries have decreased by approximately 2 days (American Hospital Association, 1988), nursing home discharges from acute care hospitals, as a percentage of all admissions, more than doubled (American Hospital Association, 1988). Fifty percent or more of admissions to skilled nursing homes in 1984 were Medicare admissions (Lewis et al., 1987; Spector et al., 1988), and these patients were the sickest in each diagnosis-related group (DRG) category of new admissions (Neu & Harrison, 1988; Shaughnessy & Kramer, 1990).

Fitzgerald, Moore, and Dittus (1988), in a study of elderly hip fracture patients residing in the community before and after implementation of PPS, found decreases in lengths of hospital stay from 15.9 days in 1983 to 8.6 days in 1985. However, discharges to nursing homes were 100 percent higher after the start of PPS. At 6 months following hospital discharge, 48 percent of those discharged to a nursing home remained in the home compared with 21 percent prior to PPS.

*Restrictions in Bed Supply and Case Mix Reimbursement.* The bed supply in nursing homes has failed to keep pace with increases in the elderly population and the increased demand created by hospitals. Nursing homes in 1984 operated at about 92 percent of capacity, a significant increase over the 1972 rate of 86 percent (National Center for Health Statistics, 1987b). The National Center for Health Statistics (1987b) reports a decline of 2.8 beds per 1000 population 65 and over between 1977 and 1988.

The high rate of bed occupancy and declines in bed supply must be viewed in the light of current and projected increases in the 85 years of age and older population who are proportionally higher users of nursing homes. Persons over 65 years old who are 85 and older increased from 40 percent in 1977 to 45 percent in 1985. Between 1990 and 2010, the age cohort 85+ will grow three to four times as fast as the general population.

In summary, there is strong and conclusive evidence that the acuity of residents admitted to nursing homes is increasing and that nursing home stays now substitute in part for hospital days. To a large degree, the overwhelming majority of residents who are appropriately placed in nursing homes are now truly "patients." This increase in acuity has substantial implications for nursing home staffing in general and utilization of registered nurses in particular.

## Nurse Staffing in Nursing Homes

Of the 1.2 million full-time equivalent employees who work in nursing homes, 700,000 provide nursing or personal care services. Nursing aides and orderlies account for over 40 percent of the total. Registered nurses, on the other hand, make up fewer than 7 percent of nursing home employees (National Center for Health

**TABLE 14–3 Number of Registered Nurses Working in Nursing Homes and Rate of Registered Nurses per 100 Nursing Home Beds, by Selected Facility Characteristics: United States, 1985***

| Facility Characteristic | Number | Registered Nurses per 100 Beds |
|---|---|---|
| Total | 103,100 | 6.3 |
| Ownership | | |
| Proprietary | 59,100 | 5.3 |
| Voluntary nonprofit | 32,000 | 8.6 |
| Government | 12,000 | 9.1 |
| Certification | | |
| Skilled nursing facility only | 25,900 | 8.4 |
| Skilled nursing facility and intermediate care facility | 55,900 | 7.7 |
| Intermediate care facility only | 14,800 | 3.6 |
| Not certified | 6,100 | 3.3 |
| Bed size | | |
| Fewer than 50 beds | 7,500 | 5.0 |
| 50–99 beds | 27,400 | 6.2 |
| 100–199 beds | 42,900 | 6.1 |
| 200 beds or more | 25,200 | 7.7 |
| Geographic region | | |
| Northeast | 32,600 | 8.8 |
| North Central | 35,300 | 6.6 |
| South | 18,100 | 3.7 |
| West | 17,100 | 7.3 |
| Place of residence | | |
| MSA† | 77,500 | 7.0 |
| Not MSA | 25,600 | 5.0 |

* From the National Center for Health Statistics. Strahan, G. *Characteristics of Registered Nurses in Nursing Homes, Preliminary Data from the 1985 National Nursing Home Survey. National Center for Health Statistics Advance Data,* 152, 1988, p. 4.
† Metropolitan statistical area.

Statistics, 1988) and less than 12 percent of the total nursing staff. Of the more than 1.6 million employed nurses in the United States, only 7 percent are employed in nursing homes (National Center for Health Statistics, 1988).

The public's perception to the contrary, minimum federal staffing requirements fail to assure an adequate professional nursing presence in nursing homes. Although the actual number of registered nurses in individual nursing homes varies considerably, only 5.6 percent of nursing homes are required to have a registered nurse on duty 24 hours a day (Jones, Bonito, Gower, & Williams, 1987). Fifty-two percent of nursing homes have no state minimum full-time registered nurse requirement. Forty-three percent have full-time but not 24-hour registered nurse requirements (Health Care Financing Administration, 1988).

In 1985 there were 6.3 registered nurses per 100 nursing home beds (National Center for Health Statistics, 1988). Medicare-certified nursing homes had 6.1 registered nurses per facility and 17.3 beds per registered nurse (Table 14–3.). Nationally, registered nurse employment evidences a high degree of variability across states, with a range of 7.7 certified beds per registered nurse in New Hampshire to 89.8 in Texas.

Consequently, because available staff is distributed over a 24-hour period, for every 100 nursing home beds the average staffing is one registered nurse (who is most likely to be the director of nursing), 1.5 licensed practical nurses, and 6.5 nursing assistants. The median amount of registered nurse time per resident per day across all nursing homes in 1985 was 12 minutes or less. Nearly 40 percent of nursing homes (7402 homes) report 6 minutes or less of registered nurse time per resident per day, and 60 percent of these report no registered nurse hours during the past week (Jones et al., 1987). In general, voluntary and government facilities and larger homes report higher ratios of registered nurses per 100 beds (Table 14–3) (Jones et al., 1987).

Logically, one would expect that if nursing home residents were sicker, professional nurse staffing would increase. In fact, however, despite increased resident acuity, the proportion of registered nurses to total nursing staff has remained relatively stable (U.S. Department of Health and Human Services, 1990). As in 1977, registered nurses still make up less than 7 percent of a nursing home's total full-time equivalent employees (National Center for Health Statistics, 1988). In a study of Pennsylvania nursing homes before and after implementation of PPS (Kanda & Mezey, 1991), despite significant increases in patient acuity, the proportion of full- and part-time registered nurses actually declined, caused primarily by a decrease in part-time registered nurses.

Because of the limited nurse-to-patient ratios, nursing practice in nursing homes is vastly different from that of hospitals. It is unusual for registered nurses in nursing homes to deliver direct patient care. Rather, their time is spent on administrative and supervisory tasks. The relative absence of physicians in nursing homes also influences registered nurses' work responsibilities. Fewer than 2 percent of nursing homes have a physician available on the premises at all times. Six percent report a physician available on the premises during weekdays. The most common coverage (48 percent of nursing homes) is physician availability on the premises but only at scheduled times (Jones et al., 1987).

Although there is strong evidence that many registered nurses working in nursing homes prefer long-term care over other areas of practice (Collings, 1986), failure to retain adequate numbers of registered nurses in nursing homes continues to be of major concern. Retention rates are the greatest for younger nurses. Registered nurses under the age of 35 have a retention rate of 77 percent in hospitals as compared with 51 percent in nursing homes. Moreover, retention is substantially linked to salary. One-year retention is 65 percent for nurses earning minimum salaries compared with 83 percent for those earning higher wages.

In 1986, almost 10 percent of registered nurses in nursing homes made less than $300 per week. Only 17 percent made $500 per week or more (Jones et al., 1987). In nursing homes, salaries for registered nurses fall substantially below those in hospitals. Fifty-five percent of registered nurses employed full time in nursing homes earn less than $400 a week compared with only 25 percent of hospital-employed nurses. Although upgrading salaries of registered nurses in nursing homes to equivalent salaries for supervisory registered nurses in hospitals would cost only

$1.00 per day per nursing home resident in 1987 dollars (Mullinex & Cornelius, 1988), the industry continues to insist that salary parity is not feasible.

Future registered nurse labor force needs in nursing homes are a factor of projected needs and the numbers needed to correct current vacancies (National Institute on Aging, 1987). There are very few data as to the registered nurse vacancy rate in nursing homes. A recent industry survey (American Health Care Association, 1988) estimated the vacancy rate to be between 20 and 27 percent. These figures do not include the 6000 registered nurses needed to comply with the Omnibus Reconciliation Act (Omnibus Reconciliation Act, 1987). Using these two figures, an estimated 21,000 to 27,000 more registered nurses are needed to staff nursing homes.

Thus, the employment of registered nurses in nursing homes continues to be a paradox. On the one hand, because of the absence of other professional providers or families of residents, their responsibilities in many ways exceed those of nurses in hospitals and home care. On the other hand, because of their limited numbers, the ability of registered nurses to assure quality care is extremely restricted. And despite evidence to the contrary, the pervasive feeling remains that the current situation is the best that can be hoped for in the face of limited fiscal and personnel resources.

## Models for Improving Quality of Care in Nursing Homes: The Role of Nurse Specialists

In contrast to this rather bleak picture of increased acuity, substandard care, and limited professional nursing presence, several innovative care models have demonstrated improvements in care of residents in nursing homes. Specialty units, such as those for residents with dementia (Wykle and Kaufmann, 1988), have been shown to be beneficial. Major improvements in the management of clinical problems, such as treatment of urinary incontinence (Collings, 1988), prevention of decubitus ulcers (Bergstrom, Braden, Laguzza, & Holman, 1987), and decreasing the use of physical restraints (Evans & Strumpf, 1989), are beginning to evolve. Improved programs for nurse aide training are now available. Most promising, however, and the focus of the remainder of this paper, is the use of nurse specialists in overseeing resident care.

With the admission of sicker patients, the health of nursing home residents is particularly compromised by the absence of on-site professional providers. A case in point is the frequency with which health problems beyond the most routine result in referral of the resident to a physician's office or the emergency room. One third of all nursing home residents are seen annually in a hospital emergency room, and many are unnecessarily admitted to the hospital. Of 765 hospital admissions generated by 27 skilled nursing facilities, one third were found to be avoidable with better nurse and physician coverage in the home (Van Buren, 1981).

Despite the frequently cited disclaimer that Medicare does not pay for nursing home care, Medicare pays virtually the full cost of these office and emergency room visits and for hospital care. The Health Care Financing Administration (1989), in a study of nursing home residents eligible for both Medicare and Medicaid in four states, estimated that in 1981 each resident used $2909 of hospital care and $1183 of physician care. Using these figures as a guide, a conservative estimate of the costs for all nursing home residents, in 1986 dollars, is at least $3 billion for hospital and $1.5 billion for physician care. Considerable cost savings could have been achieved if some of this care were provided in the nursing home.

Until recently, the lack of qualified personnel capable of providing specialized care in nursing homes precluded recommending any substitution for hospital care. Over the past 10 years, however, completion and evaluation of several large demonstration projects confirm that introducing geriatric nurse specialists in nursing homes substantially improves resident outcomes and imposes a more rationale system of care without increasing costs.

## Description of the Demonstration Projects

Geriatric nurse specialists are registered nurses who have completed a formal education program in care of the elderly. Geriatric nurse practitioners are certified for expanded practice by The American Nurses' Association and State Boards of Nursing (American Nurses' Association, 1987, 1988; Ebersole, 1985; Kane et al., 1988; Mezey & Lynaugh, 1989). In 1987, 37 academic programs prepared geriatric nurse practitioners, 27 awarding advanced degrees and 10 continuing education certificates. Approximately 1200 geriatric nurse practitioners are certified by the American Nurses' Association ("Nurse practitioner and nurse-midwifery program," 1989). The total number of nurse specialists practicing in nursing homes, however, exceeds those with geriatric nurse practitioner certification by the American Nurses' Association, since some have prepared as adult, family nurse, and geropsychiatric practitioners and clinicians and others practice in states that use criteria other than that of American Nurses' Association certification to establish practice eligibility.

Three demonstration projects, the Mountain States Health Corporation Program, the Robert Wood Johnson Foundation Teaching Nursing Home Program, and Massachusetts 1115: Case Managed Medical Care for Nursing Home Patients, "Nursing Home Connection," have tested the use of nurse specialists in nursing homes. Beginning in 1976, with funding from the Kellogg Foundation, the Mountain States Health Corporation trained, deployed, and evaluated the effectiveness of 172 geriatric nurse practitioners in over 200 nursing homes in 18 western states. Registered nurses employed by the nursing homes prepared as geriatric nurse practitioners in university-based certificate programs, returning to the nursing home for 6 months of physician-supervised preceptorship. On completion of the program, these nurses assumed newly created positions as geriatric nurse practitioners (Buchanan et al., 1990; Deitrich et al., 1990; Ebersole, 1985; Kane et al., 1988; Kane et al., 1989).

The Robert Wood Johnson Foundation Teaching Nursing Home Program encouraged faculty and students in 11 schools of nursing to practice in nursing homes (Aiken et al., 1985; Mezey et al., 1988; Mezey & Lynaugh, 1989; Shaughnessy et al., 1990; Small & Walsh, 1988). The program added approximately 1.5 full-time equivalents of nurse clinician/faculty time at each site. Faculty clinicians, who carried case loads of patients and had direct patient care responsibilities, represented different specializations, most commonly geriatric nurse and geropsychiatric nurse practitioners and clinicians. Approximately 500 undergraduate and graduate students rotated through these teaching nursing homes, further contributing to patient care activities.

In the "Nursing Home Connection" ("Case managed medical care for nursing home patients," 1987; Buchanan et al., 1989), 16 provider teams of physicians and nonphysicians, 75 percent of whom were nurse practitioners, cared for 2000 patients in 100 nursing homes (Buchanan et al., 1990). Although physicians maintained over-all responsibility for patient care, nurse practitioners and physician assistants per-formed duties and responsibilities delegated under written protocols that covered such areas as ordering diagnostic tests, special diets, rehabilitation therapy, and adjusting medications. Waivers from Medicare and Medicaid removed restrictions on billing frequency.

These three projects were similar in their use of geriatric nurse specialists to deliver care to nursing home residents. The projects differed, however, in their administrative structure. In the Mountain States project, the nursing homes were rural, freestanding facilities, one third of which had fewer than 100 beds. The great majority of nurses who were trained as geriatric nurse practitioners had worked in the participating nursing home for over 4 years prior to entering the project. With the exception of a clinical perceived experience, all educational activities were con-ducted off-site in a university setting, and the home itself was not expected to become a training site. The geriatric nurse practitioners were paid by and spent their whole time in the home, where they were responsible for a combination of direct care to residents, staff education, and some administrative tasks.

In contrast, the Robert Wood Johnson Foundation Teaching Nursing Homes were larger (all over 100 beds) and were, by virtue of the project's objectives, all linked to academic schools of nursing. The homes thus became educational sites for large numbers of undergraduate and graduate nursing students and students from other disciplines. The geriatric nurse specialists were all master's degree prepared and held combined appointments in the homes, as nurse clinicians, and as faculty in the schools of nursing. Most had not worked in the teaching nursing home prior to beginning the project. Although the greatest portion of their time in the home was spent providing direct care, faculty/clinicians also fulfilled teaching and research obligations in the schools of nursing.

In "Case Managed Medical Care for Nursing Home Patients" (1989), geriatric nurse practitioners were employed by physicians, clinics, and health maintenance organizations rather than by a nursing home. They cared for residents referred by the nursing home staff, and by virtue of a Health Care Financing Administration waiver, they were able to make unlimited visits to the nursing home, depending on the residents' need for care. These geriatric nurse practitioners had no line or staff authority within the nursing department in the nursing home but rather came into the facility as substitutes for what would otherwise have been physician visits.

Despite the differences governing their administrative framework, findings from all three projects confirm that nurse specialists in nursing homes serve a new and unique function in the delivery of care. In contrast to most registered nurses in nursing homes, these nurse specialists provided direct care to residents. A major portion of their time was spent responding to changes in residents' health status, conducting assessments, monitoring medications, giving or supervising care of residents with complex problems, and counseling residents and families (Kane et al., 1989; Shaughnessy et al., 1990). Geropsychiatric nurse clinicians worked with individual residents and groups of residents, families, and staff (McCracken-Knight, 1989; Rader, 1990; Wykle & Kaufmann, 1988). These practitioners were therefore in a position to prevent, recognize, and treat common problems and illnesses that are major causes of morbidity and transfer residents to the hospital when needed (U.S. Congress Office of Technology Assessment, 1986; Deitrich et al., 1990; Shaughnessy et al., 1990).

Assessment and management of residents took place through a process of "shared decision making" between the nurse specialists and physicians. The geriatric nurse practitioners independently obtained health histories, performed physical and mental status examinations, provided health maintenance, and counseled residents and families; jointly with physicians, they provided ongoing management, prescribed and altered medications, and ordered treatments and diagnostic tests (Deitrich et al., 1990; Kane et al., 1989; Mezey et al., 1988; Shaughnessey et al., 1990). Most states required nursing homes to have written policies with regard to the functions of geriatric nurse practitioners and their relationship to collaborating physicians (Deitrich et al., 1990).

While employees of the nursing homes, the nurse specialists provided in-service education and participated in quality assurance and infection control in addition to their patient responsibilities. Shaughnessey and coworkers (1990) attribute the significant improvements in functional status and decreased evidence of morbidity of residents in the teaching nursing homes to the assessment, planning, and staff teaching done by nurse clinicians. In some homes geriatric nurse practitioners were responsible for employee health (Kane et al., 1989; Mezey et al., 1988). Nursing home–based specialists reported to the director of nursing, the medical director, or both. They either saw all residents or only those of selected physicians. In some larger facilities they were unit based (Neubauer, LeSage, Ellor, & Roberts, 1986).

When employed by physicians or health maintenance organizations, as in the Nursing Home Connection, geriatric nurse practitioners triaged telephone calls from the home, conducted initial assessments, and made regularly scheduled visits for routine care and urgent visits for assessment and management of acute conditions (Buchanan et al., 1990; Kavesh, 1989).

Regardless of type of employment, nurse specialists increased the efficiency and satisfaction of physicians with nursing home practice. They facilitated transmittal of timely and accurate information and fostered appropriate consultation by telephone, thus allowing physicians to concentrate their time on management of complex cases; they encouraged a quicker response to acute problems and decreased unnecessary physician visits to the home (Buchanan et al., 1990; Kane et al., 1989; Mezey & Lynaugh, 1989; Shaughnessey et al., 1990).

## Demonstration Project Outcomes

Results from the evaluation studies of the three projects show that geriatric nurse specialists (1) decreased hospital admissions; (2) improved quality of care in the nursing home; (3) stabilized staff and decreased turnover; and (4) improved resident

**TABLE 14–4 Summary Contrasting Differences in Outcomes Between Participating Homes and Matched Controls in the Three Demonstration Programs Using Geriatric Nurse Practitioners**

| Desired Outcomes | Teaching Nursing Home | Nursing Home Connection | Mountain States |
|---|---|---|---|
| Fewer hospitalizations (total days) | <.001* <br> <.01† | <.02 | <.01* |
| Less use of the emergency room | NA‡ | <.005 | |
| Better functional outcomes | .001* <br> .05† | | .01–.05* |
| Better management of incontinence | .01* | <.01* | .01–.05* |
| Better management of confusion | .005 | | <.01† |
| Better management of psychotropic medications | >.05 | | <.01† |
| More discharges to the community | Modest trend | | Modest trend |
| Satisfaction with care | NA‡ | Yes | Yes |
| Cost neutral or less costly | Yes | Yes | Yes |

\* New admission samples.
† Long stay residents.
‡ NA = not assessed.

and family satisfaction. Across all three demonstrations, there is now substantial evidence that nurse specialists significantly decrease the hospitalization of nursing home residents. Hospitalizations declined significantly in all three projects. In the Robert Wood Johnson Foundation Teaching Nursing Homes, hospital admission rates declined 7 percent compared with an increase of 5 percent in matched comparison nursing homes (Shaughnessy et al., 1990). Although decreases in hospitalizations were more pronounced for residents who were newly admitted to the home, they were also evident for long-stay residents. In the Nursing Home Connection, hospitalization declined 25 percent, and the use of emergency rooms decreased significantly (Buchanan et al., 1990). In the Mountain States Health Corporation program, residents managed by geriatric nurse practitioners in the nursing home were significantly less likely to be hospitalized and had fewer hospital days when compared with matched controls (Kane et al., 1989; Buchanan et al., 1990).

Avoiding emergency room use or hospitalization required that nursing homes care for sicker residents. Yet, despite a drop in transfers to the hospital, the quality of care for residents remained unchanged or improved (Table 14–4). Specifically, the studies document that residents had better functional outcomes, less use of urinary catheters and fewer incontinent residents, and more appropriate use of medications (Buchanan et al., 1990; Deitrich et al., 1990; Kane et al., 1989; Shaughnessy et al., 1990).

Prevalence of mental disorders is a major concern in nursing homes, where more than half of the residents have serious cognitive impairments. Nurse specialists were effective in decreasing the use of physical and chemical restraints and in the management of wandering and aggressive behavior in brain-failed patients (Kane et al., 1989; Shaughnessy et al., 1990).

Improved satisfaction with care on the part of residents, families, physicians, and nursing home staff (Henderson, 1984; U.S. Congress Office of Technology Assessment, 1986; Neubauer et al., 1986, Buchanan et al., 1990), better staff morale (Deitrich et al., 1990; Kane et al., 1988), and decreased turnover of licensed and unlicensed nursing personnel were also attributed to employment of nurse specialists. Turnover among nurse's aides in nursing homes approaches 100 percent annually. One home reduced new hiring of nonlicensed staff from over 200 percent in the 6 months prior to employment of the geriatric nurse practitioner to 43 percent 6 months later (Karnowski, 1983). The Teaching Nursing Home Program relied heavily on geriatric nurse practitioners to retain staff. Decreased turnover was attributable in part to decentralization of nursing practice. With a nurse specialist readily available to verify observations by the nursing staff, clinical decisions handled on the unit and staff received prompt feedback rather than the customary practice of referral to the director of nursing. At the conclusion of the Teaching Nursing Home Program, 11 participating homes were sufficiently satisfied with the faculty/clinician role to retain 15 full-time equivalent positions for nurse specialists (Mezey & Lynaugh, 1989).

The savings achieved through the reduced hospital use totally offset the costs of employing geriatric nurse practitioners in the three demonstration projects (Buchanan et al., 1990; Shaughnessey et al., 1990). Improvements in quality of care in all three programs were cost neutral. There were no increased costs to the nursing homes in either the Mountain States or the Nursing Home Connection programs, suggesting that any nursing homes wishing to employ a geriatric nurse practitioner can afford to do so. In the Teaching Nursing Home program, the moderately higher costs in the nursing homes were balanced by lower costs associated with fewer hospitalizations. Finally, findings from the Teaching Nursing Home program show a trend toward the admission of a sicker case mix in nursing homes employing geriatric nurse practitioners.

## Reimbursement of Nurse Specialists

Because most of the cost savings achieved by geriatric nurse practitioners in nursing homes accrue to Medicare, the participants in the three demonstration projects successfully lobbied Congress to expand Medicare Part B coverage to geriatric nurse practitioners in nursing homes (Omnibus Reconciliation Act, 1987). Although similar to a 1989 amendment to Medicare (Public Law 99-509) that authorized physician assistants to recertify and to care for patients in skilled and intermediate nursing facilities, Public Law 101-239 authorizes geriatric nurse practitioners to work "in collaboration with" rather than "under the supervision of" physicians. Other than the reimbursement of nurse anesthetists, this represents the first reimbursement of nurse practitioner services under Medicare.

Employers of nurse practitioners can bill for Medicare-covered physician services and those that a nurse practitioner is legally authorized to perform in accordance with state law and state regulations. The collaboration between the nurse and physician must reflect "guidelines jointly developed by the nurse practitioner and the physician that address medical direction and appropriate supervision." Unfortunately, this legislation does not cover services of geropsychiatric nurse clinicians, who have proved to be particularly effective in nursing homes. In fact, nurses were specifically excluded from recent legislation (Omnibus Reconciliation Act, 1987) that authorizes Medicare reimbursement for the care of nursing home residents by social workers and psychologists.

This legislation has the potential to stimulate increased use of geriatric nurse practitioners in the care of nursing home residents. As currently written, the legislation authorizes reimbursement for geriatric nurse practitioner services to physicians and health maintenance organizations but not directly to geriatric nurse practitioners or nursing homes. It does, however, open the possibility for geriatric nurse practitioners in independent or group practices to contract with physicians or health maintenance organizations to provide care to nursing home residents. Until the issue of assuring a sufficient number of professional providers is resolved, substituting nursing home for hospital care will continue to generate concern as to quality of care (Kayser-Jones, Weiner, & Barbaccia, 1989). Assessment of a home's capabilities compared with those of the hospital needs to be weighed carefully when making decisions about site of treatment.

The practice arrangements for nurse clinicians have a substantial influence on quality of care. When they are in practice with physicians, employed by health maintenance organizations, or in independent contractual arrangements, geriatric nurse practitioners make clinical decisions that are unconstrained by nursing home needs or concerns. On the other hand, the presence of the geriatric nurse practitioner in the nursing home is episodic, he or she remains an outsider to the staff, and resident contacts are limited. Moreover, in such arrangements, geriatric nurse practitioners are subject to the same demands for efficiency and productivity that prevail for physicians; needless to say, this may have the opposite of the desired effect, namely, further limitations in contacts with residents.

When employed by nursing homes, nurse specialist services are available to staff and residents on a daily basis, ensuring an active role in prevention of disease and a timely response to symptoms. Nurse specialists are more readily accepted by the staff and can augment the home's supervisory, in-service, and quality assurance activities. On the other hand, nursing home–based nurse clinicians may be called on to perform tasks not specific or appropriate to their role (Kane et al., 1989). In addition, a potential source of conflict exists if the nurse clinician does not select the most cost-effective treatment option for the home. Mechanisms need to be in place that ensure that nurse specialists have sufficient independence and control of practice to make appropriate clinical decisions about treatment, irrespective of cost.

Despite demonstrated clinical benefits and cost savings, the structure of nursing homes discourages employment of nurse specialists. Although geriatric nurse practitioners enable a home to handle acute problems and manage a more complex case mix, such a caseload can increase other costs to the home. With beds in short supply, nursing homes profit from hospitalizing residents, as Medicaid programs and private patients often pay to reserve a nursing home bed (McMillan et al., 1987). Neither Medicare nor Medicaid reimbursement increases in response to maintaining residents in the home during episodes of acute illness; therefore profits are "squeezed" rather than enhanced (Mezey & Scanlon, 1988).

If Medicare is to achieve cost savings by encouraging nursing homes to care for sicker residents as a substitute for more expensive hospital care, funding options must be created that adequately reimburse the nursing homes. Nurse specialists must have the flexibility and incentive to monitor residents closely and intervene as necessary. Current rules that restrict payments solely to specified intervals and medical emergencies undermine appropriate treatment and need to be relaxed. This will not be easy to achieve because the principal payers to nursing homes are Medicaid programs and private patients, and the beneficiary of reduced hospital costs is Medicare. Fragmentation among payment sources makes it more difficult to accommodate the expanded role of nurse specialists despite the potential overall savings. On the other hand, without adequate recognition of the increased costs associated with the care of sick residents, nursing homes, which welcome the improved care provided by nurse specialists, will continue to be hampered in justifying their employment.

## Summary

It has been said that the quality of a society can be inferred from the care given to the frailest and most vulnerable of its citizens. In our society, those oldest and sickest are likely to spend some time in a nursing home. The resources we as a nation choose to invest in nursing homes reflect our beliefs about life, death, and aging and the value we ascribe to those who care for the infirm. Quality of care in nursing homes is very dependent on the active participation of professional nursing. We now know that geriatric nurse specialists can play an important role in achieving quality care at an affordable cost.

Given the weight of the evidence, nurses must advocate reimbursement policies that will provide access to professional nursing care to the hundreds of thousands of nursing home residents. Nursing is the key to ensuring quality of care in nursing homes. Public policy must encourage greater participation of nurses in nursing homes if care in this sector of the health care system, which has been inadequate for so many years, is to improve.

REFERENCES

Aiken, L., Mezey, M., Lynaugh, J.E., & Buck, C.R., Jr. (1985). Teaching nursing homes: Prospects for improving long-term care. *Journal of the American Gerontological Association, 33*(3), 196–201.
American Health Care Association (1988). AHCA manpower survey preliminary report (draft report, July, 1988). Washington, DC: American Health Care Association.
American Hospital Association (1988). Unpublished data.
American Nurses' Association (1987). *Standards of practice for the primary health care nurse practitioner.* Kansas City: American Nurses' Association.
American Nurses' Association (1988). *Standards and scope of gerontological nursing practice.* Kansas City: American Nurses' Association.

Bergstrom, N., Braden, B., Laguzza, A., & Holman, V. (1987). The Braden scale for predicting pressure sore risk. *Nursing Research, 36,* 205–210.

Buchanan, J., Bell, R., Arnold, S., Wisberger, C., Kane, R., & Garrard, J. (1990). Assessing cost effects of nursing-home-based geriatric nurse practitioners. *Health Care Financing Review, 11,* 67–78.

Buchanan J., Kane, R.L., Garrard, J., et al. (1989, October). *Results from the evaluation of the Massachusetts nursing home connection program.* RAND Publication No. JR-01. Prepared for Health Care Financing Administration. Santa Monica, CA: RAND Corporation.

*Case-managed medical care for nursing home patients* (1987). Massachusetts 1115 Waiver Program. Boston: Department of Welfare.

Collings, J. (1986, June 17). *Findings and analysis of ANA practice survey of gerontological nurses.* Presented at the American Nurses' Association Convention, Anaheim, CA.

Collings, J. (1988). Educating nurses to care for the incontinent patient. In K. McCormick (Ed.), *Incontinence in the elderly. Nursing Clinics of North America, 3,* 279–289.

Deitrich, C., Resnick, C., & Chambers, D. (1990). The effectiveness of GNPs in nursing home practice. *Journal of the American Academy of Nurse Practitioners, 2*(3), 113–120.

Ebersole, P. (1985). Gerontological nurse practitioners past and present. *Geriatric Nursing, 6*(4), 219–222.

Evans, L., & Strumpf, N. (1989). Tying down the elderly: A review of the literature on physical restraint. *Journal of the American Geriatric Society, 37,* 65–74.

Fitzgerald, J., Moore, P., & Dittus, R. (1988). The care of elderly patients with hip fracture: Changes since implementation of the prospective payment system. *New England Journal of Medicine, 319,* 1392–1397.

Harrington, C., Swan, J., & Grant, L. (1988). State Medicaid reimbursement for nursing homes, 1978–86. *Health Care Financing Review, 9,* 33–50.

Health Care Financing Administration (1989). Unpublished data.

Henderson, M. (1984). A GNP in a retirement community. *Geriatric Nursing, 5*(2), 109–112.

How each state stands on legislative issues affecting advanced nursing practice. (1990). *The Nurse Practitioner, 15*(1), 11–18.

Institute of Medicine (1986). *Improving the quality of care in nursing homes.* Washington DC: National Academy Press.

Jones, D., Bonito, A., Gower, J., & Williams, R. (1987). *Analysis of the environment for recruitment and retention of registered nurses in nursing homes.* U.S. Department of Health and Human Services, Public Health Service, Health Resources and Service Administration, Bureau of Health Professions, Division of Nursing, Washington, DC: U.S. Government Printing Office.

Kanda, K., & Mezey, M. (1991). Registered nurse staffing in Pennsylvania nursing homes: A comparison before and after the implementation of the Medicare Prospective Payment System. *The Gerontologist, 31*(3), 318–324.

Kane, R.L., Garrard, J., Skay, C., Radosevich, D., Buchanan, J., McDermott, S., Arnold, S., & Kepferle, L. (1989). Effects of a geriatric nurse practitioner on the process and outcome of nursing home care. *American Journal of Public Health, 79*(9), 1271–1277.

Kane, R.A., Kane, R.L., Arnold, S., Garrard, J., McDermott, S., & Kepferle, L. (1988). Geriatric nurse practitioners as nursing home employees: Implementing the role. *The Gerontologist, 28,* 469–477.

Karnowski, D. (1983). The GNP: An administrator's report. *Journal of Long-Term Care Administration, 11,* 41–50.

Kavesh, W. (1989). The role of geriatric nurse specialists in nursing homes: Report and findings from three demonstration projects. *The Gerontologist, 29,* 31A.

Kayser-Jones, J., Weiner, C., & Barbaccia, J. (1989). Factors contributing to the hospitalization of nursing home residents. *The Gerontologist, 29,* 502–510.

Lewis, A., Leake, B., Leal-Sotelo, M., & Clark, V. (1987). The initial effects of the prospective payment system on nursing home patients. *American Journal of Public Health, 77,* 819–822.

Lyles, Y. (1987). Impact of Medicare diagnosis related groups (DRGs) on nursing homes in the Portland, Oregon metropolitan areas. *Journal of the American Geriatric Society, 34,* 573–578.

McCracken-Knight, A. (1989). Teaching nursing homes: A project update. *Journal of Gerontological Nursing, 10,* 14–17.

McMillan, A., Gornach, M., Howell, E., Leibits, J., Prihod, R., Robey, E., & Russel, D. (1987, Winter). Nursing home costs for those dually entitled to Medicare and Medicaid. *Health Care Financing Review, 9,* 1–14.

Mezey, M., Lynaugh, J., & Cartier, M., eds. (1988). *Aging and academia: The teaching nursing home experience.* New York: Springer Publishing Company.

Mezey, M., & Lynaugh, J. (1989). The teaching nursing home program: Outcomes of care. *Nursing Clinics of North America, 24,* 769–780.

Mezey, M., & Scanlon, W. (1988). *Registered nurses in nursing homes.* Secretary's Commission on Nursing. Washington, DC: Department of Health and Human Services, 1988.

Morrisey, M., Sloan, F., & Valvona, J. (1988). Medicare prospective payment and posthospital transfers to sub-acute care. *Medical Care, 26,* 685–698.

Mullinex, C., & Cornelius, B. (1988). In Mezey, M., & Scanlon, W. (Eds.). *Registered nurses in nursing homes.* Secretary's Commission on Nursing. Washington, DC: Department of Health and Human Services.

National Center for Health Statistics (1987a). *Use of nursing homes by the elderly: Preliminary data from the 1985 National Nursing Home Survey.* Advance Data from *Vital and Health Statistics,* No. 135 (Department of Health and Human Services Publication No. [Public Health Service] 87-1250). Hyattsville, MD: Public Health Service.

National Center for Health Statistics (1987b). *Nursing home characteristics, preliminary data from the 1985 National Nursing Home Survey.* Advance Data from *Vital and Health Statistics,* No. 131 (Department of Health and Human Services Publication No. [Public Health Service] 87-1250). Hyattsville, MD: Public Health Service.

National Center for Health Statistics (1988). Strahan, G. *Characteristics of registered nurses in nursing homes, preliminary data from the 1985 National Nursing Home Survey.* Advance data from *Vital and Health Statistics,* No. 152 (Department of Health and Human Services Publication No. [Public Health Service] 88-1250). Hyattsville, MD: Public Health Service.

National Institute on Aging (1987). *Personnel for health needs of the elderly through the year 2020.* National Institutes of Health, Public Health Service, Department of Health and Human Services (National Institutes of Health Publication No. [Public Health Service] 87-2950). Bethesda, MD: National Institutes of Health.

Neglect at nursing home: In a first, suits are won (1990, July 12). *New York Times.*

Neu, C.R., & Harrison, S. (1988). *Posthospital care before and after the Medicare Prospective Payment System.* Santa Monica, CA: The RAND/UCLA Center for Health Care Financing Policy Research.

Neubauer, J., LeSage, J., Ellor, J., & Roberts, K. (1986). Family interviews: Consumer voice in long-term care. *The Gerontologist, 26,* 31A.

*Nurse practitioner and nurse-midwifery program* (1989). Rockville, MD: Division of Nursing, Department of Health and Human Services/Public Health Service/Health Resources and Services/Bureau of Health Professions.

Nursing homes costs, quality pose problems for Bush, hill (1988, December 2). *Washington Post,* p. A24.

Omnibus Reconciliation Act (1989).

Rader, J. (1987). A comprehensive staff approach to problem wandering. *The Gerontologist, 27,* 756–760.

Ray, W., Federspiel, C., Baugh, D., & Dodds, S. (1987). Interstate variation in elderly Medicaid nursing home populations. *Medical Care, 25,* 738–752.

Robert Wood Johnson Foundation (1982). *Medical practice in the United States: A special report* (pp. 34–35). Princeton, NJ: The Robert Wood Johnson Foundation.

Shaughnessy, P., & Kramer, A. (1990). The increased needs of patients in nursing homes and patients receiving home health care. *New England Journal of Medicine, 322,* 21–27.

Shaughnessy, P., Kramer, A., & Hittle, D. (1990, March). *The teaching nursing home experiment: Its effects and implications.* Study Paper 6. Center for Health Services Research, University of Colorado.

Small, N., & Walsh, M., eds. (1988). *Teaching nursing homes: The nursing perspective* (pp. 83–104). Owings Mill, MD: National Health Publishing.

Spector, M.D., Kapp, M., & Eichan, A., (1988). *Case-mix outcomes and resource use in nursing homes.* Providence: Center for Gerontology and Health Care Research, Brown University.

U.S. Congress, Office of Technology Assessment (1986, December). *Nurse practitioners, physician assistants, and certified nurse-midwives: A policy analysis* (Health Technology Case Study 37), OTA-HCS-37, Washington, DC: U.S. Government Printing Office.

U.S. Department of Health and Human Services (1990, March). *Seventh Report to the President and Congress on the status of health personnel in the United States, March 1990.* U.S. Department of Health and Human Services, Public Health Service, Health Resources and Services Administration, Bureau of Health Professions, Department of Health and Human Services Publication No. HRS-P-OD-90-1. Washington, DC: U.S. Government Printing Office.

Van Buren, C. (1981). *The acute hospitalization of residents of skilled nursing facilities in Monroe County NY, Rochester, NY.* Master's thesis. Rochester, NY: University of Rochester Department of Preventive Medicine and Rehabilitation.

Vladeck, B. (1980). *Unloving care.* New York: Basic Books.

Wykle, M., & Kaufmann, A. (1988). Case Western Reserve University Frances Payne Bolton School of Nursing and Margaret Wagner House of the Benjamin Rose Institute. In N. Small, & M. Walsh (Eds.), *Teaching nursing homes: The nursing perspective* (pp. 83–104). Owings Mill, MD: National Health Publishing.

## Chapter 15

# Psychiatric Nursing: Directions for the Future

JEANNE C. FOX

*A* MODERN HISTORY of psychiatric nursing begins with World War II. In recognition of the need for improved mental health care and education for this care, Congress passed the national Mental Health Act in 1946 (Chamberlain, 1987). Financial support for education of psychiatric nurses from the National Institute of Mental Health and Hildegard Peplau's leadership in defining psychiatric nursing theory and practice were major factors influencing the specialty's development.

Preliminary evidence suggested that psychiatric nursing would emerge as an influential professional group responsible for shaping mental health policy and quality mental health service delivery in the last quarter of this century (Krauss, 1987). On the surface, psychiatric nursing currently appears to be experiencing a serious retrenchment, with little evidence to support the expectation that responsible leadership will emerge in the near future. This chapter discusses the current psychiatric care system and issues and challenges facing psychiatric nursing. Future directions essential for the re-emergence of the specialty as a leader in mental health policy and quality psychiatric care delivery are proposed.

## Psychiatric Care Delivery

Psychiatric care differs from health care for physical illnesses. Some factors that distinguish the mental health care delivery system from physical health care delivery include

1. a history of separate facilities for treatment and care;
2. a paucity of agreed-upon standards of care and treatment;
3. an absence of agreed-upon acceptable outcomes for treatment;
4. a generally high level of public tolerance for inadequate services for the mentally ill as long as mentally ill persons are not visible in the community;

216

5. a major social movement—deinstitutionalization—resulting in major displacement of patients and disruption of services to patients;
6. inadequate public and private insurance coverage for the care of the mentally ill—coverage is insufficient and misdirected;
7. a reluctance of mental health professionals and the public to recognize and assure necessary medical, housing, and income supports essential for care of the mentally ill;
8. broad, almost universal, application of a treatment strategy (i.e., individual psychotherapy) with all variations of mental disorders despite little evidence of demonstrated effectiveness;
9. competition among core mental health professions around reimbursement for delivery of psychotherapy—competition that resulted in limited professional effort being directed toward collaborative alternative treatment and supportive and maintenance interventions;
10. a major schism between ideologies guiding care of the mentally ill in the community and inpatient care of the mentally ill—nonmedical, socially oriented professionals provide direct care in the community, whereas inpatient care is more medically oriented;
11. an absence of medical-nursing involvement in community care of the seriously mentally ill, leading to chronic difficulties for mentally ill clients in access to general health care and medical or nursing management of psychiatric-psychopharmacologic needs;
12. recent major scientific breakthroughs about psychiatric disorders that have shattered ideologic biases guiding psychiatric care for the past half-century—i.e., new evidence of neurobiologic-neurostructural abnormalities resulting in disturbed perception, cognition, information processing, social, and relationship skills—and major gaps in work force knowledge and active professional resistance to incorporating knowledge through changing practice.

The above factors significantly influence care of the mentally ill and the practice of psychiatric nursing (Aiken, 1987; Fox, 1989; Mechanic & Aiken, 1987).

Psychiatric patients in the United States moved from private institutions and alms houses to state mental hospitals in the late 1800s to early 1900s. From the mid-1800s until 1955, the number of state facilities increased, as did the number of patients admitted. Although state governments were responsible in large part for caring for the mentally ill, private facilities continued to care for private paying patients. In the 1960s criticism of custodial warehousing of mental patients in state hospitals led to rapid deinstitutionalization of the mentally ill. In 1955, there were about 565,000 patients institutionalized. In 1987, only 116,000 individuals were hospitalized in state facilities (Aiken, 1987). Concurrently, Medicare and Medicaid, as well as private insurance, emerged as major sources of reimbursement for health care (Adams, 1989; Babigan et al., 1987b; Bittker, 1988).

From the beginning of third-party reimbursement, funding of mental health services was grossly inadequate (Dulter & Fine, 1985; Cummings & Duhl, 1987; Feldman & Goldman, 1987; Frank & Lave, 1985). Further, deinstitutionalization in combination with inadequate and poorly conceptualized reimbursement systems appears to have contributed to the following current problems:

1. an increasing number of homeless persons;
2. an increasing number of nonelderly mentally ill nursing home residents;
3. an increasing readmission rate of persons to public mental hospitals;
4. a two-class system of care, with private psychiatric–general hospital psychiatric facilities serving privately insured less seriously mentally ill and public institutions serving chronically ill poor patients;
5. overutilization of inpatient care and psychotherapy;
6. underdevelopment of alternative effective organization of services required to support and maintain seriously mentally ill people in the community;
7. increasing isolation of seriously mentally ill people from the mainstream health care system and the rest of society.

Psychiatric care has historically been delivered through specialized institutions and organizations outside the mainstream of health care (Frazier & Parron, 1987). Separate facilities for the mentally ill reinforced the stigma associated with mental illness and also probably protected mental health care providers from public scrutiny of treatment practices.

Social activism of the 1960s, with accompanying concerns for civil rights, stimulated massive deinstitutionalization. However, public tolerance for inadequate services for the mentally ill remains exceptionally high even today. This tolerance in the face of increasing homelessness and serious mental illness of homeless persons may in part be explained by public ignorance about mental illness and essential mental health services.

Even among mental health professionals, there are few agreed-upon standards of treatment or expected outcomes of effective psychiatric care. Also, public and private reimbursement remains biased toward inpatient care and psychotherapy. Thus, most mental health treatment predominantly includes inpatient care and psychotherapy. Unfortunately, these treatment strategies appear to have only limited effectiveness in modifying significantly the overall course of mental illness or improving the quality of life of the seriously mentally ill.

Standards of psychiatric care and treatment outcomes tend to be related to a decrease in acute symptoms of psychiatric illness with no expectation that treatment will effect a decrease of recidivism; readmission to inpatient care; frequency or amount of psychotherapy; community adjustment problems; or long-term client discomfort and disability.

The lack of agreement among professionals about standards of care and outcome is related to the domination of psychotherapy, inpatient care, and psychopharmacology as the psychiatric methods of choice for the past half-century. This approach to care prevailed without conclusive documented effectiveness or evaluation of alternative methods of treatment. Further, a major schism of ideologies guiding community care systems and inpatient care emerged as social workers assumed leadership in community care and physicians continued to control inpatient treatment. In fact, the number of psychiatrists involved in community care of the mentally ill has actually declined since 1980.

Recent major scientific breakthroughs demonstrating neurostructural-neurochemical correlates of the psychological dysfunction associated with mental illness challenge assumptions on which current psychotherapeutic and social interventions are based.

Psychiatric care in 1990 can most accurately be described as (1) poorly reimbursed—inappropriate reimbursement for inpatient care and psychotherapy; (2) poorly organized; (3) largely directed toward inappropriate priority populations; (4) having a service delivery dominated by ineffective methods (psychotherapy), with only minimal effort directed toward stabilizing and maintaining the mentally ill in the community; and (5) having limited multidisciplinary collaboration with major competition between mental health professionals seeking reimbursement for psychotherapy (Goldman, 1987; Goldman & Lock, 1985; Gurevitz & Wallach, 1985; Fox, 1989).

The question remains, where does psychiatric nursing fit in this disrupted system of care?

## Psychiatric Nursing Care

Psychiatric nursing care in the early state asylums involved assistance with treatments and maintenance of the physical environment. Although some discussion of therapeutic nursing occurred before the mid-1900s, Peplau is credited with first articulating the interpersonal therapeutic role of psychiatric nursing (Krauss, 1987). Various nurse therapists during the past 30 years have expanded the application of psychotherapeutic ideologies to psychiatric nursing practice. Major emphasis has been placed on development of psychiatric nurses as psychotherapists. Numerous references provide anecdotal evidence of the effectiveness of psychiatric nurse psychotherapists. Unfortunately, psychiatric nurses' emphasis on psychotherapy did not include equal attention to daily client functioning or the interaction of physical, psychiatric, and social care needs of clients. The "ideal" role of the psychiatric nurse therapist was promoted, and clinical nurse specialization became the vehicle for practicing this role.

From the mid-1960s well into the late 1980s, most master's programs in psychiatric nursing were organized around psychodynamic knowledge and specific psychotherapeutic strategies: individual, group, and family therapy. With deinstitutionalization of the mentally ill, community mental health nursing emerged with some attention to community intervention. However, to a large extent, psychodynamic formulations continued to dominate psychiatric nursing education and practice (Fox, 1988).

It is understandable that psychiatric nurses sought recognition as psychotherapists as psychotherapy was accepted as the treatment of choice for psychiatric disabilities. Unfortunately, the specialty did not question the obvious failure of psychotherapy with the seriously mentally ill. Nor did psychiatric nurses actively address interacting psychiatric, physical, and social needs of these clients. Instead, psychiatric nurses organized as clinical nurse specialists to pursue third-party reimbursement for the practice of psychotherapy. Currently, certification by the American Nurses' Association as a clinical nurse specialist qualifies psychiatric nurses for third-party reimbursement in a number of states.

## Community Mental Health Care and Psychiatric Nursing

As previously mentioned, competition of mental health professions for reimbursement tied to psychotherapy has resulted in underdevelopment and underutilization of alternative community interventions and models of service delivery (Kiesler, 1987). The under-representation of psychiatric nurses and psychiatrists in community mental health service systems is well documented. The consequent failure of community mental health systems to deliver integrated services addressing physical, psychiatric, social support, and maintenance needs of psychiatric patients reflects a serious deficit largely ignored by psychiatric nurses and other mental health professionals.

The paucity of clinicians with a concern for the interaction of physical and psychiatric problems in the community system has resulted in competing ideologies and factions among practitioners in psychiatric-medically oriented inpatient facilities and community treatment clinics and psychosocial rehabilitation programs such as clubhouses and supported employment efforts. The failure of the system to provide integrated care for clients in the community also has spawned the need for new positions such as case managers.

This stopgap approach to clients' needs for quality integrated service is strongly endorsed by the public mental health system. The little research conducted on case management suggests that this approach to care is costly and not effective in avoiding frequent hospitalization for the seriously mentally ill (Franklin et al., 1987). This is not surprising, since many case management systems include the following limitations:

1. there is no clear definition of the case manager primarily as a broker of services or as a client and family advocate;
2. case managers are rarely educated with the latest information about the cognitive and behavioral limitations accompanying serious mental illness that require particular social interventions to decrease the vulnerability of seriously mentally ill clients to acute illness, nor are they educated about community action;
3. case managers have little authority, nor is their role in reference to the living environment of seriously mentally ill clients clearly enough defined to allow them to significantly increase the stability and predictability for clients in that environment;
4. treatment—psychotherapy or psychosocial rehabilitation remains outside the control of case managers;
5. case managers are not educated about physical health care needs of clients or psychopharmacology and therefore cannot attempt to evaluate

the interaction of clients' physical health status, psychopharmacologic, social, and psychological needs;

6. in general, case management has not been clearly defined as primarily a function or a process. Further, the authority and relationships of the case manager and other care providers are unclear.

Case management represents a poorly defined, narrowly conceived solution to a system in need of major changes. Imposing another position, "case manager," on a system of care already riddled with ineffective relationships among programs, care providers, and clients is not likely to significantly affect care. Little improvement in the integration or quality of care or in reduction of cost of care can be expected. A more efficient approach to the lack of integrated care would be to determine where there are gaps and how currently practicing mental health care providers could utilize their expertise to better meet clients' needs.

The introduction of psychosocial rehabilitation and psychoeducational and supported employment methodologies and programs has increased alternatives available in community care. Unfortunately, in many state systems these have been developed as separate programs that are added to a package of community services. There is little evidence that such approaches are utilized as integrating methodologies for delivering a continuum of quality inpatient and outpatient mental health services.

Psychiatric nursing roles in community mental health systems reflect the ideology of the community care system in which psychiatric nurses practice. In many community mental health programs, psychiatric nurses function as medication clinic nurses, primary therapists, or case managers. In these roles psychiatric nurses interact with clients in the medication clinic or in the community mental health center. Community mental health nurses frequently conduct education, support, and therapeutic groups, but they do not routinely provide integrated service addressing physical, psychiatric, and psychosocial health needs of clients. To date, there is little evidence that community mental health nurses routinely design and supervise health maintenance programs for clients. Further, community psychiatric nurse roles do not clearly focus on facilitating clients' daily coping, functioning, and adaptation in the community.

The advent of outreach, crisis teams, and mobile units has resulted in an increase in the participation of psychiatric nurses in home and street interventions. This movement out of community mental health centers into the lives of clients provides outstanding opportunities for quality psychiatric nursing care.

Although the problems of the community mental health system could be discussed at length, there are three areas of practice in which psychiatric nursing could make a major contribution to cost-effective quality community care for public psychiatric clients: (1) client community stabilization and prevention of unnecessary hospitalization; (2) management and monitoring of physical health care needs, psychiatric conditions, and social circumstances and the interaction of these; and (3) coordination and assurance of an integrated, coherent, supportive environment for daily living for clients with serious mental illness residing in the community.

Clients require care providers who can attend to the psychiatric disabilities that affect their perceptions, information processing, affective and behavioral responses, and daily coping, adaptation, and functioning. Clients require care providers who are knowledgeable about physical health care needs and the interaction of these with psychiatric disabilities and functional status. Clients also require care providers who will provide environmental modifications and assist them in modifying their environments to decrease their vulnerability to major psychiatric dysfunction 24 hours a day. Clients require care providers who are knowledgeable and stay informed about the effect of medications on their brain function, general health status, behavioral responses, and capacity to successfully accomplish treatment or rehabilitation goals. Clients require care providers who integrate science and caring and inquire about clients perceptions, capacities, and desires for their daily lives. Clients require care providers who collaborate with them to assure a reasonable quality of life.

In the past psychiatric nursing has not assumed the responsibility for assuring that seriously mentally ill clients are supported in their daily living environments to the degree necessary for persons with such illnesses. Nor has psychiatric nursing assumed the responsibility for assuring support for such clients as they encounter different community experiences and treatment programs in the community and in the hospital. Emerging knowledge about brain dysfunction underlying serious mental illness makes it imperative that psychiatric nursing collaborate with consumers and other health care providers to develop more effective interventions based on this knowledge.

## State Hospital Care and Psychiatric Nursing

State hospitals were the primary sites for psychiatric nursing education until the 1930s (Krauss, 1987). These institutions have been a source of continual frustration for psychiatric nursing. Many of the current problems of psychiatric nursing in the public mental health system have roots in the past status and responsibilities of nursing in state hospitals. In the past, nursing was the only core mental health profession that did not require a baccalaureate degree and advanced preparation as basic education for practice in the profession. This lack of academic preparation contributed to nursing's inferior status in the hierarchy of care delivery and in compensation for services. This inferior status was somewhat complicated because nursing was the only core mental health profession present in the hospital 24 hours a day. This 24-hour presence provided nurses with more information about patients, their strengths and weaknesses, patterns of illness, and response to treatment than that available to other professional care providers. Unfortunately, 24-hour scheduling also carried with it the responsibility for keeping the hospital system functioning. It appears that administrative requirements of keeping the system functioning consumed more and more nursing time, leaving less time for professional psychiatric nursing patient intervention.

Meanwhile, other core mental health professions provided the patient's treatment program during the 8-hour day, Monday to Friday. Nurses became and were viewed as custodial service providers and not as professionals with patient care knowledge and responsibility. Unit managers and program directors (non-nurses) emerged to coordinate the treatment program for patients. Nurses, concerned with system maintenance functions, retreated from patients and individualized treatment team participation and were consumed in ward clerk activities, scheduling, patient transportation, special services coordination, and medication documentation (Fox, 1988, 1989). Nurses in public hospitals became less and less involved in nurse-patient care activities.

Currently, a major problem in state mental health systems as a whole and state hospitals in particular is the continuing custodial system of care and view of nurses as nonprofessional and nonintegral to effective psychiatric treatment and care. To a large extent nurses are viewed as a support service to the treatment team of psychiatrists, psychologists, social workers, and activity therapists. Why have psychiatric nurses not been able to break out of this inferior position?

Unfortunately, data from a statewide survey of nurses working in public psychiatric facilities document that only 14 percent of nurses working in state hospitals have bachelor's degrees and only 3 percent are master's degree–prepared psychiatric nurses. Many state hospital nurses have worked in the system for 15 or more years. Nearly 44 percent of these nurses are over 46 years of age. Most state hospital nurses stay in their current jobs because of relationships with coworkers (18 percent) and pay and benefits (24 percent), not because they feel respected or fulfilled by their work role (5 percent) or because of opportunities for professional advancement (7 percent). In addition, nursing salaries in public inpatient facilities generally lag behind those of private care facilities, and psychiatric nurses are under-represented in top administrative positions in state mental health systems. Also, as documented by the National Institute of Mental Health Task Force on Nursing, nursing is seriously under-represented in the federal bureaucratic structure concerned with mental health research, education, and care delivery.

Within state hospitals nursing service workers are still the only group on site 24 hours of every day. This is true despite (1) the addition of new supportive and administrative positions; (2) clear evidence that public mental-hospital patients are admitted in states of much more complex illness than was true a decade ago; and (3) the fact that patients are hospitalized for much shorter periods than in the past (despite recent evidence of increasing lengths of stay).

Four overall interacting concerns related to public mental-hospital nursing today summarize the state of affairs of psychiatric nursing in the public mental health system. (1) Most practicing nurses in state hospitals have not been educated as psychiatric nurses to provide necessary nursing care to seriously ill patients admitted to these facilities. (2) Most state hospital systems still expect and reward nurses for functioning in a custodial-organizational maintenance role, which totally inhibits them from practicing quality professional patient-based care. (3) State hospital nursing practice is directly tied to specific institutions and not to stabilizing and maintaining clients in the community or to community mental health nursing practice. (4) Such nonrewarding practice environments can neither attract nor retain professional nurses committed to quality psychiatric nursing care and effective team planning and intervention.

Finally, data suggest that state hospitals do not recruit new graduates of professional nursing programs. Although the difficulties in socializing new graduates to public hospital systems are well recognized, without new graduates the nursing work force will soon largely be represented by older, retiring nurses who are less likely to be motivated to ensure that emerging knowledge about mental illness and psychiatric nursing is applied to care of public psychiatric clients (Fox, 1989).

State hospitals at this time represent one of the least desirable environments for professional psychiatric nursing practice. This is true because of nursing's continuing low status and limited opportunities for control over practice, participation in administrative decision making, collegial partnerships with other mental health professionals, and direct patient care. It is frequently argued that public care delivery systems should not be the battleground for professionalization of any care provider. This is true. However, psychiatric nurses with a professional focus on client daily functioning, adaptation, and coping and the integration of attention to physical, psychiatric, and psychosocial health needs have a responsibility for assuring public clients access to quality psychiatric nursing care. Clerical, housekeeping, transportation, and administrative services must be substituted for quality psychiatric nursing care 24 hours a day. Further, without some organized psychiatric nursing effort to significantly change the public mental health system, administrators will continue to offer public clients the lowest level of nursing services available. This is detrimental for clients. In addition, the probability that professional nurses will be recruited to the system is greatly decreased, and the future for quality nursing in state institutions appears increasingly bleak.

It is critical that psychiatric nursing leaders become actively involved in assessing how public mental health care can be cost-effectively delivered and how public clients can be guaranteed access to quality psychiatric nursing care.

Clearly, the limited participation of psychiatric nurses in community care and the dissatisfying roles for psychiatric nurses in state hospitals suggest a major gap in leadership in psychiatric nursing in public mental health. This gap is documented by the paucity of master's degree–prepared psychiatric nurses and of directors of nursing positions in the system and by an even greater absence of psychiatric nurses in systemwide leadership positions. Very few psychiatric nurses function as executive directors of hospitals or community mental health systems. Currently, no state commissioners of mental health are psychiatric nurses. Since the establishment of the National Institute of Mental Health in 1946, only one deputy director has been a psychiatric nurse. This gap in leadership is a major impediment to the development of quality public mental health care. In order for psychiatric nursing to assume professional responsibility for significantly influencing the lives of the seriously mentally ill, this void in leadership must be filled.

Given the above identified deficits in public mental health nursing, what role does psychiatric nursing play in private psychiatric hospitals and psychiatric units in general hospitals?

## *The Private Psychiatric Care System and Psychiatric Nursing*

Many authors have noted the rapid increase in the number of private psychiatric facilities and admissions of patients to these facilities that accompanied the expansion of third-party reimbursement for such services (Scherl et al., 1988; Sloan et al., 1988; Wolfe et al., 1988). This expansion occurred subsequent to the deinstitutionalization in the public mental health system. Frequently, expansion is mistakenly credited with addressing the resulting need for psychiatric care for seriously mentally ill discharged to the community. Unfortunately, there is no evidence that the needy public previously served by state mental hospitals has access to or utilizes the expanded private sector to any great degree (Cherkin, 1989; Goldman, 1987; Mahoney, 1988; Keeler et al., 1986; Katz & Trainor, 1988).

It is well documented that public mental health systems continue to serve chronic schizophrenics, organically mentally ill people, and dually diagnosed mentally ill and substance abusers. These clients routinely experience multiple readmissions and report minimal family support in the community. Only 27 percent of state hospital patients are discharged to families. In contrast, patients who are served in private psychiatric facilities and psychiatric units of general hospitals are more likely to be first admissions with less disabling disorders. Further, they are much more likely to be discharged to personal homes and families. Private hospitalization tends to be of a shorter duration, and clients admitted to private facilities are much more likely to be covered by private insurance (*Mental Health*, 1987).

Although private psychiatric facilities and psychiatric units of general hospitals do provide some acute care for nonpaying seriously mentally ill patients, the actual use of private services for acute care of the seriously mentally ill does not match the need for such service (Scheffler, 1987; Mechanic, 1989). Further, this acute care has not proved effective in improving the overall course of mental illness or quality of life of the seriously mentally ill person living in the community. Financial resources spent on private psychiatric service are increasing and those spent on public service are decreasing (*Mental Health*, 1987). However, cost-effectiveness in this area remains elusive.

Once again, reimbursement for inpatient care without an integrated system of community care, including housing, income, physical health care, and medical supervision of psychotropic interventions for community clients, results in limited success in psychiatric care delivery. It has been proposed that the cost and length of inpatient psychiatric care are more directly related to available community services than to patient characteristics or type of inpatient treatment program (Bachofer, 1988).

As the private system expanded, psychiatric nurses migrated to private care facilities. Currently, the numbers of psychiatric nurses working in general hospital psychiatric units and private psychiatric facilities is increasing at a faster rate than the numbers of psychiatric nurses in public facilities (*Mental Health*, 1987). Further, employment of nurses in partial care and outpatient facilities is actually decreasing (*Mental Health*, 1987). In contrast, the number of certified psychiatric nurses in private practice as primary or secondary employment is increasing (Fox, 1989).

There is no evidence that the increasing numbers of psychiatric nurses in private psychiatric facilities or psychiatric units of general hospitals are related to more opportunities for autonomous or meaningful practice. However, higher wages paid to nurses in these facilities do attract more nurses. Nurse shortage data suggest a higher vacancy rate of nursing positions in public mental hospitals in comparison with private facilities and psychiatric units of general hospitals (Fox, 1989).

Although psychiatric nurses appear to be seeking opportunities for expanded roles through private practice, there is little evidence that nurses employed in the private sector have been any more innovative or successful in developing new approaches to serving the seriously mentally ill than nurses employed in the public system.

Psychiatric nurses have limited influence on the nature and organization of public and private services delivered to psychiatrically ill individuals despite knowledge and nursing skills that presumably would allow them to address some of the gaps in service. Again, the questions arise—Why does psychiatric nursing fail to influence the organization of care? Why don't psychiatric nurses address serious gaps in care that their general nursing knowledge and skills prepare them to address?

Who are these nurses, where are they, and how were they educated?

## The Population of Psychiatric Nurses

Most nurses practicing in psychiatric settings are not educated as psychiatric nurses but instead are generalists. As previously noted, only about 3 percent of state hospital nurses are psychiatric nurses (nurses prepared with a master's degree in psychiatric nursing). About one sixth of all nurses practicing in psychiatric settings are educated as psychiatric nurses. In 1988, a national sample survey of master's degree–prepared nurses conducted by Moses (Mental Health U.S. 1990, DHHS) estimated that there were approximately 16,500 master's degree–prepared psychiatric nurses in the United States. Approximately 16 percent of master's degree-prepared psychiatric nurses are under 35 years of age, whereas 34 percent are 45 or older and 18 percent are over 55 years of age. Ninety-six percent of all psychiatric nurses are female, and 94 percent are white, 2.5 percent are black, less than 2 percent are Asian, 1 percent are Hispanic, and less than 1 percent are Native American. Of this number, 12,618, or 76 percent, were working in nursing and 73 percent were working 35 or more hours per week. About 45 percent of these nurses identify hospitals as their primary practice sites, whereas 14 percent are primarily employed in community mental health settings, 14 percent in academic settings, 11 percent in individual or group practice, 3 percent in health maintenance organizations, and less than 1 percent in nursing homes.

In the past, most nurses worked in one setting. Currently, about 61 percent of the full-time employed psychiatric nurses work only in one setting, whereas 39 percent work in two or more settings. Forty-two percent of psychiatric nurses report direct patient care as their primary work activity, whereas 19 percent report teaching and 21 percent report administration as their primary work activity.

Geographic distribution of psychiatric nurses across the United States is uneven. More psychiatric nurses are located in the northeast and other geographic areas where there are large numbers of other mental health professions. Further, there are more psychiatric nurses in geographic areas where the rate of inpatient care episodes is highest.

The number of master's degree–prepared psychiatric nurses relative to other master's degree–prepared nurses has been declining steadily since the National

Institute of Mental Health dramatically decreased funding of master's programs. In 1977, approximately 22 percent of all nursing master's degree graduates were prepared in psychiatric nursing. In 1987, less than 10 percent were psychiatric nurses. Approximately 53 percent of these nurses completed their master's degrees within the past 10 years, but 28 percent completed their master's degrees 16 or more years ago (Chamberlain, 1987).

Most practicing psychiatric nurses were educated in master's programs designed to prepare psychotherapists, and they have been practicing during an era of extreme competition among mental health professionals for reimbursement for psychotherapy.

## Psychiatric Nursing in the 1990s: Future Directions

Since the early 1980s there has been increasing unrest in the psychiatric nursing specialty. This turmoil appears to be related to five major factors. (1) Psychiatric nursing educators and researchers are accessing new knowledge about psychiatric illness (particularly biologic knowledge) and are recognizing the need to incorporate this knowledge in psychiatric nursing education and psychiatric nursing practice. (2) Certified clinical nurse specialists have successfully accessed third-party reimbursement for psychiatric nurses practicing psychotherapy. (3) There is increased family and consumer insistence that psychiatric nursing educators, researchers, and practitioners re-examine causal and intervention models and re-evaluate approaches to care. (4) There is increased involvement of some psychiatric nursing practitioners, educators, and researchers in the care of the seriously mentally ill, homeless, and other target populations who have suffered greatly because of ineffective or inadequate psychiatric care. (5) Funding of psychiatric nursing education is at an all-time low, and the numbers of students entering psychiatric nursing are declining.

These factors stimulate fertile opportunities for major changes and professional development of the specialty. Psychiatric nursing is emerging from an era of role blurring in psychiatric care delivery and entering a new age in which scientific knowledge about neurostructural-neurochemical, cognitive, information processing, behavioral, and social correlates of psychiatric illness will be much more rigorously integrated in effective psychiatric care. This new age provides unlimited opportunities for psychiatric nurses to utilize the complement of psychiatric, physiologic, behavioral, social, and nursing knowledge inherent in general and psychiatric nursing education.

There are psychiatric nurses who are yet to be persuaded that we must chart a new course. The hard-won victories of psychiatric nurses to practice independently and receive direct payment for services are likely to reinforce some nurses' commitment to the private practice model. Unfortunately, private practice is not likely to survive for long as the major pattern for mental health care delivery. The risk is that a major constituency of professional psychiatric nursing will be tirelessly defending a right to practice in a delivery system that is not viable because it is costly and limited in effectiveness.

The challenge for psychiatric nursing, then, is to mobilize professional energies around the development of policies and models of care delivery that cost-effectively provide quality psychiatric-mental health care services through full utilization of psychiatric nursing expertise. This shift away from the battle for the privilege of private practice toward developing cost-effective quality psychiatric and mental health care delivery systems is essential for clients and for the survival of psychiatric mental health nursing.

Psychiatric nursing's background in the biologic and psychosocial sciences and its focus on intervention in clients' daily adaptation, coping, and functioning can provide a cost-effective framework for organizing psychiatric care delivery systems.

Such a care delivery system organized around maintaining daily functioning and coping and adaptation ensures attention to physical, psychiatric, and psychosocial health needs. Reimbursement in such a system must be tied to client daily functioning and quality of life rather than to acute care episodes. Clients, families, informal care providers, or health care professionals should all be reimbursed for client daily functioning and quality daily life. This proposed framework reflects a major shift in the focus of reimbursement from inpatient acute treatment episodes to daily functioning. Psychiatric nursing could contribute cost-effectively to quality care in such a system by linking clients with resources that facilitate physical health and daily adaptation. Although capitation has not been discussed in this chapter, this proposed model is consistent with basic premises underlying capitation for services delivered to the mentally ill.

The question remains, however, whether psychiatric nurses will quickly shift their major energies away from the private practice battle to a far more critical and demanding challenge of designing new policies and model delivery systems. The private delivery system (including psychiatric nurses in private practice and psychiatric nurses employed in private care facilities and agencies) must explore new cost-effective practice models, or it seems clear that the government will impose constraints on care and practice that are not desirable for clients or practitioners. The degree to which nurses become leaders in developing policies and alternative model delivery systems to a large extent will determine the opportunities for professional practice and the opportunities available for clients to directly access nursing care in the next century.

Psychiatric nurses must develop new alliances and new partnerships with consumers and advocates, private industry, local governmental agencies, other health care providers, and state and national legislators. These alliances should assure the most cost-effective, accessible, available, efficacious health care possible for psychiatric clients. New models are necessary to link client, family, and community capacity for self-monitoring and self-maintenance with professional expertise. Professional expertise must be delivered in a manner that assures congruence of expert contribution with clients' capacities to profit from this expertise. New models that do not discriminate against and isolate individuals experiencing psychiatric illnesses from the mainstream of health care are needed. New models are required that link information about neurostructural, neurochemical, and neurofunctional deficits underlying psychiatric illnesses with treatment and environmental strategies and daily life of psychiatric clients. Increased knowledge about the information-processing deficits of psychiatric illness will require increased emphasis on the importance of home and daily life patterns in decreasing vulnerability to psychiatric crisis.

The specialty of psychiatric nursing can contribute leadership to these developments through (1) participation in policy and model system development, (2) research into effective care and care delivery systems for mental illness, and (3) collaboration with new partners to ensure these changes (Aiken, 1987).

A critical task for psychiatric nursing is the organization of the specialty to provide for clients the quality of care that the specialty has the knowledge to deliver. Psychiatric nursing has evolved from an era in which the specialty was immersed in role blurring through socialization as psychotherapists. Currently, the specialty is emerging as a major force in linking knowledge in the biologic-physiologic-psychosocial sciences with the daily coping, adaptation, and functioning of individuals and families experiencing mental disorders. This evolving theoretical and practical definition of the specialty will be facilitated by efforts to establish cohesive groups representing practice, research, and education. Currently, the primary psychiatric nursing organizations, the Society for Education and Research in Psychiatric Nursing, the Advocates for Child and Adolescent Psychiatric Nursing, the American Nurses' Association Council on Psychiatric Nursing, and the American Psychiatric Nursing Association have joined forces in the Coalition of Psychiatric Nursing Organizations in an effort to better respond to client needs and articulate the specialty to the health care system and the general public. This organizational effort is significant and should be utilized as a mechanism for establishing new alliances and coalitions to advance quality mental health care for public clients. It is critical that psychiatric nurses utilize this opportunity to ensure the most cost-effective, knowledge-based, efficacious mental health care system possible for the clients they serve.

The knowledge explosion about mental illness, particularly in the biologic sciences, requires psychiatric nursing investment in knowledge acquisition and clinical research related to care applications of this knowledge. Because quality psychiatric nursing care represents successful adaptation of biologic knowledge to social intervention and caring, the specialty must update educational programs to reflect changing knowledge and engage in clinical research to assure appropriate efficacious ethical transfer of knowledge to client care. Increasing complexity of such knowledge encourages multidisciplinary research efforts to successfully meet these objectives. Psychiatric nursing must participate in research related to (1) application of new knowledge about mental illness to care delivery, (2) development of cost-effective care interventions, and (3) ethical and philosophic concerns associated with both of the above and psychiatric nursing practice.

Psychiatric nurses, in conjunction with other mental health professionals, face an extraordinary challenge of actively participating in the design of mental health policies. These policies must provide guidelines for the development and implementation of effective mental health care delivery systems collaboratively designed and operated by care recipients and care providers. The most important task for psychiatric nursing in the 1990s is design and implementation of new policies to assure the development of system-wide mental health care integrated in a meaningful fashion with other health and social services required by mentally ill persons and their families. Procrastination and neglect of this task are likely to result in the development of policies and systems of care lacking psychiatric nurses' sensitivity and concern for clients' perceptions, daily coping, adaptation, and functioning and integrated attention to physical, psychological, and social care needs. Psychiatric nurses are responsible for representing this important perspective in the design of mental health policies and the implementation of new models of psychiatric care delivery. Psychiatric nurses in the 1990s must demonstrate the capacity and willingness to design new policies and carry out new programs solidly based on knowledge, evaluation, and collaboration among clients, families, and care providers. In the interest of our clients and the survival of the specialty, psychiatric nurses must meet this challenge.

## REFERENCES

Adams, K., Ellwood, M., & Pine, P. (1989, Fall). Utilization and expenditures under Medicaid for supplemental social security income for the disabled. *Health Care Financing, 11*(1), 1–14.

Aiken, L.H. (1990). The chronically mentally ill elderly: Financing and policy issues. In B. Fogel, G. Gottlieb, & A. Furino (Eds.), *Minds at risk: Neuropsychiatric care for the elderly.* Washington, DC: American Psychiatric Press.

Aiken, L.H. (1987). Unmet needs of the chronically mentally ill: Will nursing respond? *Image: Journal of Nursing Scholarship, 19*(3), 121–125.

Aldrich, R. (1987). The social context of change. In L. Duhl & N. Cummings (Eds.), *The future of mental health services* (pp. 15–28). New York: Springer Publishing Company.

American Psychiatric Association (1985). *Survey results on experience of psychiatric units presently operating under Medicare DRG.* Washington, DC: American Psychiatric Association, Office of Economic Affairs.

Anderson, S., & Harthorn, B. (1989). The recognition, diagnoses and treatment of mental disorders by primary care physicians. *Medical Care, 27*(9), 869–885.

Ashcroft, M., Fries, B., Nerenz, D., Falcon, S., Srivastava, S., Lee, C., Berkl, S., & Errera, P. (1989). A psychiatric patient classification system. *Medical Care, 27*(5), 543–557.

Babigian, H.M., & Reed, S.K. (1987a). An experimental model capitation payment system for the chronically mentally ill. *Psychiatric Annals, 17*(9), 604–609.

Babigian, H.M., & Reed, S.K. (1987b). Capitation payment systems for the chronically mentally ill. *Psychiatric Annals, 17*(9), 599–602.

Bachofer, H. (1988). Prospective pricing of psychiatric services. In D. Scherl, J. English, & S. Sharfstein (Eds.), *Prospective payment and psychiatric care* (pp. 9–18). Washington, DC: American Psychiatric Association.

Berwich, D. (1989). Health services research and quality of care: Assignments for the 1990's. *Medical Care, 27*(8), 763–771.

Bittker, T. (1988). Health maintenance organizations and prepaid psychiatry. In S. Sharfstein, & E.R. Brown (Eds.), *Principles for a national health program: A framework for analysis and development. Milbank Memorial Fund Quarterly, 66*(4), 573–617.

Camberg, L., & McGuire, T. (1989). Inpatient psychiatric units in non-teaching general hospitals. *Medical Care, 27*(2), 130–139.

Catalano, R. (1987). An ecological perspective on behavioral disorder. In L. Duhl, & N.

Cummings, (Eds.), *The future of mental health services* (pp. 133–148). New York: Springer Publishing Company.

Chamberlain, J. (1987). Update on psychiatric-mental health nursing education at the federal level. *Archives of Psychiatric Nursing*, 2(1), 132–138.

Cherkin, D., Grothaws, L., & Wagner, E. (1989). The effects of office co-payments on utilization in a health maintenance organization. *Medical Care*, 27(7), 669–679.

Christman, L. (1987). Who can do therapy? In L. Duhl & N. Cummings (Eds.), *The future of mental health* (pp. 99–104). New York: Springer Publishing Company.

Cummings, N., & Duhl, L. (1987). The new delivery system. In L. Duhl, & N. Cummings (Eds.), *The future of mental health services* (pp. 85–98). New York: Springer Publishing Company.

Daniels, N. (1985). *Just health care*. New York: Cambridge University Press.

DaVal, M. (1988). Changing reimbursement patterns and the realities of health care finance. In D. Scherl, J. English & S. Sharfstein (Eds.), *Prospective payment and psychiatric care* (pp. 1–8). Washington, DC: American Psychiatric Association.

Duhl, L., Cummings, N., & Hyner, J. (1987). Introduction: The emergence of the mental health complex. In L. Duhl & N. Cummings (Eds.), *The future of mental health care* (pp. 1–14). New York: Springer Publishing Company.

Dulter, J., & Fine, T. (1985). Federal health care financing of mental illness: A failure of public policy. In S. Sharfstein & A. Beigel (Eds.), *The new economics of mental health care* (pp. 17–38). Washington, DC: American Psychiatric Association.

English, J., Sharfstein, S., & Scherl, D. (1988). Diagnostic related groups and general hospital psychiatry: The American Psychiatric Association Study. In D. Scherl, J. English, & S. Sharfstein. (Eds.), *Prospective payment and psychiatric care* (pp. 19–39). Washington, DC: American Psychiatric Association.

Feldman, S., & Goldman, B. (1987). Mental health care in HMO's: Practice and potential. In L. Duhl & N. Cummings (Eds.), *The future of mental health services* (pp. 55–70). New York: Springer Publishing Company.

Fox, J. (1988). *Linking knowledge, manpower and quality care in Virginia's public mental health system*. Richmond, VA: Department of Mental Health, Mental Retardation, and Substance Abuse Services (DMHMRSAS).

Fox, J. (1989). *Final report of the Galt visiting scholar*. Richmond, VA: DMHMRSAS.

Frank, R., & Kamlet, M. (1989). Determining provider choice for the treatment of mental disorders: The role of health and mental health status. *Health Services Research*, 24, 83–103.

Frank, R., & Lave, J. (1985). The impact of Medicaid benefit design on length of hospital stay and patient transfers. *Hospital and Community Psychiatry*, 36(7), 749–753.

Franklin, J., Solowitz, B., Mason, M., et al. (1987). An evaluation of case management. *American Journal of Public Health*, 77, 674–678.

Frazier, S., & Parron, D. (1987). The federal mental health agenda. In L. Duhl & N. Cummings. (Eds.), *The future of mental health services* (pp. 29–46). New York: Springer Publishing Company.

Freiman, M., Mitchell, J., Taube, C., & Harrow, B. (1988). The 1985 National Institute of Mental Health/Health Care Financing Administration Study of Payment for Psychiatric Admissions Under Medicare: Overview and a look ahead. In D. Scherl, J. English, & S. Sharfstein (Eds.), *Prospective payment and psychiatric care* (pp. 91–106). Washington, DC: American Psychiatric Association.

Gallagher, T. (1987). Accountability and implications for supervision and future training. In L. Duhl & N. Cummings (Eds.), *The future of mental health services* (pp. 117–132). New York: Springer Publishing Company.

Goldman, H. (1987). Financing the mental health system. *Psychiatric Annals, 17*(9), 580–584.

Goldman, H. (1988). Overview of studies on psychiatric hospital care under a prospective payment system. In D. Scherl, J. English, & S. Sharfstein (Eds.), *Prospective payment and psychiatric care* (pp. 81–90). Washington, DC: American Psychiatric Association.

Goldman, H., & Gatozzi, A. (1988). Murder in the cathedral revisited: President Reagan and the mentally disabled. *Hospital and Community Psychiatry, 39*(3), 505–509.

Goldman, H., & Lock, A. (1985). Diagnostic related groups and perspective payment in psychiatric hospital care. In S. Sharfstein & A. Beigel (Eds.), *The new economics of mental health care* (pp. 105–118). Washington, DC: American Psychiatric Association.

Gudeman, J., & Shore, M. (1985). Public care for the chronically mentally ill: A new model. In S. Sharfstein & A. Beigel (Eds.), *The new economics of mental health care* (pp. 191–202). Washington, DC: American Psychiatric Association.

Gurevitz, H., & Wallach, H. (1985). Issues and choices facing psychiatry: The California experience. In S. Sharfstein & A. Beigel (Eds.), *The new economics of mental health care* (pp. 217–228). Washington, DC: American Psychiatric Association.

Harris, M., & Bergman, H. (1988). Misconceptions about use of case management services by chronic mentally ill: A utilization analysis. *Hospital and Community Psychiatry, 39*(12), 1276.

Hartwig, A., & Buss, E. (1987). The ethics of mental health practice. In L. Duhl & N. Cummings (Eds.), *The future of mental health services* (pp. 105–116). New York: Springer Publishing Company.

Herzberg, J., & Speller, J. (1985). An overview of preferred provider organizations and psychiatry. In S. Sharfstein & A. Beigel (Eds.), *The new economics of mental health care* (pp. 97–104). Washington, DC: American Psychiatric Association.

Horn, S., Chambers, A., Sharkey, P., & Horn, R. (1989). Psychiatric severity of illness: A case mix study. *Medical Care, 27*(1), 69–84.

Hurowitz, J. (1989). Meeting the medical needs in public psychiatric facilities. *Health Affairs, 8*(2), 77–83.

Hynes, J. (1987). The California mental health reform act of 1985: A case study of policy reform in the post welfare state. In L. Duhl & N. Cummings (Eds.), *The Future of Mental Health Services* (pp. 149–164). New York: Springer Publishing Company.

Katz, S., & Trainor, P. (1988). Impact of cost containment strategies on the state mental health delivery system. In D. Scherl, J. English, & S. Sharfstein (Eds.), *Prospective payment and psychiatric care* (pp. 55–66). Washington, DC: American Psychiatric Association.

Keeler, E.B., et al. (1986). *The demand for episodes of mental health services.* R 3432-National Institute of Mental Health. Santa Monica, CA: RAND Corporation.

Kiesler, C. (1987). The guilds and their organization, members and potential contributions. In L. Duhl & N. Cummings (Eds.), *The future of mental health services* (pp. 55–70). New York: Springer Publishing Company.

Krauss, J. (1987). Nursing, madness and mental health. *Archives of Psychiatric Nursing, 1*(1), 3–15.

Levenson, A. (1985). The for profit system. In S. Sharfstein & A. Beigel (Eds.), *The new economics of mental health care* (pp. 151–164). Washington, DC: American Psychiatric Association.

Mahoney, J. (1988). Future trends and emerging issues in alternative delivery systems: A purchaser's perspective. In D. Scherl, J. English, & S. Sharfstein (Eds.), *Prospective payment and psychiatric care* (pp. 139–154). Washington, DC: American Psychiatric Association.

Martin, D., Diehr, P., Price, K., & Richardson, W. (1989). Effect of a gatekeeper plan on health services use and charges: A randomized trail. *American Journal of Public Health, 79*(12), 1628–1632.

McGuire, T., & Dickey, B. (1985). Payment for mental health care: Economic issues. In S. Sharfstein, & A. Beigel (Eds.), *The new economics of mental health care* (pp. 39–52). Washington, DC: American Psychiatric Association.

Mechanic, D. (1989). *Mental health and social policy.* Englewood Cliffs, NJ: Prentice Hall.

Mechanic, D., & Aiken, L. (1987). Improving the care of patients with chronic mental illness. *New England Journal of Medicine, 317,* 1634–1638.

Miller, G. (1985). The public sector: The state mental health aging. In S. Sharfstein, & A. Beigel (Eds.), *The new economics of mental health care* (pp. 165–190). Washington, DC: American Psychiatric Association.

Muntz, R. (1985). Teaching about prospective payment systems. In S. Sharfstein & A. Beigel (Eds.), *The new economics of mental health care* (pp. 131–150). Washington, DC: American Psychiatric Association.

Musznski, I. Jr. (1985). Prospective pricing: The common denominator in a changing health care market and its implications for psychiatric care. In S. Sharfstein & A. Beigel (Eds.), *The new economics of mental health care* (pp. 1–16). Washington, DC: American Psychiatric Association.

National Center for Health Statistics (1985). *Hospital discharge survey.* Washington, DC: U.S. Government Printing Office.

National Institute of Mental Health, Mental Health United States. (1987). Mandersheid, R.W., & Barrett, S.A. (Eds.). DHHS Publication No. (ADM) 87–1518. Washington, DC: Supt. of Docs. U.S. Government Printing Office.

National Institute of Mental Health, Mental Health United States. (1987). Mandersheid, R.W., & Sonnenschein, M.A. (Eds.). DHHS Publication No. (ADM) 90–1708. Washington, DC: Supt. of Docs. U.S. Government Printing Office.

Neuerow, M.I., & Gibson, R. (1988). Prospective payment for private psychiatric specialty hospitals. In D. Scherl, J. English, & S. Sharfstein (Eds.), *The National association of private psychiatric hospitals prospective payment study* (pp. 41–54). Washington, DC: American Psychiatric Association.

Onek, J., & Glover, S. (1985). The new economics of health care: Legal issues. In S. Sharfstein & A. Beigel (Eds.), *The new economics of mental health care* (pp. 65–84). Washington, DC: American Psychiatric Association.

Patrick, D., Stein, J., Porta, M., Porter, C., & Ricketts, T. (1988). Poverty, health services and health status in rural America. *Milbank Memorial Fund Quarterly, 66*(1), 105–136.

Pomp, H., & McGovern, M. (1988). Integrating state hospital and community based services. *Hospital and Community Psychiatry, 39*(8), 553–554.

*Proceedings of National Conference on Recruitment in Psychiatric Nursing* (1981). National Institute of Mental Health.

Santos, A., Thrasher, J., & Ballenger, J. (1988). Decentralized services for public hospital patients: A cost analysis. *Hospital and Community Psychiatry, 39*(8), 827–829.

Scheffler, R. (1987). The economics of mental health care in a changing economic and health care environment. In L. Duhl & N. Cummings (Eds.), *The future of mental health services* (pp. 47–54). New York: Springer Publishing Company.

Scherl, D., English, J., & Sharfstein, S. (Eds.) (1988). *Prospective payment and psychiatric care.* Washington, DC: American Psychiatric Association.

Segal, E., & Garrett, L. (1985). The employer perspective. In S. Sharfstein & A. Beigel (Eds.), *The new economics and psychiatric care* (pp. 53–64). Washington, DC: American Psychiatric Association.

Shadoan, R. (1985). A California model of private-public cooperation delivering outpatient psychiatric care to medically indigent population. In S. Sharfstein & A. Beigel (Eds.), *The new economics of mental health care* (pp. 203–216). Washington, DC: American Psychiatric Association.

Sharfstein, S., & Beigel, A. (1985). Less is more? Today's economic climate and its challenge to psychiatry. In S. Sharfstein & A. Beigel (Eds.), *The new economics and psychiatric care* (pp. 229–240). Washington, DC: American Psychiatric Association.

Sharfstein, S. (1988). Changing insurance markets. In D. Scherl, J. English, & S. Sharfstein (Eds.), *Prospective payment and psychiatric care* (pp. 121–128). Washington, DC: American Psychiatric Association.

Sloan, F.A., Morrisey, M.A., & Valvona, J. (1988). Effects of the Medicare prospective payment system on hospital cost containment: An early appraisal. *Milbank Memorial Fund Quarterly, 66*(2), 191–220.

Stein, L.I. (1987). Funding a system of care for schizophrenia. *Psychiatric Annals, 17*(9), 592–598.

Taube, C., & Rupp, A. (1986). The effects of access to ambulatory mental health care for the poor and near poor under 65. *Medical Care, 24*(8), 677–686.

Vertrers, J., Manton, K., & Mitchell, K. (1989). Case mix adjusted analyses of service utilization for a Medicaid health insuring organization in Philadelphia. *Medicare Care, 27*(4), 397–411.

Weinstein, M., Berwich, D., Goldman, P., Murphy, J., & Barsky, A. (1989). A comparison of three psychiatric screening job tests using receiver operating characteristics (ROC). *Medical Care, 27*(6), 593–605.

Willis, P., & Langenbrunner, J. (1988). Nonpsychiatric Medicare excluded hospitals: Research studies and policy directions. In D. Scherl, J. English, & S. Sharfstein (Eds.), *Prospective payment and psychiatric care* (pp. 107–120). Washington, DC: American Psychiatric Association.

Wolfe, H., Astriachan, B., & Scherl, D. (1988). Psychiatric practice in organized health and proprietary care systems. In D. Scherl, J. English, & S. Sharfstein (Eds.), *Prospective payment and psychiatric care* (pp. 155–168). Washington, DC: American Psychiatric Association.

Wyatt, R.J., & Clark, K.P. (1987). Calculating the cost of schizophrenia. *Psychiatric Annals, 17*(9), 586–591.

## Chapter 16

# Nursing Returns to the Home Health Frontier: Markets and Trends in Home Health Care

ROSEMARY A. BOWMAN

*N*OT UNLIKE OTHER sectors of the economy, health care is driven by the prospect of business opportunity and potential profitability. Home health care is a new frontier of health services. Home health care received an injection of growth serum in the early 1980s when Medicare reimbursement policy established virtually unlimited coverage for acute/intermittent home health care services for its beneficiaries. Medicare set the precedent and stimulated the visibility that increased the demand for home care.

The Medicare benefit has narrowed in recent years as a result of federal budget cuts, and the Medicare "well" has become a less lucrative source of business for home care providers. Although Medicare has become a lesser player in the total home health care arena, its impact is still significant. Examination of the industry and its environment yields multiple factors that contribute to the growth of home health care and its opportunities for nursing.

## Growth in Home Health Care

Home health care enjoys a high level of visibility today throughout the health care industry. Although inpatient utilization in acute care settings has been decreasing, home care service revenues have increased over 68 percent since 1981. Projections through 1990 anticipate an annual average growth rate of up to 17 percent (Louden & Company, 1985). This growth will be produced by new applications of home care plus expansion of the existing frequent user market. Factors that directly contribute to the growth in home health care include changing demographics, cost-conscious payment systems, new technology, professional interest and acceptance, and increased consumer demand.

*Demographic Changes.* Historically the over-65 population has represented the vast majority of home health care patients. As this population grows, there will be

235

a corresponding need for more home health care owing to the compounding of multiple disabilities and diseases that accompany aging (Rowe, 1988).

The "old elderly" experience the greatest incidence and prevalence of acute and chronic disease. Although less than 5 percent of the 65-plus population live in nursing homes, a substantial portion of those living at large in the community report major limitations of activities of daily living owing to age-related, chronic conditions (Rowe, 1988). Approximately 5 percent of the 65- to 74-year-olds need assistance with activities of daily living, whereas approximately 35 percent of the over 85 year old population require such assistance. This combination of greater longevity and increased morbidity has led to a new phenomenon—the "young elderly" caring for the "old elderly." It is not unusual for a person of 70 years or older to have the responsibility of caring for a 90-year-old family member. A 1988 report to the United States House of Representatives noted that the average American woman spends 17 years in child rearing and 18 years caring for elderly parents (Beck, Kantrowitz, Beachy, Gordon, Hager, & Hammill, 1990). This phenomenon is intensifying with the increased longevity of the elderly and has enormous implications for home care.

*Cost-Conscious Payment Systems.*   Health care cost-containment plus deficit reduction is part of the day-to-day operating environment for all health care consumers and providers. The public sector has set the tone by limiting future expenditure increases for Medicare and Medicaid.

Legislative and regulatory changes by the federal government have had a profound effect on the entire United States health care delivery system (Rowe, 1988). The Medicare Prospective Payment System, which established payment to hospitals based on standard diagnosis-related groups, has affected the length of time all patients spend in hospitals. Private sector insurance companies, self-insured employers, and health maintenance organizations have followed the Medicare lead, adopting methods to reduce inpatient hospital stays.

One effect of shorter hospital stays for Medicare beneficiaries is that patients are discharged "quicker and sicker." Another result is that more diagnostic and treatment procedures are done on an outpatient basis on the assumption that patients can care for themselves when they return home. Home care is filling the gap left in patient care in both of these circumstances.

In the private sector, there is a concerted effort to identify cost-effective means to provide care in lieu of hospitalization. Insurance companies have employed case management companies to identify alternative ways to manage high-dollar cases, with home health care frequently identified as an option. Insurers and health maintenance organizations have demonstrated significant cost savings for many types of patients using home care (National Association for Home Care, 1986).

*Technologic Developments.*   Recent advances in technology are increasing the number of patients surviving multiple trauma, complications of pregnancy and childbirth, and complex acute and chronic illnesses. Some of these patients become dependent on technology. They may require months, years, or even lifelong nursing care up to 24 hours a day.

Technologic advances enhance the portability and simplicity of equipment, making it possible for patients to continue treatments or to be maintained in their own homes (Anderson, 1986). Portable ventilators make it possible for ventilator-dependent patients to leave the institutional setting. Total parenteral nutrition provides nutrient solutions that meet all of a patient's daily nutritional requirements infused through a central venous access by an external, minivolume infusion pump (Handy, 1988). Enteral nutrition substitutes for oral feedings by infusion of nutrients into gastroduodenal tubes or other appropriate access with support of a continuous, controlled flow pump (Berkow & Fletcher, 1987). Intravenous antibiotic therapy is administered in multiple daily doses for long-term therapy at home. Small portable infusion pumps are used for continuous infusion of controlled doses of chemotherapy agents and analgesics. Apnea monitors, phototherapy units, and fetal monitors are other types of technologic devices that are used in the home.

The features that make high-technology care available in the home include portability of equipment, composition of pharmaceutical and nutritional agents, simplicity of preparation and packaging, durability of disposables, and computerization of medical devices (Anderson, 1986). Many patients and families are taught to use high-technology equipment and to provide self-care in the home. Nurses make home visits to instruct and monitor their progress and status. Patients who are very sick may require 24-hour nursing care in the home delivered by registered nurses. The total price tag for high-technology home care can be about one third the cost of the same care in a hospital (Anderson, 1986).

*Professional Interest and Acceptance.* The Medicare home care benefit exposed many physicians to the services available from this type of care. Since the physician continues to be the gatekeeper for most payment sources, the willingness of physicians to refer patients to home care is a key to the growth of the industry.

More physicians are now educated about home care services (Anderson, 1986). Some physicians who have seen the economic viability of home care, particularly high-technology home care, have become investors in local home care companies. Medical texts also encourage the home as a formal treatment site for patients, particularly the elderly and terminally ill (Rowe, 1988).

The interest and encouragement of pharmacists in the development of home nutrition and intravenous therapy programs have also been part of the growth of high-technology home care (Harris & Mellot, 1986).

Hospitals employ discharge planners who encourage home care. Hospitals themselves have entered the home care marketplace as a means of diversification and specialization and to ensure their ongoing control of profits and referrals. Keeping patients within the hospital family has stimulated use of home care services.

Nurses are acknowledging home health care both as a practice setting and a vehicle for health care delivery. Home health care was the focus of the February, 1990, issue of *The American Nurse*, which identified the home as an important site for nursing practice (Selby, 1990).

*Consumer Demand.* Consumers have become more active decision makers regarding health care, how it is purchased, and how it is provided (Allen, 1987). Health-conscious consumers are dealing more with their health problems and are selecting wellness programs and home health care as a preferred alternative to institutionalization (Louden & Company, 1985).

With increased consumer awareness of home care, there is also an unrealistic expectation about third-party payment for home health care services. Many elderly

**TABLE 16–1 Home Health Paradigm: The Nature of Services
and *Payment Sources***

| Acute Home Care | Long-Term Home Care |
| --- | --- |
| Acute/Intermittent Care | Long-term/Custodial Care |
|   *Medicare* |   *Out of pocket* |
|   *Private insurance* |   *Medicaid* |
|   *Health maintenance organization* |   *Long-term care insurance* |
|   *Medicaid* | Long-term/Intensive Care |
| Acute/Intensive Care |   *Private insurance* |
|   *Private insurance* |   *Casualty insurance* |
|   *Health maintenance organization* |   *Health maintenance organization* |
|   *Out of pocket* | Long-term/Hospice Care |
| |   *Private insurance* |
| |   *Health maintenance organization* |
| |   *Medicare* |
| |   *Out of pocket* |

Source: Author.

and their families expect Medicare to pay for personal care assistance. The Medicare home care benefit covers acute care needs of patients who are homebound. Personal care and custodial services for an extended period are not a Medicare benefit and normally are not covered by any third-party source.

For many patients who are terminally ill, such as those with acquired immunodeficiency syndrome and terminal cancer, the home is the desired setting for care. Consumer interest plus cost savings are influencing insurers to cover private duty nursing or hospice benefits. The result is less costly to the insurance company than hospitalization and provides a better quality of life for the patient.

## Nature of Health Care Services in the Home

Home health care is made up of those services and products that enhance the physical and mental health and functional capacity of individuals confined to their homes. Home health is a vehicle for the delivery of both acute and long-term care, as illustrated in Table 16–1. Home care can be very complex or very simple. The patients may be young or very old. The nature of nursing practice in the home involves most nursing specialties. Payment sources differ with the nature of the service provided.

### Acute Care

The objective of the acute care model of home care is the recovery of the patient (Detmer, 1985). Acute care is subdivided into intermittent and intensive care.

*Acute/Intermittent Care.*   The acute/intermittent care model has evolved from the intermittent services pattern defined by the Medicare home care benefit, which has subsequently been adopted by many private insurance companies. The Medicare program finances services that promote recovery and rehabilitation of homebound beneficiaries.

Patients experiencing an acute episode of illness or injury or an exacerbation of a chronic illness receive intermittent nursing visits in their homes one or more times per week. The home care nurse promotes continuation of recovery begun in the hospital or provides care in lieu of hospitalization. The nurse supervises patients and families in self-care procedures, instructs them in diet and medication control, changes dressings, administers intravenous medication or nutrients, and performs a variety of other nursing procedures.

The literature reflects circumstances in which the efficacy of acute/intermittent care has been evaluated:

- Early hospital discharge of very low birth weight infants to the care of a nurse specialist in the home has been shown to be safe, cost-effective, and more desirable than prolonged hospitalization (Brooten et al., 1986).
- Surgical preparations at home on the day of surgery and early postsurgical discharge, both supported by home health care, reduce trauma to the patient and reduce costs to insurers and enrollees of health maintenance organizations (Drummond, Boucher, Drummond, & Geraci, 1986).
- In one study, patients with osteomyelitis, soft-tissue infections, endocarditis, and other infections received home intravenous antibiotic therapy. A multidisciplinary team of infectious disease physicians, a pharmacist, specialty nurses, and a social worker coordinated selection, education, and follow-up visits for patients. The duration of home therapy averaged 19 days, with a mean cost savings of $5728 per treatment course (Rehm & Weinstein, 1986).
- Home phototherapy for jaundiced infants who are otherwise healthy and have capable, motivated parents is a feasible, safe, and effective alternative to hospital care (Eggert, Pollary, Follamd, & Jung, 1985).

Disciplines in addition to nursing that practice in acute/intermittent home care include physical therapy, occupational therapy, speech therapy, and medical social services. A home health aide may also make visits in conjunction with a nurse or therapist to provide nominal support for patients with difficulties with activities of daily living.

The payment source for home care often defines the type of service that can or will be delivered. The most frequent payers in the acute/intermittent care model are Medicare, private insurance, health maintenance organizations, and Medicaid.

*Acute/Intensive Care.*   Acute/intensive care services address acute illness or injury experienced by patients who receive continuous nursing or personal care services provided in the home with ongoing nursing supervision and case management. These services have also been characterized as private duty home care.

Factors that determine the need for acute/intensive care include severe or debilitating illness or injury; patient inability to administer medications; limitation of mobility that threatens safety; inability to manage personal hygiene and toileting; dependency on high-technology equipment; and inability to provide for personal nutrition. Patients who have the most acute needs receive 24 hours of service daily. The duration of an episode of illness requiring acute/intensive care may be up to 4 to 6 weeks.

Examples of patients who meet one or more of the criteria for acute/intensive home care follow.

- A 92-year-old woman living alone in a retirement community falls during the night and sustains muscle strains, multiple bruises, and generalized soreness. Although no fractures occurred, she is unable to transfer into and out of bed, off a chair, or onto and off the toilet. Until the patient can safely ambulate and provide for her own nutrition, a nursing assistant is required 24 hours a day. The nursing case management focuses on determining causes for the fall for future prevention, restorative activity, and safety with nursing assistants in attendance. The nursing assistants are gradually withdrawn as independence is safely achieved.
- A young man with acquired immunodeficiency syndrome has an acute infection for which he is receiving intravenous antibiotics via a central line. While on antibiotic therapy, he is also receiving total parenteral nutrition. He is febrile, lethargic, and unable to care for himself. Neither he, his primary nurse, nor his insurance company wants him to be hospitalized. Registered nurses are required for his care around the clock. The objective is to return him to self-care after the acute exacerbation is controlled. The home care service provides the equipment and medication as well as the nursing staff.

The elderly most often pay out-of-pocket costs for acute/intensive home care services. Private insurance and health maintenance organization coverage is highly variable but often very good for services of licensed nurses in the home, either registered nurses or licensed practical nurses. Insurance coverage is rare for services of nonlicensed personnel, nursing assistants, or home health aides, although there is a beginning trend toward coverage through long-term care insurance. Medicare does not pay for acute/intensive care for elderly or disabled beneficiaries.

## Long-Term Care

Chronic illness and disability create the need for prolonged nursing care in the home in lieu of in an institution. As in acute care, the intensity of need determines the type of service that is required. The types of long-term home care are long-term/custodial, long-term/intensive, and long-term/hospice.

*Long-Term/Custodial.*   Long-term/custodial care addresses the needs of patients who have functional limitations in one or more activities of daily living, although their chronic diseases are under reasonable control. Most of the people who need long-term/custodial care are over 65 years old. Assistance with meals, medications, hygiene, dressing, shopping, mobility, and laundry is basic to long-term/custodial care.

The chronic disorders that produce the need for custodial care also require nursing monitoring and management. A nursing assistant can provide the day-to-day custodial care under the supervision of the professional nurse who defines the plan of care. If the patient has significant dementia or limitation of mobility and lives alone, staffing may be required 24 hours a day. The following are examples of long-term/custodial care.

- A 78-year-old woman with a history of seizure disorder requires supervision of her medications because of short-term memory loss. She requires observation for seizures and nominal assistance with personal hygiene. A nursing assistant is with her 8 to 9 hours daily in her son's home, where she lives. The professional nurse manages the care and provides consultation to the family.
- In a large, independent living retirement community, there are seven residents who need assistance with activities of daily living. Each one has some degree of short-term memory loss. The services provided include walking to meals, medication reminders, bathing, diet supervision, and encouragement to participate in community activities. A nursing assistant is assigned to the retirement community to assist each of these residents for brief periods during the day. The registered nurse makes regular rounds, supervising the care and status of each resident on the program.
- A teenager with a quadreplegia traumatic spinal cord injury requires a nursing assistant to get dressed each day. The process of bathing, bowel program, and dressing takes several hours of the morning. The need for daily personal care assistance will continue into adult life

The farther one gets from traditionally defined medical care, the less frequently third-party payment is available. Consistent with this premise, long-term/custodial care is usually paid out of pocket by consumers. A small percentage of consumers have long-term care insurance that covers some care at home. In some states that have a Medicaid program for home care in lieu of institutional placement, Medicaid pays for limited custodial care (Gaumer et al., 1986).

Patients who choose home care are frequently making a quality of life decision rather than an economic one. Long-term/custodial care in the home can be more expensive than nursing home care over time.

*Long-Term/Intensive Care.*   Long-term/intensive care is largely the result of the technology that saves patients who survive complex injuries and illnesses. Some of these patients become technology-dependent, relying for the rest of their lives on the equipment that saved them. Technology-dependent patients may also require daily nursing care at home because of their medical instability and the complexity of the equipment. The following are examples of long-term intensive care patients.

- A 45-year-old ventilator-dependent patient with multiple sclerosis is discharged home from an intermediate intensive care unit with a life expectancy of 6 weeks. She is subject to exacerbations accompanied by seizures, high temperatures, and a reduced level of consciousness. Her remissions allow her to leave her intensive care living room for excursions into the community. She lives at home with her family and has been supported by a 24-hour staff of licensed practical nurses for nearly 2 years. A detailed case management plan and nursing protocol directed by a primary registered nurse are the keys to her effective home care management.

• An infant born prematurely goes home after 6 months in a pediatric intensive care unit. The child has a feeding tube and is subject to periods of apnea and grand mal seizures. He was weaned from a ventilator before discharge to the home. His care is too complex for his parents to manage. A staff of registered nurses provides 24-hour private duty nursing for an undetermined period of time until the infant is stable enough to be managed, at least part time, by his parents.

There is little that is done in the hospital setting that cannot be done at home in caring for patients with very complex health problems. The site of care for patients with long-term/intensive care needs is sometimes decided by the limits of available options. If patients must be discharged from the hospital because the hospital coverage is exhausted, the choices are limited. Very few long-term care facilities accept ventilator-dependent patients. Some families learn to manage such patients at home with only intermittent help. Others must have long-term intensive nursing care for the remainder of the patient's life.

The cost of long-term/intensive home care is prohibitive for most patients unless there is insurance coverage. For an insurance company, the cost is still much less than long-term/intensive hospital care. Private health insurance or casualty insurance such as workers' compensation is the most frequent source of payment for long-term/intensive home care. Medicare does not pay for these services, and Medicaid also does not normally pay for such cases, although exceptions are sometimes made.

*Long-Term/Hospice.*   Long-term/hospice care is a nursing and palliative service for terminally ill patients and their families. The hospice concept is based on a philosophy of support and comfort for the dying. The dying patient is cared for at home by the family and nurses. Pastoral, psychological, and social services are normally included in the hospice care, in addition to nursing and medication.

Hospice services become appropriate at the point that patients and families decide that no further intervention is desired in the patient's disease process. The duration of hospice service is usually 6 months or less. The scope of service ranges from intermittent visits to 24-hour intensive nursing care. The nature of the service ranges from respite for family caregivers to assumption of the total caregiving role. Although some inpatient hospice beds are available, most hospice services have the objective that the patient will be cared for and allowed to die at home.

• A 54-year-old man has carcinoma of the large bowel with mestastasis to the liver. He and his family elected hospice services after his last hospitalization. At that time, new tumors were found, and it was agreed that chemotherapy and radiation were no longer effective. He receives total parenteral nutrition daily via central venous access. He has a morphine pump by which he receives both a continuous infusion and boluses on demand for pain control. He requires moderate assistance with ambulation. The hospice provides coverage by a registered nurse 12 hours daily when the most technical aspects of his care are executed. The family provides his night-time care. Private insurance pays 100 percent of his hospice benefit at home.

- A 4-year-old child with leukemia is sent home following her most recent exacerbation. None of her chemotherapy has had a lasting effect. Her mother has left work in order to provide most of her care. The mother manages her gastrostomy feedings, following the instructions of the hospice nurse who visits 3 days a week. A home health aide visits daily for 2 hours to help the mother with the child's bath and other personal care. The Medicaid program in her state pays for her care through a special case management program. The family has no other insurance.

Hospice is a concept that has grown in recent years. More insurance companies are including hospice coverage in order to avoid the costs of prolonged hospitalizations for terminal conditions. The Medicare benefit is somewhat narrow in coverage but it does provide for both home and inpatient hospice benefits. Medicaid coverage varies by state. The cost of hospice care is often borne or supplemented out of pocket by the patient or family.

The types of home care described above are not mutually exclusive. A patient who has received acute/intermittent care may require long-term/custodial care daily thereafter in order to prevent nursing home placement. Or a patient who has received long-term/intensive care may recover to a state of total functional independence following a period of supportive intermittent services. The pervasive element in each of these types of home care is nursing. Nursing is the key to determination of need and delivery of service.

## Organization of Home Care Services

Home health care is as organizationally diverse as the health care system itself. Nurses practice in local environments as distinct as every city block, county road, and household in the country. Nurses even deliver home health care to the homeless, finding them in community shelters or temporary group homes.

Home care providers range from small, independent businesses to large multiunit corporations. Some are very specialized, providing only a certain type of nursing care, such as pediatric services, whereas others are comprehensive, providing nursing and personal care, multidisciplinary services, complex medical equipment, medical supplies, and pharmaceuticals. Many providers of home health care are also in the business of supplemental staffing of hospitals, nursing homes, and other types of health care entities.

Classifications of home health providers include visiting nurse associations, public health departments, hospital-based agencies, local independent agencies, regional-national chains, and private duty registries. Roughly one half of all home health providers are proprietary, i.e., for-profit entities (Home health agencies and hospices by provider type, 1990).

## Regulatory Environment

Payment sources dictate much of the organizational structure and services of home health care. Medicare and Medicaid do not pay for services unless the organization is certified. Even payment for durable medical equipment requires a Medicare provider number. Providers that are certified are regulated by the conditions of participation in the Medicare program. Rules and regulations of the program are administered by state agencies and insurance companies designated as fiscal intermediaries.

Medicare providers that diversify beyond the acute/intermittent services reimbursable by Medicare typically create a separate entity or corporation through which to provide non-Medicare services. This practice is designed to avoid reimbursement problems with Medicare, but it contributes to the organizational complexity of the home care industry.

About one half of the states have license and certificate of need requirements for home health care. Definitions of home health care differ from state to state for licensing purposes. Some states regulate only acute/intermittent services, i.e., those that would be paid by Medicare and Medicaid. The certificate of need is granted if a state health planning review justifies the need for more home health services within the state. It is very difficult to get a new certificate of need approved in most states. Rate-setting bodies may also have jurisdiction relative to health care cost containment, requiring providers to go through a rate review before charges can be changed.

Companies that provide pharmaceuticals in the home must meet state pharmacy requirements, but they often do not fit definitions of home care that would require licensing or certificates of need. Rate-setting bodies may also have jurisdiction relative to health care cost containment, requiring providers to go through a rate review before charges can be changed.

## Accreditation

Accreditation is a new topic for home care, despite the fact that the National League for Nursing has had its accreditation program in place for many years. The Community Health Accreditation Program of the National League for Nursing and the Joint Commission on Accreditation of Healthcare Organizations have each developed an accreditation program for home health care providers. Both programs are voluntary. The accreditation process verifies that an organization meets prescribed operating and quality standards. Both the Community Health Accreditation Program and the Joint Commission on Accreditation of Healthcare Organizations have applied for "deemed status" with the Health Care Financing Administration of the United States Department of Health and Human Services. If and when such status is granted, accredited home health organizations will automatically be validated for Medicare certification. Accreditation is also valuable as a marketing tool.

## Referrals

Home health care is a need-driven service. Most people have little awareness of home health care options until a personal need arises. They are therefore dependent on others for recommendations, often on short notice. Referrals are made by physicians, hospital discharge planners, insurance company case managers, and other health care professionals.

Referral networks have been established by several large managed care systems, employers, and local support organizations. They are particularly useful for identifying resources for elder care (Beck et al., 1990). Knowledge about home care as an option and choice of a specific provider are frequently the result of word-of-mouth referrals from friends. Local visibility, reliability, and service are keys to having a strong referral base.

## Nurses and Home Health Care

Nurses are the principal professionals in home health care both in clinical practice and in management. The expansion of home care has increased the demand for nurses in a variety of specialties in order to meet the multiple and complex needs of patients at home. Nurses are responsible for managing very diverse populations of patients who need acute and long-term care. The home environment increases the patient care variables by the number of family and friends in attendance and the nature of the home environment itself. Unlike the hospital or nursing home, where the patient is on the provider's turf, the home is the patient's turf. The nurse is, therefore, a guest in the patient's home, delivering care at the invitation and indulgence of the patient.

The examples of care situations cited above give a sample of the types of patients and nursing requirements that are encountered in home care. Pediatric nurse specialists remove children from the relatively unfriendly hospital environment into the home, where they are comfortable. They give one-to-one care to children plus support and instruction to families. Adult nurse practitioners, infectious disease specialists, oncology nurses, geriatric nurse practitioners, and community health nurses, among other nurse specialists, each have a place in home care practice.

Acute/intermittent care patients typically receive one to three nursing visits per week. The nurse typically has an active case load of patients who will be seen for several weeks or months. The nurse sees five to seven patients daily, on average. In addition to giving direct patient care, the nurse is responsible for preparation of the care plan, coordination of care with physicians and other providers, and supervision of nursing assistants.

Except in rare circumstances, most third-party payers still require physician orders for home care before payment is made for nursing visits. If payment is out of pocket and there are no regulations to the contrary, nursing visits do not require physician authorization.

Demand for private duty nursing in the home for acute/intensive care patients is increasing. After determining the level of care required by the patient, the primary nurse, who is the case manager, defines and directs the care delivered by nursing assistants or licensed practical nurses. When a case requires staffing by a registered nurse, the primary nurse plays a coordinating role. Each registered nurse is accountable for the total care of the patient and for assuring continuity with the care plan. The nature of private duty practice is intensive in both physical and emotional care. Depth of experience and aggressive practice are essential to acute/intensive care at home. Aggressiveness is relevant to the application of nursing process for each case and to the achievement of patient care objectives by prescription of care strategies and evaluation of outcomes of care.

Long-term care and hospice patients usually have a maintenance or palliative objective as opposed to a recovery objective for care. The nurse manages the patient at home, through exacerbations and remissions of disease and finally death. If the patient is hospitalized, the nurse follows the patient while he or she is in the hospital. Adjustments in the plan of care and staffing requirements at home are made as the condition of the patient changes.

## Management

From the founding of visiting nurse associations to ownership and development of home health businesses, nurses have had a legacy of leadership in home health care (Selby, 1990). Overseeing clinical services and management within a complex regulatory environment are the nurse manager's responsibility. Vision, creativity, and coordination are essential management skills. The elderly population in need of home health is growing, although the Medicare home care benefit is narrowing. A successful nurse manager in home care has to be able to compensate for contradictions in public policy by maximizing the resources available for the patient, whether or not Medicare coverage is available.

Principles of good management should be the guide in home care as in any other business. There are, however, some issues that command the special attention of the nurse manager.

*Clinical Services.* The management of clinical services involves all aspects of patient care. Home care is a very local and a very personal business. It requires attention to detail and flexibility. Special efforts are required for communication among providers, the patient, and the family.

Case management is the process that addresses these requirements. Case management begins with the determination of whether a case is appropriate for home care. Is it possible to deliver the required care in the specific home environment? Is the family comfortable with or capable of learning complex procedures? Are there sufficient family and/or financial resources to pay for the necessary care? Will the physician support the home care program? Can staffing be arranged and put in place rapidly? How often will the registered nurse case manager visit? An objective of case management is to evaluate and provide appropriate services without breaks in the continuity of care.

Case management includes appropriate staffing. An acute/intensive care patient can be cared for by nursing assistants if they are properly instructed and supervised and are not expected to perform invasive procedures. Technology-dependent patients are best assigned to registered nurses or licensed practical nurses. Payment resources often dictate level of staffing. Matching staff to patients and maintaining consistency with preferred staff are keys to effective case management and meeting nursing care goals for patients.

The nurse manager should maintain an active clinical practice. This means being the primary nurse for a reasonable case load that is balanced with administrative demands. It is incongruous for nursing to be considered a clinical discipline when so many nurses never touch a patient. The value of clinical practice for all nurse managers is to maximize nursing skills on behalf of patients and maintain a firsthand knowledge of operations in order to facilitate assurance of quality care.

*Personnel.* One management challenge is to maintain a professional practice environment for personnel. Shortages of both professional and nonprofessional health care personnel are projected for the future (Sussman, 1990). Since home health care is a labor-intensive business, demand for personnel will grow in direct relationship to growth in number of patients. Recruitment and retention of nursing and personal care staff require creativity. Managing staff well is as important as managing patients well.

Personnel reflect the philosophy of the organization. Consistent recruitment criteria, orientation, and maintenance policies set the corporate image. Introduction of staff to patients is an effective means of communicating case management plans and corporate expectations for staff in each patient care setting.

Regulation of personnel varies from state to state. Certification of nursing assistants, referred to as home health aides, is required by a growing number of states. Medicare is in the process of implementing training and certification requirements for home health aides (Randall, 1987). Additional issues that require attention are employee policies, safety procedures, and position classification.

*Financial Issues.* Whether an organization is nonprofit or proprietary, it must have a sufficient margin and cash flow to meet operating and growth requirements. Charges for services and products have to be competitive as well as sufficient to meet operating margins. Good financial planning will address all identifiable contingencies.

Timing of collection is best from patients who pay these costs out of pocket. Payment delays of several weeks or months are not unusual with insurance companies, Medicare, and Medicaid, forcing a home care operation to carry large amounts of receivables. Slow payment plus other contingencies such as the Gramm-Rudman-Hollings cuts on Medicare payments can be devastating to such businesses (Medicare, 1990). A labor-intensive business has to meet its payroll in order to operate.

Financial statements, cost reports, and business plans are financial documents that report operating results and project the future. The nurse manager must be as conversant with these documents as with the case management plan. If a business is not financially healthy, it will not be able to continue to provide quality services to its patients.

*Pricing.* Charges for services, supplies, and equipment reflect value in the marketplace. Charges for nursing have historically been well hidden in institutional billing. Similarly, the rates paid by Medicare to home health providers are rarely known to patients, since Medicare pays 100 percent of allowable costs and providers are not permitted to bill patients if claims are denied. The public is therefore largely uneducated about the value of a professional nursing visit in the home because up to now Medicare has been the primary payer. Hourly charges in the private duty mode are better known because the patient often bears this expense out of pocket or has an insurance company policy that pays for the service.

Pricing reflects value in the marketplace, the value perceived by the payer, and the value internalized by the provider. Perception of need, convenience, competition, and relative costs all influence pricing decisions. The nature and experience of third-party payers is also a factor.

Home care companies that are providing total parenteral nutrition and other intravenous therapies are being criticized for price gouging because of their very high profit margins (Bremner, 1990a). Their pricing policy has been derived in part from comparisons with much higher hospital rates for the same service. Since the home care charge has been more attractive to insurers than the charges for comparable hospital services and patients like the convenience of being at home, the rates have not received significant attention. Recently, accusations of profiteering have been made against some providers by activists for patients with acquired immunodeficiency syndrome who are concerned about care for patients with limited or no insurance coverage.

A service must be understood in order for pricing to be set. The community nursing organization legislation supported by the American Nurses' Association and adopted by Congress in 1987 has not been implemented for two reasons. There are no existing services that are comparable that the public understands, and no one has yet determined how to set a reasonable rate to be paid for the services to be provided.

There is a crisis of value in nursing. However, it is better to be the subject of a pricing debate in the marketplace than to be invisible. Although profiteering is not advocated, home health care does present nursing with the opportunity to set competitive prices for public consumption. Nursing prices can be set for time, units of service, procedures, and the services of assisting personnel. Limitations on third-party payment should not be a deterrent to establishing a nursing service. Consumers are willing to pay for a valued service for which they have a need and whose price they understand.

*Marketing.* Determination of the scope of a product or service, definition of the market to be served, setting pricing strategies, and selling are the components of marketing. Marketing strategies will differ by location and the nature of the organization. A very specialized service will have a narrow range of target markets and options for promotion.

Like all management decisions, marketing has to be consistent with the corporate goal and, at the same time, be flexible and creative. Services need to be adjusted from time to time in order to address the inevitable changes that occur in the marketplace. The quality of service is the most important sales tool, but it will not generate more business if no one knows about it. Nursing and home care must be continually promoted to potential patients, other providers, payees, and the public at large.

*Liability.* The experience of home health care operations and nurses relative to professional liability has been good to date, as evidenced by current malpractice insurance rates. The increased acuity of patients managed at home and the dependence on equipment to aid in patient care raise the issue of increased liability exposure. Risk assessment and risk prevention are as essential to home health as to any other segment of health care.

Recruitment and screening of personnel are important to risk reduction in home care because of the unsupervised hours that staff spend in the patient's home. Meeting expectations of patients, maintaining good family relations, and effective regular supervision are essential.

## *Relationship of Nurses to Home Care Organizations*

Nurses in home care may be employees, independent contractors, or owners. Classification of employment relationships is individual to an organization. They are determined by what people actually do, how they do it, and how they are paid.

Many registered nurses practicing in home care are called independent contractors, and they are paid a flat rate per visit. This classification is advantageous to the home care company because it allows the employer to avoid variable costs, including the employer's portion of the social security tax (FICA), workers' compensation insurance, and health insurance if it is provided only to those classified as "employees." The advantage to nurses is that it promotes an independent practice model if the nurse meets all of the criteria to be an independent contractor. The criteria of the Internal Revenue Service define an independent contractor, in part, as one who has some risk of loss in doing business and one who is not performing the core business of the organization. There is serious debate regarding whether any nurse meets these criteria when practicing in home health care. It is incumbent on individual nurses themselves to keep appropriate records and operate in a way that is consistent with the Internal Revenue Service criteria if they want to be independent contractors.

If registered nurses are not independent contractors, they are classified as employees. Most home care operators have hourly positions available, particularly those providing intensive care services with private duty staff. The attractiveness of this relationship is to have flexibility and personal control over scheduling. Some companies provide benefits even to hourly staff, including insurance, paid leave time, and employee stock options.

## *Nurse Entrepreneurs*

Home care has been a good vehicle for nurse entrepreneurs. Nurses have historically been successful starting Medicare operations. Some nurses have expanded their home care operations across the country. Others have franchise operations of national companies. Most nurse entrepreneurs assume a position of owner-manager. It is also conceivable that such nurses may choose to practice nursing in their own operation, hiring someone else to be the day-to-day manager.

The capital required to start a home health care operation is estimated by projecting the cash flow needed for the expected volume of business for the start-up period, 1 to 2 years. The principal expense of a home health care business is payroll. The vehicle for making these projections is a business plan that includes pro forma financial and cash flow statements. The capital requirements for a home care operation are relatively lower than those for most other health care businesses because investment in a building is not required.

Another means of entry into the business is to purchase an existing operation. The value of an existing business may require more up-front capital. There is also the risk that there will be expensive operating problems in the business. A buyer must use "due diligence" to determine that the operation is viable and that it will not require more repair than the nurse can afford. A good existing business can be an efficient means of start-up.

All of the growth factors noted at the beginning of this chapter indicate that the future market for all types of home health care business will be good. Success is not automatic, but the opportunities are there. *Business Week* cited a home health business serving patients with acquired immunodeficiency syndrome among its 100 high growth companies in 1990 (Bremner, 1990b).

Some rules of thumb that will contribute to the success of a nurse-owned home health operation are

1. Know the local market. Do a feasibility study to determine whether there is a need for the type of service being proposed. Identify key marketing contacts.
2. Examine the competition. Who are they, and what are they doing? What do they charge? Who are their clients? Is there a niche that is not being filled?
3. Identify future trends. Success today does not spell success tomorrow if the business does not identify and adapt to changes. Be flexible.
4. Diversification requires cash and breadth of management time and skill. Acute/intermittent home care is a different business from hospital staffing. Do what you do best. Make sure expansions are timely, well financed, and fit the goals of the organization.
5. Be prepared to commit most of your time to the business. It is a 24 hour a day, 7 day a week obligation to practice nursing.
6. Promote the business constantly. Be involved in the community. Be on the lookout for new opportunities to sell.
7. Plan so that you do not run out of cash.

Once the home care business is operational, there are several opportunities for the future, depending on the objectives of the owner. It may remain a small local business, expand to other locations, diversify into related businesses, enter into a joint venture with other health care providers or related businesses, or be sold out to another company. There is a significant consolidation occurring in home health care around the country, with a few major companies acquiring many smaller operations ("KQC-parent lifetime," 1990). This process also creates new opportunities because it changes the make-up of the players in a local area.

Home care is an investment opportunity for nurses who are willing to take the risk of investing in a new home health operation by backing their nursing colleagues. Such an investment can be very attractive for an investor who is able to wait several years for the business to mature before expecting a return.

## Issues in Home Health Care

All of the indicators point to continuing growth in home health care. Both consumer demand and payment resources are expanding, including the large portion of home health expense that is paid out of pocket.

### Public Policy

Public policy for home health care has not formally changed in recent years. Coverage of the new benefits for catastrophic illness that was added to Medicare in 1988 to cover custodial services for caregiver respite was repealed in 1989 by the United States Congress. The program was to be funded by a tax on beneficiaries. The elderly rose up in protest of the user tax and succeeded in getting the bill repealed. The United States Bipartisan Commission on Comprehensive Health Care in 1990 has proposed a long-term care program that would cover home health and nursing home care for the severely disabled regardless of age or income. The proposal has a $42 billion annual price tag and little viability for passage (Beck et al., 1990).

Although there are increasing discussions of National Health Insurance, there is little likelihood that any proposal will soon be successful. There is not a broad consensus regarding what National Health Insurance should be, even though most people agree that the present health care system is inadequate in a number of ways. Medicare and Medicaid provide insufficient models on which to build National Health Insurance. In a time of continually increasing public deficit and health costs, the prospect for meaningful change in public policy is not great.

The Medicare home care benefit will continue to pay only for acute/intermittent care for beneficiaries who are homebound. Although it is possible to manipulate the benefit to make it look like a long-term/intermittent service, this is a misapplication of the program. Some home health providers are avoiding Medicare because of the difficulty of operating within its constraints. Subscribers to long-term care insurance will be among the few Medicare beneficiaries who will have resources to help pay for long-term/custodial care. Tax deductions are available for the expense of nursing or custodial care for those who itemize deductions.

Public policy will result in many people continuing to "make do" relative to the expense of health care at home. Some people will spend all of their resources and be eligible for Medicaid, although Medicaid pays less than the cost of home health care in some states (Selby, 1990). Home health operations, including visiting nurse associations and public health agencies, have limited resources to provide charity care if charity funds are available at all.

## Payment for Nursing Care

Payment by Medicare is made only to Medicare-certified home health agencies. Most third-party payers, including Medicare, require physician orders to justify payment for home health services for patient care and equipment. The only way this will change will be when nurses are able to charge directly for services provided. Meanwhile, nurses should see to it that consumers receive copies of the bill sent to Medicare from home health providers, so that they will be educated as to the value of nursing visits.

Mundinger recommended in 1983 that the Medicare home care benefit should provide for nurses to direct services and be accountable for patient outcomes and cost-effectiveness in Medicare home health operations. Nurses should be functioning as gatekeepers (Mundinger, 1983). At this writing, the Medicare-certified home health agency is not necessarily nurse-directed. In order to make Mundinger's concept work, the home health operation certified by Medicare would have to be a nursing service composed of nurses who have practice privileges in the organization and direct the care of their patients. Such a concept is far beyond the current Medicare design. This concept does work in the private sector, where nurses are both directing and providing care and being paid out of pocket. When Medicare does not cover a specific service, patients should be advised that they can purchase the services privately, paying for them out of pocket. Through these means, the value of nursing care in the home can be determined, models of comprehensive nursing service can be established, and public pressure for third-party payment will be increased.

## Quality Assurance

Home health operations are heavily regulated by some states that require licenses plus certification of personnel. Other states have no regulation at all. Home health businesses that are Medicare-certified do meet specified criteria that have quality assurance characteristics. The only quality assurance vehicle available to the home health industry across the country is accreditation. National League for Nursing accreditation gives nursing in home health care a consistent quality assurance tool regardless of the nature of the home care services provided or the sources of payment. It is a means of self-regulation for the industry that should be embraced by nurses in home health care. Professional certification of nurses practicing in home health care is another vehicle for quality assurance.

## Ethical Issues in Home Health Care

For some patients in need of home care, there are no personal or public payment sources. This is the case for many almost poor, many elderly, and patients with acquired immunodeficiency syndrome who have exhausted personal funds and health insurance. Home health providers can be of assistance by tapping into community resources or being part of the development of community resource systems that make some services available. Nurses in San Francisco are exemplars of such models for public health and care of patients with acquired immunodeficiency syndrome (American Nurses' Association, 1988).

Technology and longevity create new ethical dilemmas for nurses practicing in home health care. Allowing patients as much of a decision-making role as possible regarding the location for their care is important for all patients, even those with impaired mental function. The ethical challenge for nurses is knowing when to intervene on behalf of patients regarding ethical issues such as the best sites for care, provision of appropriate care, and preparing for death with dignity.

## Conclusion

Opportunity and change are the order of the day in home health care. Market factors are making the demand for home care increase annually at record rates. The economic environment encourages the development of new applications and delivery of health services. The experience and knowledge within nursing presents more nurses with the opportunity to create new ventures in home health care.

Nursing has a historical basis for developing the home health frontier. From the Henry Street project of the 19th century through the high-technology operations of the 20th century, nurses have been creating ways to make nursing care more accessible to their patients.

The home care operations described for the current environment will not be sufficient for the future. New means of organizing and delivering home health care will be necessary as the needs of society continue to change. This chapter has dealt only with national needs and models for health care. The future will present new opportunities internationally, where nurses can forge new home care frontiers. Nursing has the chance at this time to establish its value in the marketplace through home health care. Finally, developing national and international public policy needs the insight of nursing, so that policies regarding the delivery of quality, cost-effective home health care services are realistic, functional, and constructive.

REFERENCES

Allen, P. (1987). *Home health care products and services.* Find/SVP, New York: The Information Clearing House, Inc.

Anderson, H.J. (1986, Februrary). High-technology services help cut lengths of stay, save money. *Modern Health Care, 16*(4), 90–91.

American Nurses' Association (1988). *Nursing Case Management* (pp. 20–23). Kansas City, MO: American Nurses' Association.

Beck, M., Kantrowitz, B., Beachy, L., Gordon, J., Hager, M., & Hammill, R. (1990). Aging: Trading places. *Newsweek,* CXIV(3), 48–54.

Berkow, R., & Fletcher, A. (1987). Nutritional support. *The Merck manual of diagnosis and therapy,* 15 (p. 904). Rahway, NJ: Merck Sharp & Dohme Research Laboratories.

Bremner, B. (1990a). AIDS home care may be due for some housecleaning. *Business Week,* No. 3163, 20.

Bremner, B. (1990b). Quality home care for victims of AIDS. *Business Week.* No. 3160, 105–108.

Brooten, D., Kumar, S., Brown, L.P., Butts, P., Bakewell-Sachs, S., Gibbons, A., & Delivoria-Papadopoulos, M. (1986). A randomized clinical trial of early hospital discharge and home follow-up of very-low-birth-weight infants. *New England Journal of Medicine, 315*(15), 934–939.

Detmer, S. (1985). *The future of health care delivery systems and settings.* Aspen, CO: Presented at Nursing in the 21st Century, a Conference sponsored by the American Association of Colleges of Nursing, American Organization of Nurse Executives.

Drummond, R.C., Boucher, J.D., Drummond, L.J., & Geraci, R.C. (1986). A cost effective surgical program: Collaboration among an HMO, hospital, and home care agency. *Home Health Care Nurse, 4*(3), 37–41.

Eggert, L.D., Pollary, R.A., Follamd, D.S., & Jung, A.L. (1985). Home phototherapy treatment of neonatal jaundice. *Pediatrics, 76*(4), 579–584.

Gaumer, G.L., Birnbaun, H., Protter, F., Burke, R., Franklin, S., & Ellingson-Otto, K. (1986). Impact of the New York long-term home health care program. *Medical Care, 24*(7), 641–653.

Handy, C.M. (1988). Home care of patients with technically complex nursing needs: High-technology home care. *Nursing Clinics of North America, 23*(2), 315–328.

Harris, W.L., & Mellot, P.S. (1986). Home health care bibliography. *American Journal of Hospital Pharmacy, 43,* 699–704.

Home health agencies and hospices by provider type (1990, June). *Home Health Line, XV,* 256.

KQC-parent lifetime acquires 21 home care assets since 1987 (1990, July). *Home Health Line, XV,* 272–274.

Louden & Company (1985). *Home Care Market Outlook.* Chicago: Louden & Company.

Medicare (1990, April). *Home Health Line, XV,* 143–144.

Mundinger, M.O. (1983). *Home care controversy: Too little, too late, too costly.* Rockville, MD: Aspen Publication.

National Association for Home Care (1886, August). The cost-effectiveness of home care. *Caring, 5*(8), 27–29.

Randall, D. (1987). Home health services under Medicare: The need for organized responses to growth and change. *Pride Institute Journal of Long Term Home Health Care, 6*(4), 3–18.

Rehm, S.J., & Weinstein, A.J. (1986). Home intravenous antibiotic therapy: A team approach (abstract). *American Journal of Hospital Pharmacy, 43,* 701.

Rowe, J.W. (1988). Aging and geriatric medicine. In J. Wyngaarden & L. Smith (Eds.), *Cecil textbook of medicine* (18th ed.) (pp. 21–26). Philadelphia: W. B. Saunders Company.

Selby, T. (1990). Home health care finds new ways of caring. *The American Nurse, 22,* 12.

Sussman, D. (1990, July). Health care's sign? Help wanted. *Health Week, 4*(13), 17–34.

## Chapter 17

# Public Health Nursing: Does It Have a Future?

### CAROLYN A. WILLIAMS

SINCE THE 1970s there has been conceptual and semantic confusion surrounding the use and understanding of the terms "public health nursing" and "community health nursing." There has also been much confusion about the roles of community health nurses and public health nurses and their respective fields of practice. This has involved uncertainty about how public health nursing or community health nursing is distinct from other fields or areas of nursing practice, an issue that has led to questions about the future. These matters have been considered in a series of conferences at the national level, held over a period of years, and in the development of several position statements (American Nurses' Association, 1980; American Public Health Association, 1981; U.S. Department of Health and Human Services, 1985).

The question pursued in this chapter is: Does public health nursing have a future? In view of the increasing demand for professional nurses, uneasiness about the health status of Americans, growing concerns about access to care, increased interest in promoting health and preventing disease, and the expansion of community-based services, such a question may seem out of step with these developments. Yet, it is a matter of substance to those who view themselves as specialists in public health nursing. For example, among the leadership in the Public Health Nursing Section of the American Public Health Association, there is concern over the declining membership of the section. And the leadership of the Association of Faculty in Community Health Nursing is discussing the future of public health nursing and spearheading the formation of a coalition of interested groups and individuals to identify what needs to be done to strengthen the field and to move forward with the initiatives proposed.

The following discussion begins with a summary of the current situation in public health nursing and reasons why concerns about the future are being expressed. Included are comments regarding selected historical milestones. The second part of the discussion focuses on changes within the health care system and an identification of what is needed for the future. The discussion concludes with comments on challenges facing the field of public health nursing and a consideration of future prospects.

## Concerns About the Future

### *What Is Public Health Nursing?*

Although attempting to untangle the confusion surrounding the use of the terms "public health nursing" and "community health nursing" may seem like an exercise more appropriate for an etymologist than a health specialist, some clarification is useful. This is so for two reasons. First, what can be viewed as the future of public health nursing is determined in part by how the field is defined. Second, the difficulties associated with understanding the boundaries of the field or the key characteristics that have historically been used to distinguish it have led to some of the questions regarding the future.

In the early 1980s, both the American Nurses' Association, Division of Community Health Nursing (1980), and the American Public Health Association (1981) developed statements on how the field should be defined and the scope of practice. Because of the lack of consistency in these statements, the absence of guidelines for roles, and concerns regarding preparation, in September of 1984 the Division of Nursing held a Consensus Conference on the Essentials of Public Health Nursing Practice and Education (U.S. Department of Health and Human Services, 1985). A number of recommendations were put forward, and one of the more interesting outcomes was consensus about the terms "community health nurse" and "public health nurse." Participants agreed that "community health nurse" could be applied to all nurses who had a practice role in the community, regardless of whether they had specific preparation in public health nursing. In fact, according to the report, any nurse who did not practice in an institution could be called a "community health nurse." Unfortunately, this leads to considerable confusion, because regardless of the type of care provided (primary or tertiary), if the nurse does not work in an institution, she can be viewed as a community health nurse. And if the nurse holds either a master's or doctoral degree and practices in a community setting, the designation of community health nurse specialist can be used, independent of the specialty in which the degree was awarded. As stated in the report, "the degree may be in any area of nursing, such as maternal-child health, psychiatric-mental health, or medical-surgical nursing or some subspecialty of any clinical area" (U.S. Department of Health and Human Services, 1985, p. 4).

The key characteristic used in defining the "public health nurse" was the nature of the educational preparation as opposed to the setting in which practice occurred. It was agreed "that the term 'public health nurse' should be used to describe a person who has received specific educational preparation and supervised clinical practice in public health nursing" (U.S. Department of Health and Human Services, 1985, p. 4). The entry-level public health nurse was defined as an individual who "holds a baccalaureate degree in nursing that includes this educational preparation; this nurse may or may not practice in an official health agency but has the initial qualifications to do so" (p. 4). To be referred to as a specialist in public health nursing, the consensus was that the nurse had to have preparation at either the master's or the doctoral level, "with a focus in the public health sciences" (p. 4). There are a number of problems with these definitions, which have been detailed elsewhere (Williams, 1988). However, three clear points seem to emerge. First, that as an area of specialization, public health nursing is seen as a subset of the broader category, community health nursing. Second, specialization in public health nursing requires graduate preparation that includes the public health sciences, and, third, the setting of practice can no longer be seen as a key factor distinguishing community health nursing from other areas of specialization.

The view of public health nursing that is used in this discussion is the one expressed in the statement by the public health nursing section of the American Public Health Association (1981). Key elements of that definition are:

> Public health nursing synthesizes the body of knowledge from the public health sciences and professional nursing theories. The implicit overriding goal is to improve the health of the community. . . . Public health nursing practice is a systematic process by which:
>
> 1. The health and health care needs of a population are assessed in collaboration with other disciplines in order to identify subpopulations (aggregates), families, and individuals at increased risk of illness, disability, or premature death.
> 2. A plan for intervention is developed to meet these needs, which includes resources available and those activities that contribute to health and its recovery, the prevention of illness, disability, and premature death.
> 3. A health care plan is implemented effectively, efficiently, and equitably.
> 4. An evaluation is made to determine the extent to which these activities have an impact on the health status of the population (U.S. Department of Health and Human Services, 1985, pp. 3–4).

Although the issue may be controversial, increasingly this author believes that *specialization* in public health nursing is most appropriately operationalized in roles with administrative components, in consultant roles, in positions of professional staff to administrators (e.g., a program development specialist who is a staff member in the office of an administrator), and as nursing scientists who develop and test strategies for more effectively providing services to population groups. This is not to say that nurses in other roles do not contribute to public health programs. In fact, patients and families are nursed one at a time by nurse clinicians, whether they are staff "public health nurses," nurse practitioners, or other nurse clinicians. Although providing direct care services is necessary to the success of public health programs that have a clinical component, simply providing services is not a sufficient condition for public health nursing practice as defined above.

The remainder of the discussion deals with this more focused view of specialization in public health nursing.

## Basis of Questions About the Future

*Changes in Practice Settings.* It is suggested that one of the major concerns regarding the future of public health nursing revolves around the shifts that have occurred in the way in which business is done in nursing units in official agencies, such as health departments. Key changes include the following: a shift from generalized public health nursing or district nursing to outpatient clinic work, with very little home visiting, except for those patients served by agencies having certified home care programs; a shift from programs emphasizing prevention, health promotion, and monitoring of health to those focusing on treatment and management of acute and chronic illness of populations (indigent, Medicaid, Medicare); the hiring of individuals who have limited preparation for public health nursing practice, namely, associate degree graduates without baccalaureate level content in the field, as recommended by the recent consensus conference (Department of Health and Human Services, 1985); and the proliferation of regulatory limits on nurses working in agencies.

*Interest in Graduate Education.*   Nursing educators are concerned about declining graduate student interest in the field as contrasted with the current interest in preparation for other fields of practice, particularly critical care nursing. National League for Nursing data on nursing graduates from master's degree programs by content area show that in 1982–1983, 15.2 percent of graduates were in community health. By 1986 to 1987, the proportion of graduates majoring in community health had dropped to 8.7 percent (National League for Nursing, 1989, p. 76). The perception among graduate students that better career opportunities and higher compensation exist in hospital-based settings as compared with what is available in public health settings may be the primary factor in the declining interest in graduate education in public health nursing.

Perhaps the major source of concern regarding the future is the perception among many public health nursing educators that other areas of nursing specialization are claiming elements of what used to be defined as part of the public health nursing area of specialization. This is particularly evident among those who see the setting in which care is delivered as the key to public health nursing specialization. In the past, practice outside the home in organized official agencies and in visiting nursing services (voluntary agencies) was generally seen as the arena for public health nursing. However, in recent times, major organizational changes have occurred as a function of the vertical and horizontal administrative arrangements in the health system and, as a result, the institutional/noninstitutional distinction is less relevant. Increasingly, individuals with specialized preparation in a variety of areas, including critical care, are providing services in the homes of clients. Also, a variety of specialists who do not see themselves as public health nursing specialists are giving increased attention to the family aspects of care (although they may not be focusing on the family as a unit of care) and to issues such as prevention, patient teaching, and continuity of care. Many of these concerns are being translated into the development of clinical nursing roles within the context of hospital-based organizations or organizations that embrace both hospital inpatient and outpatient clinics and in-home services. Examples include approaches to case management that encompass discharge planning; hospital-based home care service programs that provide in-home management of clinically ill patients in need of nurse-monitored high technology care strategies; and the development of hospital-based women's care centers offering a range of services that include physicals for women executives, monitoring of health care status, prevention programs, exercise, and weight management, services that are offered by nurse practitioners and nurse clinicians who have a variety of areas of specialization and by professionals in other fields.

*Primary Care and the Emergence of Nurse Practitioners.* The emergence of national attention on primary care, beginning in the 1960s, and the concomitant development of the nurse practitioner movement may also have contributed to the perceived erosion of the specialized domain of public health nursing. The nurse practitioner movement evolved in the context of national efforts to improve access to health care for underserved populations, particularly in inner city settings and rural areas. Since the primary focus of public health nursing practice is on defining problems (assessing) and proposing solutions (treatment) for population groups or aggregates, it is not surprising that much of the nursing leadership for the development of primary care nursing came from those who were identified with the field of public health nursing. For example, it was through experiences with graduate students studying public health nursing at the University of Colorado that Loretta Ford first identified the need for additional clinical skills in ambulatory pediatrics and began preparing nurses to assume selected assessment and management decisions in the care of children. She then joined forces with Henry Silver to develop a pediatric nurse practitioner program (Ford & Silver, 1967), and the rest is history.

It is also interesting to note that the family nurse practitioner movement had its roots in the thinking and work of those involved in the preparation of public health nurses. For example, the original programs to prepare family nurse practitioners in the United States were funded by the National Center for Health Services Research beginning in 1970 and were referred to as Primex programs. The leadership for these programs was provided by individuals whose appointments were in departments of public health nursing or community health nursing or whose experience had been in community-based services. The original group of educational programs included Cornell University (Doris Schwartz), Vanderbilt University (Beverly Bowns and her successors), Indiana University (Beverly Flynn), Case Western University (Virginia Boardman, who chaired the unit in public health nursing), the Frontier Nursing Service, the School of Nursing at the University of California at Los Angeles, and the University of North Carolina at Chapel Hill (Schools of Nursing and Public Health, Margaret Dolan, and Lucy Conant). In addition to those associated with the family nurse practitioner and pediatric nurse practitioner movements, there were others in the country who were moving forward with training programs designed to meet specific health care needs in community settings. One early program was the practitioner training program at the University of Minnesota School of Public Health under the direction of Alma Sparrow, who headed the unit in public health nursing, and the activities at the University of Illinois School of Nursing within the Department of Public Health Nursing chaired by Virginia Olson.

As described in the literature (U.S. Department of Health, Education, and Welfare, 1980), some graduates of these programs and others went into what might be considered traditional public health nursing settings. However, a number chose to practice in the newly developed primary care clinics and other environments, such as outpatient clinics, community hospitals, private physicians' offices, health maintenance organizations, and institutions dealing with specialized populations, such as schools for exceptional children and nursing homes. In fact, the data indicate that only a minority of these graduates actually went into official public health nursing agencies (U.S. Department of Health, Education, and Welfare, 1980).

Looking at the primary care movement from a broad public health perspective, it can be argued that it is a clear example of how specialists in public health nursing assumed leadership for advancing new care initiatives and developed strategies for dealing with health problems based on an understanding of the needs of defined population groups. Thus, their innovation in the early days of the nurse practitioner movement can be seen as an excellent example of what specialization in public health nursing is all about. However, if one takes a narrower view, it can be argued that the emergence of the primary care movement and the commitment of training resources in the community-public health units of a number of schools of nursing and the nursing units in schools of public health to the development of direct care and primary care roles as opposed to the development of public health skills contributed to the present quandary regarding the future of public health nursing. A key point here is that the *idea* of creating nurse practitioner roles to respond to population needs can be seen as consistent with what a specialist in public health nursing should be doing. But this is not to say that nurse practitioners themselves are, in fact, "public health nurses" or are practicing public health nursing. They may or may not be practicing in a community-focused manner and providing services traditionally associated with staff public health nursing roles (teaching or counseling directed at health promotion, health protection, and disease prevention).

A recent paper on public health nursing in Canada (Matuk & Horsburgh, 1989) clearly indicates that nurses in the United States are not alone in raising questions about the future. Matuk and Horsburgh discuss the lack of pay equity in Canada between public health and hospital-based nurses. They reported that public health nurses' salaries were up to 15 percent less than those of nurses working in hospitals. Moreover, there was little public outcry during work stoppages of 1 to 6 months by public health nurses. According to Matuk and Horsburgh, the absence of obvious public concern ". . . is of great concern to many public health nurse leaders, and prompts them to question seriously the future of the profession" (p. 169).

## The Current Context for Public Health Nursing Practice

Within the last decade, a number of factors external to nursing have influenced what is going on within the world of public health nursing. These include the economic and administrative shifts that occurred in the financing and management of health care, as documented by Starr (1982), Ginzburg (1984), and Thurow (1985). Some key features of this transition include the use of private funds to capitalize health care institutions and activities; the development of corporate organizational arrangements that move control from local community boards to national headquarters; the growth of for-profit home care and the heightened attention to the profit to be returned to investors; and the increased concerns regarding the ability of potential clients to pay for services.

The increasing cost of health care has resulted in efforts on the part of the government and industry to shift more costs to other third-party payers or to consumers. Other strategies to limit costs include restrictions on which services are to be covered and which care systems are to be utilized. This has resulted in the development of managed care systems that influence the way in which decisions are made about patient care. Additional strategies include the use of preferred providers, which means that those covered by a given health plan can only use certain physicians or care institutions or pay more for other choices; the rejection of high-risk individuals by insurance companies; and defensive hiring on the part of employers who do not wish to take on employees who have negative health-related behaviors.

In the context of the changes in the cost of care and the management of health care delivery systems, new concerns about questions of access to care and equity have merged. And as observed by the Institute of Medicine's recent report on the future of public health (1988), "many state and local health agencies have become providers of last resort for uninsured persons and Medicaid clients unable to secure services in the private sector" (p. 152). Although these issues have been a matter of debate for some time (President's Commission, 1983), the emergence of a systematic effort at rationing, such as that which is occurring in the state of Oregon for those receiving public support for health care, has brought this matter to the public's attention (Daniels, 1986; Rooks, 1990).

On a more positive note, there is recent evidence of greater public and professional interest in health promotion and disease prevention. This may be due, in part, to a growing awareness of the human and economic consequences of an overemphasis on a high-technology, curative focus. Possibly, it is a function of the growing evidence that suggests that prevention does enhance well-being.

A number of developments have resulted in the beginning of a broad-based effort to focus more attention on health promotion and disease prevention. These include the creation of the United States Preventive Services Task Force in 1984 and its work (U.S. Preventive Services Task Force, 1989), the work of other groups (Amler & Dull, 1987), changes in the way in which the federal government reimburses for primary care physician services (Grimaldi, 1990), the publication of *Healthy People 2000* (U.S. Department of Health and Human Services, 1990), and the attention that segments of the general public are now giving to reducing negative health behaviors and embracing positive ones.

Questions about public health nursing in the United States have not arisen in a vacuum. In fact, national concern about the entire field of public health led to the Institute of Medicine's report (1988) on the future of public health. This study developed in response to a growing perception among a number of groups, including the Institute of Medicine's membership, that ". . . this nation has lost sight of its public goals and has allowed the system of public health activities to fall into disarray" (p. 1). In the final report, the study group stated that their analysis confirmed the original concerns that led to the development of the study. They indicated that "the current state of our abilities for effective public health action is cause for national concern and for the development of a plan of action for needed improvements" (p. 1). The study revealed that although there was widespread agreement on the overall mission of public health, little consensus was found when it came to translating broad statements into effective action. According to the report, "neither among the providers nor the beneficiaries of public health programs is there a shared sense of what the citizenry should expect in the way of services, and both the mix and the intensity of services vary widely from place to place" (p. 3).

The report set forth three main recommendations dealing with the mission of public health; the governmental role in fulfilling the mission; and the responsibilities unique to each level of government. The remainder of the numerous recommendations were defined as instrumental in implementing the three basic recommendations. The instrumental recommendations were grouped into the following categories: "statutory framework; structural and organization steps; strategies to build the fundamental capacities of public health agencies—technical, political, managerial, programmatic, and fiscal; and education for public health" (p. 7). The committee defined the mission of public health as "fulfilling society's interest in assuring conditions in which people can be healthy" (p. 7). The committee argued that the aim of public health was "to generate organized community effort to address the public interest in health by applying scientific and technical knowledge to prevent disease and promote health" (p. 7). Although it was acknowledged that the mission could be addressed by private organizations and individuals as well as public agencies, the idea was advanced that the government has a unique function and that is "to see to it that vital elements are in place that the mission is adequately addressed" (p. 7).

In clarifying what the governmental role is in fulfilling the mission, the committee stated that *assessment, policy development,* and *assurance* are the core functions at all levels of government. With regard to assessment, the committee recommended that "every public health agency regularly and systematically collect, assemble, analyze, and make available information on the health of the community, including statistics on health status, community health needs, and epidemiologic and other studies of health problems" (p. 7).

In discussing policy development, the committee recommended that "every public health agency exercise its responsibility to serve the public interest in the development of comprehensive public health policies by promoting use of the scientific knowledge base in decision-making about public health and by leading in developing public health policy" (p. 8). In the area of assurance, the committee had two major recommendations:

- "The committee recommends that public health agencies assure their constituents that services necessary to achieve agreed-upon goals are provided, either by encouraging actions by other entities (private or public sector), by requiring such action through regulation, or by providing services directly."
- "The committee recommends that each public health agency involve key policy makers and the general public in determining a set of high-priority personal and communitywide health services that governments will guarantee to every member of the community. This guarantee should include subsidization or direct provision of high-priority personal health services for those unable to afford them" (p. 8).

Of particular concern to the focus of this paper are the recommendations that deal with strategies that we developed based on the committee's analysis of problems in the field. These recommendations are referred to as "strategies for capacity building." Key points here are:

- "Public health agency leaders should develop relationships with and educate legislators and other public officials on community health needs, on public health issues, and on the rationale for strategies advocated and pursued by the health department. These relationships should be cultivated on an ongoing basis rather than being neglected until a crisis develops."
- "Agencies should strengthen the competence of their personnel in community relations and citizen participation techniques and develop procedures to build citizen participation into program implementation."
- "Greater emphasis in public health curricula should be placed on managerial and leadership skills, such as the ability to communicate important agency values to employees and enlist their commitment; to sense and deal with important changes in the environment; to plan, mobilize, and use resources effectively; and to relate the operation of the agency to its larger community role."
- "Demonstrated management competence as well as technical/professional skills should be a requirement for upper-level management posts" (Institute of Medicine, 1988, pp. 14–15).

## The Future

To frame the discussion on the future public health nursing, I would put forth three points. First, in looking at the future, a guiding concern should be responding to what is needed in the health care system. Second, are there special opportunities for nursing to make a difference in the public health field? Third, in thinking about the future, it may be more useful to consider the specialization of public health nursing broadly rather than focusing on one or two particular roles.

As we look to the future, there is no question that those responsible for health policy and the health care system need to give much more attention to dealing with preventable health problems such as high infant mortality in subgroups of the population, unwanted adolescent pregnancy, the high incidence of substance abuse, the acquired immunodeficiency syndrome epidemic, and the excessively high mortality rate among young black males. Other challenges that must be dealt with include providing adequate health and support services for especially vulnerable populations living in noninstitutionalized settings (e.g., the frail elderly, the homeless, and persons who test positive for human immunodeficiency virus), dealing with the health needs of the rapidly growing elderly population, providing adequate preventive services, and providing health services for those who are having difficulty in gaining access to the health care system and remaining within it either for financial or cultural reasons. The presence of significant problems in these areas and the growing concern about them, along with the escalation of health care costs in the United States and the spectre of rationing of health care, translate into a challenging situation in which change will be necessary and leadership very important.

A key question is, how will nursing respond? More specific to this discussion, to what extent will public health nursing provide significant leadership? In my view, the future will be influenced by the extent to which the leadership in public health nursing is able to prepare and support professionals who have the skills to *design, manage, monitor,* and *evaluate* systems of care that address population needs. Thus, whether public health nursing has a future or not is highly dependent on the extent to which attention is directed to developing nurses who are able to demonstrate these skills and assume *major* leadership roles in the *public* arena. This means that such individuals will not only be managing the nursing components of community-based services but also will have responsibility for policy and management at the top levels, in positions such as the directorship of a state or city health department. Few nurses hold such appointments now.

In order for public health nursing to be successful, it will be necessary for those in the field to be innovative in developing and demonstrating new ways to provide needed nursing services to nonhospitalized clients in community settings. In reflecting on the history of public health nursing, a common feature of those considered leaders is that they saw preventable health-related problems that were not addressed and moved forward to deal with these problems in a positive, proactive manner. This is the legacy of Lillian Wald at the Henry Street Settlement and Mary Breckinridge at the Frontier Nursing Service. This is also the legacy of individuals such as Loretta Ford, who supplied early leadership in the development of new roles for nurses providing care to the ambulatory pediatric population, and Margaret Dolan and Lucy Conant in their efforts to move forward in the development of the family nurse practitioner role in North Carolina against the "best judgment" of the majority of their associates on the nursing faculty.

Currently there are a number of examples of individuals who are continuing in this tradition and through their demonstration of innovative ways to provide services to defined community-based populations are exercising the kind of leadership that is necessary. Examples include the demonstration of a nurse-managed home follow-up program for very low birth weight infants in Philadelphia by Brooten and her colleagues (1986), Jamieson and associates' (1989) block nurse program in Minnesota for the provision of nursing services to the elderly living in their homes, the project developed by Stanhope and colleagues in Kentucky (College of Nursing, 1990) to demonstrate the impact of a nurse-managed clinic on the care of the homeless, and Flynn's work with the Health Cities project in Indiana ("Kellogg Foundation Funds," 1988), where the target population is an entire city. The reality of these efforts and of others provides considerable reason to be optimistic about the ability of nurses to provide creative leadership and about the future of public health nursing.

As mentioned in the beginning of this chapter, how one looks at the future of public health nursing is influenced in large part by how one views the contours of the field. As stated earlier and elsewhere (Williams, 1985, 1988), this author holds the view that the primary focus of public health nursing practice is on defining actual or potential health problems and proposing solutions for population groups or aggregates in community settings. I also advance the view that public health nursing as an area of specialization is a subset of the broader category of community health nursing and that specialization in it requires preparation at either the master's or doctoral level, which includes the public health sciences.

Thus, when I think about the future of public health nursing, I am thinking about the prospects for those who are specialists and who are approaching their practice with a community and population focus. I am not targeting attention to a particular clinical role such as the "traditional public health nursing" role. In fact, I would suggest that as we consider the future of public health nursing, it would be helpful to make a *distinction* between the future of the area of specialization as a whole versus the future of particular roles within the area of specialization.

There is a legitimate concern about the current status of the role of the "front line" nurse who is employed in official agencies and other settings and is referred to as a public health nurse. It is clear that more thought and attention need to be given to the kinds of clinical (direct care) roles that should be the cornerstone of models for the delivery of nursing services in community settings in the future. As Buhler-Wilkerson (1985) has pointed out, for some considerable time there has been tension regarding the scope of the nurse's role in visiting nurse associations and in official agencies. Much of this tension has revolved around the extent to which the nurse's role included both care of the sick and activities focused on prevention and health promotion. These questions and others continue: the issue is *who* will resolve them and on what basis? It is hoped that these matters will be addressed by insightful and well-prepared public health nursing specialists who are in positions to influence policy, to set agendas to demonstrate how to better provide the nursing services needed by various population groups, and to provide the leadership to design and put in place innovative nursing programs.

Over the years considerable data have been presented showing the contributions nursing can make to improving the effectiveness and efficiency of the health care system. Speaking before the American Academy of Nursing in 1981 (Fagin, 1982) and in a more recent analysis, Fagin (1986) made a particularly compelling case for the contributions nursing can make to improving the health care system. Other analyses such as that completed by the Office of Technological Assessment of the Congress (LeRoy & Solkoaitz, 1981) and those of Williams (1983), and Diers (1981) have also provided considerable information, which if acted upon could result in improved access to quality care provided by nurses at reasonable and affordable costs rather than more expensive alternatives. However, much of this information has not been acted on. After considering this situation for some time, the author is convinced that unless nurses are in positions of top leadership, the adoption of well-supported innovations in care involving nurses as primary clinicians will continue to lag.

In view of the health and health care system problems we are facing in this country, the time for new growth in public health nursing may be at hand. The report from the Institute of Medicine on the Future of Public Health argued that there is a compelling need for capacity building and for strong leadership in public health, and the prediction put forth in *Megatrends 2000* by Naisbitt and Aburdene (1990) was that the decade of the 1990s would be the decade of women in leadership. Nursing is the largest professional group in public health, but with few exceptions, nurses are not represented in major positions of leadership in the field. It can be argued that there is a substantive match between (1) what has been put forth as the focus of specialization for public health nursing, namely, dealing at the broad population level with policy and political issues and the development of strategies for health promotion, health protection, and disease prevention at the population level, and (2) what is called for by the Institute of Medicine's study as necessary to further the enterprise of public health.

The greatest need is for nurses to occupy top leadership roles, where the emphasis is on high-level management, making those decisions associated with top echelon leadership—". . . developing policy, setting priorities, allocating resources, and modifying and manipulating organizational structures" (Milbank Memorial Fund, 1976, p. 39). Currently, the majority of roles nurses occupy in organizations, whether health departments, other traditional public health structures, or hospitals, are at lower levels at which policy making is limited and the emphasis is on carrying out policy.

In order to create a future in which it is expected and accepted that nurses will occupy such leadership roles, changes need to occur in attitudes and roles, in educational programs, and in support structures. We in nursing need to develop a broader vision of what are appropriate roles for nurses. The majority of nurses and the majority of the public have a view of nurses that is fixed on "entry-level clinical roles." Such roles are the backbone of the discipline, but why should it not be expected that nurses should also serve as state or local health officers? Such positions offer superb vantage points from which to influence the health of the community and to influence which direct care providers (nurses and others) will be involved in rendering services to which specific population groups. Yet, some nurses have suggested that those who become health officers and thus are not clearly identified with public health nursing units have left public health nursing!

In addition to the need for attitudinal changes both within and outside the field of nursing, changes need to take place in the educational process. A number of these changes have been discussed in the literature, but here the need to prepare nurses for leadership roles in policy making and in the design, development, management, monitoring, and evaluation of population-focused health care systems must be emphasized. Preparation for such functions is necessary if public health nursing as defined by the American Public Health Association (1981) and described earlier in this chapter is to be practiced. And, as mentioned earlier, such functions overlap with what are being seen as administrative roles.

A number of changes have occurred in the approach to preparing nurses for administrative roles since the Institute of Medicine's 1983 study on nursing, which concluded that there was a serious scarcity of nurses with advanced education in administration and raised the question of whether graduate programs in schools of nursing can produce the quality of programs desired and the numbers of graduates needed. That report recommended the development of collaborative arrangements between schools of nursing and schools of business administration and programs in health services administration. Since that time, a number of joint master's of science in nursing and master's in business administration programs have emerged. Although such developments may be positive, from this author's observation several important things are missing from these programs that have been understood to be generic to public health, and specialization in public health nursing can be argued: ". . . the measurement and *analytical* sciences of epidemiology and biostatistics; social policy and the history and philosophy of public health; and the principles of management and organization for public health" (Milbank Memorial Fund, 1976, pp. 74–75).

The 1988 Institute of Medicine Study emphasizes the role of Schools of Public Health in preparing for leadership in public health. Yet, few linkages exist between schools of nursing—where most nurses receive their graduate preparation in public health (usually referred to as community health—and schools of public health or other academic units with programs in public health. The forging of new arrangements between schools of nursing, public health, business administration, and some medical school units (those in preventive medicine, epidemiology, and community medicine) is an area requiring attention as we prepare the nursing leaders of the future. Elsewhere, I have argued that a synthesis of selected aspects of what is referred to as nursing administration and specialization in public health nursing needs to be considered (Williams, 1985). More thought needs to be given to this idea because regardless of setting, nurse executives have a common need for certain generic leadership skills.

Although content in financial and personnel management needs to be included in the preparation of nurse executives, a primary focus should be on planning and managing the care for specific populations regardless of where those populations are located. More creative curriculum work is needed in developing the learning experiences to prepare people to design nursing care systems, to design support structures for the nurses in those systems, and to bring about positive change. Although it is clear that there is considerable overlap among skills necessary for nurse executives who deal predominantly with inpatient populations and those who deal with noninstitutionalized populations, I see specialists in public health nursing as distinct from nursing executives dealing with acute care problems. The key distinguishing features are not the setting or even the population focus but the type of populations, the strategies needed to effect change, and the broad sociopolitical context of practice. More specifically, (1) public health specialists focus on populations that are free-living in the community as opposed to those institutionalized for an acute (short-term) episode. (2) They are predominantly concerned with strategies for health promotion, health maintenance, and disease prevention. (3) Their arena of practice is a broad one—it extends beyond the confines of a given hospital or clinic; in fact, they are concerned with those in the community who are not receiving needed services (regardless of ability to pay). (4) They are also concerned with the interface between the health status and the living environment of the population (physical, biologic, and sociocultural). Last, (5) public health specialists find that influencing public policy as opposed to institutional policy is a major strategy for achieving their goals.

Additional support structures for nurses in top leadership roles need to be developed, particularly for those occupying roles that are either outside nursing units or in which a nursing executive is dealing in a broad arena. Fagin (1988) refers to such situations as "professional women at the interface" (p. 395). She is particularly interested in the nursing executive who is in "situations in which the nurse may be the only woman and nurse, a minority of one, or part of a duo or small minority in important committees, boards, and other groups dealing with a wide variety of issues that may or may not be related to nursing" (p. 395). Fagin argues that such nurses need to learn to maximize their participation so that important goals can be achieved. Clearly, much more attention needs to be given to preparing nurses with the skills needed for success in "interface" situations and for networking and other mechanisms to support their ability to function effectively. The types of dialogue initiated by Fagin need to be continued and amplified.

In conclusion, the potential for a very bright future for public health nursing exists *if* public health nursing specialists are able to move into the leadership vacuum in public health and demonstrate the kind of proactive behaviors required. For the specialty to be successful in providing such leadership, it will be necessary to have broad vision; to prepare nurses for leadership roles in policy making and in the design, development, management, monitoring, and evaluation of population-focused health care systems; and to develop strategies to support nurses in these roles. Is there a future for the specialization of public health nursing? My response is yes.

## REFERENCES

American Nurses' Association, Division on Community Health Nursing (1980). *Conceptual model of community health nursing.* Publication No. CH-10, Kansas City, MO: American Nurses' Association.

American Public Health Association, Public Health Nursing Section (1981). *The definition and role of public health nursing in the delivery of health care.* Washington, DC: American Public Health Association.

Amler, R.W., & Dull, H.B. (Eds.) (1987). *Closing the gap: The burden of unnecessary illness.* New York: Oxford University Press.

Brooten, D., Kumar, S., Brown, L.P., Butts, P., Finkler, S.A., Bakewell-Sachs, S., Gibbons, A., & Delivoria-Papadopoulos, M. (1986). A randomized clinical trial of early hospital discharge and home follow-up of very-low-birth-weight infants. *New England Journal of Medicine, 315*(15), 934–939.

Buhler-Wilkerson, K. (1985). Public health nursing: In sickness or in health? *American Journal of Public Health, 75*(10), 1155–1161.

College of Nursing, University of Kentucky (1990). *An innovative approach to health care for the homeless/very poor: A nurse managed clinic.* (Final Report on Contract #240-86-0082.) Washington, DC: Division of Nursing, Department of Health and Human Services.

Daniels, N. (1986). Why saying no to patients in the United States is so hard. *New England Journal of Medicine, 314*(21), 1380–1383.

Diers, D. (1981). Nurse midwifery as a system of care: Provider, process, and patient outcome. In L. Aiken & S. Gortner (Eds.), *Health policy and nursing practice* (pp. 73–89). New York: McGraw-Hill.

Fagin, C.M. (1982). Nursing's pivotal role in achieving competition in health care. In *From accommodations to self-determination: Nursing's role in the development of health care policy* (pp. 3–15). Kansas City, MO: American Nurses' Association.

Fagin, C.M. (1986). Opening the door on nursing's cost advantage. *Nursing and Health Care, 7*(12), 353–357.

Fagin, C.M. (1988). Professional women at the interface: The case of the nursing executive—Part II. *Journal of Professional Nursing, 4*(6), 395, 458.

Ford, L.D., & Silver, H.K. (1967). The expanded role of the nurse in child care. *Nursing Outlook, 15,* 43–45.

Ginzberg, E. (1984). The monetarization of medical care. *New England Journal of Medicine,* *310*(18), 1162–1165.

Grimaldi, P.L. (1990). Will new fee system slash physician payments? *Nursing Management,* *21*(8), 22–24.

Institute of Medicine (1983). *Nursing and nursing education: Public policies and private actions.* Washington, DC: National Academy Press.

Institute of Medicine (1988). *The future of public health.* Washington, DC, National Academy Press.

Jamieson, M., Campbell, J., & Clarke, S. (1989). The block nurse program. *The Gerontologist,* *29*(1), 124–127.

Kellogg Foundation Funds 3-year "healthy cities Indiana" Project (1988, December). *American Journal of Public Health,* *78*(12), 5.

LeRoy, L., & Solkoaitz, S. (1981). Case Study 16: The cost and effectiveness of nurse practitioners. In L. LeRoy & S. Solkoaitz, *The implications for cost-effectiveness analysis of medical technology.* Washington, DC: Office of Technology Assessment.

Matuk, L., & Horsburgh, M (1989). Rebuilding public health nursing practice: A Canadian perspective. *Public Health Nursing,* *6*(4), 169–173.

Milbank Memorial Fund (1976). *Higher education for public health.* New York: Prodist.

Naisbitt, J., & Aburdene, P. (1990). *Megatrends 2000: Ten new directions for the 1990's.* New York: William Morrow and Company.

National League for Nursing (1989). *Nursing data review.* Publication No. 19-2290, New York: National League for Nursing.

President's Commission for the Study of Ethical Problems in Medicine and Biomedical and Behavioral Research (1983). *Securing access to health care: The ethical implications of differences in the availability of health services.* Volume 1, GPO No. 040-000-00472-6. Washington, DC: U.S. Government Printing Office.

Rooks, J. (1990). Let's admit we ration health care—then set priorities. *American Journal of Nursing,* *90*(6), 39–43.

Starr, P. (1982). *The social transformation of American medicine.* New York: Basic Books.

Thurow, L.C. (1985). Medicine versus economics. *New England Journal of Medicine, 313,* 611–614.

U.S. Department of Health and Human Services (1990). *Healthy people 2000.* Washington, DC: U.S. Government Printing Office,

U.S. Department of Health and Human Services, Bureau of Health Professions, Division of Nursing (1985). *Consensus conference on the essentials of public health nursing practice and education.* Report of the conference, Sept. 5–7, 1984. Rockville, MD: U.S. Department of Health and Human Services.

U.S. Department of Health, Education, and Welfare, Bureau of Health Manpower, Division of Nursing (1980). *Longitudinal study of nurse practitioners, phase III.* Department of Health, Education, and Welfare Publication No. HRA 80-2, Hyattsville, MD: U.S. Government Printing Office.

U.S. Preventive Services Task Force (1989). *Guide to clinical preventive services.* Baltimore, MD: Williams & Wilkins.

Williams, C.A. (1983). Primary care and the cost dilemma: A case for nurse practitioners. In R. Haskins (Ed.), *Child health policy in an age of fiscal austerity: Critique of the select panel report.* Norwood, NJ: Ablex Publishing.

Williams, C.A. (1985). Population focused community health nursing and nursing administration: A new synthesis. In J.C. McCloskey & H.K. Grace (Eds.), *Current issues in nursing* (2nd ed.) (pp. 386–393). Boston: Blackwell Scientific Publications.

Williams, C.A. (1988). Population-focused practice: The basis of specialization in public health nursing. In M.K. Stanhope & J. Lancaster (Eds.), *Community health nursing: Process and practice for promoting health* (pp. 292–303). St. Louis: C.V. Mosby.

## Chapter 18

# Is Health a School Issue?
# School-Based Health Services

JUDITH B. IGOE

*T*HE 21ST CENTURY is almost 4 feet tall, weighs about 52 pounds, and is in second grade (Klein, 1988). Although this little future is now a member of the healthiest segment of our population, he or she has a one in ten chance of having a major physical, emotional, or mental disability before ever donning a cap and gown for high school graduation in the year 2001. And if this future is growing up in poverty, the chances of his or her having to struggle with adolescent health problems are even greater (Starfield, 1982).

Without prompt management of their illnesses and injuries, these students' health problems eventually exacerbate and can result in impaired learning ability as well as absenteeism. According to Klerman (1988), educators believe that students who miss more than 10 days of school in a 90-day semester (11 percent of school days) have difficulty staying at grade level. "Therefore absenteeism, like learning-related health disorders, poses a similar threat of jeopardizing a student's academic career" (Klerman, 1988, p. 1254).

If the overall 1990 school dropout rate prevails, one in twelve of today's second graders may never make it to the graduation ceremony (*Digest of Educational Statistics 1989*). Health-related factors such as teenage pregnancy, depression, physical disabilities, chronic disease, and alcohol and drug abuse are often cited as the contributing factors (Dryfoos, 1987). For black and Hispanic youth, graduation from high school is even more unlikely. By today's estimates, the national school dropout rate for black students is 15.5 percent and for Hispanics a startling 32.2 percent.

Many adolescents, however, must deal with a number of health problems that resulted from conditions at birth as well as during childhood. Drug and alcohol abuse by their mothers during pregnancy, very low birth weight, respiratory problems, and neonatal illness are recorded in the health histories of some children who manifest disorders of attention, abstract thinking, and symbolic representation (Newman & Papkalla, 1990). The Centers for Disease Control (1983) report that 2 million children have high levels of lead in their blood and that at least some of these children experience mental impairments that put them at risk for academic failure. Even those children who have healthy bodies and live in chemical-free environments are at risk of developing academic, behavioral, and language disorders by the time they reach school age if they are abused or neglected (Dubowitz, 1986).

Epidemiologic surveys confirm that adolescents make up the only age segment with mortality rates on the rise because of violence and suicide. Although the use of selected abused substances (alcohol, cigarettes, marijuana, and cocaine) among adolescents actually declined and briefly plateaued after 1979, by 1982 these behaviors, especially alcohol use, were once again on the rise (*Child Health USA, 1989*). Dryfoos (1987) has further documented that as many as one in four students between the ages of 10 and 17 are at high risk for school failure, delinquency, early unprotected sexual intercourse, and substance abuse.

According to a number of health policy analysts, statistics show a disturbing, steady decline in the well-being of America's youth, both in absolute terms and relative to other age groups and to youth in other nations (Valanis, 1986). Right now, in the 20th century, we can choose to ignore this. Or, we can go back to school, to second grade, and start helping our 4-foot, 52-pound future create a healthier 21st century.

## History of School Health Services

Using the school as a setting for the delivery of health care services is not new. Historically, it is well documented that school health concepts originated in basic public health principles and practices instituted around 1900 to identify and exclude students with contagious diseases from the classroom. A number of events were significant in the evolution of school health services and have been chronicled elsewhere (Igoe, 1991). Four time periods characterize this development: the communicable disease control era, the health guidance and consultation era, the primary care era, and the health promotion/special needs era. School health is best understood within the context of developments in education, pediatrics, nursing, and public health and within the framework of pertinent social and legislative changes (Kovar & Dawson, 1988; Lynch, 1982; Woodfill & Beyrer, 1991).

The traditional school health program that has grown out of this history consists of three core components: (1) health services, including basic care for minor complaints, general preventive screenings, and most recently primary health care and health promotion activities, (2) health education, and (3) health protection efforts, i.e., measures intended to promote a physically, socially, and psychologically healthy environment.

In the past the health services component of school health has involved school-wide screenings for sensory deficits (vision, hearing), case finding, referral, follow-up, counseling, the management of minor complaints, and liaison work with community agencies to coordinate care. With the advent of new disorders, such as early adolescent pregnancy, emotional disorders, sexually transmitted diseases, and poor lifestyle habits, many students now require psychosocial and behavioral interventions for their health problems and new types of disease prevention and health promotion services.

Schoolwide campaigns to improve diet and physical exercise habits, contraceptive advice, individual and small group counseling to reduce stress and improve self-image, and social skills training and cognitive therapies to prevent substance abuse and delay the onset of sexual activity are just a few examples of the kind of health services now available in schools.

Besides the more widely publicized maladies of the school-aged population, an increasing number of boys and girls today need to find primary health care services in their schools because they are uninsured. The 1984 National Health Interview Survey found that 4.5 million (14 percent) of students aged 10 to 18 are in this category and that those from poor and minority households are the ones least likely to have health insurance (Klein & Sadowski, 1990).

Not infrequently, some of these students have serious ear infections that, if left untreated, eventually lead to hearing loss (Flinn Foundation, 1989). Other children have repeated upper respiratory tract infections, bouts with allergies, dental decay, skin problems, and a host of other clinical disorders that may result in extended periods of absenteeism if diagnostic and treatment services are not readily available at school.

Growing numbers of acute and chronically ill and impaired students are in school today as a result of the Education for All Handicapped Children's Act of 1975 (Public Law 94:142), and they must have more complex nursing care provided at school. Among the common treatments these students require are bladder catheterization; endotracheal suctioning; colostomy, ileostomy and ureterostomy care; and nasogastric tube feedings (American Nurses' Association, 1980).

## State Requirements Regulating Health Services

Over the past 20 years there has been a transfer of state agency responsibility for school health services. Between the 1940s and 1960s, school health services became the responsibility of the education agency. However, Lovato, Allensworth, and Chan report in the 1989 edition of *School Health in America* that the picture has since changed dramatically. According to their 1987 survey findings, the department of health now exercises primary responsibility for school health services in 20 states. In another 13 states the department of education retains responsibility. In another 14 states the two agencies share this responsibility. In Alaska, the departments of social services and education share this responsibility with the department of health, and in Alabama, Idaho, and Montana, there is no designated agency responsible for school health services.

Statewide policies for school health services usually take the form of agency regulations rather than state statutes. Consequently, with the exception of immunization and child abuse laws, other policies related to school health services are neither uniform nor nationwide. This is in keeping with the "local control" principle that has been a deeply ingrained value long associated with American education. Although all states have legislation requiring immunizations for school entry and child abuse reporting by school personnel, fewer than 30 percent of states have any uniform policies for the specialized care of handicapped children.

## Various Models for Delivery of School Health Services

Given the changing needs for school health programs, the lack of uniform regulations, and the fact that school health is no longer a small change item in terms of financing, much attention has been paid to redesigning traditional school health and the services delivery system (Freeman & Heinrich, 1981; Gephart et al., 1984; Lynch, 1982). Several specific demonstration projects have informed this process and added significant information to the knowledge necessary to bring about change in this field.

### National School Health Services Program

In 1978 the Robert Wood Johnson Foundation appropriated almost 5 million dollars to fund primary health care demonstration projects using school nurse practitioners in elementary and secondary schools located in Colorado, New York, North Dakota, and Utah. Specifically, the services provided by each project included diagnosis of and treatment for acute illness and trauma, periodic health screenings (for poor vision and hearing, scoliosis, and high blood pressure), routine physical examinations, required regimens for the management of chronic illness, immunizations and vaccinations, and referrals to specialists for more complex conditions. The overall results of the project evaluation indicated that ". . . a successful comprehensive school health program *must* include a mix of primary-care, school-related health services and public health functions (Meeker, DeAngelis, Berman, Freeman, & Oda, 1986, p. 91)."

It was also found that (1) school nurse practitioners were able to independently deliver 87 percent of the care; (2) 96 percent resolution of the health problems was achieved; and (3) no significant overlap or duplication of community health services occurred.

At the end of this project new plans for funding school health were recommended. The traditional approach, which placed the entire burden for financing school health on the education system, was modified in the following way. It was proposed that schools pay for basic screening services which identify student health problems that clearly have an impact on learning (e.g., vision and hearing disabilities). Furthermore, it was proposed that local and state health departments also assume some responsibility for financing school health services, especially for the care that agency has been authorized to provide (e.g., immunizations and other communicable disease control measures). Finally, it was proposed that school health services may also encompass optional services such as primary health care, mental health counseling, and various treatments and procedures for acute illness. These are services for which some fee should be determined and some attempt made at reimbursement.

This project served as the initial prototype for school-based clinics and set the stage for further study of adolescent health services in schools.

## The Program to Consolidate Health Services for High-Risk Young People

The Robert Wood Johnson Foundation funded this nationwide program—the Program to Consolidate Health Services for High-Risk Young People—between 1982 and 1986. It was intended to provide more effective clinical services to adolescents at high risk for major health problems and to improve the training of physicians in adolescent medicine.

Each of the 20 programs involved in the project was given considerable freedom in defining and developing its comprehensive health care package for high-risk adolescents. Staff included adolescent medicine specialists, fellows in adolescent medicine, nurses (including nurse practitioners and school nurses), social workers, and counselors. Clinical facilities were located in inner city areas in hospitals, neighborhoods, and schools.

To evaluate the success of this initiative, seven of the specialized adolescent clinics were compared with three nonspecialized facilities (Earls & Robins, 1989). This evaluation found that the adolescent clinics detected and treated a wider range of medical and behavioral problems than the comparison clinics, based on self-reports of patients and confirmed by medical record documentation, and that fewer high-risk youths utilized school-based clinics. However, more males were attracted to school-based clinics than to neighborhood and hospital-based clinics.

Unfortunately, improvements in lifestyle and in specific health status outcomes were not detected during the evaluation of this project. Nevertheless, this project demonstrated the importance of specialty clinics for adolescents and also raised the question of whether medical clinics alone have the resources required to completely ameliorate the kinds of adolescent health problems that are influenced by societal and economic factors. It may be more appropriate to adjust medical treatment objectives to reflect stabilization of the risk condition rather than its actual reduction (Earls & Robins, 1989).

The project further demonstrated the viability and importance of providing a combination of clinical health services and educational and social services in clinics based at school.

## School-Based Adolescent Health Care

The School-Based Adolescent Health Care program, also funded by the Robert Wood Johnson Foundation, is an extension of earlier adolescent and school health demonstration projects. Started in 1986, School-Based Adolescent Health Care has been designed to build upon the lessons previously learned and to test the feasibility of establishing comprehensive school-based health centers for adolescents nationwide. A selection process was employed to identify 11 states in which 24 high schools that enroll nearly 40,000 students serve as demonstration sites.

This project was undertaken to address complex issues such as (1) access to care, (2) development and organization of school-based health centers, including the design of a data management health information system that interfaces with community health systems, and (3) financing mechanisms.

Each center's services were put under the direction of nonprofit private or public institutions recognized in their communities as able to lead an initiative to establish a school-based health center and eventually finance it with local health care rather than education funds. Staff include school nurse practitioners, physicians, school nurses functioning in case manager/service coordinator roles, counselors for substance abuse problems, student assistance program personnel, social workers, and health clerks.

In addition to treatment for minor illness and injuries, the project provides a variety of school-based health services, including care and referral for drug and alcohol abuse and sexually transmitted diseases; sports and employment physical examinations; immunizations; and effective preventive services aimed at pregnancy, sexually transmitted diseases, and other high-risk conditions.

An evaluation of the School-Based Adolescent Health Care program is now under way. Community endorsement has been a definite requirement for success. Despite initial controversy and misinformation concerning the distribution of contraceptives, the clinics now operate without harassment. Many factors have contributed to this outcome, including active parent participation and clear consistent communication among community leaders, school officials, and the media.

The Council on Scientific Affairs of the American Medical Association, in studying these and other school-based health centers, has acknowledged the positive results these centers have achieved in preventing teenage pregnancy and in providing essential health care to otherwise underserved populations. "The St. Paul, Minnesota program showed a decline in fertility rates in four participating high schools from 59 births per 1000 female students in 1976–1977 to 26 per 1000 in 1983–1984" (Society for Adolescent Medicine, 1988, p. 528).

In addition, based in part on the evaluation data from the model adolescent programs, the Council on Scientific Affairs issued minimal standards for school-based health centers requiring that health services be supervised by a physician and that on-site services be provided by a professionally prepared school nurse.

## Disabled Children

Perplexing questions about the needs of school children and youth with handicaps, disabilities, and chronic illness have also captured the interest and attention of school officials, parents, and health professionals over the past decade and influenced the restructuring of school health services. Several national projects have attempted to determine what is required and how best to formulate policies on behalf of these students and their families.

The first of these nationwide studies was the Collaborative Study of Children with Special Needs directed by John Butler at Boston Children's Hospital in the early 1980s (Butler, Rosenbaum, & Palfrey, 1987). This study involved profiling the experiences of students eligible for special education under Public Law 94:142. Patterns of school placement, health care use, expenditures, and service coordination difficulties were identified in various school districts throughout the United States.

Among the findings from this study were reports of parents and teachers having insufficient understanding of the real and potential side effects of medications taken by the children, gaps as well as overlap in community health service delivery, and general confusion about health care among the teaching staff, who had limited understanding of the students' conditions. Unfortunately, this study did not investigate the school health services available to these students, but the findings from this project provided a substantial data base for planning purposes and led to the development of policy and procedure manuals for specialized school health services.

The most extensive investigation of the needs of chronically ill students was a national project initiated in the early 1980s by the Center for the Study of Families and Children of the Vanderbilt University Institute for Public Policy Studies under the leadership of James Perrin, M.D., and Henry Ireys, Ph.D. (Walker, 1987). At that time students with chronic illnesses did not qualify for special education services unless they were academically below grade level. This study was extremely important because it provided a framework for developing policies that eventually guaranteed these children and youth access to related health and other special education services.

As a result of the Vanderbilt project, a composite profile of the students with chronic disease was established for the first time. In addition, the need to improve homebound policies for schools and the need to establish national guidelines for medication administration in the schools were just two of the many important outcomes of this project that subsequently produced concrete results.

## Child-Initiated Care

In 1971, Charles and Mary Ann Lewis began a study at the University of California at Los Angeles to test the effects of having elementary school children actively participate in decision-making activities related to their own health complaints during the school day (Lewis & Lewis, 1989). Children in the experimental intervention were allowed to visit the school nurse without seeking teacher permission. Although the study produced numerous results, its desired goal of shaping more appropriate health care use behavior was not achieved in those situations in which the family was not involved. It found, therefore, that family-centered school health services are most important.

Another important finding with special implications for school nursing practice was the discovery of a close association between frequent visits to the nurse and academic difficulties. In fact, an early warning sign of school problems and risk behaviors related to dropping out of school may be frequent visits to the school nurse.

## Nursing's Various Roles

The delivery of care in the nontraditional health setting of the school as well as the evolution in school-based service delivery models have presented many challenges and opportunities for nurses. Currently, there are approximately 26,000 registered professional nurses working in 15,577 public school districts (*Digest of Educational Statistics 1989*).

The majority of these nurses function in staff positions as school nurses. Their educational preparation in nursing varies. Some have nursing diplomas. Others have associate degrees in nursing. Many are prepared at the baccalaureate level with degrees in education or counseling. A small number have doctoral degrees. However, it is impossible to be any more precise in describing their positions or credentials because there are no universal tracking systems to provide this at either federal or state levels. Health officials tend to aggregate this information with public health nursing data, whereas schools factor it into other categories such as "classified staff."

With such diversity in terms of nursing preparation, the role of the school nurse is neither clear-cut nor standardized. The frequent absence of any infrastructure to support a school health program, limited supervision, and the tremendous variations in the ratios of students to nurses and nurses to school buildings only add to the confusion and reduce the likelihood that all school nurses function according to an established framework of practice, although many certainly do.

Fortunately, some positive change is under way. The professional school nurse associations have adopted joint practice standards, and the state school nurse consultants (N = 29) are attempting to orient school nurses to these standards. However, the complexity of the health problems they face and the organizational difficulties they encounter in attempting to function in the nontraditional health system of the school clearly warrant better educational preparation and further role clarification. There are several major roles nurses have held in school health. They are summarized as follows:

*School Nurse–Teacher.* From the 1940s until the 1960s, the role of the nurse as school nurse–teacher was prominent in this country, especially on the East Coast. With dual credentials in health and education, these nurses represent the opposite end of the role spectrum from school nurse practitioners, described below, who are academically prepared specifically to provide primary health care, clinical services in schools to individual clients.

School nurse–teachers were primarily found in the classroom, not the clinic, where they served a very useful function as health teachers. However, since their educational preparation usually took a different route than that of most classroom teachers, it is doubtful that the school nurse–teachers were viewed as genuine teachers.

Professionally, school nurse–teachers closely aligned themselves with teachers' associations rather than nursing organizations. Indeed, the National Association of School Nurses is an affiliate of the National Education Association, although it has strengthened its affiliation with nursing organizations in recent years.

A combination of circumstances led to a decline in the popularity of the school nurse–teacher role beginning in the late 1970s and culminating in the 1980s, when the New York school system (the largest employer of school nurse–teachers) virtually eliminated the position, replacing the school nurse–teacher with diploma-prepared nurses who had clinical skills. This change was largely the result of budgetary problems (health education was viewed as a "luxury item") and the growing need to have clinically skilled nurses in schools who could evaluate the increasing numbers of students who had no other source of health care.

*School Nurse Practitioner.*   The school nurse practitioner role originated in 1969 as a collaborative effort between the University of Colorado Schools of Nursing and Medicine and the School Health Services Division of the Denver Public Schools. The school nurse practitioner's role is focused on the delivery of primary health care services to individual students and encompasses a number of tasks and functions, as summarized in the following list:

1.  is an advocate for children/adolescents and their families in the health arena and helps them to gain access to community health services beyond the school setting;
2.  provides primary health care to school-aged children, especially those who have no other access to care, are disabled, or who have handicaps and/or chronic health conditions;
3.  accurately obtains and maintains a thorough, systematic, age-appropriate data base that includes health, social history, physical assessment, developmental appraisal, and screening information on school-aged youth and evaluates the child's health status based on data collected;
4.  participates with other health and educational professionals in the evaluation and management of children with disabilities and chronic health conditions;
5.  interprets student health status for school personnel, emphasizing abilities as well as disabilities, and provides guidance regarding management and readjustments of students' educational and health programs; and
6.  counsels and guides school-aged children, adolescents, and parents in assuming personal responsibility for their own health and in learning how to negotiate the health care delivery system effectively.

*Community Health Nurse Specialist for School-Aged Youth.*   The community health nurse specialist for school-aged youth is a new role for school nurses and is based on the following assumptions. First, it is considered advantageous for nurses working with school-aged youth to hold managerial roles in community health. Second, it is projected that nursing centers for school-aged youth will develop in school and community settings in the near future, and nurses will be needed to administer, plan, and operate these organizations.

The knowledge and competencies required for these types of responsibilities are compatible with but different from the role of the school nurse practitioner, who could provide the bulk of the primary health care in schools. Although the two roles, school nurse practitioner and school-aged youth specialist, share a common interchangeable conceptual framework of practice (Igoe, 1987), the functions of the community health nurse specialist working with school-aged youth are more managerial than clinical. The school-aged youth specialist in effect is the school's epidemiologist, program planner, and manager for school health; case manager/coordinator; and facilitator for disease prevention and health promotion services. The graduate degree plan for this school nurse role was developed at the University of Colorado

School of Nursing, and 20 graduates are now participating in an evaluation of this role.

## Implications for Nursing's Policy Agenda

In spite of a 100-year history, there is still debate on whether or not to provide school-based clinical services for children and adolescents, and, even among those who support service provision, there is disagreement on how to define, configure, and staff the school health program in general.

The most frequently cited advantages of providing school-based health care are the following.

### Economies of Scale in Service Delivery

The school setting is an ideal location for wide-scale health screenings, provided the testing is worthwhile, screeners are qualified, salaries are reasonable, and referral and follow-up efforts produce results.

Using this same theory of economy of scale, the delivery of primary health care in school-based clinics by certified school nurse practitioners may also prove to be worthwhile. The services are readily accessible and frequently utilized, failed appointments are rare, and problem resolution rates have been reported to exceed 90 percent (Meeker et al., 1986). However, actual cost savings resulting from this arrangement have yet to be specifically demonstrated.

### School Health Services Enhance the Student's Ability to Learn

Although the connection between learning and health status needs further exploration, there is some indication that students need to be healthy to learn. In a study of elementary school students in Arizona, the children most frequently in the nurse's office with complaints of illness also had the lowest achievement scores (Harris, 1989). Other studies of school-aged youth have demonstrated an association between low blood glucose levels midmorning, no breakfast, and diminished mental alertness and processing capabilities (Kolbe, 1984). As findings such as these accumulate, school officials are becoming increasingly willing to acknowledge the benefits of providing health and nutrition services in the schools.

### School Health Services Are Meeting the Health Needs of Uninsured and Underinsured Students

It is estimated that there are over 37 million Americans who lack health insurance coverage, with children representing the largest segment of the uninsured population (Oberg, 1990). For these students, the only source of health care may be the school health program. Despite the fact that there are reportedly hundreds of school-based clinics for adolescents and some for elementary, middle, and junior high schools, the demand far exceeds the supply when one considers that there are 15,577 public school districts in the country (*Digest of Educational Statistics 1989*).

## School Health Services Are Essential and Legislated for Chronically Ill and Medically Fragile Students

Currently about 10 percent of all students receive some degree of special education. With the enactment of Public Law 94-142, the "Education for All Handicapped Children Act of 1975," and the passage of the related "Education of the Handicapped Act Amendments of 1986" (PL99-457, Part H), school health as well as educational services has become available to infants, toddlers, preschoolers, and school-aged youth who are disabled. For these students as well as those who are chronically ill and apparently eligible for services under the requirements of Section 504 of the Rehabilitation Act of 1973 (29 USC 794) and its implementing regulations (34 CFR Part 104), the school system is required to assume the cost of providing the related health services that are needed.

## Helping to Attain the "Year 2000 Health Objectives" for the Nation

The "Year 2000 Health Objectives" establish a specific disease prevention and health promotion agenda for the schools (Allensworth et al., 1988). It is anticipated that school health services will expand to include screenings for sensory deficits, nutritional and physical fitness and endurance, cardiovascular risk factors, substance abuse, and other high-risk behaviors. Special attention for those students who are vulnerable must be a part of this initiative and will require the expertise of school health personnel who have not only clinical skills and knowledge of pediatrics and public health but also a background in disease prevention and health promotion.

## School Health Services Can Become an Extension of Other State Supported Community-Based Child Health and Service Programs and Thereby Benefit from New Financing Mechanisms

Since 1983, when the Tatro case legally established the difference between medical care and health service (*Tatro v. Texas, 1980 & 1983*) in reference to a child with spina bifida, there have been efforts to coordinate and combine various nonmedical health services with other types of child care programs. The main purpose of this was to improve the quality and efficiency of service delivery by consolidating funding streams from health, education, and social services agencies, especially in the areas of early childhood education and services to students who are disabled.

To illustrate, the Minnesota state legislature and public administrators from the Departments of Human Services, Education, and Health developed a coordinated plan to provide the Title XIX Early Periodic Screening Diagnosis and Treatment program in schools as part of their early childhood screening program. Not only are these combined school-based screenings more comprehensive than previously but the funding reimbursement to schools is much more generous and therefore provides an added incentive for "buy-in" from school administrators.

The Early Periodic Screening Diagnosis and Treatment program in schools represents perhaps the best example of a community-based health initiative introduced into a school system in order to ensure success (Stenmark & Igoe, 1984). Today, a number of states, including Arkansas, Connecticut, California, Minnesota, Mississippi, and Louisiana, have implemented this preventive health care program by itself at various grade levels. Significant increases in the enrollment of Title XIX-eligible children have been documented in these school-based screening programs.

Although the number of participating states is limited, some school systems also have Title XIX Medicaid privileges that entitle the district to offer medical services for low-income families who qualify in school-based clinics. Connecticut is a state in which schools receive Medicaid reimbursement. In addition, the Omnibus Budget Reconciliation Act of 1989 (OBRA89) includes provisions whereby schools are now entitled to reimbursement for costs associated with the delivery of related health services to students eligible for Medicaid who are disabled, handicapped, or medically fragile. Since schools must bill for these services, school officials now must learn about third-party billing. Early reports indicate school personnel have been somewhat reluctant to enter the health field to this extent. However, recently, the rate of success in processing claims for one school district in Illinois was over 25 percent, which amounted to literally thousands of dollars. Since they are desperately in need of financing for school health services, it is likely that schools will tolerate the difficulties encountered in setting up the data management systems they need to bill Medicaid and other insurers for related services.

The generally recognized disadvantages of providing health services in schools include the following.

*Bureaucratic Turf Issues and Limited Infrastructure in Schools for the Delivery of Expanded School Health Services.* Survey data from school health programs at the University of Colorado, the National Association of School Nurses, and the American School Health Association indicate that although school health supervisors report the existence of procedure manuals and job descriptions, there is a shortage of resources to plan, develop, and effectively manage the school health services component of school health programming. Over 50 percent of school health managers, for example, are technically not prepared to supervise the delivery of clinical services in schools. Rather, their educational backgrounds and experience are in other fields, such as physical education, administration, and guidance and counseling (Slaughter, Igoe, & Nelson, 1984).

It is also rare for school districts to have separate school health budgets. This situation limits the extent to which school health programs can plan for the future and places control for these funds in the hands of others who may not understand the clinical implications of various budget requests.

Finally, there is an uneven distribution of school nursing staff from school system to school system. Almost 50 percent of the school districts in this country have a total student enrollment of 2500 students or less. This student body is then subdivided into a high school, some junior high schools and/or middle schools, and elementary schools. These circumstances create professional staffing problems because the ratio of students to nurses can be as low as 300:1 when the nurse remains in one building. If the nurse is assigned to several schools, services get diluted and professional nursing care becomes so overextended that it soon becomes meaningless.

Some school nurse supervisors have begun to experiment with various criteria to assist with staffing assignments, such as making assignments based on needs assessments and the severity of health problems within certain buildings. In other instances, school health services are regionalized, and nurses are organized into education service districts or boards of cooperative services, where they relate to individual schools as members of consulting teams rather than as direct providers of service. In general, uneven distribution of school health resources within school systems creates major delivery system problems.

*Unresolved Nurse Practice Issues.* One final barrier to providing health services in schools has recently come to light. It concerns the limitations of some state nurse practice acts that prevent the delegation of nursing care responsibilities and supervision of others. School nurse groups in Colorado and Iowa report their nurse practice acts have actually hindered their efforts to improve the quality of care offered to disabled youth and weakened their attempts to include ancillary health personnel (e.g., health clerks) in the care of students.

## Toward a New Agenda

Numerous conferences and heated debates, plus the expenditure of millions of dollars, have produced very little in the way of specific policy for transforming school health into an organized and integrated system of student health. It is no wonder when one considers that this constantly questioned and variously defined and staffed program straddles the boundaries of three very powerful and complex public agencies: public health, education, and, most recently, social services. Adding to this confusion is the fact that the components of school health—health services, health education, and a healthy environment—are rarely consolidated into one formalized program, at either state or local levels, for purposes of program administration and management. In terms of policy development, school health therefore may be the responsibility of all three agencies, no one's business, or somewhere in-between.

With the 1990s in progress and the year 2000 on the horizon, conservation of resources is uppermost in the minds of public policy makers. "Currently there are 93 programs operated by 13 federal agencies that provide a variety of services to children and their families. The total expenditure for fiscal year 1986 was 118 billion dollars, which represents 12 percent of total fiscal year 1986 outlays" (Garwood, Phillips, Hartman, & Zegler, 1989, p. 434).

Given this moderately sufficient treasure chest—at least in the minds of conservative lawmakers—and their hesitancy in having the government interfere with parents' rights and responsibilities, it is very likely that child-related services will not be expanded significantly in the near future. Consequently, the one other alternative is to restructure public services for children, adolescents, and their families into community-based multiservice agencies, called family support centers. This strategy may offer a new environment for interagency collaboration and cooperation and actually improve the school health delivery system for children and youth (Kagan, 1989).

Family support centers could, under one roof, combine a number of social, legal, education, and health services such as parenting classes, social services, nutrition and health services, job training, legal aid services, and career counseling. Simultaneously the centers could provide case management for those in need. Such an arrangement takes into account single parents' busy lifestyles and offers people a "one-stop shopping" approach with a family focus.

In order to succeed, these facilities must be centrally located, easily accessible, and more economical and efficient to operate than the single-purpose agencies that currently provide these services (i.e., health department, social service agency, school systems). Furthermore, bureaucratic turf issues must be minimized, and the role of the consumer—the family—must be strengthened and expanded.

Reforming the service delivery system in this way opens the door for center management to become a shared responsibility between public agencies and families. Local broad-based coalitions including children, adolescents, and parents could join with the professionals in designing these school-based family centers.

The school has repeatedly been identified as the logical site for this type of activity, and the "lighted schoolhouse" concept referred to by Klein and Sadowski (1990) advances the idea of schools as community centers. Unlike the community center of the 1960s, which had a commitment to social action, the emphasis of the new school-based family center would be on improving the family's strength and functioning, not the least of which would include the family's health.

Indeed, although the emphasis is limited to early childhood services, a legislative basis already exists for providing family support services in schools through Public Law 99-457, Education for the Handicapped Amendments of 1986 (Part H), Head Start, Title V Social Security Act, Chapter 1 of the Elementary and Secondary Education Act, the Family Support Act, the Child Development Act, and the Even Start Act (Garwood et al., 1989). However, in order to develop a wider basis for improving school-based family services in general, new Title V maternal and child health regulations must be enacted that support school health services specifically.

It is also time for the governors of each state to identify a lead agency to take responsibility for bringing together all the state and federal resources available for school health services and for providing leadership in establishing plans and policies for school health.

Contrary to long-held beliefs that Americans insist on "home rule" (local control) over any matters concerning their schools, a 1989 annual Gallup education poll sponsored by the professional educational fraternity Phi Delta Kappa showed a surprising preference for national standards.

State health and education coalitions must be convened by a lead agency to frame overall school health policy in order to address school health services, health education, and environmental health issues. It is important that these policies be balanced and take into consideration the needs of all students to have adequate disease prevention, health promotion, and health protection (environmental) services as well as the need of some students with special health problems to have complex nursing care available at schools. At the same time, health professionals must deal with the growing demand for more primary health care at school, including diagnostic and treatment services. Again, the maternal and child health division of the state health department should be actively involved in these endeavors as well as other agencies responsible for disease prevention, health promotion, and health protection services and care for students with handicaps, disabilities, and chronic illness.

Professional associations for nursing and education need to continue to meet and deliberate some important professional issues and common concerns, including the blurring and blending of roles between nurses and teachers that have come to light since the enactment of the Education for All Handicapped Children's Act. A recent survey of 150 Kansas teachers, for example, identified that 70 percent of the teachers were performing complex health-related procedures in the classroom and 21 percent of them were doing this without benefit of any guidelines. Contact with the school nurse appeared to be on an inconsistent basis (Mulligan-Ault, 1988).

It is time for nursing leaders in community health, school health, occupational health, home health, and college health to begin a dialogue about the similarities in their roles and the need to further strengthen their positions within public health circles by integrating some of their functions into broader specialty areas.

Changes also must be made in the provisions of the Medicaid expansion bill of 1989 (OBRA, 1989) that enables pediatric nurse practitioners and family nurse practitioners to receive direct third-party reimbursements for the primary care services they provide to Medicaid recipients. Certified school nurse practitioners who practice in comprehensive school-based clinics with adequate data management systems deserve similar privileges.

As the trend emerges in higher education to involve universities in the overall management of elementary and secondary school systems, schools of nursing should consider becoming actively involved in the design, administration, and management of school-based family support centers (Bailey, 1990). School nurses, in any one of the roles described above, are well prepared to make a valuable contribution to family support centers as either health coordinators or clinicians or both. However, they need the support and technical assistance of other nursing colleagues, which an affiliation with a nursing school would provide.

The National Center for Nursing Research has as one of its areas of concentration the study of health promotion for children and youth. A knowledge base specific to health promotion nursing interventions for school-aged youth in the aggregate is sorely needed and also deserves attention.

As nursing shapes its policy agenda for the year 2000, the needs of vulnerable children and youth must not be overlooked. Realizing that most students need school health services and that nurses are well qualified to manage school health programs, priority must be given to support policy-making efforts that improve school health services. Hayes, as quoted in Klein and Sadowski (1990), explains why and offers a fitting conclusion to this discussion:

> We live in a society with such great inequities, unfairness and trauma, particularly for those persons trapped in poverty, that anger and rage is a constant reality for young people. . . . Most of us yearn for the schools that we experienced that did not require the provision of all the services necessary today. But that was a different time and a different world . . . (p. 168).

REFERENCES

Allensworth, D., Eberst, R., Hertel, V., Igoe, J., Neill, C., Olsen, L., Ross, J., & Seffrin, J. (1988). *Year 2000 health objectives for the nation: Recommendations for the school health program.* Testimony presented before the U.S. Public Health Service and the American Alliance for Health, Physical Education, Recreation and Dance, Kansas City, MO.

American Nurses' Association (1980). School nurses working with handicapped children. Kansas City, MO: American Nurses' Association Publication No. NP-60.

Bailey, K. Pueblo school system comes under the management of the Southern Colorado University (1990, October 14). *Rocky Mountain News, 132*(175), 24.

Butler, J.A., Rosenbaum, S., & Palfrey, J.S. (1987). Ensuring access to health care for children with disabilities. *New England Journal of Medicine, 317,* 162–165.

Centers for Disease Control (1983). Lead poisoning. MMWR—Annual Summary 31(54). Washington, DC: Public Health Service, Department of Health and Human Services Publication No. (CDC) 84-8241.

*Child health 1989.* (1989, October). U.S. Department of Health and Human Services Publication No. (PH5) Bureau of Maternal and Child Health and Resource Development, Office of Maternal and Child Health, HRS-M-CH8915. Washington, DC: U.S. Department of Health and Human Services.

*Digest of educational statistics 1989* (25th ed.) (NCES 89-643) (1989). Washington, DC: U.S. Department of Education Office of Educational Research and Improvement.

Dryfoos, J.G. (1987). *Youth-at-risk: One in four in jeopardy.* New York: Report to the Carnegie Corporation.

Dubowitz, H. (1986) *Child maltreatment in the United States: Etiology, impact and prevention.* Washington, DC: Office of Technology Assessment, U.S. Congress.

Earls, F., & Robins (1989). Comprehensive health care for high risk adolescents: An evaluation study. *American Journal of Public Health, 79,* 999–1005.

Flinn Foundation Special Report (1989). The health of Arizona's school children: Key findings of two surveys by Louis Harris and Associates, Inc., and the UCLA School of Medicine. Phoenix: Flinn Foundation.

Freeman, R.B., & Heinrich, J. (1981). *Community health nursing practice.* Philadelphia: W.B. Saunders Company.

Garwood, G.S., Phillips, D., Hartman, A., & Zegler, E. (1989). As the pendulum swings, federal agency programs for children. *American Psychologist, 44*(2), 434–440.

Gephart, J., Egan, M.C., & Hutchins, V.L. (1984). Perspectives on health of school age children. *Journal of School Health, 54*(1), 11–17.

Harris, L. (1989). *The health of Arizona school children, key findings of two surveys* (Flinn Foundation Special Report). Phoenix: Flinn Foundation.

Igoe, J.B. (1987). *The role of the community health nurse specialist working with school age youth.* Unpublished manuscript. Denver: University of Colorado Health Sciences Center, School Health Programs.

Igoe, J.B. (1991). The community health nurse in schools. In M. Stanhope, & J.L. Lancaster (Eds.), *Community health nursing: Process and practice for promoting health.* 3rd ed. St. Louis: C.V. Mosby.

Kagin, S. (1989). Family-support programs and the schools. *Education Week, 8*(17), 33, 40.

Klein, G. (1988, August 30). Class of 2001. *Rocky Mountain News, 130*(130), 27.

Klein, J., & Sadowski, L. (1990). Personal health services as a component of comprehensive health programs. *Journal of School Health, 60*(4), 164–169.

Klerman, L. (1988). School absence: A health perspective. *Pediatric Clinics of North America,* 35(6), 1253–1269.

Kolbe, L. (1984). Improving the health of children and youth: Frameworks for behavioral research and development. In *Proceedings of the British Conference on Health Education Research.* London: Forbes.

Kovar, M.G., & Dawson, D. (1988). The health status of pre-school and school age children. In H. Wallace, G. Ryan, & A. Oglesby (Eds.), *Maternal and child health practices.* (3rd ed.) (pp. 427–439). Oakland, CA: Third Party Publishing Company.

Lewis, C.E., & Lewis, M.A. (1989). Educational outcomes and illness behaviors of participants in a child-initiated care system: A 12-year follow-up study. *Pediatrics, 84*(5), 845–850.

Lovato, C., Allensworth, D., & Chan, F. (1989). *School health in America. An assessment of state policies to protect and improve the health of students* (Publication No. G005). Kent, Ohio: American School Health Association.

Lynch, A. (1982). *Redesigning school health services.* New York: Human Science Press.

McCune, S. (1989). *Guide to strategic planning for educators.* Alexandria, VA: Association for Supervision and Curriculum Development.

Meeker, R.J., DeAngelis, C., Berman, B., Freeman, H.E., & Oda, D. (1986). A comprehensive school health initiative. *Image: Journal of Nursing Scholarship, 18*(3), 86–91.

Mulligan-Ault, M., Guess, D., Struth, L., & Thompson, B. (1988). The implementation of health related procedures in classrooms for students with severe multiple impairments. *Journal of the Association for Persons with Severe Handicaps, 13*(2), 100–109.

National Council on Patient Information and Education (1989). *Prescription for safety: Improving prescription medicine use among children and teenagers.* Washington, DC: National Council on Patient Information and Education.

Newman, L., & Papkalla, N. (1989, November). Health related learning disorders. *Brown University Newsletter, 5*(11), 1.

Oberg, C. (1990). Medically uninsured children in the United States: A challenge to public policy. *Pediatrics, 85*(5), 824–831.

Ransom-Kuti, D. *The health of youth* (1989). World Health Organization (WHO) Technical Discussion. Geneva: World Health Organization.

Slaughter, E.L., Igoe, J.B., & Nelson, N. (1984). *Report of a national survey of school nurse supervisors.* Unpublished manuscript. Denver: University of Colorado Health Sciences Center, School Health Programs.

Society for Adolescent Medicine (1988). Position paper on school-based health clinics. *Journal of Adolescent Health Care, 9,* 526–530.

Starfield, B. (1982). Family income, ill health and medical care of U.S. children. *Journal of Public Health Policy, 3,* 244–259.

Stenmark, S., & Igoe, J. (1984). *School health programs: Does Medicaid have a role in financing?* Unpublished manuscript. Denver: University of Colorado Health Sciences Center, School Health Programs.

*Tatro v. Texas,* 625 F. 2d 557 (5 Cir. 1980); 703 F. 2d 823 (5 Cir. 1983).

Valanis, B. (1986). *Epidemiology in nursing and health care.* Norwalk, CT: Appleton-Century-Crofts.

Walker, D.K. (1987). Chronically ill children in schools: Programmatic and policy directions for the future. *Rheumatic Disease Clinics of North America, 13,* 113–121.

Woodfill, M., & Beyrer, M. (1991). *The role of the nurse in the school setting: An historical view as reflected in the literature.* Kent, OH: American School Health Association.

## Chapter 19

# Advanced Nursing Practice: Future of the Nurse Practitioner*

LORETTA C. FORD

*T*HE NURSE PRACTITIONER movement is one of the finest demonstrations of how nurses exploited trends in the larger health care system to advance their own professional agenda and to realize their great potential to serve society. All health institutions have been influenced and changed by this innovation: nursing education, practice, research and credentialing; health care delivery patterns; state and federal legislation; health care financing and reimbursement policies; and professional organizations and health literature. Nurse practitioners have revolutionized the way nurses think and act, feel about themselves, and are perceived by others. The movement has been one of the most significant events in nursing history. Amazingly, it began just a little over two decades ago.

From a perspective of 25 years in the nurse practitioner movement, this chapter traces the significant historical aspects of the movement and projects future directions. Two salient observations arise from this analysis. The concept of the nurse practitioner first flourished and later thrived for different reasons, one political and the other professional. Policy makers and some physicians quickly embraced the idea of the nurse practitioner. They perceived the nurse practitioner as a physician substitute in a context of a national shortage of physicians and problems in access to care. Nurses were not enthusiastic about the concept early on. However, the movement thrived because the foundation of the nurse practitioner was deeply rooted in the enduring values and goals of professional nursing.

In 1965, the American Nurses' Association had issued its position paper on Educational Preparation for Nursing (American Nurses' Association, 1965). The Western

* The author gratefully acknowledges the prompt and generous responses to requests for data and information from Dr. Ada Davis, Ms. Evelyn Moses, and Ms. Edith Whitley, Division of Nursing (Department of Health and Human Services, Washington, DC: U.S. PHS and HRS); Dr. Nancy J. Macintyre, New York State Coalition of Nurse Practitioners; Dodie Downey Russell, Chair of The National Alliance of Nurse Practitioners; the American Nurses' Association Council of Clinical Nurse Specialists and Council of Primary Health Care Nurse Practitioners; and Karen Forbes; and the American Nurses' Association Credentialing Center.

Interstate Council on Nursing Education had completed a study on the clinical content of graduate nursing programs (Ford, Cobb, & Taylor, 1967). Discussions about the nature of nursing and the scope of practice were on the agenda of every nursing organization. The time was ripe for change.

The first pediatric nurse practitioner program was a demonstration project inaugurated at the University of Colorado in 1965, by public health nurse Loretta C. Ford and pediatrician Henry K. Silver, Professors of Nursing and Medicine, respectively (Ford & Silver, 1967). The social and professional ferment of the decade provided both the cultural context and the opportunity to educate nurses for an expanded role in child health care. This preparation was seen as a strategy to gain autonomy and self-determination in practice, to energize nursing education curricula, and to fulfill nursing's social mandate to serve humankind.

The Colorado pediatric nurse practitioner program was a model created from the values and expressed direction of professional nursing. Academically and scientifically grounded, the program was health-oriented and clinically focused. The nurses were prepared for autonomy in clinical judgment and collegiality and collaboration in team care. The primary care needs of children identified from family health surveys and from the practice of public health nurses helped in determining the educational content, processes, and goals of the program.

One of these goals was to expand the nurse's scope of practice by increasing her depth of knowledge of the growth and development and conditions of health and illness in children, structuring the data collection format on physical and psychological phenomena, and emphasizing clinical judgment and management. The program stressed the autonomy, authority, and accountability of the professional nurse in practice. Role preparation also emphasized the nature of nursing, which was defined later in the Social Policy Statement of the American Nurses' Association: to diagnose and treat actual or potential health problems, to teach, counsel, and guide, and to return the person served to informed self-care or if that was impossible, to a peaceful, dignified death (American Nurses' Association, 1980).

The codirectors of the first pediatric nurse practitioner program sought to demonstrate that qualified nurses prepared in a specialized, educational program could deliver community-based, high-quality health care and supervision of well children safely, competently, confidently, and acceptably. Collegiate schools of nursing could benefit from the findings and integrate nurse practitioner competencies and skills into their curricula, thereby assuring institutionalization of the concept into nursing education. Only then could the children and families of the nation receive the kind of care, promised as a "right" in the social ferment of the 1960s. Although the perceived shortage of primary care physicians was not the rationale for our efforts, it gave nurses the opportunity to reclaim ground they had lost in the 1930s when the American Academy of Pediatrics claimed all of well child care for pediatricians. Before that, public health nurses were the primary providers in well baby clinics, milk stations, and homes (DeMaio, 1981).

But the reclaiming of ground was to be done cognitively, academically, and scientifically through study and demonstrations, not by fiat or political maneuvers. Our work and that of many other investigators and the emergence of the concept of primary care provided an extensive proving ground for research (Alpert & Charney,

1973). Paradoxically, the idea of the nurse practitioner was so timely, so responsive to immediate social needs, and so attractive to individuals and institutions that before the first 4 years of test data were available, many programs for the preparation of nurse practitioners sprang up. Coincidentally, mutations of the original model occurred. Established academic standards were not always maintained. The focus of some programs shifted from a nursing to a medical model. Legal authorization and specialty certification outside of nursing were sought, mostly for the protection of the practitioner. Also, organized nursing was slow to address the needs of nurse practitioners for recognition and affiliation. As a result, new and more responsive organizations emerged.

In spite of some of these problematic variations, the outcomes of the nurse practitioner movement constitute a modern success story (Mezey & McGivern, 1986).

No professional role has been more thoroughly discussed, described, studied, and reported than that of the nurse practitioner. Thousands of publications are in the public domain on the preparation, practice, performance, and placement of nurse practitioners and the public policy affecting them. A recent comprehensive review of two decades of research on the nurse practitioner was published by the Office of Technology Assessment in 1986. The study concluded that nurse practitioners in primary and ambulatory care "within their areas of competence . . . provide care whose quality is equivalent to that of care provided by physicians." Further, nurse practitioners are "more adept than physicians at providing services that depend on communication with patients and preventive action (U.S. Congress, Office of Technology Assessment, 1986).

Other studies, some of which are cited in the Office of Technology Assessment report, show that the nurse practitioner is

- Clinically safe, competent, and confident in caring for a large percentage (some say 70 to 80 percent) of all ambulatory patients (Komaroff et al., 1976; Record et al., 1980; Sackett, 1974; Sox, 1979);
- Well accepted by patients, nurses, and many other professionals, including the physicians with whom they collaborate (American Nurses' Association, 1983; Levine et al., 1976; Lewis & Resnick, 1967; Mitchell, 1986; Spitzer et al., 1974);
- Well satisfied with her role and relationships but less pleased with some work environments and rewards (Weill, 1989);
- Cost effective in both preparation and practice (American Medical Association, 1983; U.S. Department of Health and Human Services, 1984);
- An attractive model for recruiting potential students into the profession;
- Becoming institutionalized in most master's education programs and in a variety of practice settings (see Table 19–1);
- An influential political force in shaping health policy (*The Nurse Practitioner*, 1989);
- Struggling to secure reimbursement for services and to be free from unnecessary controls to practice;

**TABLE 19-1 Nurse Practitioner Master's Programs, United States, 1989**

| | |
|---|---|
| Number of schools | 71 |
| Number of programs | 168 |
| Specialties: | |
| Family | 53 |
| Pediatrics | 27 |
| Adult Health | 28 |
| Gerontology | 26 |
| Obstetrics/gynecology and women's health | 20 |
| Other | 14 |

Note: Twenty-eight continuing education nurse practitioner programs are offered, 17 of which are in universities.
Source: *Directory of Nurse Practitioner Programs in USA*, National Organization of Nurse Practitioner Faculties, May 1989 (Washington, D.C.).

- Increasingly legally authorized in state practice statutes. Forty-three states have special nurse practitioner legislation, and 34 states have laws that provide for prescriptive privileges ("How each state," 1990);
- Professionally credentialed (see Table 19–2);
- Enjoying an enhanced public image as a professional nurse;
- Expanding into new settings and new specialties as needs, demands, and opportunities arise (Ford, 1986);
- A political force within professional organizations, forming new organizations and alliances and assuming leadership positions in them (the National Alliance of Nurse Practitioners is a conglomerate of 13 specialty nurse practitioner organizations with a membership of 15,000 nurse practitioners);
- Recruited widely for many positions around the world for community-based care, institutional services, and special health projects and programs;
- Influential in academic settings, introducing faculty practice and altering graduate and undergraduate nursing education curricula (Forbes, 1990); and
- Flexible in responding to the emerging health needs of changing populations, such as persons infected with human immunodeficiency virus, the chronically ill, the homeless, the elderly, and the urban and rural poor.

Nurse practitioners are positioned by history and performance to meet the challenges of the 1990s and beyond. In a short quarter of a century, they have established themselves as a norm along with clinical nurse specialists in advanced practice today.

A recent survey by two American Nurses' Association councils on core curriculum content of nurse practitioners and clinical nurse specialist programs noted "striking similarities between them." Nurse practitioner programs have "greater focus on history, physical assessment and pharmacology content." The authors conclude: "Still, it cannot be denied that all advanced practitioners must have these skills [physical assessment] highly developed to fully evaluate and treat all clients. Today, both roles are strongly and equally rooted in nursing as evidenced by the nursing

**TABLE 19–2 Nurse Practitioner Certification Data**

| | |
|---|---|
| American Nurses' Association total (10/88) | 12,276* |
| Family nurse practitioners | 5595 |
| Adult nurse practitioners | 4460 |
| Pediatric nurse practitioners | 1384 |
| School nurse practitioners | 431 |
| Gerontologic nurse practitioners | 247 |
| General nurse practitioners | 159 |
| National Certification Board[†] | |
| Pediatric nurse practitioners | 3726 |

Note: 137 members of the National Association of Pediatric Nurse Associates and Practitioners are certified by both the National Association of Pediatric Nurse Associates and Practitioners and the American Nurses' Association.
  * Source: American Nurses' Association, Center for Credentialing Services, *Professional Certification*, 1990.
  † Source: National Association of Pediatric Nurse Associates and Practitioners, *Membership Survey*, 1989, Cherry Hill, NJ.

theory component" in both the nurse practitioner and clinical nurse specialist programs (Forbes, 1990).

Over the years, about half of the funding for nurse practitioner programs has come from the Division of Nursing and recently has been earmarked almost exclusively for master's level preparation. The most recent allocation for both nurse practitioner and nurse midwifery programs is almost 13.5 million dollars, similar to previous annual allowances.

Although the future of the nurse practitioner was predicted by some to be rather bleak (Spitzer, 1984; Weston, 1975) because of the projected glut of physicians and other factors, history is proving otherwise. The demand for them has risen dramatically, as it has for all nurses.

The changing demographics and disease patterns, the complexity and costs of the health care services, and the failures of the current system to contain health service costs constitute opportunities for nurse practitioners to grow. The aging population, with its specific needs to maintain vigor and functional independence, including the small percentage of elderly in nursing homes, has found the nurse practitioner to be the practitioner of choice. As lifespan, chronic illnesses, and diseases spread by lifestyle increase, a continuing demand for nurse practitioners is created. Nurse practitioners will also be needed to assist in restructuring our failing health care system. Once again, as nurse practitioners found in the early 1960s, an enabling environment sets the stage and provides opportunities for their leadership in a new order of meeting people's needs for health care.

W.D. Ruckelshaus (1989), former administrator of the Environmental Protection Agency and now chief executive officer of a large corporation, gave a formula recently for getting things done in a free society. He wrote:

> First, there has to be agreement on a set of values, some public consensus that there is a goal worth pursuing. Next must come a set of incentives, by which society can be seen to reward those who pursue the values and sanc-

tion those who do not. In market economies, incentives usually involve money. Finally, institutions must be able to adopt the values and administer the incentives (Ruckelshaus, 1989).

As society's values for health change and demands rise to increase access and reduce costs, the nurse practitioner will become more highly valued as a primary care provider. Each of the three steps identified by Ruckelshaus is not fully accomplished in orderly progression, but there is growing awareness that society's values for health and its health-seeking behaviors are changing. Health is no longer considered just the absence of disease. Nor is there widespread expectation that health professionals are solely responsible for the cure and care of people. Today, there is more recognition that health determinants are in the hands of the people themselves, as are some of the solutions to today's health problems. The United States Public Health Service objectives for the year 2000 address these determinants: genetic endowment, environmental factors, lifestyle, and health services. A sample of the draft objectives, which are under review, provides telling evidence of national health concerns and offers myriad opportunities for nurse practitioners.

United States Public Health Service Draft Objectives to Promote Health and Prevent Disease include the following:

- To maintain the vitality and independence of older people.
- To reduce HIV [human immunodeficiency virus] infection and sexually transmitted diseases.
- To increase immunization and infectious disease control.
- To improve maternal and child health.
- To reduce the toll from cancer . . . (and) other chronic disorders.
- To reduce high blood cholesterol and high blood pressure.
- To improve health education and preventive services (Public Health Service, U.S. Department of Health and Human Services, 1989).

These and other objectives related to lifestyle patterns, work site risks, and environmental health will carry recommendations for education, practice, and research for nurse practitioners, who will be primary care providers in a host of settings in the 1990s.

The next step that Ruckelshaus identified—incentives—although it takes the positive form of public recognition and status, lacks a secure monetary base. However, 19 states have third-party reimbursement legislation for nurse practitioners and 15 others are exploring legislative authorization. Insurance companies in seven states without legislative requirements reimburse nurse practitioners ("How each state," 1990). Federal health policy is changing also, although slowly.

In late 1989, President George Bush signed legislation that allows direct payment to certified pediatric and family nurse practitioners providing Medicaid services; employers of nurse practitioners can receive direct Medicare payments for nurse practitioner services given in nursing homes; and nurse practitioners and clinical nurse specialists collaborating with a physician are authorized under Medicare to certify and recertify a nursing home patient's need for skilled nursing care (American Nurses' Association News Release, 1989c).

These are indeed victories, as is the extensive evidence of institutionalization of the role occurring through graduate degree education programs, legislative and credentialing mechanisms, advertised positions, civil service and military job descriptions, and the establishment of specialty professional organizations.

Additionally, other challenges will arise as United States Public Health Service objectives focus public attention on the promotion of health, prevention of disease, education, and self-care. These elements are basic components of the nature and function of nursing and within the scope of practice of nurse practitioners. The opportunities will abound for nursing, nurse practitioners, and all nurses in advanced practice to step up and take charge through innovative patterns of entrepreneurship and intrapreneurship, through participation in capitated systems of care, and through political maneuvers to influence state and national health policies.

## Practice Expansions

### Entrepreneurship

Nurse practitioners are demonstrating that they can offer services as independent entrepreneurs delivering health care to defined populations, operating managed care facilities, consulting, and creating group practice arrangements. Although the roster of nurse entrepreneurs is small—perhaps 3 percent of nurses in the United States— in many areas nurse practitioners have led the way. Carlson, a nurse-owner of a consultant corporation, cited a study by Adeylotte on the characteristics of a typical nurse entrepreneur as "female, 40–49 years old, married with 1–3 children, a member of the State Nurse's Association, has a master's degree in nursing, is certified by ANA in a specialty, and has 10–15 years of nursing experience" (American Nurses' Association, *The American Nurse*, 1989b). More liberal reimbursement benefits and consumer choices will encourage nurse practitioner entrepreneurship, although the numbers are expected to remain small.

### Intrapreneurship

Although most nurse practitioners work within the organized systems of ambulatory health care, health maintenance organizations, clinics, and physicians' offices, there are indications of the predicted spread of nurse practitioners into hospital inpatient services. Additionally, nursing homes are seeking to employ nurse practitioners, and as the traditional patterns of nursing practice (e.g., unit-bound, standard hours, inflexible rules, lack of professional autonomy) change, inpatient services will become attractive to nurse practitioners; they will become intrapreneurs. With their creativity, competence, commitment, and courage, nurse practitioners will bring new ideas, insights, and enlightenment to the total system of care. Best of all, nurse practitioners will influence the quality of care provided to patients and their families in institutions, although the trends and opportunities will probably be organized into capitated systems, possibly created by public-private partnerships.

As concerns about access, quality, and costs of health care are raised by governments, industry and labor, and the general public, there is increasing interest in universal health insurance coverage for all Americans. Calls for a national health plan are heard in every quarter, and some states—California, New York, Oregon, and others—are investigating options for statewide insurance coverage for the uninsured. The full use and reimbursement of nurse practitioners in any such plan is crucial to the success of the enterprise and offers great hope for the future, not only for nurse practitioners but for society. Past history of nurse practitioner experience in capitated systems is worth repeating. Nurse practitioners have proved themselves to be cost-effective deliverers of primary care, improving access and assuring quality care in health maintenance organizations (Barham & Steiger, 1982). Occasionally, difficulties arise when health maintenance organizations deviate from their original goal to offer comprehensive, preventive health care and begin to function as traditional narrow, technical medical services. Under these conditions, nurse practitioners are expected to serve as physician substitutes. Some studies comparing nurse practitioners with physicians on medical productivity, such as time required for episodic visits, show that nurse practitioners are less productive (Barham & Steiger, 1982). Other studies have reported different findings (Fagin, 1981). However, in either case, nurse practitioner productivity should be measured longitudinally with indices of health outcomes in patients and their overall cost of health resources. Nurse practitioners have been shown to use fewer resources, and over time behavioral changes in patients can offer greater cost savings for society and less pain and fewer problems for the patients and their families.

Since capitated health care systems are likely to be introduced, especially for some targeted populations—the uninsured, underinsured, chronically ill, and elderly—nurse practitioners should be prepared educationally and politically to meet these challenges.

## Education

The content and processes of nurse practitioner programs are generic to all nursing education programs. At the undergraduate level, comprehensive physical and mental assessment skills should be taught and linked to clinical decision making. At the master's level, the fusion of the clinical specialist and nurse practitioner roles and programs should occur, allowing for more depth in assessment, training in pharmacology, and advanced management skills for all who aspire to advanced practice in nursing. Increased attention needs to be given in all programs to care of the chronically ill, the elderly, and those with mental health problems. Additionally, consideration needs to be given to internships or residencies to accommodate advanced learning of clinical skills for which graduate credit is inappropriate. The current proliferation of separate specialty programs, each with low enrollments and high costs, needs to be carefully examined and the inefficiencies of these programs eliminated. Creative educational designs and innovative teaching strategies will need to be employed to attract and retain future student populations.

Although only a few post-master's continuing education nurse practitioner programs are offered for nurses prepared as clinical specialists, this trend is likely to escalate and then recede as the merging of the two programs occurs.

Education and service must forge closer ties in order to reap the benefits of both skilled clinicians in service and the teaching and research competencies of faculty. Faculty practice plans for those who can skillfully combine the three aspects of practice, education, and research need to be developed along with reward systems that recognize the triple competencies.

Nursing faculty should give much more attention to the needs of mature women students and the predicted new type of college student who will be older, less affluent, and from varied ethnic backgrounds and whose cultural roots and life experience strengths are so desirable and needed in nursing practice.

Some schools of nursing have created their own clinical resources, such as wellness and lifestyle centers and case management services to use for teaching and research purposes. Other existing sites for teaching and research, such as centers for the homeless, nursery schools, industries, nursing homes, and others should be pursued. The teaching hospital and teaching nursing home concept could be extended to a host of community-based services.

Paramount to the success of any such venture is a sound fiscal plan. Reimbursement for nursing services is a major hurdle for the profession generally and has local, state, and national implications for the development of a sound financial policy for accessible health care.

## Financing

Reimbursement for nurse practitioner services is not only a fiscal problem per se but also a political problem. Concerns about the numbers of uninsured in this country and the rising health costs suggest that some type of universal health plan with a strong prevention component will come into being. The United States Public Health Service objectives mentioned earlier are congruent with the nature of professional nursing and the scope of practice of the nurse practitioner. Nurse practitioners are the most well-positioned providers of primary care in both rural and urban areas in both community-based services and homes.

The strategies, logistics, and tactics for the reform movement must be politically generated and implemented. Currently, California is exploring a statewide insurance plan to increase access to health care for its uninsured and minority populations. Other state governments are considering programs to address specific health problems, such as child health needs, care of patients with acquired immunodeficiency syndrome, and rural elderly populations. As states lead the way, their proposed laws need to be carefully monitored for opportunities to call to legislators' attention the need to reshape reimbursement policy in the interest of serving all people. Recently, New York State authorized Medicaid reimbursement to nurse practitioners after one pediatric nurse practitioner, Cheryl Martin-Schroeder, working in collaboration with a pediatrician, was first paid and then denied payment for her services to an underserved child population. Her cause was championed by the New York State Nurses' Association (1989), and eventually, its persistence paid off. The law was changed to authorize payment to all nurse practitioners. In New Mexico last year, the Aetna Life and Casualty Insurance Company denied previously paid Medicare claims by physicians for nurse practitioner services to elderly rural people (Ready, 1989). The refusal was based on a technicality citing that nurse practitioners were not "directly supervised" by physicians in their offices. The nurse practitioners were located in satellite clinics.

The most effective state legislative political force consists of hometown folks and local and state political action groups. Nurse practitioners who are committed, alert, tuned in to local trends, and persistent know this and have successfully used strategic approaches to influence political decisions. Social times are changing. Although different parts of the country are moving at different rates, with the information technology available and with their own organizational collaboration, cooperation, and communication, nurses are now showing the way to make nationwide movement possible and effective.

The underlying data base for political action must be continually gathered, evaluated, analyzed, reported, and used judiciously. A research agenda must include past, current, and projected information on nurse practitioner resources—preparation, placement, performance, progress, payment, and practices. One national data bank, initiated in 1990 under a federal contract with UNISYS Corporation, "will collect information on adverse action against health care practitioners—including nurses." However, if past history is any predictor of the future, for nurse practitioners there will be little to report on litigation (Quinlan & Bodenhorn, 1990).

A central repository of comprehensive data on nurse practitioners is sorely needed. Additionally, clinical nursing research on outcomes in patient health status is vital to validate the quality of care, to establish standards of care, to add to the fund of general knowledge, and to provide the scientific base for educational programs. Studies of structure and organizational designs and financing could yield vital information and help to identify the barriers to access and quality in the system. Identifying qualified practitioners, however, is another matter.

## Credentialing

The growth of specialties and credentialing has been dramatic: 210,000 nurses are certified in specialties by the American Nurses' Association and 25 other organizations. Without a common definition of a credential, confusion and chaos can result; the public, the practitioner, and the profession will not be well served. As American Nurses' Association President Lucille Joel (1989) noted recently, "Specialization and advanced practice are most properly regulated internally by a profession through the peer review process and by subsequent conferring of a credential which can be easily interpreted by the public." Currently, the Josiah Macy Foundation is sponsoring a program on the definition of specialties with a view toward identifying some common designations and credentials. These and other efforts to clarify credentialing should resolve some of the issues of reimbursement, recognition, and rewards in advanced practice.

## Conclusion

The nurse practitioner movement was born at a most propitious time in the nation's history. The sociopolitical upheaval, the professional ferment in nursing, the shortage of physicians in primary care, and a growing, vocal, demanding populace enabled the movement first to survive and eventually to thrive. The early fears in nursing that nurse practitioners would be exploited by physicians and policy makers for the delivery of medical care have not been realized. Indeed, it has been the nurse practitioners who have led the way to successfully integrate the nurse practitioner concept into all of society's major institutions. Nurse practitioners have initiated changes not only in nursing education and practice but also in legislation and in the organization and financing of health care delivery. The challenge ahead for nurse practitioners is once again to take advantage of an enabling environment and move professionally and politically to help solve the problems of access, quality, and cost in health care. Nurse practitioners are well positioned to lead the way.

The internal tensions of the profession are resolving. Professional nurses realize that the struggle for public recognition and rewards requires internal unity, a solid political power block, coalitions of likeminded people (especially lay people), and the use of appropriate strategies, logistics, and tactics.

Reflecting on these 25 years of social change and the evolution and solid success of the nurse practitioner brings to mind Ferguson's parallel experience in another social movement (1980). She reflected:

> At first the idea of creating a new order by perturbation seems outrageous. . . . Yet our traditional wisdom contains parallel ideas. We know that stress often forces new solutions, that crisis often alerts us to opportunity; that the creative process requires chaos before form emerges; that individuals are often strengthened by suffering and conflict, and that societies need a healthy airing of dissent.

Today, society's disenchantment with its health care offers another unique opportunity for nurse practitioners. Now is the time for them to exploit, once again, perturbations in the larger health care system to accomplish professional agendas, and at the same time fulfill nursing's social mandate to serve humankind.

REFERENCES

Alpert, J., & Charney, E. (1973). *The education of physicians for primary care.* Rockville, MD: U.S. Public Health Service.

American Medical Association (1983). Center for Health Policy Research. Reynolds, R.A., Abram, J.B. (Eds.), *Socioeconomic characteristics of medical practice 1983*. Chicago: American Medical Association.

American Nurses' Association (1965). *ANA, A Position Paper 1965*. New York: Educational Preparation for Nurse Practitioners and Assistants to Nurses. Kansas City, MO: American Nurses' Association.

American Nurses' Association (1980). *Nursing: A social policy statement*. Kansas City, MO: American Nurses' Association.

American Nurses' Association (1983). *Nurse practitioners: A review of the literature*. Kansas City, MO: American Nurses' Association.

American Nurses' Association (1989a). *ANA 1990 Certification Catalogue*. Kansas City, MO: American Nurses' Association.

American Nurses' Association (1989b, September 7). Directions. *The American Nurse*, p. 16.

American Nurses' Association News Release (1989c, December 5). Washington, DC: American Nurses' Association.

Barham, V.Z., & Steiger, N.J. (1982). Health maintenance organizations and nurse practitioners: The Kaiser experience. In L.H. Aiken (Ed.), *Nursing in the 1980s, crises, opportunities, challenges*. American Academy of Nursing, Philadelphia: J.B. Lippincott.

DeMaio, D.J. (1981). Health services for children: A descriptive analysis of an urban program. In L. Aiken (Ed.), *Health policy and nursing practice* (pp. 158–182). American Academy of Nursing, New York: McGraw-Hill Book Company.

*Directory of nurse practitioner programs in USA* (1989, May). Washington, DC: National Organization of Nurse Practitioner Faculties.

Fagin, C.M. (1982). Nursing's pivotal role in American health care. In L.H. Aiken (Ed.), *Nursing in the 1980s: Crises, opportunities, challenges* (pp. 459–473). Philadelphia: J.B. Lippincott.

Ferguson, M. (1980). *The acquarian conspiracy* (p. 313). Los Angeles: T.P. Tarcher, Inc., and New York: St. Martin's Press.

Forbes, K.E., Rafson, J., Spross, J.A., & Kozlowski, D. (1990, April). The clinical nurse specialist and nurse practitioner core curriculum survey. *The Nurse Practitioner Journal, 15*(43), 46–48.

Ford, L.C. (1986, January). The nurse practitioner in surgical nursing practice. *Surgical Rounds, 9*(9), 94–96.

Ford, L.C., Cobb, M., & Taylor, M. (1967). *Defining clinical content, graduate nursing programs, community health nursing*. Boulder, CO: Western Interstate Council on Nursing Education, Western Interstate Commission for Higher Education.

Ford, L.C., & Silver, H.K. (1967, September). Expanded role of the nurse in child care. *Nursing Outlook, 15*(9), 43–45.

How each state stands on legislative issues affecting advanced nursing practice (1990, January). *The Nurse Practitioner, 15*(1), 11–18.

Joel, L. (1989, November/December). In search of a rational future for certification. *The American Nurse, 21*(10), 8.

Komaroff, A.L., Sawayer, K., Flatley, M., & Browne, C.M. (1976, March/April). Nurse practitioner management of common respiratory and genitourinary infections, using protocols. *Nursing Research, 25*(2), 84–89.

Levine, D.M., Morlock, J.J., Mushlin, A.I., Shipiro, B.S., & Malitz, F.E. (1976, April). The role of new health practitioners in prepaid group practice: Provider differences in process and outcomes of medical care. *Medical Care, 14*(4), 326–347.

Lewis, C.E., & Resnick, B.A. (1967, December 7). Nurse clinics and progressive ambulatory patient care. *New England Journal of Medicine, 277*(23), 1236–1241.

Mezey, M.D., & McGivern, D.O. (Eds.) (1986). *Nurses, nurse practitioners: The evolution of primary care.* Boston: Little, Brown & Co.

Mitchell, J. (1986, April 14). *Medicare reimbursement for physician services.* Hearings Before the Subcommittee on Health, House Committee on Ways and Means, United States Congress.

New York State Nurses Association (NYSNA) Report (1989, October/November). *The Official Newsletter, 20*(9), 1.

Public Health Service, U.S. Department of Health and Human Services (1989, September). *Promoting health/preventing disease, year 2000 objectives for the nation draft for public review and comment* (pp. 483). Washington, DC: PHS.

Quinlan, D.S., & Bodenhorn, K.A. (1990, Winter). Update: The national practitioner data bank. *Specialty Nursing Forum, 2*(1), 8.

Ready, T. Nurse practitioners protest coverage denial. (1989, October 10). *Health Week, 3*(20), 9, 44.

Record, J.C., McCally, M., Schweitzer, S.O., Blomquist, R.M., & Berger, B.D. (1980, Fall). New health professions after a decade and a half: Delegation, productivity and costs in primary care. *Journal Health Political Policy Law, 5*(3), 470–497.

Ruckelshaus, W.D. (1989, September 5). The politics of waste disposal. *Wall Street Journal,* sec. A, p. 18.

Sackett, D.L. (1974, February). The Burlington randomized trial of the nurse practitioner: Health outcomes of patients. *Annals of Internal Medicine, 80*(2), 137–142.

Sox, H.C., Jr. (1979, September). Quality of patient care by nurse practitioners and physician's assistants: A ten-year perspective. *Annals of Internal Medicine, 91*(3), 459–468.

Spitzer, W. (1984). The nurse practitioner revisited—slow death of a good idea. *New England Journal of Medicine, 310*(16), 1049–1052.

Spitzer, W.O., Sackett, D.L., Kergin, D.J., Hackett, B.C., & Olynich, A. (1974). The Burlington randomized trial of the nurse practitioner. *New England Journal of Medicine, 290*(5), 251–256.

U.S. Congress, Office of Technology Assessment (1986, December). *Nurse practitioners, physician's assistants, and certified nurse midwives: A policy analysis* (Health Technology Case Study 37), OTA-HCS-37 (p. 5). Washington, DC: U.S. Government Printing Office.

U.S. Department of Health and Human Services (1984). Public Health Service, Bureau of Health Professions. *Report to the President and Congress on the status of health personnel in the United States.* Vols. I and II. (Department of Health and Human Services Publication No. HRS-P-OD 84-4.) Washington, DC: U.S. Government Printing Office.

U.S. Department of Health and Human Services (1990). *Healthy people 2000: National health promotion and disease prevention objective.* DHHS Publication No. (PHS) 91-50213. Washington, D.C.: Public Health Service.

Weill, V.A., Love, M., Pron, A.L., Tesoro, T.A., Grey, M., Hickel, M., Teti, B., & Serota, J. (1989, March-April). Future potential, phase I: Nurse practitioners look at themselves. *Journal of Pediatric Health Care, 3*(2), 76–82.

Weston, J.L. (1975). Whither the nurse in the nurse practitioner? *Nursing Outlook, 23*(3), 148.

# PART IV

Caring for Vulnerable Groups

## Chapter 20

# Strategies to Reduce Infant Mortality

LAUREN S. ARNOLD
RAE K. GRAD

*I*NFANT MORTALITY has long been considered an accurate indicator of the overall health of a community, and, as such, has been closely followed as a marker of the health of the nation. Over the course of the past century, efforts to decrease infant mortality have resulted in drastic reductions in infant death and illness rates. However, during the 1980s, progress toward improving pregnancy outcomes and infant survival came to a virtual standstill and in some populations actually deteriorated. In response, national attention in the legislative and health care arenas has recently focused on infant mortality, its causes and its consequences.

The purpose of this chapter is to examine the issue of infant mortality from a health care as well as a sociologic perspective. The intent is to provide a better understanding of the causes and consequences of infant mortality in order to more effectively target efforts in the 1990s to promote those strategies that are most likely to be effective in improving the health and well-being of the nation's children.

## Infant Mortality: Definition of the Problem

Infant mortality statistics are sensitive to social factors influencing the quality of life and overall health of a population. Infant mortality statistics reflect access of the general population to such basic elements as housing, food, sanitation, employment, education, and health care. Because infant mortality statistics are sensitive to such complex social and health factors, they are widely used at local, state, national, and international levels for measuring the health status of populations.

The infant mortality rate for any year is defined as the number of deaths in infants under 1 year of age per 1000 live births occurring in the same year (National Center for Health Statistics, 1989b). Infant deaths are further divided into two categories according to age: neonatal deaths are those that occur during the first 27 days of life, and postneonatal deaths are those that occur between 28 days and 1

303

year of age (National Center for Health Statistics, 1989b). The infant mortality rate encompasses both neonatal and postneonatal mortality.

In 1987 (the most recent year for which final data were available), the overall national infant mortality rate was 10.1 per 1000 live births (National Center for Health Statistics, 1989b). The black infant mortality rate of 17.9 per 1000 live births was nearly twice the white rate of 8.6 per 1000 live births (National Center for Health Statistics, 1989b). In comparison to other industrialized nations, the United States lags behind in caring for its mothers and infants. In 1987, the United States' infant mortality rate ranked only 20th worldwide. According to UNICEF (1988), the United States ranked behind first place Japan (whose rate is 5.0) and other industrialized nations, including Canada, France, Spain, and Great Britain. Even less developed countries such as Singapore have lower infant mortality rates.

Infants born in the nation's urban communities are at the highest risk of death during infancy. In 1987, 17 of the 22 cities with populations over 500,000 had overall infant mortality rates higher than the national average (National Commission to Prevent Infant Mortality, 1990, unpublished data). In fact, the cities with the highest rates (Detroit, Washington, D.C., Baltimore, and Memphis) have infant mortality statistics similar to those of such underdeveloped countries as Costa Rica, Rumania, Yugoslavia, and Cuba (Table 20–1) (National Commission to Prevent Infant Mortality, 1990, unpublished data).

Progress toward reducing infant mortality has been uneven. In some communities, rather than improving, infant mortality has actually increased during the 1980s. In Indianapolis the infant mortality rate increased by more than 10 percent between 1980 and 1986 (Hughes, Johnson, Rosenbaum, & Liu, 1989). In six other cities (Baltimore, Memphis, New Orleans, Philadelphia, San Diego, and San Jose), a similar trend persisted through the year 1987. It has been suggested that this downward trend in progress is associated with increases in conditions such as poverty among children; substance abuse; child abuse and neglect; and inaccessibility of appropriate health care (Hughes et al., 1989). Infant mortality trend data reveal that over time, progress in reducing infant mortality has been substantial. However, periods of decline have occurred, during which major national efforts were launched to re-establish the pattern of progress. Such an effort may once again be required in the 1990s.

## Infant Mortality Trends Over Time: A Historical Analysis

In order to understand the current issues surrounding infant mortality and to identify strategies that hold the most promise for addressing the problem, an analysis of historical trends related to infant mortality is important. This analysis will provide some insight into the social and health care perspectives of the issue and guidance for identifying effective strategies to be implemented in the future.

Substantial progress in reducing infant mortality was made in the first half of the decade. In 1900, data from ten states and the District of Columbia indicated an

**TABLE 20–1 Infant Mortality Rates, Ranking of the Developed Countries, 1988\*†**

| Rank | Country | Infant Mortality Rate‡ |
|---|---|---|
| 1 | Japan | 4.8 |
| 2 | Finland | 5.3 |
| 3 | Sweden | 5.8 |
| 4 | Netherlands | 6.8 |
| 4 | Switzerland | 6.8 |
| 6 | Singapore | 7.0 |
| 7 | Canada | 7.2 |
| 8 | Hong Kong | 7.4 |
| 9 | Federal Republic of Germany | 7.5 |
| 10 | Denmark | 7.6 |
| 11 | France | 7.7 |
| 12 | Norway | 8.0 |
| 13 | Austria | 8.1 |
| 13 | German Democratic Republic | 8.1 |
| 15 | United Kingdom | 9.0 |
| 16 | Australia | 9.2 |
| 16 | Ireland | 9.2 |
| 16 | Spain | 9.2§ |
| 19 | Italy | 9.5 |
| 20 | Belgium | 9.7‖ |
| 21 | Israel | 10.0 |
| 21 | New Zealand | 10.0‖ |
| 21 | United States | 10.0 |
| 24 | Greece | 11.0 |

\* Source: The *State of the World's Children,* United Nations Children's Fund (UNICEF). Oxford: Oxford University Press, 1991.
† Singapore and Hong Kong, not defined as "developed" by the United Nations, are included in the ranking since they have infant mortality rates below the United States rate.
‡ Number of infant deaths per 1000 live births.
§ Rate is for 1986.
‖ Rate is for 1987.

infant mortality rate of 150 per 1000 live births (Starfield, 1985). By 1940, through tremendous national efforts in which nurses played a significant role, the rate had declined to 47 per 1000 live births (Pratt, 1982). These reductions were attributable in large part to improved sanitation, pasteurization of milk supplies, development and implementation of coordinated health services for mothers and infants, improved nutrition, health education, and advances in the education and practices of health professionals. However, these gains were not sustained. In 1954 the rate was 26.4, and there it stayed until 1960 (Pratt, 1982). This break in progress has been attributed to the increase in birth rate, now commonly known as the postwar baby boom, and the migration of severely disadvantaged families into northern cities where maternity health care systems were unprepared for the demand (Arnold, Brecht, Hockett, Ampacher, & Grad, 1987). A reversal of this pattern of decline in progress was initiated in the 1960s, when new programs were introduced, but it was to be repeated again in the 1980s.

## The Great Society Programs

During the 1960s, major changes were made in maternal and child health programs. A national plan to combat mental retardation was launched by President John F. Kennedy. The President's Panel on Mental Retardation stated that mental retardation was most closely associated with premature birth and inadequate prenatal care. In a speech to the nation, the President emphasized the importance of prenatal care in reducing the likelihood of neurologic damage in infants. Subsequently, major changes were made in maternal and child health programs. In 1963, Title V of the Social Security Act was amended to create the Maternity and Infant Care Program to provide comprehensive maternity and infant care for low-income, high-risk women. The Medicaid program was established in 1965 and served as the financing mechanism for the Maternity and Infant Care program and other maternity and newborn services. Other programs were established during the 1960s, such as The Medicaid Early and Periodic Screening, Diagnosis, and Treatment program for children; the Special Supplemental Food Program for Women, Infants, and Children; the Comprehensive Neighborhood Health Centers program; and Migrant Health programs. The rather depressing infant mortality statistics of the 1950s and early 1960s improved later in the decade. The rate dropped to 22.4 by 1967 from the 1966 rate of 23.7. In those two years, the infant mortality rate decreased twice as much as it had in the entire previous decade (Pratt, 1982).

Reductions in the infant mortality rate continued so that by 1970, the rate was 19.8 (Pratt, 1982). Optimism about progress, however, was tempered by the wide disparity between white and nonwhite rates. The white rate of 17.9 was nearly half the nonwhite rate of 31.8 (Pratt, 1982). A federal report was published, *Towards a Comprehensive Health Policy for the 1970's* (U.S. Department of Health Education and Welfare, 1971), noting that despite improvements in the overall health status of Americans, the United States ranked behind 12 other industrialized countries in infant mortality with a rate of 19.8. The report cited the causes of unnecessary infant deaths as inadequate geographic distribution of health services, unorganized systems of health care, insufficient availability of financing for prenatal care, and excessively high costs of medical care.

Developments in maternal and child health services during the 1970s were led by the proliferation of high-technology approaches to clinical care. The virtual technology explosion in maternal-fetal science made it possible to diagnose and treat conditions previously thought to be not amenable to clinical intervention. Sophisticated specialized services for mothers and infants at risk for complications were established, combining technology with highly trained health care providers. As a result, survival rates of premature infants improved substantially. However, the high operating cost of high-risk perinatal services made it fiscally imperative to limit their development to areas of high population density. As a result, many communities were left without access to services for their high-risk mothers and infants. Efforts were made to develop regionalization plans that delineated referral patterns for high-risk mothers and infants. With no federal coordination, the success of these efforts was spotty, and many states remain without a formalized regionalization plan to date (Table 20–2).

**TABLE 20–2  Infant Mortality Rates\* for Cities of 500,000+ Population, 1987**

| CITY | Total INFANT MORTALITY RATE | RANK | White INFANT MORTALITY RATE | RANK | Black INFANT MORTALITY RATE | RANK |
|------|------|------|------|------|------|------|
| Baltimore | 19.2 | 20 | 14.0 | 21 | 21.1 | 13 |
| Boston | 11.9 | 10 | 7.6 | 1 | 18.2 | 8 |
| Chicago | 16.6 | 17 | 10.9 | 17 | 22.9 | 17 |
| Cleveland | 15.5 | 15 | 10.5 | 15 | 20.0 | 9 |
| Columbus | 9.5 | 4 | 8.0 | 4 | 13.9 | 2 |
| Dallas | 10.3 | 6 | 7.9 | 2 | 15.7 | 4 |
| Detroit | 19.7 | 22 | 9.0 | 8 | 23.0 | 18 |
| Houston | 11.4 | 9 | 9.8 | 14 | 15.6 | 3 |
| Indianapolis | 13.3 | 14 | 9.6 | 12 | 23.7 | 20 |
| Jacksonville | 12.7 | 12 | 9.0 | 8 | 20.3 | 11 |
| Los Angeles | 10.5 | 8 | 8.5 | 5 | 21.1 | 13 |
| Memphis | 17.7 | 19 | 10.6 | 16 | 21.5 | 15 |
| Milwaukee | 12.2 | 11 | 7.9 | 2 | 17.9 | 7 |
| New Orleans | 15.8 | 16 | 12.8 | 20 | 17.4 | 6 |
| New York City | 12.7 | 12 | 11.3 | 19 | 16.2 | 5 |
| Philadelphia | 17.3 | 18 | 11.2 | 18 | 23.6 | 19 |
| Phoenix | 10.4 | 7 | 9.7 | 13 | 20.6 | 12 |
| San Antonio | 9.3 | 3 | 8.5 | 5 | 20.1 | 10 |
| San Diego | 9.6 | 5 | 9.4 | 11 | 13.5 | 1 |
| San Francisco | 7.7 | 1 | 8.7 | 7 | † | — |
| San Jose | 8.7 | 2 | 9.2 | 10 | † | — |
| Washington, D.C. | 19.3 | 21 | † | — | 22.8 | 16 |

Source: Adapted from National Center for Health Statistics (1990). Vital statistics of the United States, 1987. Volume II, Mortality, Part A. Washington, D.C.: Public Health Service.
 \* Rates are deaths per 1000 live births.
 † Fewer than 20 deaths.

## 1990 Health Goals for Mothers and Infants

At the beginning of the 1980s, the United States Surgeon General published health goals to be met by 1990 (U.S. Department of Health and Human Services, 1980). The following goals related to maternal and child health were established:

1. Infant health will improve, and by 1990, infant mortality will be reduced to fewer than nine infant deaths per 1000. No county and no racial or ethnic group of the population should have an infant mortality rate in excess of 12 (at present 10.1 overall and 17.9 for black infants) (Children's Defense Fund, 1989).

2. The neonatal death rate should be reduced to no more than 6.5 per 1000 live births (at present 6.5 overall) (Children's Defense Fund, 1989).

3. Low birth weight babies should constitute no more than 5 percent of all live births; no county and no racial or ethnic group of the population should have a rate of low birth weight infants that exceeds 9 percent of all live births (at present 6.9 percent overall and 12.7 percent for black infants) (Children's Defense Fund, 1989).

4. Virtually all women and infants should be served at levels appropriate to their need by a regionalized system of primary, secondary, and tertiary care for prenatal, maternal, and perinatal health services.

5. The proportion of women in any county or racial or ethnic group who obtain no prenatal care during the first trimester of pregnancy should not exceed 10 percent (at present about 10 percent for black women) (Children's Defense Fund, 1989).

6. Virtually all newborns should be provided with neonatal screening for metabolic disorders for which effective and efficient tests and treatments are available.

7. Virtually all parents of infants should be able to participate in primary health care that includes well child care; growth and development assessment; immunization; screening, diagnosis, and treatment for conditions requiring services; and appropriate counseling regarding nutrition, automobile safety, and prevention of other accidents such as poisoning.

8. At least 90 percent of all children should have completed their basic immunization series by age 2 for measles, mumps, rubella, polio, diphtheria, tetanus, and pertussis (approximately 85 percent in 1985) (Children's Defense Fund, 1989).

The 1990 health objectives, established in 1980, are appropriate markers against which progress in reducing infant mortality can be measured.

## Current Infant Mortality Trends

Until recently the United States had made remarkable progress in reducing infant mortality. Substantial progress was made in the 17-year period from 1968 to 1985, during which the infant mortality rate declined by approximately 50 percent, from 21.8 to 10.6. By 1980, the infant mortality rate had dropped to approximately 13 percent of its rate in the early 1990s (Brooks-Gunn, McCormick, & Heagerty, 1988).

However, after two decades of sustained progress (1960 to 1979), the infant mortality rate has come to a virtual standstill, and the curve of decline has actually flattened out (Fig. 20–1). The 1987 rate of 10.1 is down from the 1986 rate of 10.4 (National Center for Health Statistics, 1989b). For the first time in several years, this change is statistically significant (National Center for Health Statistics, 1989b). However, although it is encouraging that the direction of the curve is downward, it is doubtful that the 1990 goal of 9.0 will be reached (Hughes et al., 1989).

Racial disparities in progress continue to exist. In 1987, the black infant mortality rate of 17.9 was more than twice the rate for white infants (8.6) (National Center for Health Statistics, 1989b). This gap represents the widest black versus white gap since 1940, when infant mortality data were first collected by race. Not since the period preceding the establishment and expansion of the maternal and child health programs in the mid-1960s has there been such a sustained lack of progress in lowering the black infant mortality rate (Hughes et al, 1989). At the current rate of progress, it is unlikely that the 1990 goal of 12 black infant deaths per 1000 live births will be met before the year 1996 (Children's Defense Fund, 1989).

From 1986 to 1987, the overall neonatal mortality rate (infant deaths under 28 days) declined from 6.7 to 6.5 per 1000 live births, a statistically significant change.

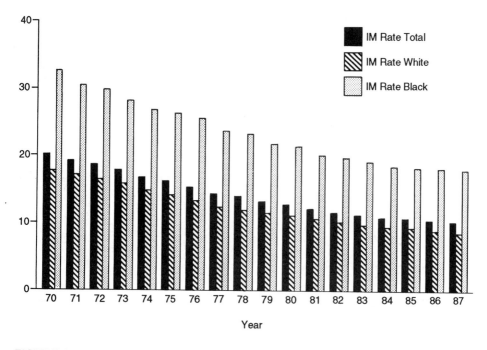

**FIGURE 20–1.** Infant mortality rate by race, 1970–1987

Source: Adapted from National Center for Health Statistics. (1990). Health, United States, 1989. Hyattsville, MD: Public Health Source.

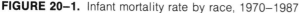

The white rate in 1987 was 5.5 compared with the black rate of 11.7. Neonatal mortality rates have declined since 1960 for both races, but the white rate has declined faster than the black rate: an average annual decrease of 4 percent compared with 3 percent for black infants (National Center for Health Statistics, 1989b).

The postneonatal rate (deaths of infants from 28 days to 1 year old) remained unchanged from 1986 to 1987, at 3.6 per 1000 live births. For white infants, the postneonatal death rate was 3.1, unchanged from 1986. For black infants, the rate was 6.1, down from the 1986 rate of 6.3 (National Center for Health Statistics, 1989b). This decrease, although not statistically significant, follows a period of increase between 1984 and 1985 (Hughes et al., 1989).

## Causes of Infant Mortality

Studies have delineated the specific causes of infant mortality by timing of infant death. The leading cause of postneonatal mortality is sudden infant death syndrome, followed by congenital anomalies, and then accidents and infectious diseases (National Center for Health Statistics, 1989b). The postneonatal mortality rate is higher among populations of low socioeconomic status, who are more likely to live with poor sanitation, inadequate and unsafe housing, and in households in which the mother has had little formal education (Miller, 1985; National Center for Health Statistics, 1989b).

The increase in postneonatal mortality that occurred in the mid-1980s may be explained by deaths of unhealthy infants who survived the first 27 days of life as a result of newly developed technology (Office of Technology Assessment, 1988). Another explanation is the increase in accidents, the third leading cause of death in this age group (National Center for Health Statistics, 1989b). Infectious disease also remains a major cause of postneonatal mortality. Immunization rates have dropped during the 1980s, making the Surgeon General's goal of a 90 percent immunization rate for 2 year olds virtually unattainable (Children's Defense Fund, 1989).

Neonatal deaths are closely linked to prenatal and intrapartum conditions, including congenital anomalies and disorders relating to a short gestation and low birth weight (infants born weighing under 2500 g or 5 pounds, 8 ounces).

## Low Birth Weight

Low birth weight (under 2500 g) results from preterm birth (fewer than 37 completed weeks of gestation) or from intrauterine growth retardation (Pritchard & MacDonald, 1980). Infants born at low birth weights are 40 times more likely to die within the first month of life than their normal weight counterparts, with the incidence rising to 200-fold for infants in the very low birth weight category (under 1500 g) (McCormick, 1985). Low birth weight survivors are at greater risk of developing long-term disabilities such as cerebral palsy, mental retardation, neurodevelopmental delays, and hearing and vision disabilities (Hack & Fanaroff, 1989; McCormick, 1985). They are also at risk for exposure to altered family functioning ranging from physical abuse to extreme overprotectiveness (Escalona, 1982).

During the 1980s the percentage of infants born at low birth weights remained essentially unchanged. In 1987, the rate was 6.9 percent, the same as in 1979 (National Center for Health Statistics, 1989a). Racial disparity exists here as well. The proportion of white infants born at low birth weights was 5.7 percent, an increase over the 1986 rate of 5.6. For black infants, the proportion changed from 12.5 percent in 1986 to 12.7 percent in 1987, a change that is not statistically significant (National Center for Health Statistics, 1989a). Infants born to teenage mothers (31.8 per 1000, a 4 percent increase over 1986) and to mothers in their forties are at greatly elevated risk of low birth weight, with proportions ranging from 7.9 to 13.7 percent (National Center for Health Statistics, 1989a). At the current rate of progress, the 1990 goal of reducing the proportion of low birth weight infants to 5 percent will not be met until 2031. The goal for black infants of 9 percent will not be met until the year 2055 (Children's Defense Fund, 1989).

The risk of delivering a low birth weight infant increases for women living in poverty with associated characteristics, such as single marital status; fewer than 12 years of completed education; unemployment; and inadequate access to health care (Binsacca et al., 1987; Institute of Medicine, 1985). Medical conditions associated with low birth weight include abnormalities of the reproductive tract, low hematocrit levels (under 34 ml/dl), and medical complications of pregnancy (Lieberman, Ryan, Monson, & Schoenbaum, 1987).

Lifestyle practices suspected of increasing the incidence of low birth weight include cigarette smoking, exposure to stressful conditions, inadequate sleep and rest, and drug and alcohol abuse (Meis, Ernest, & Moore, 1987). Cocaine and crack, in particular, are increasingly associated with low birth weight infants because of the related obstetric complications, unhealthy lifestyle practices, and sociodemographic characteristics connected with their use. Recognition of the effects of cocaine use on infant health has just begun and is now an area of intense investigation.

## Prenatal Care

The factor most closely associated with low birth weight is inadequate prenatal care. Prenatal care appropriate to a woman's level of risk that begins in the first trimester of pregnancy and continues regularly throughout pregnancy is associated with improved pregnancy outcomes, especially for women at increased medical or social risk or both (Institute of Medicine, 1988; Moore et al., 1986). In 1987, 76 percent of all women initiated prenatal care in the critical first trimester of pregnancy, a rate that has remained essentially unchanged since 1979. This period of stagnation for prenatal care follows a decade of sustained progress during which the proportion increased from 68 to 75 percent (National Center for Health Statistics, 1989a). Racial disparity in the timing of prenatal care increased in 1987, with 79 percent of white women and only 61 percent of black women initiating care in the first trimester. The situation among black women has actually deteriorated, with a slight decline in the proportion of black women receiving first trimester care from 62 percent in 1986 to 61 percent in 1987. Moreover, the percentage of women receiving late (initiated in the third trimester of pregnancy) or no prenatal care increased in most age groups by 2 to 5 percent (National Center for Health Statistics, 1989a). At the current rate of progress, the 1990 prenatal care goal of 90 percent enrollment in the first trimester will not be met until the year 2094, and for black women not until the year 2153 (Hughes et al., 1989).

Women at greatest risk for receiving inadequate prenatal care include those who are ethnic minorities, teens, single, multiparous, living in poverty, living in inner city or isolated rural communities, and without a high school education (Institute of Medicine, 1988). Not surprisingly, recognized barriers to prenatal care include financial inaccessibility, inadequate health system capacity, nonsupportive practices and environments, and attitudinal and knowledge deficits regarding the importance of prenatal care (American Nurses' Association, 1987; Institute of Medicine, 1988; U.S. General Accounting Office, 1987).

Despite the well-documented benefits of prenatal care, for many women access to it remains difficult, if not impossible. The marked slowdown in progress toward reducing infant mortality has been attributed to the declining use of prenatal care by populations at risk and the resulting consequences.

## Slowdown in Progress Toward Reducing Infant Mortality

The decline in progress during the 1980s is a subject of great concern to many. Why the deterioration? As is usual in complex social issues, a number of contributing factors have been identified, including birth weight distribution, lifestyle practices, and economic factors.

Changes in birth weight distribution play a significant role in the slowdown in progress (Office of Technology Assessment, 1988). Infant mortality reductions in early years were attributable, in large part, to declines in postneonatal deaths, which early in this century accounted for 60 percent of all infant deaths. These reductions in early loss of life were attributable to declines in infectious diseases, improved sanitation, and improved nutrition. However, comparable decreases in neonatal mortality have not been forthcoming, and by midcentury the ratio shifted so that approximately 60 percent of all infant deaths occurred in the neonatal period (Brooks-Gunn et al., 1988).

Although mortality rates for infants in the lowest birth weight categories have improved, the birth weight distribution has actually deteriorated. Between 1977 and 1984, the percentage of infants born at normal birth weights (greater than 2500 g) increased slightly, but the distribution of low birth weight infants shifted toward the lowest birth weight category (under 1000 g) (Office of Technology Assessment, 1988). The progress that has been made in birth weight–specific mortality has been attributed to recent advances in technology and clinical care for very low birth weight infants, and the possibility that this care is postponing the death of some infants who earlier would have appeared in the vital statistics as spontaneous abortions has been proposed (National Center for Health Statistics, 1989b). The ability of technology to save infants born at ever-decreasing birth weights is questionable. It has even been suggested that the maximal benefit derived from advances in neonatal care has been reached, and future gains in infant mortality resulting from technology will be limited (Office of Technology Assessment, 1988).

Another possible factor in the slowdown of progress is the changing demographics of pregnancy, with shifts toward either end of the age spectrum. Infant mortality is highest among women in their teen and later reproductive years, who represent an increasing proportion of births (National Center for Health Statistics, 1989b). Also, unhealthy lifestyle practices, including the use of alcohol, tobacco, and recently, the skyrocketing use of illegal drugs by pregnant women, play a significant role in the deterioration of the health status of women and infants. Drug abuse, particularly cocaine, has been associated with recent increases in infant deaths. The overwhelming proportion of crack cocaine abuse among pregnant women has become problematic. Preliminary, unpublished data indicate that in some centers, close to one third of women screen positively for cocaine use within 24 hours of giving birth. In many cities, cocaine use is seriously threatening the health of infants. In the first 6 months of 1989, the District of Columbia's infant mortality rate increased by nearly 50 percent to 32.3 from a 1988 rate of 23.2. The major reason cited for the increase is the epidemic use of crack cocaine and the concomitant breakdown of the family structure (Abramowitz, 1989).

Economic factors have been cited as influencing progress in infant mortality. Reductions in funding of several federal programs for women and children occurred in the early 1980s. Miller (1985) suggests that these reductions in funding have weakened national policies for the care and protection of pregnant women and children, leaving many without access to the care they need. Furthermore, it has been suggested that the system of health care for mothers and children is incapable of meeting the increasing and ever-changing needs of the populations it serves (National Commission to Prevent Infant Mortality, 1988).

Another possible explanation is the erosion of the employer-paid health insurance system. Between 1980 and 1986, the number of medium-sized and large firms providing family health coverage dropped by 33 percent (Alan Guttmacher Institute, 1987). As a result, many women of childbearing age and their children have been left without health insurance. In 1985, 17 percent of women of childbearing age had no health insurance, and another 8 percent had private insurance but no maternity benefits. During that same period, approximately 20 percent of children under age 18 had no health insurance (Torres & Kenney, 1989).

Another economic variable contributing to the deterioration of maternal and child health is the growth of poverty among children. Children living in poverty have a greater risk of exposure to harmful environmental conditions and inadequate access to health care. The percentage of children living in poverty increased from 16 percent in 1979 to 20.0 percent in 1987 (Children's Defense Fund, 1989). Among infants and toddlers, the proportion is 25 percent. One and a half million more children live in poverty today than in 1980 (Children's Defense Fund, 1989). Among children in families headed by young women, one in three is poor, and among black children, nearly one-half live in poverty. The income levels for many of the families of these children fall far below the federal poverty line. In 1987, almost half lived in households with incomes below half the federal poverty line ($4528 for a family of three in 1987 dollars) (Children's Defense Fund, 1989).

The combination of these simultaneously occurring economic variables has created a situation in which many mothers and infants are denied financial access to needed health services. Consequently, the nation is faced with paying the high economic and human costs of infant mortality.

## Consequences of Infant Mortality

The consequences of infant morbidity and mortality are numerous. The human tragedy associated with poor pregnancy outcome and infant death can be emotionally debilitating to a family and can lead to maladaptive behaviors among its members. The economic consequences can be staggering as well.

The annual bill for neonatal intensive care (the most expensive form of care in the health care system) exceeds 2.5 billion dollars (Office of Technology Assessment, 1988). The inpatient costs for initial hospitalization of a low birth weight infant may range from $14,000 to $30,000 (Office of Technology Assessment, 1988). The lifetime cost to care for a child born at a low birth weight can reach $400,000 (Office of

Technology Assessment, 1988). Those high costs stand in contrast to the low cost of prenatal care, which is about $600.00 (Institute of Medicine, 1988). It has been estimated that for every $1.00 invested in prenatal care, $3.30 can be saved in neonatal care costs (Institute of Medicine, 1985).

Much of this steep neonatal bill is generated by the uninsured population. Maternity care and newborn care account for the largest single source of uncompensated care, approximately 27 percent of the 7.4 billion dollars in unpaid hospital bills in 1985 (Alan Guttmacher Institute, 1987). Of this total, 1.1 billion dollars were covered by state and local tax appropriations, 1.7 billion dollars were allocated by hospital budgets for charity care, and 4.6 billion dollars represented uncollectible bills (Alan Guttmacher Institute, 1987). Consequently, low birth weight infants contribute to the ever-increasing rise in insurance premiums and tax bills paid by corporations, small businesses, and private citizens.

## Strategies to Reduce Infant Mortality

The disturbing trends in infant mortality and the unmet potential of reducing preventable infant deaths present important challenges to public policy makers and health care providers. Recognizing this challenge, Congress established the National Commission to Prevent Infant Mortality in 1987. The bipartisan Commission, composed of 16 members representing both houses of Congress, state government, and health care providers, was led by its Chairman, Governor Lawton Chiles (Democrat from Florida). The Commission's charge was to develop a national plan to reduce infant mortality. At the completion of its first year, a report was issued defining the issue and outlining recommendations to reduce infant mortality (National Commission to Prevent Infant Mortality, 1988). Recommendations were generated by many sources. A historical analysis of federal initiatives revealed that, over time, three major strategies were effective: increasing access to prenatal care; providing comprehensive health and social services to mothers and infants in appropriate facilities; and coordinating care at the federal level to reduce duplication and eliminate gaps. Strategies were also derived from public hearings and surveys of providers and administrators of maternal and child health services.

The plan outlined by the Commission recommends two broad-based initiatives: providing universal access to health care for every mother and infant, and reordering national priorities so that the health and well-being of the nation's mothers and infants receive high level attention.

### Universal Access to Care

The Commission declared that "every mother and every baby must be able to get the health care they need (National Commission to Prevent Infant Mortality, 1988, p. 14). Furthermore, no financial, geographic, or administrative barriers to care should exist. Health care should be initiated early, be of high quality, and be readily accessible and appropriate to the health risks presented. The action plan for providing universal access includes the following strategies.

*Financing Care*

1. The Medicaid program should be expanded to cover all pregnant women and infants who have family incomes at or below 200 percent of the federal poverty level. Recent federally mandated expansions of Medicaid eligibility allow for pregnant women and infants with increases up to 133 percent of the federal poverty level to be covered (effective April 1, 1990). Further expansion is still needed to cover many low-income, uninsured families.

2. Assets tests for pregnant women applying for Medicaid should be eliminated. In many states, a family's possessions (including the family car and house) are considered when determining eligibility for Medicaid. This procedure is cumbersome and excludes many needy families.

3. Eligibility for Medicaid for pregnant women and infants should be continuous throughout the infant's first year of life.

4. The private sector should make available prenatal and pediatric health care. All employment-based health insurance should include maternity and well-baby care coverage for employees, their spouses, and their dependents.

5. Self-employed and unincorporated businesses should be allowed to deduct the full cost of health insurance as a business expense.

6. To increase the availability and affordability of private group health insurance for small employers, insurance pooling mechanisms should be established.

*Access to Care.* Limited financial resources on the part of the public are not the only barriers to care. There is also a formidable array of obstacles within the system that make it difficult, if not impossible, to obtain needed health care. Not the least among these is the fact that the United States lacks a national health policy. "The Commission maintains that no pregnant woman or infant should go without preventive health care because the system currently prevents them from doing so. Maternity and early infant care are too important to allow anyone to fall through the cracks" (National Commission to Prevent Infant Mortality, 1988, p. 19). The plan of action outlined to address nonfinancial barriers to care includes the following:

1. Women must be made aware of the full array of available services as soon as they become pregnant. It would be best if pregnant women and infants could secure all necessary services at one location. At a minimum, there must be coordination of programs including Medicaid; Title V Maternal and Child Health Programs; the Special Supplemental Food Program for Women, Infants, and Children; Community and Migrant Health Centers; social and welfare services; and family planning services. In a recent study, the major reason given by women for not initiating prenatal care was lack of knowledge about its importance in improving pregnancy outcomes (U.S. General Accounting Office, 1987). Health care providers and public health officials have been creative over the recent past in designing outreach programs to educate women about the importance of prenatal care and assisting them in obtaining it (Institute of Medicine, 1988). Unfortunately, to date, few data exist about the effectiveness of these programs. However, as was demonstrated in the early part of this century, community outreach may hold promise for reducing infant mortality in the future.

2. Congress should require that all Medicaid-eligible infants be automatically enrolled at birth in the Medicaid Early and Periodic Screening, Diagnosis, and Treatment program. Currently, fewer than half of all eligible children receive any of these services. States should also be required to offer follow-up services for any problems identified in screenings.

3. The Medicaid application forms must be simplified, and states should adopt a streamlined eligibility process, such as "presumptive eligibility," under which all pregnant women applying for Medicaid would be immediately eligible for services for up to 45 days or until the formal application is denied or accepted.

4. The number of providers willing to serve high-risk pregnant women and infants must be increased and the malpractice crisis addressed.

5. In order to encourage more maternity and pediatric providers to participate in the Medicaid program, states should examine ways to adjust their Medicaid reimbursement rates and simplify the administrative requirements. The combination of low reimbursement rates and administrative difficulties turns many providers away from accepting Medicaid patients. As a result, many pregnant women and children have difficulty finding health care practitioners to provide needed care.

6. A home visitors program for pregnant women and new mothers, particularly those in high-risk populations, should be established. Several home visiting programs employing nurses and trained lay visitors have been evaluated. Olds and coworkers (1986) found positive outcomes in a system of prenatal and postnatal home visits by nurses. Similarly, in a study of hospital-based transitional follow-up care for very low birth weight infants, Brooten and colleagues (1986) achieved positive outcomes and cost savings through early discharge and nurse specialist follow-up.

## Reordering National Priorities

The Commission stated that "this nation must make the health and well-being of mothers and babies a top priority" (National Commission to Prevent Infant Mortality, 1988, p. 22). Before our nation can devote the resources needed to succeed in the fight against infant mortality, we must first make the public aware of the extent—and the seriousness—of the problem. Unfortunately, the existing federal structure does not provide sufficient exposure for maternal and child health issues. It fails to provide the kind of unified leadership supplied by the Children's Bureau prior to its dissolution in 1969. The Commission suggests that a single entity, such as a permanent council on children's health and well-being, be reinstated to serve as a national focal point for developing and executing a public awareness campaign on infant mortality. The Commission recommends that the council:

1. Develop and distribute to every pregnant woman a maternal child health handbook to encourage early prenatal care and serve as an infant's health record.

2. Design and implement a national awareness campaign to promote maternal and child health using an expert panel representing the media, marketing and advertising, health care, and the private sector.

3. Encourage coordination of the many federal agencies having jurisdiction over maternal and child health programs.

4. Serve as a liaison between public and private sector initiatives and collaborative efforts for mothers and children.

## Goals for Future Progress in Reducing Infant Mortality

Goals for reducing infant mortality by the year 2000 have been proposed by the Department of Health and Human Services. In order to make the needed improvements in maternal and infant health proposed by the Department of Health and Human Services, a concerted effort must be launched. Such an effort requires full participation by all: providers, payers, policy makers, business leaders, and consumers. From a public policy perspective, the political landscape for pushing maternal and child health issues has not yet been sufficiently developed to make a big difference. Raising these issues to the top of political agendas is needed to make further progress. In addition, each and every citizen must consider the issues of healthy children and what can be done to make a difference. The strategies recommended by the National Commission to Prevent Infant Mortality can serve as a national blueprint for action.

Nurses, as individuals, and groups can be influential in planning and implementing the necessary changes in the health care system so that improvements in maternal and child health are achievable. Through the effective use of nursing's innate power, progress in reducing unnecessary infant deaths can be realized. To succeed, individual nurses and nursing groups should use:

- The power of the pen—write what you see and know. Communicate with those in policy-making positions.
- The power of the spoken word—get out and communicate with lay and consumer groups.
- The power of your education—you are an authority figure in places where you least expect it. Take advantage of your knowledge and expertise.
- The power of your vote—make an issue of infant mortality in local, state, and federal elections.
- The power of collaboration—forge alliances and networks and foster therapeutic environments where needed.
- The power of believing in your convictions—act on your beliefs that children deserve the best chance in life we have to give them.

REFERENCES

Abramowitz, M. (1989, September 30). Infant mortality soars here. *The Washington Post*, 1, A13.
Alan Guttmacher Institute (1987). *The financing of maternity care in the United States.* New York: Alan Guttmacher Institute.

American Nurses' Association (1987). *Access to prenatal care: Key to preventing low birthweight.* Kansas City, MO: American Nurses' Association.

Arnold, L. (1989). *A vision for America's future.* Washington, DC: Children's Defense Fund.

Arnold, L., Brecht, M., Hockett, A., Amspacher, K., & Grad, R. (1989). Infant mortality: Lessons from the past. *American Journal of Maternal Child Nursing, 14*(2), 75–82.

Binsacca, D., Ellis, J., Martin, D., & Petitti, D. (1987). Factors associated with low birthweight in an inner city population. The role of financial problems. *American Journal of Public Health, 68,* 645.

Brooten, D., Kumar, S., Brown, L., Butts, P., Finkler, S., Bakewell-Sachs, S., Gibbons, A., & Delivoria-Papadopoulos, M. (1986). A randomized clinical trial of early hospital discharge and home follow-up of very-low-birth-weight infants. *New England Journal of Medicine, 315,* 934–939.

Brooks-Gunn, J., McCormick, M., & Heagerty, M. (1988). Preventing infant mortality and morbidity: Developmental perspectives. *American Journal of Orthopsychiatry, 58*(2), 288–296.

Escalona, S. (1982). Babies at double hazard: Early development of infants at biologic and social risk. *Pediatrics, 70*(5), 670–676.

Hack, M., & Fanaroff, A. (1989). Outcomes of extremely low birthweight infants between 1982 and 1988. *New England Journal of Medicine, 321*(24), 1642–1647.

Hughes, D., Johnson, K., Rosenbaum, S., & Liu, J. (1989). *The health of America's children: Maternal and child health data book.* Washington, DC: Children's Defense Fund.

Institute of Medicine (1985). *Preventing low birthweight.* Washington, DC: National Academy Press.

Institute of Medicine (1988). *Prenatal care: Reaching mothers, reaching infants.* Washington, DC: National Academy Press.

Lieberman, E., Ryan, K., Monson, R., & Schoenbaum, S. (1987). Risk factors accounting for racial differences in the rate of premature birth. *New England Journal of Medicine, 317*(12), 743–748.

McCormick, M. (1985). The contribution of low birthweight to infant mortality and childhood morbidity. *New England Journal of Medicine, 312*(2), 82–90.

Meis, P., Ernest, J., & Moore, M. (1987). Causes of low birthweight births in public and private patients. *Obstetrics and Gynecology, 156,* 1165–1168.

Miller, C. (1985). Infant mortality in the U.S. *Scientific American, 253*(1), 31–38.

Moore, T., Origel, W., Key, T., & Resnik, R. (1986). The perinatal and economic impact of prenatal care in a low socioeconomic population. *American Journal of Obstetrics and Gynecology, 145,* 797–801.

National Center for Health Statistics (1989a). Advance report of final natality statistics, 1987. *Monthly Vital Statistics Report, 38*(3), 6–12.

National Center for Health Statistics (1989b). Advance report of final mortality statistics, 1987. *Monthly Vital Statistics Report, 38*(5), 8–9.

National Center for Health Statistics (1990). Health, United States, 1989.

National Commission to Prevent Infant Mortality (1988). *Death before life: The tragedy of infant mortality.* Washington, DC: National Commission to Prevent Infant Mortality.

Office of Technology Assessment (1988). *Healthy children: Investing in the future* (Report No. OTA-H-345). Washington, DC: U.S. Government Printing Office.

Olds, D., Henderson, D., Tatelbaum, R., & Chamberlin, R. (1986). Improving the delivery of prenatal care and outcomes of pregnancy: A randomized trial of nurse home visitation. *Pediatrics, 77,* 16–28.

Pratt, M. (1982). The demography of maternal and child health. In H. Wallace, E. Gold, &

A. Oglesby (Eds.), *Maternal and child health practices: Problems, resources, and methods of delivery.* New York: John Wiley.

Pritchard, J., & MacDonald, P. (1980). *Williams Obstetrics.* New York: Appleton-Century-Crofts.

Starfield, B. (1985). Giant steps and baby steps: Toward child health. *American Journal of Public Health, 12,* 497–501.

Torres, A., & Kenney, A. (1989). Expanding Medicaid coverage for pregnant women: Estimates of the impact and cost. *Family Planning Perspectives, 21*(1), 19–24.

UNICEF (1988). *The state of the world's children.* Oxford, England. Oxford University Press.

U.S. Department of Health and Human Services (1980). *Healthy people: The Surgeon General's report on health promotion and disease prevention.* Washington, DC: U.S. Government Printing Office.

U.S. Department of Health, Education, and Welfare (1971). *Towards a comprehensive health policy for the 1970's.* Washington, DC: U.S. Government Printing Office.

U.S. General Accounting Office (1987). *Medicaid recipients and uninsured women obtain insufficient care* (Report No. HRD-87137). Washington, DC: U.S. Government Printing Office.

## Chapter 21

# Low Birth Weight: Practice and Policy Issues

DOROTHY BROOTEN
HELEN KNAPP

Infant mortality is an indicator of the overall health status of nations. It is closely linked to poverty and related social factors, including funding for family planning, abortion; social support for pregnant women, new mothers, and infants; and access to health care. Unfortunately, the United States currently ranks 20th in infant mortality among industrialized countries (UNICEF, 1988). The nation's high infant mortality rate is due largely to its high low birth weight (LBW) rate, a factor staggering in its economic and human costs. Lowering the LBW rate and ultimately the nation's infant mortality rate will require substantial efforts in preventing LBW as well as further gains in the care of LBW infants whose preterm births cannot be avoided. This chapter will review the magnitude of the problem, a synthesis of what is known about prevention of LBW, issues on the care and cost of LBW infants, alternatives to high cost neonatal intensive care, and barriers to implementation of these alternatives.

## Magnitude of the Problem

Currently over 270,000 LBW infants (less than 2500 g) are born annually in the United States, with 48,000 of them born at very low birth weights (less than 1500 g) (National Center for Health Statistics, 1990). Low birth weight results from infants being born prematurely (less than 37 weeks' gestation) or from infants experiencing intrauterine growth retardation, or both. Low birth weight is a major determinant of infant mortality, with the risk of mortality increasing with decreasing birth weight. Low birth weight infant survivors have a greater incidence of handicaps, poorer general health in the first year of life, and projected lower lifestream earnings over a lifetime, and the financial and human costs of their care are staggering.

The contribution of LBW to infant mortality in the United States is relatively greater now than it was in the past. Early in this century, two thirds of infant deaths occurred in the postneonatal period (between 28 days and 12 months of age) (Institute of Medicine, 1985). Most were normal weight infants (greater than 2500 g) at birth who died of infections, diarrhea, or respiratory illness due to environmental factors. Over the first half of the century, infant mortality rates declined by half from 100 to 50 deaths per 1000 live births, with most of the decrease occurring among postneonatal deaths. Observers attributed this largely to reductions in infectious diseases and improved nutrition (Institute of Medicine, 1985). Despite these changes, which can also affect birth weight, there appeared to be relatively little change in the distribution of birth weights of infants (Institute of Medicine, 1985; National Center for Health Statistics, 1980).

By 1950, two thirds of all infant deaths were occurring in the neonatal period (first 28 days of life) largely because of prematurity (less than 37 weeks' gestation) (Shapiro, Schlesinger, & Nesbitt, 1968). Since the mid-1960s, the nation's infant mortality rate declined rapidly, with only a modest decline in the proportion of LBW infants born. In the 15 years from 1970 to 1985, for example, the infant mortality rate decreased by 50 percent and the LBW rate decreased by 15 percent (Centers for Disease Control, 1988). However, from 1980 to 1986, the LBW rate remained the same (6.8 percent) (Centers for Disease Control, 1988; Hughes et al., 1989), and most recent statistics indicate that it is increasing (National Center for Health Statistics, 1989a). As a proportion of all births, very LBW births have increased steadily since 1979 (Hughes et al., 1989). Thus, most of the progress in reducing infant mortality over the 16-year period (1970 to 1986) resulted not from a reduction in LBW but from improved survival of LBW infants, a situation attributed to technologic improvements in perinatal and neonatal care (Hughes et al., 1989).

Although overall infant mortality has improved somewhat since 1960, differences in mortality rates among subgroups in the population remain. Black infants, for example, are twice as likely to be born LBW and very LBW as white infants. They are also twice as likely to die as white newborns in the neonatal period, and the disparity between the death rates of the two groups is increasing (National Center for Health Statistics, 1989). The incidence of LBW is also greater among poor, less educated, and unmarried women (Binsacca et al., 1987; Institute of Medicine, 1985; Kleinman & Kessel, 1987; Wise et al., 1988).

While it increases infant mortality, LBW is also associated with increased, often devastating and costly morbidity. Low birth weight infants are twice as likely to suffer one or more handicaps such as mental retardation, deafness, blindness, physical limitations, learning disabilities, delayed speech, autism, cerebral palsy, epilepsy, or chronic lung problems (Brecht, 1989; Institute of Medicine, 1985; McCormick, 1989). Low birth weight infants remain three times as likely as those of normal weight to have adverse neurologic sequelae (McCormick et al., 1981). The risk increases with decreasing birth weight, with 8 to 19 percent of very LBW infants severely affected (McCormick, 1985; Papile et al., 1983). Compared with normal weight infants, those with LBW are twice as likely to have a serious anomaly, and those with very LBW are three times as likely to have such an anomaly (Christianson et al., 1981; McCormick, 1985).

The cost of providing care to LBW infants is among the most expensive of any patient group, with mean hospital charges for some groups of very LBW infants exceeding $160,000 (Walker, Feldman, Vohr, & Oh, 1984). Initial hospitalization of LBW infants is lengthy, especially that of the very LBW infant group, for whom lengths of stay may average between 47 and 70 days or more (Office of Technology Assessment, 1987; Walker et al., 1984). The lengthy hospitalization and complex care needed for these infants often result in iatrogenic problems for the infants and increased stress on families.

Following hospital discharge, the general health of LBW infants is also poorer than that of infants with birth weights greater than 2500 g. In the postneonatal period, LBW infants are five times and very LBW infants 20 times more likely than normal weight infants to die in the first year of life (McCormick, 1985). Reports indicate that between 25 to 50 percent of very LBW infants are rehospitalized within the first year of life, compared with a 19 percent rate for LBW infants and an 8.4 percent rate for infants weighing 2500 g or more (McCormick et al., 1980; Mutch et al., 1986; Termini et al., 1990). Additionally, LBW infants' mean length of stay during rehospitalization exceeds that of normal weight infants (McCormick et al., 1980). The average number of physician visits in the first year of life is also higher, with 14 to 16 visits for very LBW infants compared with 10 for normal weight infants. Low birth weight infants account for 20 percent of all postneonatal deaths (McCormick, 1985).

In summary, although the infant mortality rate in the United States has declined over the past two decades, the rate of LBW infants has declined far less. The LBW rate then stabilized, and currently it is increasing. The very LBW rate as a proportion of all births has been rising since 1979. The nation's decline in infant mortality over two decades is largely the result of increased survival of LBW infants in costly, specialized care units. Technology, however, is now reaching the limit of its ability to save smaller and more premature infants. Current statistics suggest that further substantial reductions in infant mortality, especially in neonatal mortality, will require prevention of the birth of LBW infants.

## Prevention

A belief that prevention of any substantial number of LBW infants is possible in the United States requires accepting three basic assumptions. First it assumes that the cause of LBW is known. Second, it assumes that an investment of resources will be made to ameliorate the cause. Third, it assumes that solutions will be accepted and acted upon by all or most pregnant women. The inability over many decades to substantially reduce the LBW rate, particularly the very LBW rate, highlights the fallacy of assuming that prevention of LBW can or will occur easily or readily in the United States.

### Causes of Low Birth Weight

As noted by the Institute of Medicine (1985), despite important new research findings and improvements in the science of obstetrics, understanding of the basic causes of preterm labor and intrauterine growth retardation is limited. However, a variety of factors and conditions have been associated with preterm onset of labor, including abruptio placentae, amnionitis, congenital malformation, placenta previa, pre-eclampsia, premature rupture of membranes, multiple pregnancy, and urinary tract infections. In many cases of premature birth, no association with pathologic factors can be identified (Institute of Medicine, 1985). Some research indicates that idiopathic premature labor resulting in a premature infant is significantly greater in private, more affluent populations (Meis, Ernest, & Moore, 1987). Intrauterine growth retardation is associated with conditions that interfere with placental circulation (e.g., separation and infarctions); development or growth of the fetus (e.g., maternal chronic hypertension or renal disease); or the general health and nutrition of the pregnant woman (e.g., cardiac or pulmonary disease, smoking, substance abuse) (Institute of Medicine, 1985). For many growth-retarded infants, no relevant pathogenic factors can be identified. Additionally, prematurity and intrauterine growth retardation occur together in 30 percent of LBW infants, in some instances due to factors mentioned previously and in some instances without a demonstrable association with a suspected pathogenic factor (Institute of Medicine, 1985).

In the absence of adequate knowledge regarding etiology, a large body of information has developed about individual risk factors associated with LBW. These factors include demographic risk, medical risks predating the pregnancy or with the current pregnancy, behavioral and environmental risks, and health care risks (Table 21–1). Inadequate prenatal care is a major factor associated with LBW. Several points are clear in examining risk factors and the scales that were subsequently developed to identify women at high risk for LBW infants. First, the risk factors are widely distributed in the population. Second, the predictive ability of the risk scales developed subsequently is somewhat limited. Although the scales are helpful in distinguishing between high- and low-risk women, the significant incidence of LBW delivery in low-risk women and groups suggests further work is needed to improve the predictive capabilities of these instruments and assessment systems. Third, when risk factors are identified through screening, most are amenable to interventions (Institute of Medicine, 1985). However, identification of risk factors and interventions to reduce these risks are dependent on early (first trimester) and regular (9 or more visits for 36 weeks' gestation) prenatal care (Kessner et al., 1973).

It has been estimated that nationally, LBW deliveries could be reduced by 15 percent among whites and 12 percent among blacks if all women began prenatal care in the first trimester and if they continued to receive care throughout pregnancy (Institute of Medicine, 1985). Additionally, women who receive adequate prenatal care and still deliver LBW infants have infants who have significantly better perinatal survival and less respiratory distress and intraventricular hemorrhage (Leveno, Cunningham, Roarke, Nelson, & Williams, 1985). Approximately 30 percent of pregnant women in the United States receive insufficient or no prenatal care for a variety of reasons (Gold, Kenney, & Singh, 1987).

## Insufficient Prenatal Care

Factors associated with insufficient prenatal care include demographic, structural, cultural, and personal factors. Demographic risk factors include ethnicity,

**TABLE 21–1  Principal Risk Factors for Low Birth Weight**

I. Demographic Risks
  Age (less than 17; over 34)
  Race (black)
  Low socioeconomic status
  Unmarried
  Low level of education

II. Medical Risks Predating Pregnancy
  Parity (0 or more than 4)
  Low weight for height
  Genitourinary anomalies/surgery
  Selected diseases such as diabetes,
    chronic hypertension
  Nonimmune status for selected infections
    such as rubella
  Poor obstetric history, including previous
    low birth weight infant, multiple
    spontaneous abortions
  Maternal genetic factors, such as low
    maternal weight at own birth

III. Medical Risks in Current Pregnancy
  Multiple pregnancy
  Poor weight gain
  Short interpregnancy interval
  Hypotension
  Hypertension/pre-eclampsia/toxemia
  Selected infections such as
    symptomatic bacteriuria, rubella, and
    cytomegalovirus
  First or second trimester bleeding
  Placental problems such as placenta
    previa, abruptio placentae

  Hyperemesis
  Oligohydramnios/polyhydramnios
  Anemia/abnormal hemoglobin
  Isoimmunization
  Fetal anomalies
  Incompetent cervix
  Spontaneous premature rupture of
    membranes

IV. Behavioral and Environmental Risks
  Smoking
  Poor nutritional status
  Alcohol and other substance abuse
  Diethylstilbestrol exposure and other
    toxic exposures, including
    occupational hazards
  High altitude

V. Health Care Risks
  Absent or inadequate prenatal care
  Iatrogenic prematurity

VI. Evolving Concepts of Risk
  Stress, physical and psychosocial
  Uterine irritability
  Events triggering uterine contractions
  Cervical changes detected before onset
    of labor
  Selected infections such as *Mycoplasma*
    and *Chlamydia trachomatis*
  Inadequate plasma volume expansion
  Progesterone deficiency

Source: Institute of Medicine (1985), *Preventing Low Birthweight.* Washington, D.C., National Academy Press, p. 51.

age, education, parity, marital status, income, and geographic location. Nonwhites (blacks, Hispanics, Native Americans) are less likely to receive care early or to receive sufficient care compared with whites. Black women, for example, are twice as likely to receive late or no care as compared with white women (10.1 percent versus 4.7 percent) (Institute of Medicine, 1988). Pregnant women under 15 are at high risk of obtaining late or no prenatal care, as are women over age 40 (Institute of Medicine, 1988). Women with less than a high school education and women with two or more children tend to receive late or no care. Unmarried women are more than three times as likely as married women to obtain late or no prenatal care (13 percent versus 3.4 percent) (Hughes, Johnson, Rosenbaum, Simons, & Butter, 1988). Women with incomes below the federal poverty level consistently show lower rates of early care and higher rates of late or no care than women with higher incomes. Women receiving insufficient prenatal care are concentrated most often in inner cities and isolated rural areas (Singh, Torres, & Forret, 1985).

Over the past decades, a number of structural barriers to care have been identified, including financial barriers, inadequate capacity of prenatal care systems, and problems in the organization, practices, and atmosphere of prenatal services. Financial barriers have been cited as the major problem in most studies. An estimated 26 percent of women of reproductive age have no insurance to cover maternity care (Alan Guttmacher Institute, 1987). Thirty-five percent of poor women are completely uninsured (Alan Guttmacher Institute, 1987). Although the Medicaid program has been important in increasing access to prenatal care, the enrollment process may be lengthy, clinics are overburdened and unable to schedule appointments promptly, and reimbursement rates to physicians are low and some physicians will not provide care to women on Medicaid. These factors, combined with the decrease in obstetricians and reduced obstetric practices owing to growing concerns about malpractice, add to the inadequacy of prenatal care systems to provide care for pregnant women, especially low-income women (Institute of Medicine, 1985). Other classic barriers to prenatal care include service hours that do not accommodate schedules of women who work or go to school, long waits, transportation and child care problems, and communication problems between providers and clients (Institute of Medicine, 1985).

The use of prenatal care can also be limited by a woman's attitude toward her pregnancy, toward prenatal care, and by her cultural beliefs, lifestyle, and other psychologic attributes. Women who had not planned the pregnancy and who view it negatively tend to seek care late or not at all. Recent pilot work by York and colleagues indicates that lower socioeconomic status urban women who received little or no prenatal care reported that reasons for doing so were personal. In this retrospective study of women who received insufficient prenatal care, it was found that all pregnancies were unplanned. Stated reasons for not receiving care were not wanting the pregnancy and not wanting to invest in it (Ruth York, personal communication, June 14, 1990).

Not all women value prenatal care and see it as important. For some groups who view pregnancy as a normal event, prenatal care is considered necessary only if they have an illness (Warneke et al., 1975; Poland, 1989; Warrick, 1986). Dysfunctional lifestyles, including transience, homelessness, abuse, and family violence, are also associated with insufficient prenatal care, as is maternal depression, anxiety, fear, and denial (Chao et al., 1984; Poland, 1989). Despite these many factors associated with inadequate prenatal care, national efforts to recruit pregnant women into care and to keep them in care are essential in reducing the incidence of LBW infants or even in improving the upward distribution of birth weights (Institute of Medicine, 1988). Additionally, the cost-effectiveness of prenatal care has been underscored by the Institute of Medicine. In a 1985 report, the Institute calculated that for each additional dollar spent on providing more adequate prenatal care to low-income, poorly educated women, prenatal care could reduce total expenditures for direct medical care of their LBW infants by $3.38 during the first year of life; the savings would result from a reduced rate of LBW deliveries (Institute of Medicine, 1985).

## Prenatal Care Programs

Recently the Institute of Medicine's committee on prenatal care reported that a number of programs have been successful in improving women's participation in prenatal care (Institute of Medicine, 1988). Programs the committee reviewed were grouped according to major emphases, which were as follows: (1) reducing financial obstacles to care; (2) increasing the basic capacity of the system used by low-income women; (3) making services more accessible and acceptable to clients; (4) identifying women in need of prenatal care (case finding); and (5) provision of social support (Institute of Medicine, 1988).

The committee concluded that each of the five types of programs can succeed not only in bringing women into care but in maintaining their participation in care as well. The success of many of the programs was modest, and the committee was struck by the amount of effort these programs involve, the degree of personal dedication required of their leaders, and the difficulties many had to overcome to make progress. In reviewing the program types, the committee reported that few programs attempted to remove financial barriers (Institute of Medicine, 1988). Most attempted to reduce financial barriers by enlarging clinic systems used by low-income women rather than enabling them to use provider systems already in place, such as physicians in private practice.

Increasing the capacity of the services used by low-income women did, however, improve prenatal care use among this population. Nurse practitioners, certified nurse midwives, and other practitioners were often central to this approach. Programs that improved internal policies and procedures regarding how clients were treated and the atmosphere of the setting also demonstrated improved participation in prenatal care. Although case finding improved participation in care, data from programs that used case finding with outreach workers and similar personnel suggest that the number of clients recruited is often low and that the cost per client enrolled can be very high, particularly in highly mobile urban settings. The committee reported that nonetheless, outreach workers can sometimes find the women who are hardest to reach. Program managers reported that outreach workers can be difficult to recruit, train, supervise, and motivate, and that only the most skilled and persistent are likely to succeed. Case finding using telephone hotlines, however, appears to be successful; it is less expensive and meets a real need. The committee found little evidence that cash incentives brought women into care. Programs emphasizing social support indicate that this approach can result in increased numbers of prenatal visits, especially among populations at greatest risk of insufficient care such as young teens and low-income minority women (Institute of Medicine, 1988).

The committee reported that many program leaders face major problems in implementing and maintaining programs. Problems include planning programs, finding financial and community support, dealing with bureaucracies, recruiting and keeping personnel, and sustaining momentum. Virtually all programs struggle with problems of program evaluation, including what data to collect, how to get it collected, and adequate money, staff, and time to do quality evaluation studies (Institute of Medicine, 1988).

The committee reviewed programs that evaluated their effectiveness in terms of the month of pregnancy in which prenatal care was begun or the number of visits or both. Programs that evaluated impact on birth outcome (length of gestation, birth weight, Apgar score, or infant mortality) were excluded from the review. Reports of program effectiveness using the latter outcome measures have been mixed (Alexander & Cornely, 1987; Gortmaker et al., 1987; Grassi, 1988; United States General Accounting Office, 1990; Rivara et al., 1985; Schramm, 1985). Although some programs have reported improved rates of LBW deliveries, they have tended to be improvements in the upper birth weight distribution of LBW. Few studies report improvements in the rate of very LBW infants born (Covington, Carl, Daley, Cushing, & Churchill, 1988), and as with the previous set of programs, quality evaluation studies of these programs are rare.

## Social and National Funding Factors

Apart from individual risk factors and programs focused on their improvement, LBW has historically been associated with a number of national, social, and funding factors. Reduction of poverty and increased social support programs have been associated with reduction in LBW and infant mortality. Increases in legal abortions have been reported as the single most important factor in reducing neonatal mortality, followed by use of organized family planning services by low-income women (Grossman & Jacobowitz, 1982). An example of these factors at work was provided in the decade of the 1970s, which also saw the sharpest decline in infant mortality (Miller, 1985). During that period there was an expansion of social support programs, including Aid to Families with Dependent Children, food stamps, and Medicaid, and development of special programs to improve access to maternity-related services. There was a decrease in the proportion of unwanted childbearing through provision of easier access to family planning and abortion services, an improved economy, a reduced poverty rate, nutrition supplements for pregnant women, and dramatic advances in care of high-risk newborns (Miller, 1985). Since 1981, federal support for family planning and abortion has been sharply reduced, as have many national programs of social support. During that same period, the LBW rate, which had been decreasing, stabilized at 6.8 percent (Hughes et al., 1989) and is now increasing (National Center for Health Statistics, 1989a). The LBW rate for blacks, a subgroup at greater economic disadvantage, increased during this period (Hughes et al., 1989).

Although the cause of LBW is not known, women at risk can be identified through adequate prenatal care and interventions carried out to decrease the risk of LBW deliveries. However, over 30 percent of pregnant women receive inadequate prenatal care for financial, delivery system, or personal reasons, and the many social and funding factors associated with inadequate prenatal care and high infant mortality remain the same or have worsened (Gold et al., 1987). It is improbable that the LBW rate will decrease in the near future unless a major reallocation of resources occurs in this country in favor of family planning and abortion services, pregnant women, infants, and family life. In view of current circumstances, continued efforts to improve care to LBW infants and their families are warranted.

## Care and Cost of Low Birth Weight Infants

Given the trends of the past decade and the current increases in LBW and very LBW rates, further efforts are needed in the care of this vulnerable group to ensure they have every opportunity for healthy and productive lives. Although technologic advances of the last several decades have increased the survival of this group, problems in caring for these infants remain. The high technology treatment itself imposes iatrogenic problems on the infants and increased stress on their families. Despite extremely high total treatment costs, investment strategies to date have been concentrated in the acute care phase, with few resources being devoted to follow-up care. Much attention has focused on the development and implementation of medical interventions for premature infants. Alternate models of care delivery that have the potential of decreasing stress on families and reducing costs as well as improving infant outcomes have not received comparable attention or funding.

## Care—Iatrogenic Problems

Although neonatal intensive care has increased the survival of LBW infants and reduced the incidence of handicaps, not all intensive care interventions appear to be therapeutic. A number of studies suggest that the intensive care environment, with its bright lights and din of machinery, may be causing permanent damage to infants' hearing, vision, and motor coordination. The noise levels in some neonatal intensive care units have been found to be comparable to those of a factory interior, automobile traffic, or a busy office. Microphones placed in the incubators have revealed noise levels exceeding 80 decibels—levels that over time are associated with hearing loss (Gottfried et al., 1981). Average decibel levels inside an isolette obscure certain frequencies and enhance others. Telephones, public address announcements, monitors, and human voices are obscured. An infant attempting to locate the origin of a human voice may inadvertently lean to look away from the speaker because of deflection of sounds (Weibley, 1989). Sounds penetrating most clearly and loudly are from nonhuman mechanical or metallic devices, including high-frequency sounds made by slamming and squeaking doors, trash cans, and addressograph machines. These sounds coincide with startle, jerk, and jump activities in the infants (Hilton, 1987; Newman, 1981; Weibley, 1989). The excessive noise may also be responsible for elevated blood pressure found among some infants in these nurseries (Gottfried et al., 1981).

Prolonged exposure to cool white fluorescent lights in both children and adults has led to depletion of calcium, among other negative biochemical and physiologic effects. Growth could be hindered in infants exposed to this type of lighting 24 hours a day (Gottfried et al., 1981). In many neonatal intensive care units, there is typically no diurnal rhythmicity of light, which some investigators believe may interfere with the infants' development of normal biologic rhythms (Gottfried & Gaiter, 1985). In utero, a 28- to 32-week-old fetus sleeps approximately 80 percent of the time. These sleep periods are thought to be important for neuronal maturation. Several studies have documented the repeated intrusions in infant rest, with one study reporting an average of 132 disturbances a day for care or treatment. The mean duration of undisturbed rest was 4 to 10 minutes (Duxbury et al., 1984; Korones, 1976).

Other complications originate with treatments and equipment. Position deformities such as the characteristic narrow, flattened heads of preterm infants are common. The infant's fragile skin is traumatized from monitor leads, tape, or restraints (Gottfried & Gaiter, 1985). Low birth weight infants are particularly susceptible to accidental trauma because they lack the means to avoid it. If positioned against a heat source, for example, the infant does not have the strength or coordination to shift his or her body away (Weibley, 1989). Additionally, the longer the infant is hospitalized, the greater the opportunity for contracting infections. Infants in intensive care may also suffer a kind of primary social deprivation. They are separated from parents, most interactions with staff members are painful rather than comforting, and near normal social interactions are almost absent (Linn, Horowitz, & Fox, 1985).

## Cost of Care

The high cost of delivering neonatal care to LBW infants is an area of concern for those making public policy decisions as well as for health care providers, insurers, and families. The costs are both direct and indirect. Although data exist to substantiate direct costs of health care for LBW infants, indirect economic or human costs are less well documented.

*Direct Costs.* The cost of providing direct care to LBW infants is extremely high. Establishing and maintaining a neonatal intensive care unit is costly, with mean annual equipment costs of $70,000 or more (Bajo, 1983). Highly skilled staff (physician, nurse, various therapists) is required, and high stress levels in these units result in burnout and high turnover. Among high cost hospitalizations, neonatal hospitalizations are one of the most expensive of any type (Institute of Medicine, 1990; Office of Technology Assessment, 1987; Schroeder et al., 1979). Reported hospital charges for care of LBW infants range from means of $20,000 to in excess of $167,000, with charges increasing as gestational age and birth weight decrease (Fuchs & Perreault, 1986; Schroeder et al., 1979; Walker et al., 1984). The costs are borne by private insurance plans, the government, the family, and hospitals. Allocation of the actual costs of this care is difficult because of the diversity and complexity of hospital billing and third-party reimbursement practices (Kaufman & Shepard, 1982). Through cross-subsidies, the high costs of caring for some neonates are borne by others. Neonatal intensive care charges are often not fully reimbursed by Medicaid or by insurance plans that pay only for "allowable" costs. Because it is difficult for a hospital to adjust charges continuously as a patient moves from one level of care to another, cross-subsidies are based on variations in length of stay. The costly days at the beginning of an infant's stay are clearly subsidized by the much less expensive growth and recovery period at the end of the stay. Cross-subsidies resulting from fixed per diem reimbursement create economic incentives for hospitals to admit less costly borderline cases in the neonatal intensive care unit unnecessarily or to prolong the recovery period at the end of an infant's stay when the excess of revenue over cost is greatest (Kaufman & Shepard, 1982).

The initiation of diagnosis-related groups (DRGs) has added to the complexity of determining the costs of care for this group. In this system, patients with exceptionally long lengths of stay or exceptionally high costs compared with most patients discharged in the same DRG are considered outliers. The Health Care Financing Administration determined that 6 percent of discharges paid by Medicare would qualify as outliers and that days of care beyond the outlier threshold would be reimbursed at the uniform rate of 60 percent of the DRG-specific per diem rate of payment in all DRGs, regardless of the reason for the extended stay (Berki & Schneier, 1987).

The number of DRGs for newborns is very limited, with wide variation in severity of infant illness possible within some categories. DRGs 385 (Neonates Died or Transferred), 386 (Extreme Immaturity) and 387 (Prematurity with Major Problems) are illustrative. In one study of hospitals in Maryland, 31 percent of all newborns in DRG 386 and 16 percent of all newborns in DRG 387 were outliers (Berki & Schneier, 1987). Although the mean length of stay of outliers in the normal newborn category was 9.7 days, the mean length of stay of outliers in DRGs 386 and 387 was more than 2 months. The mean charge per outlier discharge in DRG 386 was five times the mean for inliers; in DRG 385, the mean charge for outliers was 18 times the mean for inliers. Within DRGs 385, 386, and 387, 50 percent of patient days were devoted to outliers. The 418 newborn discharges in these three DRGs represented less than one hundredth of the newborn discharges in the study but generated more than one quarter of hospital charges for all newborn discharges. In 1985 prices, the mean charge for these outliers was $33,762, generating hospital charges of $14.1 million. Of all newborn outliers, 85 percent were discharged from teaching hospitals with 200 or more beds.

Teaching hospitals tend to receive infants requiring more complex care who are often transferred from community or nonteaching hospitals (Berki & Schneier, 1987). The latter institutions may keep less severely ill neonates within the same DRGs in their own institutions. The difference in severity of infant illness and need for resource-intensive care demonstrates that teaching hospitals in particular may bear a disproportionate financial burden under the current DRG system, whereas nonteaching hospitals, especially small ones, may be overcompensated. It also explains a major incentive in the establishment of neonatal intensive care units in many community hospitals and the resulting deregionalization of care.

*Indirect Costs.*   Indirect costs of caring for LBW infants result from stresses on the family unit. Although clinicians have long been aware of stresses on families of LBW infants, relatively little research has been conducted on the needs of these families. Harper and associates (1976) reported that 76 percent of parents with infants in the neonatal intensive care unit developed a level of emotional difficulty that required treatment ranging from the use of tranquilizers to hospitalization for hypertension.

Mothers of LBW infants have been documented to have more anxiety and depression the week following birth than mothers of term infants (Brooten et al., 1988; Gennaro, 1988). How long anxiety and depression last in mothers of LBW and very LBW infants is not clear, nor is it clear how these psychologic stress responses differ over time. Some investigators report that maternal anxiety may persist for months after delivery (Jeffcoate, Humphrey, & Lloyd, 1979), whereas other investigators have failed to find continued anxiety or depression after the initial postpartum period (Brooten et al., 1988; Gennaro, 1988; Trause & Kramer, 1983). Discrepancies in research findings may stem in part from inadequate differentiation between responses of mothers of LBW and very LBW infants or from failure to examine variables of infant birth weight and morbidity. Blumberg (1980), for example, found that mothers of ill preterm infants were more stressed (measured by anxiety and depression) than mothers of less sick babies. Mothers of sicker preterm infants have been found to be more depressed and less interactive even after the infant has made a full medical recovery than mothers of less ill preterm infants (Minde, Whitelaw, Brown, & Fitzhardinge, 1983). In other studies, however, mothers appeared equally stressed regardless of how ill their infant appeared to health care professionals (Benfield, Leib, & Reuter, 1976), and mothers of sicker preterm infants were found to have enhanced rather than diminished caregiver-infant interactions (Beckwith & Cohen, 1978).

Little information is reported on the effects of high risk infants on family function. Related studies of children with chronic or catastrophic illness suggest that the usual patterns of family function may be disrupted substantially. Serious and/or chronic illness in children has been associated with marital instability (Pless & Pinkerton, 1975), changed parental employment opportunities and family income (Salkever, 1980), decreased social contacts and vacations as a result of the burden of care for the child and the lack of alternate caregivers (Stein & Riessman, 1980), problems in other children in the family (Breslau, Weitzman, & Messenger, 1981), and increased workload for the mothers (Breslau, 1983). Data on the effects of LBW infants on families are beginning to emerge. Work by Gennaro and colleagues (1990) on the care and cost burden of LBW infants on families is demonstrating that mothers of very LBW infants who were employed are being forced to reduce their employment hours or quit work entirely following hospital discharge of their infant in part because of lack of caregivers prepared to provide care to high-risk infants. At the same time that employment is reduced for these families, out-of-pocket health care costs for the infant are increased. McCormick and associates (1986) also reported higher out-of-pocket expenses for hospitalization, ambulatory care, and medical equipment for families who have very LBW infants compared with those with normal weight infants.

At the time of discharge from the hospital, parents express fear and feelings of inadequacy and desire more information, instruction, and help in caring for the LBW infant at home (Butts et al., 1988; Desmond et al., 1980; Jeffcoate et al., 1979; Victor, 1977). Work with families after discharge of their LBW, premature, or sick newborn has been identified as important in preventing failure to thrive, child abuse, and accidents as well as in improving the developmental levels of these children (Barnard et al., 1982; Barrera et al., 1986; Chapman & Pike, 1988; Resnick et al., 1988). Why some LBW infants are poorly parented has been of considerable interest to numerous investigators.

When compared with full-term normal weight infants, LBW infants have different behavioral responses, which can affect caregiving. The behaviors of preterm infants reveal limitations of interactional capacity, including global responses, difficulty sustaining attention to meaningful stimuli, narrow range of tolerance to stimulation, decreased ability to be soothed, and reduced integration of behavior patterns. Consequently, the preterm LBW infant demonstrates arousal to seemingly innocuous types of stimulation, disorganized responses, decreased availability for social interaction with parents or caregivers, reduced time spent in the restorative stage of quiet sleep, and uneven transitions between states of consciousness. This inability to organize behavior and give cues makes it difficult for parents and caregivers to receive direction in providing appropriate care and in validating their caregiving competence.

Studies have documented that developmental outcomes can be improved and the cost of hospitalization reduced if caregivers are assisted with interpreting the infant's behavior and instructed in developmentally appropriate responses. Evaluations of programs that encourage parent-child contact during the hospital stay and provide in-home parental guidance, support, and infant stimulation found that home environments were more conducive to normal infant development: maternal-infant relationships were stronger; fewer infant feeding problems were present; fewer accidents occurred; and infants achieved higher developmental levels by 3 years of age (Barrera et al., 1986; Hayes, 1980; Larson, 1980; Resnick et al., 1988). Additionally, very LBW infants appear to gain most from programs of intervention.

## Alternatives to High-Cost Hospitalization

Despite the obvious direct and indirect economic burdens a LBW infant places on the family as well as on society, health care investment strategies and efforts to control costs to date have been directed largely toward the acute hospital phase of care. This is true despite a growing number of studies that indicate that earlier discharge of LBW infants at discharge weights averaging from 1830 g to 2079 g with follow-up care in the home can be safe, therapeutic, and cost-effective (Bauer & Tinklepaugh, 1971; Berg et al., 1969; Davies et al., 1979; Derbyshire et al., 1982; Dillard & Korones, 1973; Lowry et al., 1978; Lefebvre et al., 1982; Singer & Wolfsdorf, 1975; Singh, 1979). In Great Britain, for example, infants have been discharged earlier from the hospital through the established system of home follow-up, which provides the family with continued professional contact after discharge (Davies et al., 1979; Derbyshire et al., 1982). In a recent report, LBW infants were discharged early from the hospital and visited at home a mean of 11 times by community neonatal nurses, who monitored infant well-being, parental coping, and environmental adequacy. Four percent of the infants were rehospitalized while under the care of the specialist nurses. When compared with the cost of providing continuing inpatient neonatal care, earlier discharge was estimated to have saved approximately £250,000 in 1985 (Couriel & Davies, 1988).

In the United States a similar approach was tested by Brooten and colleagues. In this randomized clinical trial, one group of very LBW infants was discharged earlier than the hospital routine. For families in the early discharge group, instruction, counseling, home visits, and daily on-call availability of a hospital-based nurse specialist were provided. In the early discharge group, the majority of whom were undereducated and poor, infants were able to be discharged a mean of 11 days earlier, 200 g less in weight, and 2 weeks younger than in the control group. Hospital charges were 27 percent less and physician charges 22 percent less in the early discharge group compared with the control group. There were no differences in number of rehospitalizations, acute care visits, or growth and developmental outcomes of infants in both groups. On a national scale, the group estimated that if only half of very LBW infants born in the United States each year were provided with this service, the possible savings using conservative estimates would be $167 million (Brooten et al., 1986).

In addition to this approach, a variety of models are providing follow-up for the LBW and very LBW infant after hospital discharge. These follow-up services include the traditional hospital-based high-risk follow-up clinic, the community or public health nurse follow-up, and follow-up services provided by health maintenance organizations and entrepreneurial groups. Although some of these models incorporate earlier hospital discharge and provide a comprehensive approach to monitoring the physical and developmental outcomes of the infant and parental coping and parenting, most do not (Gennaro et al., 1991). Even though earlier hospital discharge of LBW infants with adequate home follow-up has been demonstrated to be safe, cost-effective, and a service valued by parents, several problems currently stand in the way of its fuller implementation.

First, earlier hospital discharge of LBW infants can either be a negative or a positive cost factor for hospitals, depending on reimbursement plans and patient mix, as described previously. Second, in many patient groups, follow-up services may not be available or the quality of the service may be such that neonatologists are reluctant to use them for fear of increased risk to the infant and malpractice claims. Third, establishing follow-up services requires convincing third-party payers of the economic gain. However, insurance companies reportedly are willing to negotiate coverage in order to reduce their costs. Health maintenance organizations and private payer organizations that have not had home care and equipment benefits have authorized payment for providers of follow-up services and for equipment as an alternative to expensive hospital care (Block, Davis, Huebner, & Sutherland, 1989). Last, there is a need for greater direct reimbursement for nurses to provide follow-up services for high-risk infants and their families.

This is an opportune time for nurses to assume more of a leadership role in improving the LBW rate and in improving outcomes of LBW infants and families as well as controlling health care costs. Currently, with an unacceptable infant mortality rate and a reduced national employment pool for the future, there is a national refocusing on pregnant women, children, and their well-being. In 1990, Medicaid coverage was extended to all pregnant women and children up to 1 year of age with family incomes of 133 percent or less of the federal poverty level. States have the added flexibility of expanding the coverage to women and infants in families with incomes up to 185 percent of the poverty level (Roper, 1989). Other legislative changes are focused on child health with early and periodic screening and treatment. It is a prime time for nurses to provide a greater proportion of direct primary care services to pregnant women, infants, and children and to be directly reimbursed for these services.

## Summary

In summary, as we enter the 1990s, the challenge of reducing the LBW rate and subsequently the infant mortality rate sharpens. Several points are clear. First, more research into the causes of LBW is needed. Second, the LBW rate is not likely to be reduced significantly unless major resource allocation occurs to improve access to and the content of prenatal care. Recruiting pregnant women into prenatal care through enhanced access and maintaining them in care will remain difficult and expensive. The effect on LBW rates will probably remain small, reflecting an equal or greater effect of poverty and other social problems such as substance abuse and acquired immunodeficiency syndrome. Programs of enhanced access to prenatal care will not affect the incidence of LBW infants in women who do not wish to be pregnant or who have no investment in the outcome of the pregnancy but who have no alternative but to be pregnant because funds for family planning and abortion services are being cut or eliminated. This situation is most acute for lower income women, those with substance abuse, and similar high-risk groups. These groups are also those with the fewest resources to care for LBW infants after birth.

In the next decade care for LBW infants will continue to improve as we gain an even greater understanding of the developmental needs of these infants and families. Treatment costs will remain high, and the debate on where to cease interventions will continue. Earlier hospital discharge of LBW infants will remain a problem in many areas of the country barring changes in reimbursement policies and establishment of adequate follow-up services. Nursing's greatest contribution in the care of mothers at high risk for LBW infants and the care of these infants and their families will be made through provision of direct care, research to improve that care, and advocacy for this group.

## REFERENCES

Alan Guttmacher Institute (1987). Blessed events and the bottom line: Financing maternity care in the United States. New York: The Alan Guttmacher Institute.

Alexander, G.R., & Cornely, D.A. (1987). Prenatal care utilization: Its measurement and relationship to pregnancy outcome. *American Journal of Preventive Medicine, 3*(5), 243–253.

Bajo, K. (1983). Equipment costs: The neonatal intensive care unit and the modern obstetric unit. *Clinics in Perinatology, 10*(1), 175–187.

Barnard, K., Booth, C., Mitchell, S., & Telzrow, R. (1982). *Newborn nursing models.* Seattle: University of Washington, Department of Parent and Child Nursing.

Barrera, M.E., Rosenbaum, P.L., & Cunningham, C.E. (1986). Early home intervention with low birthweight infants and their parents. *Child Development, 57,* 20–33.

Bauer, C., & Tinklepaugh, W. (1971). Low birthweight babies in the hospital. *Clinical Pediatrics, 10,* 467.

Beckwith, L., & Cohen, S. (1978). Preterm birth: hazardous obstetrical and postnatal events as related to caregiver behavior. *Infant Behavior and Development, 1,* 403–411.

Benfield, D.F., Leib, S., & Reuter, J. (1976). Grief responses to parents after referral of the critically ill newborn to a regional center. *New England Journal of Medicine, 294,* 975–978.

Berg, R.B., Salisbury, A.J. (1971, November). Discharging infants of low birthweight reconsideration of current practice. *American Journal of Diseases of Children, 122,* 414–417.

Berg, R., Salisbury, A., & Kahan, R. (1969). Early discharge of low birthweight infants. *Journal of the American Medical Association, 210,* 1892.

Berki, S.E., & Schneier, N.B. (1987). Frequency and cost of diagnosis-related group outliers among newborns. *Pediatrics, 79*(6), 874–881.

Binsacca, D., Ellis, J., Martin, D., & Petitti, D. (1987). Factors associated with low birthweight in an inner city population: The role of financial problems. *American Journal of Public Health, 77*(4), 505–506.

Block, C., Davis, J., Huebner, S., & Sutherland, A. (1989). Home care for high-risk infants: The first year. *Caring, 8*(5), 11–17.

Blumberg, N. (1980). Effects of neonatal risk, maternal attitude, and cognitive style on early postpartum adjustment. *Journal of Abnormal Psychology, 89,* 139–150.

Brecht, M.C. (1989). The tragedy of infant mortality. *Nursing Outlook, 37*(1), 18–22.

Breslau, N. (1983). Care of disabled children and women's time use. *Medical Care, 21,* 620–629.

Breslau, N., Weitzman, W., & Messenger, K. (1981). Psychological functioning of siblings of disabled children. *Pediatrics, 67,* 344–353.

Brooten, D. (1988). Influencing health care public policy decisions: A model for determining cost effectiveness of health care delivery services provided by nurses. *Proceedings of the Second Invitational Conference, National Commission on Nursing Implementation Project* (pp. 149–163). Milwaukee, WI: National Commission on Nursing Implementation Project.

Brooten, D., Gennaro, S., Brown, L., Butts, P., Kumar, S., Bakewell-Sachs, S., & Gibbons, A. (1988). Anxiety, depression and hostility in mothers of preterm infants. *Nursing Research, 37,* 213–217.

Brooten, D., Kumar, S., Brown, L., Butls, P., Finkler, S., Bakewell-Sachs, S., Gibbons, A., & Delivoria-Papadopoulos, M. (1986). A random clinical trial of early discharge and home followup of very low birthweight infants. *New England Journal of Medicine, 315,* 934–939.

Butts, P.A., Brooten, D., Brown, L., Bakewell-Sachs, S., Gibbons, A., & Kumar, S. (1988). Concerns of parents of low birthweight infants following hospital discharge: A report of parent-initiated telephone calls. *Neonatal Network, 7*(2), 37–42.

Centers for Disease Control (1988). Progress toward achieving the 1990 objectives for pregnancy and infant health. *Morbidity and Mortality Weekly Report, 37*(26), 405–408, 413.

Chao, S., Imaizumi, S., Gorman, S., & Lowenstein, R. (1984). *Reasons for absence of prenatal care and its consequences.* New York: Department of Obstetrics and Gynecology, Harlem Hospital Center.

Chapman, J., & Pike, R. (1988). *Effects of hospital and home standardized intervention programs for prematurely born infants: Evidence of detrimental outcome.* Paper presented at the Nurses Association of the American College of Obstetrics and Gynecology (NAACOG) Research Conference, Toronto, Canada.

Christianson, R.E., van den Berg, B.J., Milkovich, L., & Oechsli, F.W. (1981). Incidence of congenital anomalies among white and black live births with long-term follow-up. *American Journal of Public Health, 71,* 1333–1341.

Couriel, J.M., & Davies, P. (1988). Costs and benefits of a community special care baby service. *British Medical Journal, 296,* 1043–1046.

Covington, D.L., Carl, J., Daley, J.G., Cushing, D., & Churchill, M.P. (1988). Effects of the North Carolina prematurity prevention program among public patients delivering at New Hanover Memorial Hospital. *American Journal of Public Health, 78*(11), 1493–1495.

Davies, D., Herbert, S., Haxby, V., & McNeish, A. (1979). When should preterm babies be sent home from neonatal units? *Lancet, 1,* 914.

Derbyshire, F., Davies, D., & Bacca, A. (1982). Discharge of preterm babies from neonatal units. *British Medical Journal, 284*, 233.

Desmond, M., Vorderman, A., & Salinas, M. (1980). The family and the premature infant after neonatal intensive care. *Texas Medicine, 76*, 60.

Dillard, R., & Korones, S. (1973). Lower discharge weight and shortened nursery stay for low birthweight infants. *New England Journal of Medicine, 288*, 131.

Duxbury, M.L., Henly, S.J., Broz, L.J., Armstrong, G.D., & Wachdorf, C.M. (1984). Caregiver disruptions and sleep of high-risk infants. *Heart & Lung, 13*(2), 141–147.

Fuchs, V.R., & Perreault, L. (1986). Expenditures for reproduction-related health care. *Journal of the American Medical Association, 255*(1), 76–81.

Gennaro, S. (1988). Postpartal anxiety and depression in mothers of preterm infants. *Nursing Research, 37*, 82–85.

Gennaro, S., Brooten, D., Bakewell-Sachs, S. (1991). Post discharge services for low birthweight infants. *JOGN, 201*(1): 29–36.

Gennaro, S., Brooten, D., & Hornberger, K. (1990). Nonmedical costs associated with having a low birthweight infant. Manuscript submitted for publication.

Gold, R.B., Kenney, A.M., & Singh, S. (1987). Paying for maternity care in the United States. *Family Planning Perspectives, 19*(5), 190–193, 195–206.

Gortmaker, S.L., Clark, C.J.G., Graven, S.N., Sobol, A.M., & Geronimus, A. (1987). Reducing infant mortality in rural America: Evaluation of the Rural Infant Care Program. *Health Services Research, 22*(1), 91–115.

Gottfried, A.W., & Gaiter, J.L. (Eds.) (1985). *Infant stress under intensive care: Environmental neonatology.* Baltimore: University Park Press.

Gottfried, A.W., Wallace-Lande, P., Sherman-Brown, S., King, J., Coen, C., & Hodgman, J. (1981). Physical and social environment of newborn infants in special care units. *Science, 214*, 673.

Grassi, L.C. (1988). Life, money, quality: The impact of regionalization on perinatal/neonatal intensive care. *Neonatal Network, 6*(4), 53–59.

Grossman, M., & Jacobowitz, S. (1982). Variations in infant mortality rates among counties of the United States: The roles of public policies and programs. In J. Vandre Graag, W. Neenan, & T. Tsukahara (Eds.), *Economics of health care.* New York: Praeger Special Studies.

Harper, R., Sia, C., & Sokal, S. (1976). Observation on unrestricted parental contact with infants in the neonatal intensive care unit. *Journal of Pediatrics, 89*, 441.

Hayes, J. (1980). Premature infant development: The relationship of neonatal stimulation, birth condition and home environment. *Pediatric Nursing, 6*, 33.

Hilton, A. (1987). The hospital racket: How noisy is your unit? *American Journal of Nursing, 87*, 59–61.

Hughes, D., Johnson, K., Rosenbaum, S., & Liu, J. (1989). *The health of America's children: Maternal and child health data book.* Washington, DC: Children's Defense Fund.

Hughes, D., Johnson, K., Rosenbaum, S., Simons, J., & Butter, E. (1988). *The health of America's children. Maternal and child health data book.* Washington, DC: Children's Defense Fund.

Institute of Medicine (1985). *Preventing low birthweight.* Washington, DC: National Academy Press.

Institute of Medicine (1988). *Prenatal care: Reaching mothers, reaching infants.* Washington, DC: National Academy Press.

Institute of Medicine (1990). *Science and babies: Private decision, public dilemmas.* Washington, DC: National Academy Press.

Jeffcoate, J., Humphrey, M., & Lloyd, J. (1979). Disturbances in parent relationships following preterm delivery. *Developmental Medicine and Child Neurology, 21,* 534–538.

Kaufman, S.L., & Shepard, D.S. (1982). Costs of neonatal intensive care by day of stay. *Inquiry, 19,* 167–178.

Kessner, D.M., Singer, J., Kalk, C.E., et al. (1973). Infant death: An analysis by maternal risk and health care. In *Contrasts in health status,* vol. 1. Washington, DC: National Academy Press.

Kleinman, J.C., & Kessel, S.S. (1987). Racial differences in low birth weight: Trends and risk factors. *New England Journal of Medicine, 317*(12), 749–753.

Korones, S.B. (1976). Disturbance and infants' rest. In T. Moore (Ed.), *Iatrogenic problems in neonatal intensive care, Report of the 69th Ross Conference on Pediatric Research.* Columbus, OH: Ross Laboratories.

Larson, C. (1980). Efficacy of prenatal and postpartum home visits on child health and development. *Pediatrics, 66,* 191.

Lefebvre, F., Veilleux, A., & Bard, H. (1982). Early discharge of low birthweight infants. *Archives of Disease in Childhood, 57,* 511.

Leveno, K.J., Cunningham, F.G., Roark, M.L., Nelson, S.D., & Williams, M.L. (1985). Prenatal care and the low birth weight infant. *Obstetrics and Gynecology, 66*(5), 599–605.

Linn, P.L., Horowitz, F.D., & Fox, H.A. (1985). Stimulation in the NICU: Is more necessarily better? *Clinics in Perinatology, 12,* 407–422.

Lowry, M., Jones, M., & Shanahan, M. (1978). Discharge of small babies from hospital. *Archives of Disease in Childhood, 106,* 101.

McCormick, M.C. (1985). The contribution of low birthweight to infant mortality and childhood morbidity. *New England Journal of Medicine, 312,* 82–90.

McCormick, M.C. (1989). Long-term follow-up of infants discharged from neonatal intensive care units. *Journal of the American Medical Association, 261,* 1767–1772.

McCormick, M.C., Shapiro, S., & Starfield, B.H. (1980). Rehospitalization in the first year of life for high-risk survivors. *Pediatrics, 66*(6), 991–999.

McCormick, M.C., Stemmler, M.M., Bernbaum, J.C., & Farran, A.C. (1986). The very low birth weight transport goes home: Impact on the family. *Developmental and Behavioral Pediatrics, 7*(4), 217–223.

McCormick, M.C., Wessel, K.W., Krischer, J.P., Welcher, D.W., & Handy, J.B. (1981). Preliminary analysis of developmental observations in a survey of morbidity in infants. *Early Human Development, 5,* 377–393.

Meis, P.J., Ernest, J.M., & Moore, M.L. (1987). Causes of low birth weight births in public and private patients. *American Journal of Obstetrics and Gynecology, 156,* 1165–1168.

Miller, C.A. (1985). Infant mortality in the U.S. *Scientific American, 253*(1), 31–37.

Minde, K., Whitelaw, A., Brown, B., & Fitzhardinge, P. (1983). Effect of neonatal complications in premature infants on early parent-infant interaction. *Developmental Medicine & Child Neurology, 25,* 763–777.

Morris, J.N., & Heady, J.A. (1955). Social and biological factors in infant mortality. *Lancet, 1,* 343–349.

Mutch, L., Newdick, M., Lodwick, A., & Chalmers, I. (1986). Secular changes in rehospitalization of very low birth weight infants. *Pediatrics, 78*(1), 164–171.

National Center for Health Statistics (1980). *Factors Associated with Low Birthweight: United States, 1976* (Department of Health, Education, and Welfare No. [Public Health Service] 80-1915). Washington, DC: U.S. Government Printing Office.

National Center for Health Statistics: Vital Statistics of the United States, 1988, Vol. 1. Natality. DHHS. Pub. No. (PHS) 90–11100. Public Health Service. Washington, U.S. Government Printing Office, 1990.

National Center for Health Statistics (1989a). Advance report of final natality statistics, 1987. *Monthly Vital Statistics Report, 38*(3), 6–12.

National Center for Health Statistics (1989b). Advance report of final mortality statistics, 1987. *Monthly Vital Statistics Report, 38*(5), 8–9.

Newman, L.F. (1981). Social and sensory environment of low birth weight infants in a special care nursery: An anthropological investigation. *Journal of Nervous and Mental Disease, 169*(7), 448–455.

Office of Technology Assessment (1987). *Neonatal intensive care for low birthweight infants: Costs and effectiveness* (Office of Technology Assessment-HCS-38). Washington, DC: U.S. Government Printing Office.

Papile, L.A., Munsick-Bruno, G., & Schaefer, A. (1983). Relationship of cerebral intraventricular hemorrhage and early childhood neurologic handicaps. *Journal of Pediatrics, 103*, 273–277.

Pless, I.B., & Pinkerton, R. (1975). *Chronic childhood disorder: Promoting patterns of adjustment.* London: Henry Kimpton.

Poland, M. (1989). Ethical issues in the delivery of quality care to pregnant indigent women. In L. Whileford & M. Poland (Eds.), *New approaches to human reproductive, social and ethical dimensions.* Boulder, CO: Westview Press.

Resnick, M., Armstrong,. S., & Carter, R. (1988). Developmental intervention program for high-risk premature infants: Effects on development and parent-infant interactions. *Developmental and Behavioral Pediatrics, 9*, 73–78.

Rivara, F.P., Culley, G.A., Hickok, D., & Williams, R.L. (1985). A health program's effect on neonatal mortality in eastern Kentucky. *American Journal of Preventive Medicine, 1*(3), 35–40.

Roper, W.L. (1989). From the health care financing administration. *Journal of the American Medical Association, 261*(2), 197.

Salkever, D. (1980). Children's health problems: Implications for parental labor supply and earnings. In V.R. Fuchs (Ed.), *Economic aspects of health* (pp. 221–251). Chicago: University of Chicago Press.

Schramm, W.F. (1985). WIC prenatal participation and its relationship to newborn Medicaid costs in Missouri: A cost benefit analysis. *American Journal of Public Health, 75*(8), 851–857.

Schroeder, S., Showstack, J., & Roberts, H. (1979). Frequency and clinical descriptions of high-cost patients in 17 acute care hospitals. *New England Journal of Medicine, 300*, 1306.

Shapiro, S., Schlesinger, E.R., & Nesbitt, R.E.L. (1968). *Infant, perinatal, maternal and childhood mortality in the United States.* Cambridge, MA: Harvard University Press.

Singer, B., & Wolfsdorf, J. (1975). Early discharge of infants of low birthweight: A prospective study. *British Medical Journal, 1*, 362.

Singh, M. (1979). Early discharge of low-birthweight babies. *Tropical and Geographical Medicine, 31*, 565.

Singh, S., Torres, A., & Forret, J.D. (1985). The need for prenatal care in the United States. Evidence from the 1980 National Natality Survey. *Family Planning Perspectives, 17*(3), 118–124.

Stein, R.K., & Riessman, C.K. (1980). The development of an impact-on-family scale: Preliminary findings. *Medical Care, 18*, 465–472.

Termini, L., Brooten, D., Brown, L., Gennaro, S., & York, R. (1990). Reasons for acute care visits and rehospitalizations in very low-birthweight infants. *Neonatal Network, 8*(5), 23–26.

Trause, M.K., & Kramer, L. (1983). The effects of premature birth on parents and their relationship. *Developmental Medicine and Child Neurology, 25,* 459–465.

UNICEF (1988). *The state of the world's children.* Oxford, England: Oxford University Press.

United States Accounting Office (1990). Home Visiting: A promising early intervention strategy for at risk families (GAO/HRD–90–83) Washington, D.C.: U.S. Government Printing Office.

Victor, Y. (1977). Caring for parents of high risk infants. *Medical Journal of Australia, 2,* 534.

Walker, D.J.B., Feldman, A., Vohr, B.R., & Oh, W. (1984). Cost-benefit analysis of neonatal intensive care for infants weighing less than 1,000 grams at birth. *Pediatrics, 74*(1), 20–25.

Warneke, R., Graham, S., Mosher, W., Montgomery, E., & Schotz, W. (1975). Contact with health guides and use of health services among blacks in Buffalo. *Public Health Reprints, 90,* 213–222.

Warrick, L. (1986, October). *Barriers to prenatal care in Maricopa County, Arizona.* Paper presented at the 114th Annual Meeting of the American Public Health Association, Las Vegas, Nevada.

Weibley, T. (1989). Inside the incubator. *American Journal of Maternal Child Nursing, 14,* 96–100.

Wise, P.H., First, L.R., Lamb, G.A., Kotelchuck, M., Chen, D.W., Ewing, A., Hersee, H., & Rideout, J. (1988). Infant mortality increase despite high access to tertiary care: An evolving relationship among infant mortality, health care, and socioeconomic change. *Pediatrics, 81*(4), 542–548.

## Chapter 22

# Adolescents: Improving Life Chances

ANN O'SULLIVAN
JEANNE BROOKS-GUNN
DONALD F. SCHWARZ

*I*MPROVING THE LIFE chances of adolescents is one of the greatest challenges for health professionals both now and in the coming decade. The number of single teenage mothers and the rates of injuries and deaths caused by violence among teenaged males are particularly high among underclass youth.

This chapter reviews the adolescent experience in terms of the determinants of health-related behaviors, with special emphasis on teenage pregnancy and violence as health problems of particular concern to the individual and to society. Trends in the United States are compared with those in other developed countries. Our aim is to call attention to these complex and controversial public health problems, since their solution requires prevention, research, and understanding by health care professionals.

## The Adolescent Experience

The transition from childhood to adolescence is remembered by most adults as exciting but often embarrassing and terrifying. What makes adolescence so important, and for some, so difficult, are the many decisions to be made and the many developmental tasks to be mastered. These tasks include accommodation to pubertal changes and acceptance of a new body shape in a society with strict standards of attractiveness, standards that the majority cannot meet (Attie & Brooks-Gunn, 1987, 1989; Attie et al., 1989). It is a time when childhood ties to parents must be renegotiated, and yet teenagers' demands for more autonomy and a larger role in family decision-making sometimes exceed their ability to act maturely (Brooks-Gunn & Zahaykevich, 1989, Smetana, 1988; Steinberg, 1987). As direct parental control lessens, most adolescents turn to their parents for advice but also begin to seek the advice of others, particularly their peers. However, this broadening social network is full of conflicting messages, which the teenager must learn to sift and weigh (Feldman & Elliott, 1990, chaps. 7 & 11).

Entry into middle school poses an overwhelming challenge for a significant subset of teenagers, namely, those who cannot master the new academic skills and those who are having difficulty in other developmental tasks of adolescence, and their school performance declines (Simmons et al., 1988; Simmons & Blyth, 1987). Learning-disabled adolescents also find the transition from elementary school problematic (Blum, 1986; Levine, 1988).

Approximately 25 percent of high school students work part time (Greenberger, Steinberg, Vaux, & McAuliffe, 1980). These part-time jobs may offer students the opportunity to learn about the workplace and to acquire new skills. In some cases, the jobs may adversely affect the students' school performance and expose them to negative adult behaviors, such as the use of drugs or alcohol.

During adolescence, many teenagers exhibit negative or labile mood states, whereas those who experience multiple life events are at high risk of depression (Baydar, Brooks-Gunn, & Warren, 1990). It is also a time when out of control behavior such as conduct disorders, juvenile delinquency, and aggression, especially in boys, reaches its apex (Cairns et al., 1989; Feldman & Elliott, 1990, chap. 16). It should be noted that depression and aggression during adolescence are associated with problems in adulthood (Kandel et al., 1989; Robins, 1974). Finally, adolescence is a time when teenagers must learn to deal with sexual arousal and relationships with the opposite sex.

There is no orderly sequence to the above challenges. Often, teenagers must confront a number of tasks simultaneously, and they have little control as to when these tasks will present themselves (see Adams et al., 1989; Brooks-Gunn & Petersen, 1983; in press, 1990; Brooks-Gunn et al., 1985; Feldman & Elliott, 1990; Gunnar & Collins, 1988; Lerner & Foch, 1987; Lerner et al., 1991; and Simmons & Blyth, 1987; for reviews of the most current literature on adolescent development).

## *Establishing Positive Health-Related Behaviors in Adolescence*

A major task of adolescence is the development of healthy behaviors. Yet experimentation with adult behaviors such as drinking, smoking, and sex is so common as to be considered a rite of passage for many teenagers. For some, particularly disadvantaged youth, these high-risk behaviors can have dramatic impact on the teenager's current and future well-being.

The extent to which adolescents succeed in establishing healthy behaviors is associated with several important factors: parental, peer, social cognitive, and emotional influences, and societal constructions of adolescent behavior. In this respect, there is increasing evidence that younger teenagers generally have more difficulty engaging in health behaviors than do older adolescents and adults (Brooks-Gunn, 1990; Paikoff & Brooks-Gunn, in press). For example, compared with older teens and adults, younger diabetic teens are less likely to regulate their diets and younger sexually active teens are much less likely to use contraceptives (Brooks-Gunn & Furstenberg, 1990; Hofferth & Hayes, 1987; Sonenstein, Pleck, & Ku, 1989). The many developmental challenges that the younger adolescent faces, coupled with an added difficult variable, may be too much for the less mature individual to handle.

*Parental Influences.*   In a recent study, students in fifth through twelfth grades and their parents were asked to determine whether parental authority was legitimate in a variety of situations. The teenagers identified more situations as those in which they had personal jurisdiction, whereas the parents identified more situations as those in which social conventions should dictate behavior. The teens understood their parents' perspective but nevertheless rejected it (Smetana, 1988).

These findings are pertinent to health behavior in that teenagers perceive sexual and substance use behavior to be under personal jurisdiction, whereas their parents perceive such behavior as subject to social convention (see Brooks-Gunn, 1990). Parent-child conflicts also arise over appropriate health behaviors, as in eating disorders (Attie & Brooks-Gunn, 1989) and chronic illnesses (Johnson, Silverstein, Rosenbloom, Carter, & Cunningham, 1986). Gender also is a factor in adolescent reaction to parental control of health behaviors: there is more passive opposition by girls and more active opposition by boys (Brooks-Gunn & Zahaykevich, 1989).

*Peer Influences.*   Peer networks are an important influence on adolescent health behaviors. Although the values of peer groups are widely divergent, not all are antithetical to parental values (Feldman & Elliott, 1990, chap. 7). At the same time, sex, substance use, and smoking are not isolated acts but are part of the peer culture. Little is known about how peers actually encourage or discourage one another from engaging in unhealthy behaviors. What the teenagers themselves report is that they do what they think or know their friends are doing (Hofferth & Hayes, 1987).

*Social Cognitive Influences.*   During adolescence, the social cognitive constructions of decision making are in flux (Feldman & Elliott, 1990, chap. 3; Paikoff & Brooks-Gunn, in press). Issues associated with social cognitive and cognitive processes include perceived costs and benefits of certain behaviors; understanding future consequences and probable risk; knowledge of role-governed behavior; and refinement of interpersonal negotiation strategies (Brooks-Gunn, 1990; Irwin & Millstein, 1991; Paikoff & Brooks-Gunn, in press). For example, over time teenagers are able to view situations from multiple perspectives and to think more consistently and systematically (Damon & Hart, 1982; Feldman & Elliott, 1990, chap. 14).

*Emotional Influences.*   Emotional functioning changes in adolescence, particularly in the early to middle years when negative affect increases because of multiple life events (Baydar et al., 1990; Petersen et al., 1991; Simmons et al., 1988). Negative feelings such as depression or loneliness increase the likelihood that adolescents will engage in high-risk behaviors. The work on drug use and depression by Kandel and coworkers (1989) is a case in point.

*Social Constructions of Adolescent Behavior.*   Societal beliefs concerning certain health behaviors may take on new meaning for young adolescents who are making decisions about their own health, perhaps for the first time. We believe that society's views of health behaviors are extremely important; they largely determine the nature of the debate as to whether and when a particular behavior is deemed appropriate.

But societal views are often contradictory. For example, substance use is frowned upon but tacitly accepted as part of adult behaviors, and teenagers emulate their elders (Bachman, Johnson, O'Malley, & Humphrey, 1988). Similarly, teenage sexual behavior is not condoned but is tolerated. In this, the societal views of the United

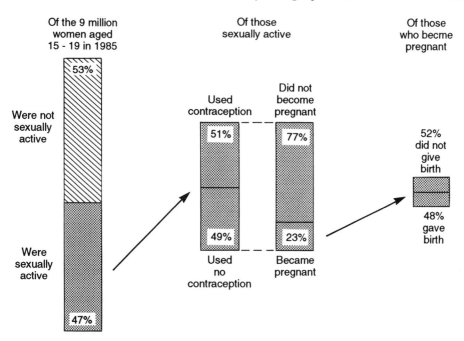

**FIGURE 22–1.** Pregnancy and the American teenager.

*Source:* "500,000 a year; Fewer teen mothers but more unmarried" by L. Tamar, 1988 (March). *New York Times,* p. 50. Copyright 1988 by *New York Times*. Reprinted by permission.

States differ markedly from those of most Western European nations, which seem more accepting of youthful sexuality and stress regular contraceptive use rather than abstinence (Jones, Forrest, Henshaw, Silverman, & Torres, 1988).

Teenage pregnancy and violence, high-risk behaviors that are of acute concern, particularly among underclass youth, are discussed in the following sections.

## Teenage Pregnancy: Defining the Problem

Adolescent pregnancy is widely recognized as a complex and serious problem in our society. The National Research Council Panel on Adolescent Pregnancy and Childbearing titled their exhaustive study *Risking the Future* (Hayes, 1987), a telling indication of the magnitude of the problem.

The statistics are alarming: more than a million teenage girls in the United States become pregnant each year, just over 400,000 teenagers obtain abortions, and nearly 470,000 give birth. The majority of these births are to unmarried mothers, nearly half of whom have not yet reached their 18th birthday (Hayes, 1987). Of the 9 million women aged 15 to 19 years in 1985, 47 percent were sexually active, and of these, 49 percent used no contraception. Twenty-three percent became pregnant, and 48 percent gave birth (Fig. 22–1).

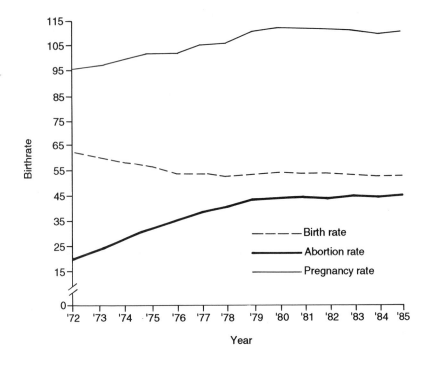

**FIGURE 22–2.** Birth rate, abortion rate, and pregnancy rate per 1,000 women aged 15–19, 1972–1985.

*Source: Teenage pregnancy in the United States* (p. 42) by S.K. Henshaw, A.M. Kenney, D. Somberg, & J. Van Vort, 1989. New York: Alan Guttmacher Institute. Reprinted by permission.

Trends in the rates for teenage pregnancies, abortions, and births appear to have stabilized. As seen in Figure 22–2, pregnancy rates in women aged 15 to 19 years rose from 95 per 1000 in 1972 to a peak of 111 per 1000 in 1980 and 110 per 1000 in 1985. Birth rates for this cohort decreased over time from 62 births per 1000 in 1972 to 52 per 1000 in 1978, increased slightly to 53 per 1000 in 1980, and decreased to 51 per 1000 in 1986 (National Center for Health Statistics, 1988). Abortion rates for this cohort increased during the 1970s to 43 per 1000 in 1980, leveling out at 44 per 1000 in 1985.

*One trend that is not stable is the relationship between the birth rate and the marital status of the adolescent.* Of the teenagers who currently carry their pregnancies to term, half are unmarried, whereas in 1960 only 15 percent of teenage mothers were unmarried (Bureau of Census, 1983). One explanation for this more than 300 percent increase in the rate of single adolescent mothers may have to do with society's attitude toward sex outside of marriage. Figure 22–3 depicts the growth in premarital conception among adolescent women. In the early 1960s, 46 percent, in the early 1970s, 66 percent, and in the early 1980s, over 70 percent of teens conceived when they were single.

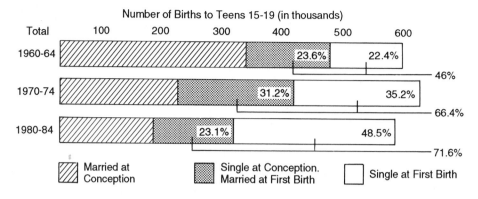

Number of Births to Teens 15-19 (in thousands)

**FIGURE 22–3.** Percentage of first-born babies conceived out of wedlock by year of baby's birth and mother's marital status.

*Source:* "Out of wedlock births, premarital pregnancies, and their effect on family formation and dissolutions" by M. O'Connell and C. Rogers. *Family Planning Perspectives*, 16, p. 159 (1984), The Alan Guttmacher Institute. Reprinted by permission.

## United States Rates Compared with Those of Other Developed Countries

Compared with Europe, Australia, Canada, New Zealand, and Japan, the United States has the highest pregnancy, abortion, and birth rates for women aged 15 to 17 years (Tietze & Henshaw, 1986). The pregnancy rate of this age group is over twice that of Canada, England, and Wales and over ten times that of the Netherlands. The most striking contrast is among the youngest teenagers: American girls under age 15 are at least five times more likely to give birth than young adolescents in any other country for which data are available (Hayes, 1987).

For women aged 15 to 19 years, pregnancy, abortion, and birth rates in the United States are among the highest in the world (Henshaw, Kenney, Somberg, & Van Vort, 1989). Birth rates in developed countries (except for Czechoslovakia and Hungary) range from 50 percent to 12 percent of the United States rate. Recent population studies have also shown that adolescent birth rates are declining more rapidly in most developed countries than in the United States (United Nations Adolescent Reproductive Behavior, 1988). The United States abortion rate in 1983 for this age cohort was the highest of any developed country and more than twice that of any published rate.

## Determinants of Early Sexual Behavior

Teenage pregnancy is a health-related behavior that must be considered within the context of early sexual activity. The likelihood that an adolescent will be sexually active outside of marriage depends on a number of factors, including sex, race or ethnicity, age, and socioeconomic status.

*Sex Differences and Parental Communication.* Some studies have found that parental communication about sexuality has no effect on adolescents' behavior (Cvetkovich & Grote, 1983; Furstenberg et al., 1984; Kahn, 1984). There have also been some findings where parental communication has had an effect, but they are qualified by the sex of the teenager. For sons, communication about sexuality with the mother was found to be associated with less sexual activity, whereas communication with the father was associated with greater sexual activity (Kahn, 1984). A study by the Office of Adolescent Pregnancy Prevention found no relationship between frequency of communication about sexuality and the subsequent sexual activity of the daughter.

A national survey of young adults found that 64 percent of the males were sexually active by age 18 compared with 44 percent of the females (Hayes, 1987).

*Race and Ethnicity.*   Data for the period 1970 to 1982 indicated that black adolescents, compared with white adolescents, had significantly higher levels of sexual intercourse outside of marriage (Hayes, 1987). Between 1979 and 1982, however, levels of sexual activity among black girls declined substantially, whereas they increased in white girls. In 1983, the 13 percent difference between blacks and whites was the lowest since data were made available and was significantly less than the 31 percent difference reported in 1976 (Hayes, 1987).

Similar data are not available for Hispanic teenagers, but estimates from the 1982 National Survey of Family Growth indicate that levels of premarital sexual activity among Hispanic teenagers are closer to the levels for whites than to those for blacks.

*Age.*   Data from the 1982 National Longitudinal Survey of Youth (Zelnik & Shah, 1983) showed that 17 percent of boys and 6 percent of girls under the age of 15 reported having had intercourse. About one third of boys who were younger than 15 years old when they became sexually active used contraception at first intercourse compared with almost 60 percent of those who were older than 18 when they initiated sexual activity. Race differences in the proportion who are sexually active are especially pronounced among the younger teenagers. At age 15 years, 42 percent of blacks reported that they were sexually active compared with 12 percent of whites and 19 percent of Hispanics (Hayes, 1987).

*Socioeconomic Status and Mother's Educational Level.*   Data from the 1982 National Longitudinal Survey of Youth (Zelnik & Shah, 1983) indicate that lower socioeconomic status is associated with the initiation of sexual activity at earlier ages. When young people are differentiated by their mother's educational attainment, clear differences emerge by race and sex. Teenagers with well-educated mothers are more likely to postpone initiation of sexual activity. Among boys, the percentage having had intercourse by age 18 increases from 56 to 62 to 72 percent, respectively, as the mother's education declines from a level beyond high school, to high school graduate, to dropout. Among girls, the comparable proportions are 34, 41, and 54 percent. Nevertheless, the incidence of premarital sex remains higher among blacks at all ages, even when maternal educational attainment is controlled (Hayes, 1987).

## Consequences of Becoming an Unmarried Teenage Mother

A substantial body of research now exists indicating that teenage mothers and their families are more likely to experience lower social and economic attainment and are at considerable developmental and health risks. The consequences are even greater for unmarried disadvantaged teens.

## Consequences for the Mother

*Poverty.* Teenage mothers are disproportionately poor and dependent on public assistance for their economic support. Their grants from Aid to Families with Dependent Children are also larger than women starting their families after 21 years of age because this population has a higher than average number of infants. (Burt, 1986). The majority of families require two wage earners to maintain a reasonable standard of living. Thus, single mothers are disadvantaged from the outset by having only one income source.

*Lack of Education.* A number of studies conclude that teenage mothers complete fewer years of school and are less likely to earn a high school diploma or attend college compared with those who delay motherhood until their twenties (Haggstrom et al., 1983; Moore & Hofferth, 1980; Mott & Marsiglio, 1985). Dropping out of school is common among teenage mothers. Not until the mid-1970s were schools required to provide programs of study for pregnant teens. Previously, schools had discriminated against such students on the basis of pregnancy. Recent findings from a 17-year follow-up study of teenage mothers found that those who were not themselves children of teenage mothers gained more than half of their educational attainment 6 or more years after the birth of their first child (Furstenberg, Brooks-Gunn, & Morgan, 1987).

*Health Risks for Teen and Infant.* Pregnant teenagers under age 15 are at increased risk of complications such as toxemia, anemia, and cesarean section. Their risk of maternal morbidity and mortality is 2.5 times that of pregnant women aged 20 to 24, and their infants are twice as likely to be premature or of low birth weight (Alan Guttmacher Institute, 1981).

*Marital Status.* The majority of adolescent marriages are unstable and end in divorce. Yet those teenage mothers who marry before rather than after the birth of their child may be less likely to separate from their husbands in later years (McLaughlin et al., 1986). In their 17-year follow-up, Furstenberg and coworkers (1987) found that three quarters of the sample teen mothers from Baltimore married, but a substantial proportion divorced. Other studies have found that remarriage after divorce is less likely among blacks than among whites.

*Employment and Income.* Working teenage mothers, particularly those who have several children who are close in age, are generally employed with low wages and less job satisfaction (Haggstrom & Morrison, 1979). But the differences in employment between teen and older mothers vary over time. At intervals of 1 year and 5 years after high school, teenage mothers are less likely to be working. At intervals of 11 years and 17 years after high school, teen mothers who is taking time out to raise children. Women with poorly paying jobs (such as teen mothers) also face difficulties in finding jobs that offer fringe benefits such as comprehensive health and dental coverage for themselves and their children (Moore & Burt, 1982).

## Consequences for the Children

*Lower Academic Achievement.* Findings indicate that children of teenage mothers score lower in academic achievement tests and that their retention in grade and teacher evaluation of their school performance are also negatively reflected. Whether these findings are related to the teen mother's lack of ability, motivation, discipline, encouragement, or support of her child is not known (Furstenberg et al., 1987; Moore, 1986).

*Emotional Development.*   Children of teenage mothers are characterized as socially impaired. Sons have been described as impulsive and overactive (Moore, 1986). Furstenberg and coworkers (1987) found a high incidence of school behavior problems such as suspension, running away, or violence toward others in the adolescent children of teen mothers.

*Increased Risk of Becoming a Teenage Parent.*   Moore (1986) found that white adolescents with teenage mothers show a greater risk of becoming teen parents. The work of Furstenberg and associates (1987) challenges this finding, given the wide diversity of outcomes they encountered in their 17-year follow-up study.

## Current Policies and Programs

The number and variety of interventions aimed at preventing teenage pregnancy and childbearing have grown dramatically over the past 15 years. Many have been promoted by the federal government, such as those implemented by the Office of Adolescent Pregnancy Prevention (Stahler, DuCette, & McBride, 1989). Others such as the Teen Parent Education and Employability Program (1986–1989) and those programs evaluated by JRB Associates, such as New Haven Young Mother Program, have been initiated by states and local communities. Still others have been developed as a result of investments by private foundations and philanthropic groups. Among these programs are Project Redirection, funded by Manpower Demonstration Research Corporation (Polit, Quint, & Riccio, 1988); Too Early Childbearing, funded by Charles Stewart Mott Foundation (Polit, 1986); and Five Model Program (JRB Associates, 1981).

The most troublesome finding is that few programs have proved successful (Polit, 1986; Polit et al., 1988; Stahler et al., 1989). Even more distressing is the finding that those that have been successful either in delaying first-time pregnancies among their clients, such as the Baltimore Self Center (Zabin, Hirsch, Smith, Street, & Hardy, 1986), or in delaying second-time pregnancies, such as the Teen-Tot program (O'Sullivan & Cone, 1986), are not maintained when they do not meet the primary goals of the institution despite positive evaluation. Both programs were very similar in that they offered on-site medical services, counseling, and education and dispensed contraceptives.

An extensive review of teen parent care programs found only three models (Elster et al., 1987; Olds, 1988; O'Sullivan, 1990) that demonstrated positive outcomes for the teen mother or her infant.

Elster's comprehensive care model provided medical, psychosocial, and nutritional services to pregnant adolescents, young mothers, and their infants. Follow-up at 12 months showed little difference in pregnancy outcomes, but at 12 months and 26 months the intervention group scored significantly higher on measures encompassing medical, psychosocial, and parenting events than did the comparison group.

Olds' model provided an intensive program of prenatal and postnatal nurse home visits for socially disadvantaged adolescents bearing first children. Follow-up during the first four years showed that the intervention group had a significant 82 percent increase in number of months of employment; a year longer interval between first and second births; and 43 percent fewer subsequent pregnancies though insignificant changes from the comparison group.

O'Sullivan's model, a cost-effective health care program for infants of first-time adolescent mothers, in addition to routine well-baby care provided innovative strategies designed to break the cycle of repeat pregnancies. These included rigorous follow-up when the young mother missed an appointment for well baby care; ongoing talks with the mother about her plans for returning to school and her use of family planning; and reinforcement of family planning through additional history taking from the mother during each well baby visit.

At 18-month follow-up, the repeat pregnancy rate was 12 percent in the intervention group and 28 percent in the control group ($P < .01$). Infants in the intervention group were more likely to be fully immunized (33 percent) than were those in the control group (18 percent) ($P < .02$). Although emergency room use for infant problems remained high for both groups, those in the intervention group who continued to attend clinic used the emergency room less often ($P < .03$).

These significant findings suggest that an innovative comprehensive health care program can be a cost-effective way to bring about better outcomes for both adolescent mothers and their infants.

Innovations in the O'Sullivan model extend the practice to include working with the teenage mother's mother and the teen's siblings between the ages of 11 to 17 years of age. Additional goals of the model include (1) increasing the number of teen mothers who return to school or work by helping them find day care for their infants after their first pregnancy, and (2) counseling the siblings of the teenage mothers, who are at twice the risk of becoming teen parents themselves, to delay their first pregnancy.

The newest waiting room innovations, in addition to the use of audiovisual tapes and film strips, are to include a star chart noting the program goals and each mother's progress toward being a model mother by delaying future pregnancies, returning to work or school, and having her infant immunized appropriately for age. A wall-sized zoning street map (with each home outlined) is now available to foster networking among the teens, who can become "neighbors" by seeing each other's map pins and noting each other's address.

After continued intensive follow-up and outreach for at least eight weeks after a missed appointment, more informal networking among the teens, and more praise for their progress in the program, the results suggest that a comprehensive health care program is one way to bring about better outcomes for both adolescent mothers and their infants.

## Implications of the Problem for Nursing in the 1990s

Presentation and/or modification of the negative outcomes of unplanned sexual activity is one of the most important areas of intervention for nurses and other health care providers in the 1990s.

In the United States during the past two decades, there has been no coherent policy toward adolescent pregnancy and childbearing. American teenagers receive conflicting messages about sexuality, sexual behavior, and sexual responsibility. Premarital sex, cohabitation, and nonmarital sexual relationships are common ways of life among the adults teenagers see and hear about, often including their own parents or the parents of peers. Yet they receive little open and informed advice about sexuality, contraception, or the harsh realities of early pregnancy and childbearing (Hayes, 1987).

Nurses and health care providers must campaign for a change in our nation's attitude toward sexuality. The problem is of such magnitude that we can no longer tolerate a "hands-off—this is a family issue"—policy. We would not hesitate to speak up if a child ran out into a busy street without looking, and yet children are engaging in unprotected sexual activity and no one is speaking up. Protecting children from the negative outcomes of unplanned sexual activity goes beyond the issue of family—it is a community and a public health issue as well.

There is intense debate over what would constitute effective solutions to the problem of teenage pregnancies, particularly because of conflicting moral, political, and social concerns.

Those who believe that parents should have the final authority and responsibility for their children under 18 years of age oppose any publicly funded program that addresses issues of premarital sexual activity, contraceptive advice, or counseling regarding options in pregnancy.

Those who believe that society's norms of sexual behavior have changed readily support such publicly funded programs. Others who advocate adoption as the only acceptable alternative to early parenthood lobby for more social service facilities. Finally, there are those who believe that teenage childbearing creates long-term stress that requires special programs, supports, and services to foster growth-promoting environments for both teens and their infants.

The role of abortion as a societal approach to teenage pregnancy is probably the most controversial issue of all. Regardless of individual beliefs, the differences in law and public policy among states mean that the issue of legal and safe abortion will continue to be debated throughout the 1990s.

The Center for Population Options filed an amicus brief in November, 1989, arguing that the laws in Ohio and Minnesota that require parental consent and notification "unduly burden" an adolescent's right to a safe and legal abortion (Senderowitz, 1990). The National Research Council (Hayes, 1987) panel had already concluded that there is no scientific basis for restricting the availability of abortion to adolescents. Moreover, some data have shown that requiring parental consent often causes an adolescent to delay an abortion, leading to second-trimester abortions and increased health risk. Yet it seems likely that programs that help adolescents make decisions about the resolution of an unintended pregnancy may become less accessible because of federal funding cutbacks.

Nursing must also be prepared to deal with the realities that face today's teenagers in the inner city:

- Many are the offspring of teenage mothers.
- The pregnant teen who looked to the father of her child for her support is usually abandoned by him.

- Many teenagers have neither a room of their own where they can escape from violence or drugs nor a sense of anything else they can call their own. A new baby is "their own."
- Many do not value education because success in school is not held in great esteem by their class.
- Because of the pervasiveness of the drug culture, many do not have their mothers available for family-supported role modeling. A startling finding is that the grandmothers are more heavily involved in the drug culture than are the teenage mothers under 17.
- Few teenage mothers view preventive health care, primary care, prenatal visits, and well baby visits as important to themselves and their children (Slap & Schwartz, 1989; Slap 1988).

## Violence as an Adolescent Health Problem

The problem of teenage violence differs fundamentally from that of teenage pregnancy. Pregnant adolescents are of concern primarily because of their age, unmarried state, and perceived and actual cost to society. This is cultural determination. In those societies in which childbearing occurs early, adolescent parenting is accepted and supported.

Violence is a much different concern. Becoming pregnant at age 15 is considered an imprudent but not illegal act. Inflicting injury on another at age 15 is considered both dangerous to society and a criminal act.

The psychodynamics of these two high-risk behaviors also differ (Blum, 1989; Jessor & Jessor, 1977). It should be noted, however, that violent teenagers are often sexually active and that pregnant teenagers, like other women, are at relatively high risk of being victims of violence (Adams-Hillard, 1985).

The differences between these two high-risk health behaviors must be clearly understood if health care professionals are to develop and implement appropriate interventions.

## Defining the Problem

Violence is a major adolescent health problem and a leading cause of adolescent death in the United States. Homicide accounts for 10 percent of mortality before age 24 (Centers for Disease Control, 1989). Among the United States population under age 18, four to five teens are murdered and three to four are arrested for murder every day.

Among those aged 15 to 24 years, mortality rates for homicide increased almost 300 percent between 1950 and 1980 (Blum, 1987). The rate for white males aged 15 to 19 years was 2.7 per 100,000 in 1959 and 10.0 per 100,000 in 1986 (United States Department of Health, Education, and Welfare, 1974; United States Department of Health and Human Services, 1988). Although rates declined slightly between

1980 and 1984 (O'Carroll, 1988), they are again climbing, and the increase is associated with increased use of cocaine and crack. In 1984, there were 3.584 deaths per 100,000 due to homicide in this age group.

Homicide represents only a small part of this adolescent health problem, as the ratio of violence-related injuries to death is greater than 100:1 (Rosenberg & Mercy, 1986). A statewide study in Massachusetts showed that 44.4 per 10,000 adolescents, aged 10 to 14 years, and 164.9 per 10,000 adolescents, aged 15 to 19 years, came to an emergency room for a violence-related injury in one year (Guyer, Leschoier, Gallagher, Hausman, & Azzara, 1989).

Violence is a common event in the lives of the nation's teenagers. In 1987 the National Adolescent Health Survey found that for the year 1986, 49 percent of boys and 28 percent of girls reported having been in at least one fight; 34 percent of respondents were physically threatened, and 14 percent were robbed. Thirteen percent were attacked at school and 16 percent were attacked outside of school. Twenty-three percent of the boys reported carrying a knife at least once, and 64 percent of the boys and 19 percent of the girls reported shooting a gun (Centers for Disease Control, 1989).

A second survey of an urban teenage population revealed similar rates to those found nationally for robbery and assault in general. Four percent of the teenagers reported having been shot, and 10 percent had been stabbed. Forty-two percent had witnessed a shooting, 24 percent a knifing, and 23 percent a murder (Gladstein & Slater, 1988).

Data from the National Crime Survey indicate that 1 in 13 boys and 1 in 28 girls between the ages of 12 and 15 were victimized by violence in 1985. These proportions increased by 22 percent for adolescents aged 16 to 19 years (United States Bureau of Justice Statistics, 1987).

At Harlem Hospital, after nearly 20 years of constant rates of child and adolescent gun trauma (Barlow, personal communication), emergency room cases of gun injury in those under age 19 tripled between 1986 and 1987, with a 10 percent increase in 1988. A similar pattern (doubling) has been found for 1987 versus 1988 in Philadelphia (Philadelphia Injury Prevention Program, personal communication).

## Determinants of Adolescent Violence

Rates of homicide and injuries attributable to violence increase sharply during adolescence (Guyer et al., 1989). Factors associated with this high-risk behavior include age, gender, race, socioeconomic status, family systems, and psychiatric and psychological problems.

*Age.*     Adolescents are a population at high risk for violence. The transition to adulthood involves not only rapid psychological and physiologic changes but also many developmental tasks that must be mastered. The behaviors associated with these tasks, e.g., individuation from family, development of sexual identity, and development of a moral and personal value system through experimentation, predispose teenagers to violence (Friedman, 1989). Adolescents are intensely self-conscious, particularly when subject to strong peer pressures and sexual tensions; they are also easily embarrassed, and a perceived insult can cause them to over-react. As separation from family grows and the desire for independence increases, an adolescent with an injured ego may lash out and inflict injury.

*Gender.* Two thirds of adolescent homicide victims are males (Centers for Disease Control, 1982). A similar proportion has been found for intentional injuries (Guyer et al., 1989). Lower rates for homicide and violence-related injuries among adolescent females may be due to differences in weapon-carrying behaviors and role modeling. However, as gender stereotypes continue to change in our society, we can expect to see the gap narrow between male and female rates for adolescent homicide and violent injuries.

*Race.* Homicide rates for black males, ages 10 to 14, are 3.7 times those for white males, and the rates for black males, ages 15 to 19, are 5.7 times those for white males (Centers for Disease Control, 1986). Homicide is the leading cause of death among black adolescents (Centers for Disease Control, 1985) and the third leading cause among white adolescents.

Nationwide data on homicide and violent injury are not available for Hispanics, but one study of homicide rates in five Southwestern states found that among males ages 15 to 19, Hispanics were at intermediate risk (27.4 deaths per 100,000) compared with whites (8.6 deaths per 100,000) and blacks (36.5 deaths per 100,000). Of the Hispanic homicide victims, 65.1 percent had been shot and 23.8 percent stabbed. Percentages for white victims were 58.75 percent and 17.5 percent; for black victims, 70.3 percent and 18.5 percent, respectively (Centers for Disease Control, 1986).

Although violence is commonly perceived as being inter-racial in nature, recent analyses of national crime and homicide data indicate that 80 percent of homicides occur between individuals of the same race (Centers for Disease Control, 1982).

*Socioeconomic Status.* Homicide rates and risk of violent deaths are higher among populations at or below the poverty level. The link between poverty and homicide has been discussed in several recent studies (Loftin & Parker, 1985; Williams, 1984). In his study of poverty and homicide in Detroit for the period from 1926 to 1978, McDowall (1986) found that increases in the level of poverty paralleled increases in homicide rates.

It is unclear whether crowding, hopelessness, racial anger, unemployment, urban life, or other stresses are the key factors that put economically disadvantaged adolescents at increased risk of death or injury caused by violence.

*Family Factors.* "Love deprivation" (Walsh & Beyer, 1987) and abuse as a child (Lewis et al., 1989; Straus, 1979; Widom, 1989) have been associated with criminal violence and domestic abuse at a later age. However, no studies to date have examined whether noncriminal violent behavior in a child's home is a predictor of violent behavior later in adolescence.

Some studies, based on children's responses to television violence, have suggested that violence is a learned behavior (Liebert, 1986; Roscoe & Callahan, 1985; Strasburger, 1989), but other work has been contradictory (Singer, 1989). Several studies have examined the immediate responses of children to violent events (Payton

& Krocker-Tuskan, 1988; Pynoos & Nader, 1988). They have found a "post-traumatic stress disorder," with disturbances in aggression and sexuality, alterations in the sense of security and vulnerability, challenged self-esteem, stress in family and peer relationships, and changes in future orientation. Longer follow-up is necessary to confirm or measure the impact of witnessed violence in childhood on adolescent behavior.

*Psychiatric and Physiologic Disorders.*   Several studies have found that those who commit homicides often have serious brain disorders (Bell, 1986; Kwentus et al., 1985; Lishman, 1973) or a history of congenital problems (Kandel et al., 1989). Bell (1986) has suggested a link between physical brain disease and violence, whereas others have associated serious psychiatric disorders with aggression and delinquency (Lewis et al., 1989; Taylor & Brooks-Gunn, 1984).

Kashini and colleagues (1987), in interviews with 150 adolescents ages 14 to 16, found that those with Diagnostic and Statistical Manual of Mental Disorders or DSM-III–defined psychiatric diagnoses (18.7 percent) were more likely to use physical violence and verbal aggression in resolving conflicts. They were also more likely to have been abused as children.

To date, there have been no studies of the relationship of psychological problems such as depression to violent behavior in adolescence. And no data are available on the incidence of psychological/neurologic problems among adolescent victims of injuries due to violence.

*Drugs and Alcohol.*   Research with adult substance users has shown an association between alcohol and drugs and crime (Collins & Schlanger, 1988; Wish & Johnson, 1986), but little is known specifically about adolescents (Dembo et al., 1987). The adult literature supports the association of violence and substance abuse, based on the assumption that alcohol and drugs loosen inhibitions and increase aggressive behavior. The lay press has widely reported the rapid increase in cocaine use and its association with violence (Moore, 1988). However, workers in the field are careful to distinguish between drug *use* and drug *trading*. Anecdotal information indicates that illegal drug trading increases the likelihood of violent injury.

## Preventing Teenage Violence: Whose Problem Is It?

The statistics on adolescent homicides are staggering, and yet we have few hard data on adolescent rates in violent injuries. The reason is that the problem of violence has long been considered the domain of criminal justice and mental health professionals. Each of these disciplines approaches the problem of violence in a different way.

The criminal justice system seeks to punish or rehabilitate the perpetrator (Currie, 1985) and defines a case of violence as one in which a law is broken and a crime is committed. For example, criminal justice professionals become involved in cases of domestic violence and child abuse only when injuries are reported and charges are pressed. As a result, the focus of the criminal justice system has been on the threat of force and use of coercion rather than on the outcomes of force and injury.

The literature in criminology reflects this focus through its emphasis on recidivism, deterrence, and retaliation.

The mental health profession seeks to understand the psychodynamic phenomena associated with antisocial behavior and to identify appropriate behaviors. Traditionally, mental health professionals have attempted to define violence in terms of aggressiveness and psychopathy. More recently, the profession has begun to explore the emotional effect of violence on victims. There is also a growing literature on the impact of violence in childhood on child imagery and behavior (Kratcoski, 1985), but the primary interest continues to be the prediction of which children are more likely to be violent as adults (Lewis et al., 1989; Widom, 1989).

The health care profession has come rather late to the study of violence. Traditionally, health care professionals have been concerned with the effects of violence rather than with the threat or psychology of violent behavior. It is only within the past 15 years that the health care profession has begun to explore its role in the field of adolescent violence.

## The Role of Health Care Professionals

For adolescents with self-inflicted injuries, we have clear protocols; we know the right questions to ask, and school systems, emergency rooms, mental health providers, and human service workers know how to respond.

But for the thousands of teenagers who are being injured by the violence of others each day or are inflicting injuries on others, we have no clear protocols, no right questions, no ready responses. For example, those of us in acute care settings question teenagers about the cause of an injury only when it is their chief complaint, perhaps because we would not know what to do for these adolescents once our question was answered.

A review of the literature from 1983 to 1989 identified only four articles with suggestions for violence prevention/intervention strategies. Each focused on a different professional group: public health (Spivak, Prothrow-Stith, & Hausman, 1988); medicine (Stringham & Weitzman, 1989); mental health (Bell, 1987); and nursing (Newell-Withrow, 1987). The suggested strategies included public health education, outreach, counseling, parent education, and changes in societal acceptance of violence. Only Newell-Withrow suggested a developmental approach to the problem of violence. Of the strategies suggested, none has the rigor of a protocol and none has been evaluated.

Nor do we have the tools to measure violence (other than after an injury has occurred), to predict violence, to teach about violence, or to raise public awareness of violence.

Violence in America has become a daily phenomenon: one that we see on television and read about in the newspapers and one that our children witness, experience, and learn. The alarming rate of violence-related injuries among adolescents will not decline until the patterns of violent behavior are broken. These patterns will not be broken unless there is rigorous research, consistent application of research findings, and public pressure for social change. In each of these tasks, nursing has a critical role. We must play our role exceedingly well if the problem of adolescent violent behavior is to be solved.

## Improved Life Chances for Adolescents

Improving life chances for teenagers must begin in the preteen years rather than in adolescence. Risk-taking and experimentation during the teen years are considered normal behaviors because they help adolescents achieve independence, identity, and maturity. Many adolescents, however, have a sense of invulnerability to the consequences of their behavior (Blum, 1987).

Nurses must, therefore, begin to develop models for parents, grandparents, teachers, troop leaders, and others that give concrete example of what to say to young children regarding sexuality and violent behavior. Nurses must also be aware of the determinants of health-related behaviors so that they may counsel preteens and give them appropriate guidance or protect themselves from the negative outcomes of sexual experimentation or violent behaviors.

Nurses must also take note of changes in public opinion. In 1987, the proportion who considered premarital sex to be wrong increased by 7 percent, the first increase since 1969 (Gallup, 1988). This change in public opinion is likely to have a ripple effect on funding policies such as AFDC-WIC (Aid to Families with Dependent Children—Women, Infants, Children).

When primary prevention programs fail, nurses must be prepared to offer support, education, and rehabilitation to the pregnant teenager, the teenage perpetrator of violence, and the teenage victim of violence. These special nursing initiatives must include continuity of outreach and follow-up. Nurses must also be advocates for these troubled teens within the health, education, and human services systems, government funding agencies, and policy planning boards at the local, state, and national levels.

A generation is at risk. The nation cannot afford to fail them.

REFERENCES

Adams, G.R., Montemayor, R., & Gullotta, T.P. (1989). *Advances in adolescent development: Biology of adolescent behavior and development.* Newbury Park, CA: Sage Publications.
Adams-Hillard, P.J. (1985). Physical abuse in pregnancy. *Obstetrics and Gynecology, 66,* 185–190.
Alan Guttmacher Institute (1981). *Teenage pregnancy: The problem that hasn't gone away.* New York: Alan Guttmacher Institute.
Attie, I., & Brooks-Gunn, J. (1987). Weight-related concerns in women: A response to or a cause of stress? In R.C. Barnett, L. Biener, & G.K. Baruch (Eds.), *Gender and stress* (pp. 218–254). New York: Free Press.
Attie, I., & Brooks-Gunn, J. (1989). The development of eating problems in adolescent girls: A longitudinal study. *Developmental Psychology, 25*(1), 70–79.

Attie, I., Brooks-Gunn, J., & Petersen, A.C. (1989). The emergence of eating problems: A developmental perspective. In M. Lewis & S. Miller (Eds.), *Handbook of developmental psychopathology*. New York: Plenum Publishing Corporation.

Bachman, J.G., Johnston, L.D., O'Malley, P.M., & Humphrey, R.H. (1988). Explaining the recent decline in marijuana use: Differentiating the effects of perceived risks, disapproval, and general lifestyle factors. *Journal of Health and Social Behavior*, *1*(29), 92–112.

Baydar, N., Brooks-Gunn, J., & Warren, M.P. (1990). *Determinants of depressive symptoms in adolescent girls: A four-year longitudinal study*. Manuscript submitted for publication.

Bell, C.C. (1986). Coma and the etiology of violence, Part 1. *Journal of the National Medical Association*, *78*, 1167–1176.

Bell, C.C. (1987). Preventive strategies for dealing with violence among blacks. *Community Mental Health Journal*, *23*, 217–228.

Blum, R. (1986). Developing with disabilities in early adolescence. *Early adolescent transitions: An interdisciplinary symposium*. Charleston, SC.

Blum, R. (1987). Contemporary threats to adolescent health in the United States. *Journal of the American Medical Association*, *257*, 3390–3395.

Blum, R. (1989). Executive summary. *Journal of Adolescent Health Care*, *11*, 86–90.

Brooks-Gunn, J. (1990). *Why do young adolescents have difficulty adhering to health regimes?* Manuscript to be published.

Brooks-Gunn, J., & Furstenberg, F.F. Jr. (1990). Coming of age in the year of AIDS: Sexual and contraceptive decisions. *Milbank Quarterly*, *68*(suppl. 1): 59–84.

Brooks-Gunn, J., & Petersen, A.C. (Eds.) (1983). *Girls at puberty: Biological and psychosocial perspectives*. New York: Plenum Press.

Brooks-Gunn, J., & Petersen, A.C. (Eds.) (1991, April). Special issue: The emergence of depression in adolescence. *Journal of Youth and Adolescence*, *20*(2).

Brooks-Gunn, J., Petersen, A.C., & Eichorn, D. (Eds.) (1985). Special issue: Time of maturation and psychosocial functioning in adolescence. *Journal of Youth and Adolescence*, *14* (3–4).

Brooks-Gunn, J., & Zahaykevich, M. (1989). Parent-child relationships in early adolescence: A developmental perspective. In K. Kreppner & R.M. Lerner (Eds.), *Family systems and life-span development* (pp. 223–246). Hillsdale, NJ: Erlbaum.

Bureau of the Census (1983). *Marital status and living arrangements*. Current Population Reports. (Series p. 20, No. 389.) Washington, DC: Bureau of the Census.

Burt, M. (1986). *Estimates of public costs for teenage childbearing*. Unpublished paper prepared for the Center for Population Options, Washington, DC.

Cairns, R.B., Cairns, B.D., Neckerman, H.J., Ferguson, L.L., & Gariepy, J.L. (1989). Growth and aggression: 1. Childhood to early adolescence. *Developmental Psychology*, *2*(25), 320–330.

Centers for Disease Control (1982). Homicide—United States. *Morbidity and Mortality Weekly Reports*, *31*, 599–602.

Centers for Disease Control (1985). Homicide among young black males: United States, 1970 to 1983. *Morbidity and Mortality Weekly Reports*, *32*, 629–633.

Centers for Disease Control (1986). *Homicide surveillance: High-risk racial and ethnic groups—blacks and Hispanics, 1970–1983*. Atlanta: Centers for Disease Control.

Centers for Disease Control (1989). Results from the national adolescent health survey. *Morbidity and Mortality Weekly Reports*, *38*, 147–150.

Collins, J.J., & Schlenger, W.E. (1988). Acute and chronic effects of alcohol use on violence. *Journal of Studies on Alcohol*, *9*, 516–521.

Cvetkovich, C., & Grote, B. (1983). Adolescent development and teenage fertility. In W. Byrne and J. Fisher (Eds.), *Adolescents, sex and contraception*. Hillsdale, NJ: Lawrence Erlbaum.

Currie, E. (1985). *Confronting crime: An American challenge*. New York: Pantheon Books.

Damon, W., & Hart, D. (1982). The development of self-understanding from infancy through adolescence. *Child Development, 53*, 841–864.

Dembo, R., Washburn, M., Wish, E.D., Schmeidler, J., Getreu, A., Berry, E., Williams, L., & Blount, W.R. (1987). Further examination of the association between heavy marijuana use and crime among youths entering juvenile detention center. *Journal of Psychoactive Drugs, 19*, 361–373.

Elster, A.B., Lamb, M.E., Tavare, J., & Ralston, C.W. (1987). The medical and psychosocial impact of comprehensive care on adolescent pregnancy and parenthood. *Journal of the American Medical Association, 258*, 1187–1192.

Feldman, S.D., & Elliott, G. (Eds.) (1990). *At the threshold: The developing adolescent*. Cambridge: Harvard University Press.

Friedman, H.L. (1989). The health of adolescents: Beliefs and behavior. *Social Science and Medicine, 29*, 309–315.

Furstenberg, F.F., Brooks-Gunn, J., & Morgan, S.P. (1987). *Adolescent mothers in later life*. Cambridge: Cambridge University Press.

Furstenberg, F.F., Herceg-Baron, R., Shea, J., & Webb, D. (1984). Family communications and teenagers' contraceptive use. *Family Planning Perspectives, 16*(4), 163–170.

Gallup, G., Jr. (1988). The Gallup Poll: Public Opinion, 1987. Wilmington, DE: Scholarly Resources, Inc.

Gladstein, J., & Slater, E.J. (1988). Inner city teenagers' exposure to violence: A prevalence study. *Maryland Medical Journal, 37*, 951–954.

Greenberger, E., Steinberg, L., Vaux, A., & McAuliffe, S. (1980). Adolescents who work: Effects of part-time employment on family and peer relations. *Journal of Youth and Adolescence, 9*, 189–202.

Gunnar, M.R., & Collins, W.A. (Eds.) (1988). *Transitions in adolescence: Minnesota symposia on child psychology* (Vol. 21). Hillsdale, NJ: Erlbaum.

Guyer, B., Leschoier, I., Gallagher, S.S., Hausman, A.J., & Azzara, C.V. (1989). Intentional injuries among Massachusetts children and adolescents. *New England Journal of Medicine, 321*, 1584–1588.

Haggstrom, G.W., Kanouse, D.E., & Morrison, P.A. (1983). *Accounting for the educational shortfalls of young mothers*. Unpublished manuscript. Santa Monica, CA: RAND Corporation.

Haggstrom, G.W., & Morrison, P.A. (1979). *Consequences of parenthood in late adolescence: Findings from the national longitudinal study of high school seniors*. Santa Monica, CA: The RAND Corporation.

Harter, S. (in press). Adolescent self and identity development. In S. Feldman & G. Elliott (Eds.), *At the threshold: The developing adolescent*. Cambridge: Harvard University Press.

Hayes, C.D. (Ed). (1987). Risking the future. *Adolescent Sexuality, Pregnancy and Childbearing Volume 1*. Washington, DC: National Academy Press.

Henshaw, S.K., Kenney, A.M., Somberg, D., & Van Vort, J. (1989). *Teenage Pregnancy in the United States*. New York: The Alan Guttmacher Institute.

Hofferth, S.L., & Hayes, C.D. (Eds.) (1987). *Risking the future: Adolescent sexuality, pregnancy, and childbearing, Volume II*. Washington, DC: National Academy of Sciences Press.

Irwin, C.E., & Millstein, S.G. (1991). Risk-taking behaviors during adolescence. In R.M.

Lerner, A.C. Petersen, & J. Brooks-Gunn (Eds.), *Encyclopedia of adolescence*. New York: Garland Press.

Jessor, R., & Jessor, S. (1977). *Problem behavior and psychosocial development: A longitudinal study of youth*. New York: Academic Press.

Johnson, S.B., Silverstein, J., Rosenbloom, A., Carter, R., & Cunningham, W. (1986). Assessing daily management in childhood diabetes. *Health Psychology, 6*(5), 545–564.

Jones, E., Forrest, J.D., Henshaw, S.K., Silverman, J., & Torres, A. (1988). Unintended pregnancy, contraceptive practice and family planning services in developed countries. *Family Planning Perspectives, 2*(20), 53–67.

JRB Associates (1981). Final report on national study of teenage pregnancy. McLean, VA: JRB Associates.

Kahn, J.R. (1984). *Familial communications and adolescent sexual behavior*. Final report to Office of Adolescent Pregnancy Prevention. Office Population Affairs. Cambridge: American Institutes for Research.

Kandel, E., Brennan, P.A., Mednick, S.A., & Michelson, N.M. (1989). Minor physical anomalies and recidivistic adult violent criminal behavior. *Acta Psychiatrica Scandinavica, 79*, 103–107.

Kashini, J.H., Beck, N.C., Hoeper, E.W., Fallahi, C., Corcoran, C.M., McAllister, J.A., Rosenberg, T.K., & Reid, J.C. (1987). Psychiatric disorders in a community sample of adolescents. *American Journal of Psychiatry, 144*, 584–589.

Kratcoski, P.C. (1985). Youth violence directed toward significant others. *Journal of Adolescence, 8*, 145–157.

Kwentus, J.A., Hart, R.P., Peck, E.T., & Kornstein, S. (1985). Psychiatric complications of closed head trauma. *Psychosomatics, 26*(1), 8–17.

Lerner, R.M., & Foch, T.T. (Eds.) (1987). *Biological-psychosocial interactions in early adolescence: A life-span perspective*. Hillsdale, NJ: Erlbaum.

Lerner, R.M., Petersen, A.C., & Brooks-Gunn, J. (1991). *Encyclopedia of adolescence*. New York: Garland Press.

Levine, M.D. (1988). Transitional capacities overdue or exceeded: The phenomenology of academic underachievement in early adolescence. In M.D. Levine & E.R. McAnarney (Eds.), *Early adolescent transition* (pp. 193–208). Lexington, MA: Lexington Books.

Lewis, D.O., Lovely, R., Yeager, C., & Della-Femina, D. (1989). Toward a theory of the genesis of violence: A follow-up study of delinquents. *Journal of the American Academy of Child and Adolescent Psychiatry, 28*, 431–436.

Liebert, R.M. (1986). Effect of television on children and adolescents. *Journal of Developmental Behavior in Pediatrics, 7*, 43–48.

Lishman, W.A. (1973). The psychiatric sequelae of head injury: A review. *Psychological Medicine, 3*, 304–318.

Loftin, C., & Parker, R.N. (1985). An errors-in-variable model of the effect of poverty on urban homicide rates. *Criminology, 23*, 269–287.

McDowall, D. (1986). Poverty and homicide in Detroit, 1926–1978. *Victims and Violence, 1*(1), 23–34.

McLaughlin, S.D., Grady, W.R., Billy, J.O.G., Landale, N.S., & Winges, L.D. (1986). The effects of the sequencing of marriage and first birth during adolescence. *Family Planning Perspectives, 18*, 12–18.

Moore, K.A. (1986). *Children of teen parents: Heterogeneity of outcomes*. Final report to the National Institute of Child Health and Human Development. Washington, DC: Child Trends.

Moore, T. (1988, August). The black-on-black crime plague. *U.S. News & World Report,* pp. 48–55.

Moore, K.A., & Burt, M.R. (1982). *Private crisis, public cost: Policy perspectives on teenage childbearing.* Washington, DC: Urban Institute.

Moore, K.A., & Hofferth, S.L. (1980). Factors affecting early family formation: A path model. *Population and Environment, 3,* 73–98.

Mott, F.L., & Marsiglio, W. (1985). Early childbearing and completion of high school. *Family Planning Perspectives, 17,* 234–237.

National Center for Health Statistics (1988). Advance report on final natality statistics—1986. *Monthly Vital Statistics Report, 3* (3, Suppl.).

Newell-Withrow, C. (1987). Observations of children, youth, violence. *Journal of Pediatric Health Care, 1,* 77–84.

O'Carroll, P.W. (1988). *Homicide among black males 15–24 years of age, 1970–1984.* Centers for Disease Control Surveillance Summaries, *Morbidity and Mortality Weekly Reports, 37*(SS-1), 53–60.

O'Connell, M., & Rogers, C.C. (1984). Out of wedlock births, premarital pregnancies and their effect on family formation and dissolutions. *Family Planning Perspectives, 16*(4), 157–162.

Olds, D.L., Henderson, C.R., Tatelbaum, R., & Chamberlin, R. (1988). Improving the life-course development of socially disadvantaged mothers: A randomized trial of nurse home visitation. *American Journal of Public Health, 78*(1), 1436–1445.

O'Sullivan, A.L. (1990). Tertiary prevention with adolescent mothers: Rehabilitation after first pregnancy. In S. Humenick (Ed.), *Adolescent pregnancy: Nursing perspectives and prevention* (pp. 1–23). White Plains, NY: March of Dimes.

O'Sullivan, A.L., & Cone, K.L. (1986). A special health care program for adolescent mothers and their infants. *American Journal of Diseases of Children, 140*(4), 295.

Paikoff, R.L., & Brooks-Gunn, J. (in press). Taking fewer chances: Teenage pregnancy prevention programs. *American Psychologist.*

Payton, J.B., & Krocker-Tuskan, M. (1988). Children's reactions to loss of parent through violence. *Journal of the American Academy of Child and Adolescent Psychiatry, 27*(5), 563–566.

Petersen, A.C., Sarigiani, P.A., & Kennedy, R.E. (1991, April). Adolescent depression: Why more girls? [Special issue]. *Journal of Youth and Adolescence, 20*(2), 247–271.

Polit, D.F. (1986). *Comprehensive programs for pregnant parenting teenagers: An assessment.* Unpublished paper. Jefferson City, MO: Humanalysis.

Polit, D.F., Quint, J.C., & Riccio, J.A. (1988). *Challenge of serving teenage mothers—lessons from project redirections.* New York: Manpower Demonstration Research.

Pynoos, R.S., & Nader, K. (1988). Children who witness the sexual assaults of their mothers. *Journal of the American Academy of Child and Adolescent Psychiatry, 27,* 567–572.

Robins, L.N. (1974). *Deviant children grown up: A sociological and psychiatric study of sociopathic personality.* (Reprinted from Baltimore: Williams & Wilkins.) Huntington, NY: Robert E. Krieger Publishing.

Roscoe, B., & Callahan, J.E. (1985). Adolescents' self-report of violence in families and dating relations. *Adolescence, 20,* 545–553.

Rosenberg, M.L., & Mercy, J.A. (1986). Homicide: Epidemiologic analysis at the national level. *Bulletin of the New York Academy of Medicine, 62,* 376–399.

Senderowitz, J. (1990). CPO files amicus brief with supreme court. *Options, 2,* 3.

Simmons, R.G., & Blyth, D.A. (1987). *Moving into adolescence: The impact of pubertal change and school context.* New York: Adline De Gruyter.

Simmons, R.G., Burgeson, R., & Reef, M.J. (1988). Cumulative change at entry to adolescence. In M. Gunnar & W.A. Collins (Eds.), *Development during transition to adolescence: Minnesota symposia on child psychology, 21,* 123–150. Hillsdale, NJ: Erlbaum.

Singer, D.G. (1989). Children, adolescents, and television—1989: I. Television violence: A critique. *Pediatrics, 83,* 445–446.

Slap, G.B. (1988, November 1). The periodic health examination and adolescent pregnancy: 1988. *Annals of Internal Medicine, 109*(9), 692–694.

Slap, G.B., & Schwartz, J.S. (1989, July). Risk factors for low birth weight to adolescent mothers. *Journal of Adolescent Health Care, 10*(4), 267–274.

Smetana, J.G. (1988). Concepts of self and social convention: Adolescents' and parents' reasoning about hypothetical and actual family conflicts. In M. Gunnar & W.A. Collins (Eds.), *Development during transition to adolescence. Minnesota symposia on child psychology* (vol. 21, pp. 79–122). Hillsdale, NJ: Erlbaum.

Sonenstein, F.L., Pleck, J.H., & Ku, L.C. (1989). Sexual activity, condom use and AIDS awareness among adolescent males. *Family Planning Perspectives, 21*(4), 152–158.

Spivak, H., Prothrow-Stith, D., & Hausman, A.J. (1988). Dying is no accident: Adolescents, violence, and intentional injury. *Pediatric Clinics of North America, 35,* 1339–1347.

Stahler, G.J., Du Cette, J., & McBride, D. (1989). The evaluation component in adolescent pregnancy care project: Is it adequate? *Family Planning Perspectives, 21,* 123–126.

Steinberg, L.D. (1987). The impact of puberty on family relations: Effects of pubertal status and pubertal timing. *Developmental Psychology, 23,* 451–460.

Strasburger, V.C. (1989, March). Children, adolescents, and television—1989: II. The role of pediatricians. *Pediatrics, 83*(3), 446–448.

Straus, M.A. (1979). Measuring intrafamily conflict and violence: The conflict tactics (CT) scales. *Journal of Marriage and the Family, 41,* 75–81.

Stringham, P., & Weitzman, M. (1989). Violence counseling in the routine health care of adolescents. *Journal of Adolescent Health Care, 9,* 389–393.

Tamar, L. (1988, March). 500,000 a year; Fewer teen mothers but more are unmarried. *New York Times,* p. 6.

Taylor, P.J., & Brooks-Gunn, J. (1984). Violence and psychosis, I. Risk of violence among psychotic men. *British Medical Journal, 288,* 1945–1949.

*Teen parent education and employability program* (1986–1989). Philadelphia: Southeastern Pennsylvania Private Industry Council.

Tietze, C., & Henshaw, S.K. (1986). *Induced abortion: A world review.* New York: Alan Guttmacher Institute.

United Nations Adolescent Reproductive Behavior (1988). Evidence from developed countries. *Population Studies, 1*(109).

United States Bureau of Justice Statistics (1987). *Criminal victimization in the United States.* Washington, DC: U.S. Department of Justice.

United States Department of Health, Education, and Welfare (1974). *National vital statistics system: Mortality trends for leading causes of death, United States, 1959–1969.* (Department of Health, Education, and Welfare Publication No. HRA 74-1853:51.) Washington, DC: U.S. Government Printing Office.

United States Department of Health and Human Services (1988). *Vital statistics of the U.S., 1986.* (Department of Health and Human Services Publication No. Public Health Services 88-1122:32.) Washington, DC: U.S. Government Printing Office.

Walsh, A., & Beyer, J.A. (1987). Violent crime, sociopathy and love deprivation among adolescent delinquents. *Adolescent, 22,* 705–717.

Widom, C.S. (1989). The cycle of violence. *Science, 224,* 160–166.

Williams, K.R. (1984). Economic sources of homicide: Reestimating the effect of poverty and inequality. *American Sociology Review, 49,* 283–289.

Wish, E., & Johnson, B.D. (1986). The impact of substance abuse on criminal careers. In A. Blumstein, J. Cohen, J.A. Roth, & C.A. Visher (Eds.), *Criminal careers and career criminals* (pp. 52–88). Washington, DC: National Academy Press.

Zabin, L.S., Hirsch, M.B., Smith, E.A., Street, R., & Hardy, J.B. (1986). Evaluation of a pregnancy prevention program for urban teenagers. *Family Planning Perspectives, 18,* 119–126.

Zelnick, M., & Shah, F.K. (1983). First intercourse among young Americans. *Family Planning Perspectives, 15*(3), 64–73.

# Chapter 23

# Victims of Rape and Sexual Abuse

ANN W. BURGESS
CAROL R. HARTMAN

He came in through the window, through Uncle Bobby's window. I thought it was Uncle Bobby coming home. The man hit me and told me to shut up. I don't want to talk about it any more.

This statement by a four-year-old girl was made on behalf of her mother who was being evaluated for the impact of a forcible rape. The rape occurred in the early evening. The mother had fallen asleep on the couch watching the evening news, and the child was playing in her bedroom. Two assailants had entered through a back window of a first floor apartment. The child was hit, ordered to be quiet, and forced to witness the robbery, rape, and beating of her mother.

## The Problem of Rape

Rape and abuse affect the lives of thousands of people each year. Contrary to popular belief, they are not uncommon events. Since 1977, the rate of forcible rape has increased by 21 percent, which is the largest increase in all violent crimes. The 1988 Federal Bureau of Investigation Uniform Crime Report cites 92,486 cases of forcible rape of females of consenting age (Federal Bureau of Investigation, 1988). And although an estimated 250,000 cases of child sexual abuse are reported annually (Finkelhor, 1987), many sexually abusive acts are never reported (Fuller & Bartucci, 1988).

There are also statistics on the subject of "hidden rape." Mary Koss, who studied the incidence and prevalence of sexual aggression and victimization on college campuses, argues that because of the inadequacies in the methods used to measure sexual assault, national crime statistics, criminal victimization studies, and conviction or incarceration rates fail to reflect the true scope of rape (Koss, 1985).

Historically, the realization of rape as a violent act committed in a sexual context signaled the beginning of national efforts to address the problems inherent in this traumatic life event (Largen, 1985). Prior to the resurgence of the women's movement, avoidance and silence dominated professional and societal reactions to victims of rape. Given this pattern, the first efforts of feminist women's groups and professionals were to raise the awareness of others that rape was a criminal act not desired by the victim. Furthermore, the victim was not responsible for the behavior and choices of the predator. The rapist was acting out of his own intentions and patterns of belief. Previously, the act of rape and victim response were strongly linked to social discrimination and oppression surrounding the sex role attributes ascribed to women.

Compared with other types of serious crime, rape has a number of unique characteristics. First, it is difficult to know how frequently rape occurs because of the low reporting rate for this crime. Accurate estimates of the incidence and prevalence of rape are not readily available because the majority of rape victims do not report the crime to the police, do not receive medical attention from hospitals, or do not seek help from service agencies such as rape crisis centers (Kilpatrick et al., 1985a). Second, unlike the case in other crimes, there is considerable variation in what constitutes a "real" rape (Holmstrom & Burgess, 1978; Sanders, 1980; Williams, 1984). Law enforcement agents and child protective service workers use the term "unfounded" when there is insufficient evidence or to dismiss the complaints of a "nonbelievable" victim. Third, rape is the only serious crime in which victims are generally held responsible for their own assault. It is believed by many that people like to be overpowered sexually, that women say "no" but mean "yes," and that women issue false reports regarding rape to "save face," "get even," or conceal pregnancy (Burt, 1980). Fourth, rape is treated distinctively in the courtroom, for example, as a property crime (Brownmiller, 1975; Sanders, 1980). Further, rules of evidence have been unique and stringent (e.g., signs of resistance required as a proof of nonconsent, the need for third-party corroboration). Fifth, rape and sexual abuse are selectively perpetrated by the male segment of the population and are selectively borne by the female segment of the population. And sixth, rape instills fear in women and serves to limit their freedom by placing constraints on their activities (Griffin, 1971; Riger & Gordon, 1988; Warr, 1985).

## Definitions

Part of the problem inherent in understanding rape and sexual assault is derived from an equivocal definition. From a legal perspective, rape is a criminal act. Although there are variations among states, rape, as legally defined, generally refers to forced sexual penetration of a victim by an offender who is not the victim's spouse. Because the legal definition of forcible rape is so restrictive, sexual assault has been used to cover a wider range of sexual crimes, including attempted rape, indecent assault and battery, and sodomy. Most statutes define as illegal any type of sexual behavior with a child, irrespective of the use of force or threat of force or consent of the victim. Statutory rape may also be charged in those cases in which the victim is legally unable to give consent by virtue of mental deficiency, psychosis, or altered state of consciousness induced by sleep, drugs, illness, or intoxication.

## Causes of Rape

Theories used to explain rape focus on factors inherent in the victim, society, and the rapist.

### Victim Factors

The underlying belief of the victim model is that rape is a primarily sexual act and that the victim in some way provoked the offender. That is, for the offender to have been sexually aroused, something in the victim must have triggered this arousal. Thus, statements attributing seductive or sexual behaviors or dress or life-style to the victim are commonly heard when this model prevails. Brownmiller (1975) outlined common beliefs perpetuated by society, such as "all women want to be raped," "women falsely accuse innocent men of rape," "women provoke rape by their physical appearance," "women secretly enjoy being raped," and "nice girls don't get raped."

Criminology and psychiatry occasionally follow this theme of "victim precipitation"and victim participation. It was von Hentig's observation (1948) that the victim in many instances "led the evil-doer actively into temptation."

### Societal Factors

Social control/social conflict models maintain that perpetrators adhere to a belief system that allows them to both engage in and justify rape. This belief system is thought to be the result of enculturation in a society that legitimizes violence (of which sexual aggression is one form) against women. The results of numerous studies (Malamuth & Donnerstein, 1984) have supported this model by showing a relationship between certain attitudes (e.g., acceptance of rape myths, sex role stereotyping) and various measures of aggression.

Traditional socialization patterns, argued feminists, encourage males to associate power, strength, and dominance with masculinity and passivity, submission, weakness, and inferiority with femininity. As Weiss and Borges (1973) note, socialization prepares women to be "legitimate" victims. Feminists emphasized that rape served the social control function of keeping women "in their place" (Brownmiller, 1975; Griffin, 1971; Reynolds, 1974). The end result of this is that social practices and beliefs that legitimize sexual aggression against women do so as a way of maintaining the inequitable distribution of power in our society.

Scully and Marolla (1984) argue that rape has become a "medicalized" social problem. They suggest that the notion of rape as a nonutilitarian act committed by a few "sick" men is too limited a view of sexual violence because it excludes culture and social structure as predisposing factors. Scully and Marolla's analysis of 114 incarcerated rapists revealed that rapists used sexual violence as a method of revenge and/or punishment; a means of gaining access to unwilling or unavailable women; a bonus added to burglary or robbery; a recreational activity; and a form of impersonal sex that gained the offender power over his victims.

## Rapist Factors

In a major contribution to offender research, Prentky and coworkers (1985) designed a classification system based on clinical understanding of the motives of over 1500 men observed at the Massachusetts Treatment Center for Sexually Dangerous Persons. These researchers suggest that all rapes clearly include a mixture of motivations, but for some rapists the need to humiliate and injure through aggression is the most salient feature of the offense, and for others the need to achieve sexual dominance is more prominent.

Prentky and associates describe four categories of men who sexually assault adult women. (1) For the *sexual nonsadistic rapist*, the assault is primarily an expression of his rape fantasies. There is usually a history of sexual preoccupation typified by the living out or fantasizing of a variety of perversions, and there is often a high level of sexual arousal accompanied by a loss of self-control, causing a distorted perception of the victim/offender relationship. In psychological terms, this rapist is "compensating" for acutely felt inadequacies as a male. (2) For the *opportunistic* rapist, sexual behavior is expressed as an impulsive, predatory act. For him, the sexual component is less integrated into fantasy life and has far less psychological meaning. These assaults often occur within some particular and characteristic context such as driving down a dimly lit street and noticing a woman walking toward her car. The assault may be understood as a man looking for a woman to exploit sexually. This offender is the most frequently described subtype of rapist in both clinical and popular literature. (3) For the *vindictive rapist*, sexual behavior is an expression of anger and rage. Sexuality is primarily aggressive in its aim, with the victim representing the hated individual(s). This type of rapist is a misogynist, and therefore the aggression may span a wide range of behaviors from verbal abuse to brutal murder. (4) For the *sadistic rapist*, sexual behavior is an expression of sexually aggressive (sadistic) fantasies, with an apparent fusion of these feelings. Murder may well be the outcome of the assault.

Empirical studies have shown that violence and sex are intertwined in a multiplicity of ways in our society even in normal males. It has been suggested that rape exists on a continuum with what many people regard as "normal" heterosexuality (Holmstrom & Burgess, 1983). Evidence for this position has come from studies demonstrating a proclivity to rape among normal males (Malamuth, 1981).

## The Aftermath of Rape

The consequences of rape and sexual assault are serious and long-lasting. Rape and sexual assault are public health problems of major importance. Not only is a large number of the population affected but also the rate of recovery of rape victims is slower than that for victims of other types of crimes (Resnick, 1987). The increasingly distressing fact is that for some victims, recovery may not be as complete as once thought. Kilpatrick and coworkers (1987) found that 16.5 percent of assessed rape victims were diagnosed with post-traumatic stress disorder an average of 17 years after the assault.

As demonstrated in the opening case example, when we think of victims of rape and sexual abuse, we need to recognize that the assaults claim indirect victims as well. Children may witness the assault and distress of a parent and thus be traumatized (Pynoos & Eth, 1985). In the case of children who are sexually abused outside the family, parental response to knowledge of the abuse has been very disruptive to the parents' lives, suggesting the development of a post-traumatic stress disorder in the parents themselves (Burgess et al., 1990; Kelley, 1990).

Although it has been shown that most types of crime have a psychological impact on victims (Kilpatrick et al., 1987a), sexual assault has been shown to be particularly deleterious (Burgess & Holmstrom, 1974; Burgess et al., 1984; Kilpatrick et al., 1985a). Long-term problems in the areas of psychological functioning, social adjustment, and sexual behavior have been identified (Ellis, 1983; Finkelhor et al., 1989; Holmes & St. Lawrence, 1983; Steketee & Foa, 1987).

Clinical research on the emotional outcomes of rape generally describes a staging or progression of emotional responses (Sutherland & Scherl, 1970; Symonds, 1976) with a focus on a rape trauma syndrome (Burgess & Holmstrom, 1974). Research has identified specific symptoms such as fear, anxiety (Kilpatrick, Vernon, & Resnick, 1979), depression (Frank & Stewart, 1983), or post-traumatic stress disorder (American Psychiatric Association, 1987) in victim response to rape.

## Organization of Victim Care

### History of Care

The organization of victim care may be viewed through its two decades of existence. The decade of the 1970s saw the first service programs established. Within this time period two important forces were responsible for bringing the problem of rape to the attention of the United States in the late 1960s. First, primary credit must be given to the re-emergence of the women's movement for initiating the consciousness-raising groups and then the "speak-outs," where women began saying publicly what they had not dared to before about rape. Second, in response to a rising crime rate and the growing community concern over the problem of rape, Senator Charles Mathias of Maryland introduced a bill in September, 1973 to establish the National Center for the Prevention and Control of Rape. The purpose of this bill was to provide a focal point within the National Institute of Mental Health from which a comprehensive national effort would be undertaken to research, develop programs, and provide information leading to aid for the victims and their families, to rehabilitation of offenders, and, ultimately, to curtailment of rape crimes. The bill was passed by overwhelming vote in the 93rd Congress, vetoed by President Ford, and successfully reintroduced. The National Center was established through Public Law 94-63 in July, 1975.

Concurrent with governmental efforts to focus on the problem of sexual violence, researchers were beginning to explore how victimization may have hidden consequences for both the individual and society as a whole. Victimization surveys conducted by the United States Census Bureau provided a wealth of data on the extent of crime in the United States, and early research focusing on rape (Burgess & Holmstrom, 1974, 1978), domestic violence (Bard & Sangrey, 1979; Walker, 1979), child victims (Burgess et al., 1978), and elderly victims (Young, 1976) began to give depth to the nascent reform effort.

The second decade, the 1980s, witnessed a series of governmental responses to the public's awareness of victim issues and the translation of the ideas of victim harm, treatment, and rights into tangible reforms.

In 1982, a Task Force on Victims of Crime was established by President Reagan to investigate the plight of victims, and it issued a final report that presented 68 recommendations on how the treatment of victims should be improved. In the same year, the United States Congress finally seized on the victim issue and signed into law the Victim and Witness Protection Act. To victims of federal crime, it provided improved protection from intimidation and harm, almost mandatory restitution payments from convicted federal offenders, and a set of fair standards for treatment of victims in the federal criminal justice system.

States began to pass victims "bills of rights" that provided a rapid growth of victim assistance programs. That growth was accelerated by passage of the capstone legislative achievement of this era, the Victims of Crime Act of 1985. Fashioned by a bipartisan group of sponsors in the Congress, the Victims of Crime Act called for the creation of a Crime Victims' Fund, derived from the collection of all federal criminal fines, forfeited bail bonds, and penalty assessments imposed on federal offenders. Funds so collected in one year are expended the next year as grants to support state victim compensation programs and local victim assistance programs (Young, 1988).

## Institutional Response

The institutional response to rape victims has been most organized around the initial crisis period. There are organized citywide services if the victim reports the crime. The report triggers a multiagency approach that is legally but not health-directed. That is, police officers begin an investigation and transport the victim for a rape examination that is usually paid for by the state. The county prosecutor directs the criminal investigation and trial. The roles and responsibilities are fairly clearly delineated in cases of adult victims.

Accountability of services is at the crisis level of care. That accountability of care varies in the attention it pays to the physical evidence of rape, the evaluation of potential sexually transmitted diseases, and psychological interventions.

Continuity of care is a function of (1) economics, (2) views regarding rape and the needs of victims, and (3) issues of confidentiality.

*Economics.* The policies directing the services are idiosyncratic to the institution. They depend on the structure for supporting services to rape victims, and these services are one of three types: (1) a fee-for-service and follow-up mental health services; (2) a combination of fee-for-service, in which the evidentiary examination is paid for by the state but the cost of psychological services is borne by the victim; and (3) reimbursement through the Victims of Crime Act of 1985. In order to receive federal funds, states must offer mental health counseling to victims. Each state must decide how to implement this requirement. Thus, the type of service depends on the interface between the hospital and the legal system.

This reimbursement method results in an uneven and at times fragmented response to the physical and emotional health needs of sexual assault victims. This is also true of the types of legal assistance available to the victim. There is less organization for follow-up services beyond the crisis period. Primarily victims of sexual assault either utilize the rape crisis services or finance their own extended care. Nurses who are knowledgeable regarding reimbursement issues for victim services can play a critical role in the organization and reimbursement of victim care for their agency.

*Stereotypes About Victim Care.* The beliefs about victim care are predicated on what people know to be the response and consequences of sexual abuse. These beliefs are influenced by prevailing myths and some factual information. Although most health care providers acknowledge the immediate trauma of rape, variability exists in the belief and recognition that there are potentially long-term negative consequences that extend beyond the crisis period. In some settings there may even be a tendency to discount the severity of the immediate response. This is particularly true when victims present themselves in a controlled or numb, detached manner (Burgess & Holmstrom, 1974).

*Confidentiality.* Both from the legal standpoint and the stigma aspect of rape, there is a propensity for people to blame the victim and take an enabling attitude toward the offender. This point is extremely important in understanding the perpetuation of problems that emerge from sexual assault and abuse. It is difficult for some health providers to deal with offender behavior and societal norms that justify sexual violence. These cases often involve young people, such as in acquaintance rape cases. Emphasis can, in such cases, be placed on protecting, explaining, and minimizing the behavior of the offender. This reality places any victim in double jeopardy when she makes rape and sexual assault public.

## Essential Health and Legal Services for Victims

Victims of rape and sexual assault need access to acute health services and legal resources. Nurses, as part of a multidisciplinary team, can supervise the paraprofessional workers who work on the crisis hotline and accompany the victim through the health and legal systems. Clinical nurse specialists are providing gynecologic examinations, crisis counseling, and follow-up mental health services.

*Emergency Clinical Services.* Crisis services include a 24-hour rape hotline staffed by trained paraprofessional personnel who can provide assistance, information, and referrals for additional needed services.

Victim accompaniment is provided by trained paraprofessional staff available to accompany victims to the hospital following an assault. This step can ensure that rape victims are adequately informed regarding hospital procedures (including procedures for the collection of evidence). Because many initial police interviews are conducted at the hospital, accompaniment provides trained advocates who can help victims make informed choices regarding prosecution.

Health and gynecologic examinations are essential for victims. Depending on the hospital protocol, both nurse practitioners and physicians conduct the health and evidentiary examinations and testify in court on their findings. Several states have specially designated sexual assault nurse examiners (SANEs) who are trained in examination procedures and the collection of forensic evidence. State training programs provide certification for this role.

*Crisis Counseling.*   Crisis counseling is generally provided by emergency department or psychiatric nurses after the medical and nursing emergency services have been completed. In some settings, the psychiatric liaison nurse or clinical nurse specialist in psychiatric mental health nursing provides this service. The basic assumptions underlying this type of intervention include: (1) the rape represents a crisis in that the victim's style of life is disrupted; (2) the victim is regarded as "normal" or functioning adequately prior to the external stress event; (3) crisis intervention aims to return the victim to her prerape level of functioning as quickly as possible. The crisis model is issue-oriented treatment designed to ameliorate symptoms of anxiety, fear, depression, loss of control, and decreased assertiveness (Burgess & Holmstrom, 1974; Burgess & Holmstrom, 1986). The objective of the model is to validate the crisis nature of the event, review the details of the rape, and focus on issues raised by the crisis. This focus is on the assault and its aftermath; with an emphasis on (1) assisting the person to achieve mastery over the life-threatening anxiety caused by the rape, (2) identifying a supportive social network, and (3) seeking self-enhancing ways of solving problems related to the rape and the subsequent events that occur (e.g., criminal investigations, court proceedings).

*Criminal Justice Services.*   Criminal justice services are offered through the victim witness staff of the prosecutor's office. These include keeping the victim informed of the charges filed and any bail considerations. Prior to any court appearance, the victim is given an orientation to the courthouse and the courtroom and told what to expect in a hearing or a trial. After trial, many states allow the victim to be involved in the sentencing process by providing a victim impact statement. After sentencing, the victim needs to be kept informed about probation, revocation hearings, parole hearings, escapes, appeals, and other issues related to the criminal justice system.

*Follow-Up Services.*   Mental health services for victims are provided by clinical specialists in psychiatric mental health nursing. Some victims require short-term counseling; others may be in need of longer term therapy from a nurse experienced in working with victims of sexual assault. Several effective treatment procedures have been developed to target specific rape-induced symptoms (Burgess & Holmstrom, 1986; Koss & Harvey, 1987; Ochberg, 1988).

Nurse-therapists skilled in family therapy provide intervention for members of the victim's family network who may develop post-trauma symptoms. In hearing of the victimization, family members often recreate the victim's experience in their own minds. This process has its own arousal phenomenon and encoding capacity that trigger symptoms, depending on how this information is received, stored, and regulated.

## Case Discussion

To return to the brief case example at the beginning of the chapter, the impact of the rape, abuse, and robbery was extensive for the victim, her child, and other family members. The mother not only suffered physical lacerations to her head and body but she contracted herpesvirus from the rape. Health care follow-up was important because the herpes infection became exacerbated when she was under stress. She developed post-trauma symptoms of mood swings, exaggerated startle reflex, flashbacks to the rape, anxiety, fears, and depression. The assault, which occurred in her apartment, disrupted her sense of security. In addition, her inability to physically protect her child from being abused had been great, and she had struggled between fears for her own life and that of her child. Knowing her child had been hit left her searching for strategies that would divert the assailants from further assault on the child. The aftermath of all this was the mother's sense of self-recrimination and of helplessness, which were not readily amenable to counseling. This put the mother at risk for substance abuse, a prior coping mechanism that she had used to deal with her problems. The self-recrimination mechanism impaired the mother's capacity to deal with and resolve the terror inherent in the assault. This was further complicated by the disturbing behavior of her child. The little girl, confused by what she had witnessed, manifested many symptoms of fear: night terrors, being easily startled, headaches, and stomach aches. She vacillated between being clinging and frightened of separation from her mother and impulsive destructive outbursts. Further, she developed sexualized behavior patterns that were distressing and alarming to her mother. It was difficult for the mother to cope with her own victimization and at the same time be constructive in her support and understanding of her child. In addition to this outcome, the trauma of the rape was intensified by the development of new fears at work. The mother resigned from her employment to seek work in a less public setting. There was also the legal process to endure. Although she had been an eyewitness to the crime, the child was not judged competent to give testimony, which distressed both the mother and the child. The criminals were not identified.

To mitigate some of the negative consequences, it is important for nurses to understand the need for care beyond the emergency room. Using a nurse-to-nurse referral system between clinical nurse specialists and community health nursing services, a nurse could aid this mother and child and could interface with social services and the school system to provide important support for the child as well as for the mother. Contact with advocates for victims can be used to support the mother and child through the legal phase of the case. A referral to a self-help group can support the mother while she is going to work. This type of plan, case management and intervention, is possible when professionals have a framework and policies established to work together to provide services.

## Prevention Efforts

Nurses assume a variety of roles in the assessment and treatment of rape and sexual assault victims, including that of educator, case finder, clinician, and researcher.

They play a role in advocacy and legislative activities and in the development of services.

Nursing can support all forms of *primary* prevention programs that teach children, women, and exploited groups about their rights and responsibilities in personal safety. There have been efforts by nurses to address the needs of children and adolescents through school-based programs. These programs address childrens' rights to assert and protect themselves from unwanted, inappropriate sexual advances from older children and adults. Nurses also take a leadership role in promoting focused types of prevention programs, such as self-education groups and stress inoculation programs that prepare people for a potentially traumatic event and how they might respond (e.g., self-defense courses, appropriate response to sexually dangerous situations).

*Secondary* prevention requires casefinding for rape and sexual assault. Nurses need to routinely assess for victimization history. In institutionalized populations such as the elderly, mentally handicapped, mentally ill, and incarcerated, nurses need to be alerted to the symptoms of sexual assault and abuse and to the behaviors of staff who care for patients at all levels. Understanding some of the types of problems inherent in this area includes being aware of the impact of sexual abuse on handicapped, mentally retarded, and psychotic patients. People who are unable to defend themselves physically or verbally are vulnerable. Nurses are in a particularly strategic position to both prevent abuse within institutions and to develop insight into how people present themselves when abused. This information is needed not only for therapeutic purposes but also to support patients in their right to justice. Casefinding can be done in institutions (e.g., clinics, emergency rooms) as well as in community settings.

Nurses should be assigned to the various internal review committees that deal with professional conduct and with developing policies for reporting and investigating sexual abuse. Nursing can be held accountable for the monitoring and conduct of people who have access to patients, whether they are staff or nonstaff. The following case illustrates this point (Mertz, 1986).

Community residents were shocked when a prominent anesthesiologist was arrested for sex acts with anesthetized female patients. The physician had orally copulated women in the operating room, while surgery was in process, many times during a two-year period. Citizens found it incredible that this activity had continued undetected. Immediate community response was disbelief and outrage. It became apparent that although the behavior had been reported by nurses, the hospital had taken no action.

As nurses began their grand jury testimony, the community learned that two years earlier, a circulating nurse had observed the anesthesiologist, standing behind opaque drapes at the head of the operating table, with his penis in the patient's mouth. Stunned, the nurse asked another circulating nurse to verify what she saw. Both nurses reported the incident to the operating room nursing supervisor; after the operation all three talked with the surgeon and examined the stain on the drapes. The surgeon did not believe their account, did not order laboratory tests on the stained material, and told the nurses not to discuss the matter.

The supervising nurse then reported the incident to the head of anesthesiology.

When the nursing supervisor, the anesthesiology chief, and the surgeon confronted the anesthesiologist, he denied the charges. No further reports were made. After the charges filed through hospital channels failed to bring results, the operating room nurses decided to gather evidence and take it directly to the hospital administrator. Approximately two years after the initial incident and after observing suspicious movements by the anesthetist with a 12-year-old patient, the nurses collected a specimen of secretions from the patient's suction tubing to test for the presence of semen. They prepared a report and submitted it to the administrator but received no response. The nurses then presented their report to the state medical licensing board. The physician was suspended from the hospital staff, and when this action was reported to the licensing board and investigated, the district attorney was notified. Charges were filed against the anesthesiologist, who attempted suicide and was hospitalized. When the abuse became public, the state nurses' association held a press conference to urge nurses to speak out regardless of a hospital gag order. An editorial in the local newspaper observed that a complaint whose seriousness would have been recognized instantly if it had come from a physician was dismissed because it came from a nurse.

Soon after public disclosure, the hospital executive director was suspended and later fired. Medical staff bylaws were changed to tighten procedures, and the composition of the board of trustees was altered so that physicians no longer constituted a majority of members. The Joint Commission on Accreditation of Hospitals revoked the hospital's accreditation but later reinstated it. The state medical quality assurance board and the board of registered nursing moved to suspend the licenses of two doctors and three nurses for "gross negligence and unprofessional conduct" in failing to investigate and report the offenses. On appeal, only the operating room nurse supervisor had her license revoked, and a judge later ruled that she should have a new hearing because she was denied due process of law in the previous revocation proceedings.

## Public Policy and Legislation

### Public Policy Recommendations

Public attention to the problem of rape often correlates with media reports of crimes. Two highly publicized cases in the late 1980s of sexual violence in New York City, the "preppie murder" and the "jogger in Central Park," resulted in an outcry from women's organizations in that city. The outcome of this pressure was that the Governor of New York, Mario M. Cuomo, appointed a multidisciplinary task force to develop recommendations relevant to rape. In addition to the task force members, 23 state agencies designated liaisons to the task force to assist in research and review of the issues. These recommendations, issued in the spring of 1990, represent the current thinking on ways to improve addressing victims' needs.

1. Develop a statewide public campaign to combat stereotypes about victims of sex crimes and involve the media and advertising industries.

2. Develop new training requirements for professions that work with the victims of sexual assault and with sex offenders.
3. Encourage colleges and universities to establish policies addressing rape and sexual assault on campus.
4. Expand efforts to ensure the confidentiality of communication between sex crime victims and crisis counselors.
5. Develop an evidence collection kit that addresses the needs of adult and child victims of rape and sexual assault.
6. Develop a policy regarding human immunodeficiency virus/acquired immunodeficiency syndrome infection for victims of sex offenses.
7. Develop guidelines to ensure that any sex offense is referenced when plea-bargained to a non-sex offense.
8. Develop new programs for sex offenders.

## Public Legislation

Some current legislative issues include the Victims of Crime Act, rape/incest/abortion and pregnancy, child abuse reporting, laws, rape and sexual assault training, hospital protocols, human immunodeficiency virus testing, and a sex offender registry.

### Victims of Crime Act

During the first nine months of fiscal year 1989, federal judges ordered 331 million dollars in criminal fines to be paid by those convicted in federal courts. This fund, as mentioned earlier, helps pay for services for victims. However, only 133.5 million dollars was paid into the federal Crime Victims' Fund. And, because of spending limitations imposed on the Fund by the Congress in 1988, only $125 million of that sum will be dispersed to states for crime victim assistance and compensation in fiscal year 1990. Of the remainder, 2.2 million dollars will go to the Administrative Office of the Courts for use in creating a new computerized fine collection system, and 6.3 million dollars will be returned to the federal treasury (Largen, 1990).

The history of the Victims of Crime Act teaches us that public policy and legislation are only one stage. The next stage is implementation. The discouraging executive response to the legislation requires that advocacy play a role in monitoring effective implementation. This requires the professional organizations in nursing to devise strategies on local, state, and national levels to keep processes in action that help offset the traumatic aftermath of rape.

### Rape/Incest and Abortion

In October, 1989, the Congress approved a fiscal year 1990 appropriations bill for the Departments of Education, Labor, and Health and Human Services that included a provision allowing Medicaid funding for abortion in cases of rape, incest, and life-threatening pregnancy. The legislation was vetoed by President Bush, and the veto was sustained by the House of Representatives in a 231 to 191 vote. Since 1981, the only exception Congress has allowed has been abortion to save the life of the woman. Representative Barbara Boxer (Democrat of California), sponsor of the abortion funding measure, vowed to "keep coming back" (Largen 1990).

Two cases (*Hodgson v. Minnesota, Nos. 88-1125 and 88-1309* and *Ohio v. Akron Center for Reproductive Health, No. 88-805*) with implications for minors who become pregnant as a result of sexual assault will be reviewed by the Supreme Court in 1990. Both cases involve states with parental notification laws but no "judicial bypass" procedures. This procedure of judicial bypass allows for minors who feel they cannot inform their parents before they receive health care. The Hodgson case, in particular, will provide the Court with its first opportunity to study the application of such laws rather than their facial constitutionality. Previous court decisions have established that states cannot require parental consent without setting up a bypass procedure. In current cases, the states argue that such a procedure is not needed because only parental notification, not consent, is required (Largen 1990).

## Child Reporting Laws

Nurses, like all health professionals, are mandated to report child sexual abuse. Because the content of state reporting provisions and reform initiatives varies, nurses need to follow the reporting law in their state. Legislation is needed in some states to clarify to whom the report should be made and to require that agencies assigned responsibility in cases of child abuse share information with all other agencies with case responsibility (the police, social workers, nurses, mental health workers).

## Rape and Sexual Assault Training

States vary as to their requirements for training of health professionals in the area of rape and sexual assault. Policy for mandated training ensures that principles and concepts of victim trauma are translated into practice. New York and Texas are examples of states with requirements for recertification.

## Hospital Protocols

A survey of New York hospitals that have treated rape victims revealed that not all hospitals have protocols for dealing with victims of rape and sexual assault. There were no specialized staff members for dealing with victims and no staff training in evidence collection in hospitals. There are often long waiting periods before victims receive care and treatment. Not all staff who deal with victims are knowledgeable about victims' rights, e.g., many hospitals routinely call police to report a rape, in violation of patient confidentiality. Not all hospitals are willing to provide care to victims. Many victims suffer additional victimization in court, where they find their case is hindered by lack of evidence or incorrectly handled, collected, or stored evidence. This survey led to the recommendation for uniformity of sexual assault examinations and evidence collection (Avener, 1990).

## Human Immunodeficiency Virus Testing

*Victim Testing.*   In the aftermath of sexual assault, the threat of becoming infected with the human immunodeficiency virus that causes acquired immunodeficiency syndrome has become a serious concern for victims. This virus, which can be sexually transmitted, is known to be carried by asymptomatic individuals who may have acquired infection through sexual contact or sharing needles for drug injection. The potential for transmission of human immunodeficiency virus may be increased when trauma to the tissues of the genital tract occurs. At the present time, data from which to estimate the likelihood of becoming infected with human immunodeficiency virus after a sexual assault are lacking; however, the *British Medical Journal* reports that seroconversion to human immunodeficiency virus occurred in the three months after a rape in a woman who had no other identifiable risk factors for human immunodeficiency virus infection (Murphy, Kitchen, Harns, & Forster, 1989).

Rape counselors are divided about whether or not counseling concerning acquired immunodeficiency syndrome should be included in the routine crisis care of victims. In one study, 26 percent of rape victims spontaneously identified the possibility of human immunodeficiency virus infection as a health concern (Baker, Burgess, Davis, & Brickman, 1989). Many rape counselors refer victims for human immunodeficiency virus anonymous testing if they initiate the issue.

*Offender Testing.*   Two testing issues relate to the offender. One is the DNA testing of sex offenders. During its 1989 session, the Arizona legislature enacted legislation that would require DNA testing of convicted sex offenders and toughen the penalties for repeat sex offenders. Results of DNA testing would be retained by the Arizona Department of Public Safety for possible later use in linking repeat offenders to other or future crimes. The penalty charge would require life imprisonment for recidivist offenders who use or show a deadly weapon or cause serious physical injury to a victim (Largen, 1990).

The second issue is offender testing for human immunodeficiency virus and is being addressed in several states. Legislation was filed in Oregon to require those convicted of sex crimes to be tested for infection with human immunodeficiency virus if such a request is made by the crime victim. In Florida, a police officer may require human immunodeficiency virus testing on a rape suspect if the officer has reasonable cause to believe the suspect is infected.

Policies are needed to protect the rights of both offender and victim, but ones that do not ignore the fact that victims can be infected with acquired immunodeficiency syndrome and other sexually transmitted diseases (Murphy et al., 1989). Counseling and monitoring systems need to be set up if this is to be done in a humane and constructive manner.

## Sex Offender Registry

Child protection from sex offenders is a major societal concern. It has been recommended by several national organizations that legislation be enacted to facilitate a comprehensive, relevant information-sharing system for the purposes of child protection. Specifically, existing statutes should be amended to permit the Federal Bureau of Investigation National Crime Information Center to provide conviction and wanted information to a state or local law enforcement or criminal justice agency on behalf of an agency empowered by state law to receive criminal history information in employee screening. Such a system would allow for national screening instead of the piecemeal methods currently in place. It would provide a useful tool for child service agencies around the country working with law enforcement services. And it would be limited to conviction information, not the more constitutionally problematic arrest information.

## Conclusion

There are many critical areas for further research and policy recommendations, but none as critical as the area of the prevention of sexual violence. Although services to crime victims have increased in quantity and improved in quality in the last decade, Swift (1985) observes that no breakthroughs have been achieved in preventing sexual assault. In fact, reported rates of these crimes keep increasing (Uniform Crime Report, 1988).

A goal of primary intervention is to eliminate rape from our society. If rape is fostered by certain social structures and beliefs, preventive efforts should focus on those sociocultural structures and beliefs. There are both optimistic and pessimistic implications from this interpretation. The encouraging implication is that high rates of rape are not inevitable. It is possible for a society to be rape-free or at least have a very low rape rate (Sanday, 1981). The discouraging point is that to eliminate rape one would have to make radical changes in the ideology and social structure of a society such as ours. If Burt (1980) is correct in stating that "the task of preventing rape is tantamount to revamping a significant portion of our social values" (p. 229), then the time to begin is now, and nurses, as critical health care providers, can take a leadership role.

REFERENCES

American Psychiatric Association (1987). *Diagnostic and statistical manual of mental disorders* (3rd ed., revised). Washington, DC: American Psychiatric Association.
Avener, A. (1990). Governor's task force on sexual assault. Final report. New York.
Baker, T., Burgess, A.W., Davis, R., & Brickman, E. (1989). Rape victims' concern about possible exposure to AIDS. *Journal of Interpersonal Violence, 5*(2), 49–60.
Bard, M., & Sangrey, D. (1979). *The crime victim's book.* New York: Basic Books.
Brownmiller, S. (1975). *Against our will: Men, women and rape.* New York: Simon and Schuster.
Burgess, A.W., Groth, A.N., Holmstrom, L.L., & Sgroi, S.M. (1978). *Sexual assault of children and adolescents.* Lexington, MA: Lexington Books.

Burgess, A.W., Hartman, C.R., Kelley, S.J., Grant, C.A., & Gray, E.B. (1990). Parental response to child sexual abuse trials involving day care settings, *Journal of Traumatic Stress, 3*(1), 395–405.

Burgess, A.W., Hartman, C.R., McCausland, M.P., & Powers, P. (1984). Response patterns in children exploited in sex rings and pornography. *American Journal of Psychiatry, 141*(5), 656–662.

Burgess, A.W., & Holmstrom, L.L. (1974). Rape trauma syndrome. *American Journal of Psychiatry, 131*, 981–986.

Burgess, A.W., & Holmstrom, L.L. (1978). Recovery from rape and prior life stress. *Research in Nursing and Health, 1*(4), 165–174.

Burgess, A.W., & Holmstrom, L.L. (1986). *Rape: Crisis and recovery*. West Newton, MA: Awab, Inc.

Burt, M.R. (1980). Cultural myths and supports for rape. *Journal of Personality and Social Psychology, 38*(2), 217–230.

Ellis, E.M. (1983). A review of empirical rape research: Victim reactions and response to treatment. *Clinical Psychology Review, 90*, 263–266.

Federal Bureau of Investigation (1988). *Crime in the United States: Uniform crime reports.* Washington, DC: U.S. Department of Justice.

Finkelhor, D. (1987). The sexual abuse of children: Current research reviewed. *Psychiatric Annals, 17*(4), 233–241.

Finkelhor, D., Hotaling, G., Lewis, I., & Smith, C. (1989). Sexual abuse and its relationships to later sexual satisfaction, marital status, religion, and attitudes, *Journal of Interpersonal Violence, 4*(4), 379–399.

Frank, E., & Stewart, B.D. (1983). Treating depression in victims of rape. *The Clinical Psychologist, 36*, 95–98.

Fuller, A.K., & Bartucci, R.J. (1988). HIV transmission and childhood sexual abuse. *Journal of the American Medical Association, 259*, 2235–2236.

Griffin, S. (1971). Rape: The all-American crime. *Ramparts, 10*, 28.

Holmes, M.R., & St. Lawrence, J.B. (1983). Treatment of rape-induced trauma: Proposed behavioral conceptualization and review of the literature. *Clinical Psychology Review, 3*, 417–433.

Holmstrom, L.L., & Burgess, A.W. (1978). *The victim of rape: Institutional Reactions.* New York: John Wiley. New edition 1983, New Brunswick, NJ: Transaction.

Holmstrom, L.L., & Burgess, A.W. (1983). Rape and everyday life. *Society, 20*(5), 33–40.

Kelley, S.J. (1990). Parental stress response to sexual abuse and ritualistic abuse of children in day care centers. *Nursing Research, 39*(1), 25–29.

Kilpatrick, D.G., Best, C.L., Veronen, L.J., Amick, A.E., Villeponteaux, A., & Ruff, G.A. (1985). Mental health correlates of criminal victimization: A random community survey. *Journal of Consulting Clinical Psychology, 53*, 866–873.

Kilpatrick, D.G., Saunders, B.E., Veronen, L.J., Best, C.L., & Von, J.M. (1987). Criminal victimization: Lifetime prevalence, reporting to police, and psychological impact, *Crime and Delinquency, 33*, 468–478.

Kilpatrick, D.G., & Veronen, L.J. (1983). Treatment for rape-related problems: Crisis intervention is not enough. In L.H. Cohen, W. Claiborn, & G. Specter (Eds.), *Crisis Intervention.* New York: Human Sciences Press.

Kilpatrick, D.G., Veronen, L.J., & Best, C.L. (1985). Factors predicting psychological distress among rape victims. In *Post-traumatic therapy and victims of violence* (pp. 113–141). New York: Brunner/Mazel.

Kilpatrick, D.G., Veronen, L.J., & Resnick, P.A. (1979). The aftermath of rape: Recent empirical findings. *American Journal of Orthopsychiatry, 49*(4), 658–669.

Kilpatrick, D.G., Veronen, L.J., Saunders, B.E., Best, C.L., Amick-McMullen, A., & Padu-hovich, J. (1987). *The psychological impact of crime: A study of randomly surveyed crime victims*. National Institute of Justice, Grant No. 84-IJ-CX-0039, Final Report. Washington, DC.

Koss, M.P. (1985). The hidden rape victim. Personality, attitudinal, and situational character-istics. *Psychology of Women Quarterly, 9*, 193–212.

Koss, M.P., & Harvey, M. (1987). *The rape victim: Clinical and community approaches to treatment*. Lexington, MA: Stephen Greene Press.

Largen, M.A. (1985). The anti-rape movement. In A.W. Burgess (Ed.), *Rape and sexual assault: A research handbook*, Vol. 1. New York: Garland Publishing Co.

Largen, M.A. (1990). *NNVSA network news*. Ivy, VA: P.O. Box 409.

Malamuth, N.M. (1981). Rape proclivity among males. *Journal of Social Issues, 37*, 138–157.

Malamuth, N.M., & Donnerstein, E. (Eds.) (1984). *Pornography and sexual aggression*. Orlando, FL: Academic Press.

Mertz, A.W. (1986). Sexual abuse of anesthetized patients. In A.W. Burgess & C.R. Hart-man (Eds.), *Sexual exploitation of patients by health professionals* (pp. 61–65). New York: Praeger.

Murphy, S., Kitchen, V., Harris, J.R.W., & Forster, S.M. (1989). Rape and subsequent seroconversion to HIV. *British Medical Journal, 299*, 718.

Ochberg, F.M. (Ed.) (1988). *Post-traumatic therapy and victims of violence*. New York: Brunner/Mazel Psychosocial Stress Series.

Prentky, R.A., Cohen, M.L., & Seghorn, T.K. (1985). Development of a rational taxonomy for the classification of rapists: The Massachusetts Treatment Center. *Bulletin of the American Academy of Psychiatry and the Law, 13*, 39–70.

Pynoos, R.S., & Eth. S. (1985). Children traumatized by witnessing acts of personal violence: Homicide, rape, or suicide behavior. In S. Eth & R.S. Pynoos (Eds.), *Post-traumatic stress disorder in children* (pp. 17–44). Washington, DC: American Psychiatric Press.

Resnick, P.A. (1987). Psychological effects of victimization: Implications for the criminal jus-tice system. *Crime and Delinquency, 33*(4), 468–478.

Reynolds, J.M. (1974). Rape as social control. *Catalyst, 8*, 62–67.

Riger, S., & Gordon, M.T. (1988). The impact of crime on urban women. In A.W. Burgess (Ed.), *Rape and sexual assault*, Vol. 2 (pp. 293–312). New York: Garland Publishing Co.

Sanday, P.R. (1981). The socio-cultural context of rape: A cross-cultural study. *Journal of Social Issues, 37*, 25.

Sanders, W.B. (1980). *Rape and women's identity*. Beverly Hills, CA: Sage Publications.

Scully, D., & Marolla, J. (1984). Convicted rapists' vocabulary of motive: Excuse and justifica-tion. *Social Problems, 31*, 530–544.

Steketee, G., & Foa, E.B. (1987). Rape victims: Post-traumatic stress responses and their treatment: A review of the literature. *Journal of Anxiety Disorders, 1*, 69–86.

Sutherland, S., & Scherl, D. (1970). Patterns of response among victims of rape. *American Journal of Orthopsychiatry, 40*, 503–511.

Symonds, M. (1974). The rape victim: Psychological patterns of response. *American Journal of Psychoanalysis, 35*, 19–25.

Swift, C. (1985). The prevention of rape. In A.W. Burgess (Ed.), *Rape and sexual assault*, Vol. 2 (pp. 413–426). New York: Garland Publishing Co.

*Uniform crime report by FBI*. (1988). Washington, DC: Government Printing Office.

von Hentig, H. (1948). *The criminal and his victim*. New Haven: Yale University Press.

Walker, L.E. (1979). *The battered woman*. New York: Harper & Row.

Warr, M. (1985). Fear of rape among urban women. *Social Problems, 32,* 238–250.

Weiss, K., & Borges, S.S. (1973). Victimology and rape: The case of the legitimate victim. *Issues in Criminology, 8,* 72.

Williams, L.S. (1984). The classic rape: When do victims report? *Social Problems, 31,* 460–467.

Young, M. (1976). *Older Americans crime prevention project final report.* Portland, OR: Multanomah County Division of Public Safety.

Young, M. (1988). The crime victims' movement. In F.M. Ochberg (Ed.), *Post-traumatic therapy and victims of violence.* New York: Brunner/Mazel.

# Chapter 24

# Health Care for the Homeless

ADA M. LINDSEY

$W$HO ARE THE homeless? Why has homelessness emerged as a sociopolitical, economic, and public health phenomenon? What is the magnitude of the problem? What are the health care problems of the homeless? What has been done? What are the implications for future action? Do nurses and nursing have a contribution to make in determining needs and in providing health care to homeless individuals? In considering deliberative responses to these questions, it is possible to begin to understand the complexities involved in planning for and in providing health care for homeless people.

## Characteristics of the Homeless

Many definitions of the homeless have been proposed. One common element in these definitions is that the person lacks a stable, adequate residence or has no regular place to live. The Stuart B. McKinney Homeless Assistance Act of 1987 (U.S. Congress, House, 1987 P.L. 100-77) defines a homeless person as "one who lacks a fixed, permanent nighttime residence or whose nighttime residence is a temporary shelter, welfare hotel, transitional housing for the mentally ill, or any public or private place not designed as sleeping accommodations for human beings" (Institute of Medicine, 1988, p. 137).

The demographic characteristics of the homeless have changed from the previous decades when older men suffering from chronic alcoholism accounted for most homeless persons (U.S. Department of Housing and Urban Development, 1984). Although males still remain the largest majority of homeless, the age of that population has decreased to an average of 34 to 37 years (U.S. Department of Housing and Urban Development, 1984; Institute of Medicine, 1988). Perhaps the most dramatic change in the composition of the homeless is the appearance of families. In fact, families are currently the largest growing subgroup of the homeless, usually women with dependent children (U.S. Conference of Mayors, 1987a; 1989; Wright & Weber, 1987). From a survey conducted in 25 cities, the U.S. Conference of Mayors (1986) reported that 56 percent of the homeless are single men, 25 percent are single women, and the remaining 19 percent are families with children or adolescents. The 1989 27-city survey reported by the U.S. Conference of Mayors (1989) shows a change in the composition of the homeless; 36 percent were families with children. Within all subgroups, minorities are over-represented.

Single homeless women and homeless women with children are less likely to have a history of mental illness than are single homeless men, and they rely more on shelters for sleeping and food than do homeless men (Burt & Cohen, 1989). Homeless families most often are headed by individual adult females. These women have few or no supportive relationships, and many have been victims of family violence. Homeless families with both parents are found more often in rural areas.

Bassuk and Rosenberg (1988) compared 49 homeless families with 81 families housed in public or private subsidized housing, all single female-headed families; both groups were poor and had been on welfare for a long time. The housed families had extended families and relatives whom they saw frequently and sometimes lived with, in contrast to the homeless mothers, whose support networks were fragmented. A major factor that differentiated housed welfare families from homeless families was the option to share housing with others. Because of weak support networks, homeless families do not have as many options for shared living arrangements. The homeless mothers also reported a higher frequency of abuse when they were children and of battering as adults, and a higher frequency of psychiatric problems, including drug and alcohol abuse, than did the housed mothers. Descriptions of homeless families and characteristics of homeless mothers are summarized in the Institute of Medicine report (1988).

In comparison to their representation in the general population, there are fewer elderly among the population who are homeless. Rossi and colleagues (1987) reported 19 percent of Chicago's homeless as being elderly compared with 30 percent of domiciled people who are elderly. Farr and colleagues (1986) reported 5 percent of the Los Angeles skid row homeless population as being over 61 years old compared with 17 percent of those domiciled in Los Angeles county who were over 61. In the Robert Wood Johnson Foundation-Pew Memorial Trust–funded Health Care for the Homeless projects, only 3 percent of those who came to health care clinics were over 65 years old compared with 12 percent of the general United States population who are over 65 (Wright & Weber, 1987). There are several plausible explanations for the relatively low numbers of elderly among the homeless. (1) The elderly are eligible for Social Security benefits at age 62 and Medicare at 65 among other benefits, including subsidized housing. (2) Homeless individuals may not survive long enough to become elderly. (3) Sampling techniques of counting the homeless used in research may not capture the homeless elderly (Institute of Medicine, 1988). Also, fewer elderly persons may participate in the various programs for the homeless.

Homeless people are found in urban, suburban, and rural areas. Because so little information was available on the rural homeless population, the Institute of Medicine Committee on Health Care for Homeless People commissioned a special study. Several important differences between the rural and the urban homeless populations were found (Institute of Medicine, 1988). Many rural homeless live as part of an extended family network or live in substandard housing and are less likely to receive assistance. Homeless people are less visible in rural communities, and as a result the population is virtually unidentified.

When plans to establish or expand services for homeless individuals are made public, many people who have homes or businesses in these areas protest such plans, maintaining that homeless individuals pose a threat to property, business, and life. Snow and colleagues (1989) examined the criminal records of a random sample of homeless people in Austin, Texas, for a 27-month period and compared the findings with those for domiciled adult men from the same community. They found that homeless men had a higher arrest rate, but the majority of offenses were for public intoxication, theft, burglary, and violation of city ordinances rather than for violent crimes. The domiciled adult men were arrested for more serious violent crimes. When data were adjusted for age, they determined an arrest rate for violent crime of about 24 per 1000 versus approximately 12 per 1000 for domiciled adult men and homeless men, respectively. Homeless men have a higher arrest rate for burglary and theft. Arrests were made for breaking into buildings primarily to find shelter, and arrests for shoplifting showed the homeless attempting to obtain cigarettes, food, drink, and items that could be sold on the street. Snow and colleagues (1989) suggest that what prompts the criminal activity of many homeless people is the lack of or inaccessibility of alternatives for survival. The profile developed from these findings show that homeless men who were arrested were under 35 years of age, had been homeless longer, and had had some contact with the mental health system.

Homeless individuals have very little privacy and therefore are constantly in the public view, which possibly increases their chances of being arrested. Some of their behaviors, such as begging or panhandling, bring attention to them. Homeless individuals are often subjects of negative attention because of their lifestyle and consequent behaviors. Snow and others (1989) describe this scenario as a criminalization process that leads to increased opportunity for arrests. They provide evidence of a "stigmatization bias" against homeless men. All these factors influence political support or resistance on the part of the public to providing and locating services greatly needed by the homeless populations.

As is evident from these brief descriptions, the homeless population is quite heterogeneous. Thus, the reasons for people becoming homeless also are varied (U.S. House of Representatives Select Committee on Children, Youth, and Families, 1987; Wright, 1989).

## Reasons for Increased Homelessness

There were 33 million people in the United States in 1985 classified as living in poverty; this represented an increase of 10 million people since 1973 (Institute of Medicine, 1988). The Institute of Medicine Committee on Health Care for Homeless People concluded that the major reason for the number of homeless people in the United States is the lack of "decent, affordable housing" (Institute of Medicine,

1988, p. 26). Although the cost of housing has escalated, since 1980 there has been a tremendous decline (60 percent) in direct federal subsidies for low-income housing construction and maintenance. Urban areas have undergone revitalization in the course of which development projects removed low-income housing and replaced it with more expensive housing. During the past 30 years, the number of single room occupancy accommodations has decreased by half. There clearly is a lack of affordable housing. Rent control also has been cited as contributing to homelessness (Tucker, 1987). The economic recessions in the late 1970s and early 1980s contributed to continued low or minimum wages, to plant closures, and to unemployment. There has been a decrease in the demand for low-skilled workers, and the national minimum wage is not sufficient to enable people to rent or purchase housing. The decline in availability of low-income housing and the increase in housing costs have led to overcrowded housing (as individuals and families double up) and to homelessness. The young males who now are the greatest proportion of the homeless population are not eligible for most of the existing social service (public assistance programs) benefits. For those who do qualify for public assistance, cutbacks in financial support for the provision of services have eroded their availability, and general assistance benefits in many states are not sufficient to cover minimally adequate housing (Institute of Medicine, 1988).

Some suggest that the increase in homelessness is a reflection of further disintegration of our family structure. Bassuk suggests that "lack of a home is symptomatic of total disconnection from supportive people and institutions" (Bassuk, 1984, p. 43). Many of the homeless are indeed social isolates and are alienated from society. The homeless are different from those who are poor in that they are alone and lack the social connections or relationships with friends and family (Bassuk & Rosenberg, 1988; Burt & Cohen, 1989; Lockhead, 1988b; Rossi et al., 1987; Whitman, 1988). Adult homeless males, in particular, are more likely never to have been married and lack close family relationships.

Reasons why adolescents run away and become homeless include abuse from parents or guardians, being forced to move out of their homes, and behavioral problems including psychiatric disturbances and substance abuse. The questionable legal status of homeless adolescents as minors presents problems in providing services to them. They cannot give legal consent, and without documentation they may not qualify for public assistance.

Health problems such as a major mental illness or acquired immunodeficiency syndrome or chronic degenerative disease may result in homelessness, particularly if there is a lack of supportive or alternative housing facilities. Individuals with these kinds of health problems may become unable to work and thus eventually are unable to pay for housing.

The plan in the 1960s for the deinstitutionalization of the mentally ill from the large state hospitals included development of small community-based mental health centers. Slightly more than one quarter of those anticipated centers were ever opened (Institute of Medicine, 1988). Thus, implementation of the plan for deinstitutionalization was flawed. Only mentally ill persons who are judged to be dangerous to themselves or others can be involuntarily committed to a mental hospital. Most communities do not have adequate treatment resources for the mentally ill who do not require hospitalization but who need assistance. These individuals do not have access to the care they need, and if they are unable to obtain shelter, they may become homeless. It has been estimated that 30 to 40 percent of the homeless are mentally ill (Lockhead, 1988b; U.S. Department of Health and Human Services, 1986; Wright & Weber, 1987). With the enactment of the Stewart B. McKinney Homeless Assistance Act of 1987, funds have been allocated for demonstration grants to provide new mental health care service approaches for homeless individuals (Salem & Levine, 1989).

Alcohol abuse and drug abuse also contribute to the increasing number of homeless. There are many fewer arrests for vagrancy and drunkenness as a result of the decriminalization of public drunkenness over the past 20 years (Whitman, 1988). Without a support system, incidence of personal problems such as chemical dependency, mental illness, or physical health problems increases the likelihood of an individual's becoming homeless. Some homeless individuals are too confused or unable or unwilling to indicate their needs; others may not be able to take advantage of social services that are available.

Three patterns of homelessness have been described: temporary (situational), episodic, and chronic (Institute of Medicine, 1988). Those who are temporarily homeless often have been displaced because of some calamity such as fire or eviction. With favorable economic and housing conditions and the absence of compounding factors such as mental illness, it is likely that rehousing for this group of homeless can be accomplished rather quickly. Episodically homeless refers to the pattern in which people alternate between being homeless and finding housing. Examples of those who are episodically homeless include individuals who lack sufficient resources to pay a full month's rent or who are chronically mentally ill and periodically exhibit behavior that is intolerable to those with whom they live. Episodic homelessness also may result from spousal and/or child abuse. Individuals who are mentally ill or are substance abusers or both are those who most typically are the chronically homeless. These people spend one or more years on the street without stability of residence, although some do have brief periods of shelter, including institutionalization.

## Size of the Homeless Population

It is difficult to count the homeless, and those who do count them use varying definitions of homeless. For example, are those who are temporarily housed in shelters or in single-room occupancy units or voucher hotels for a few nights counted with those who are on the streets, in the parks, in tents, under scrap material covers, and under viaducts? Are those who spend the night in transportation terminals or in all-night movie theaters and those who live in abandoned cars or their own cars included? There also are the hidden, marginal, or borderline homeless (prehomeless), who are tenuously housed with friends or relatives. There is a turnover of homeless; some move into a residence, whereas others shift into the category of temporarily without housing.

In 1984, the United States Department of Housing and Urban Development estimated the number of homeless in this country to range from 250,000 to 350,000 (U.S. Department of Housing and Urban Development, 1984). Advocates for the homeless place the number closer to a range of 2 to 3 million; they use a more inclusive definition that covers persons at high risk for becoming homeless as well as those who are actually homeless (Lockhead, 1988a). The National Alliance to End Homelessness recently has estimated that in the United States, there are 735,000 people who are homeless on any given night and that in 1988 from 1.3 to 2 million people would be homeless for one or more nights (Alliance Housing Council, 1988). Based on a reinterpretation of the U.S. Department of Housing and Urban Development (1984) study, they estimated a 20 percent annual growth rate in homelessness (Alliance Housing Council, 1988). According to surveys from the 25 representative cities included by the U.S. Conference of Mayors (1987a), there was a reported range of 15 to 50 percent annual increase in the homeless population in the sampled cities. The suburban homelessness rate is estimated to be one third of the urban rate. Very few data exist about homeless adolescents and runaway youths (Council on Scientific Affairs, 1989). Estimates of the numbers of youths vary, ranging from 500,000 to over 2 million; most do not receive social services and thus may be lost for counting purposes.

One example of counting the homeless is a study done for the city of Chicago. The size and composition of the homeless population in that city were estimated using two samples; one sample was taken from those housed in shelters and the other was from an enumeration of homeless found in places outside of dwelling units between midnight and 6:00 A.M. (Rossi et al., 1987). Both groups were interviewed to obtain demographic information and data about their employment and living patterns. The surveys were conducted in early fall (sample selected from 22 shelters and 168 census blocks) and late winter (sample selected from 27 shelters and 245 census blocks), with a total of 722 homeless people being interviewed. Of their sample, 76 percent were male, and the average age was 40 years. Those under 25 or over 65 years of age were under-represented, and blacks and Native Americans were over-represented. Young black women with children constituted 14 percent of the sample. Three characteristics were found to be prevalent in this sample: extreme poverty, disability resulting from poor health (physical and mental), and social isolation and lack of ties to others. Rossi and coworkers found that the Chicago homeless survive on less than half the poverty level income. The average person surveyed had been homeless for 22 months but without a steady job for more than 4 1/2 years. The estimated size of the Chicago homeless population was 2722 on an average night and about 6000 people over a 1-year period. Estimates of numbers of homeless also were derived from those using other special purpose shelters such as detoxification centers, shelters for battered women, and facilities for chronically mentally ill; those who were in some temporary housing arrangement on the nights of the interviews were also included. This, at best, still represents an estimate of the size of the homeless population in Chicago in 1985. There continues to be considerable discussion about the definition of homeless and who should be counted.

A variety of problems in estimating the size, composition, and selected characteristics of the homeless population have been cited (Institute of Medicine, 1988; Piliavin, Westerfelt, & Elliott, 1989). For example, Piliavin and colleagues (1989) present a case for sample selection bias and the effects of choice-based sampling as used by Wright and Weber (1987) in estimating mental illness among the homeless. They suggest that the large data set reported by Wright and Weber (1987), which was based only on homeless clinic users, may not be representative of or generalizable to the homeless population as a whole, and thus utility of the data for policy and program determinations may be limited. The reported figures, representing the number of homeless people nationally, have been based mostly on estimation techniques, and the range of these estimates across studies is relatively great (Institute of Medicine, 1988). Regardless of the real number, homelessness is increasingly apparent, and these individuals have urgent needs.

## Health Status and Health Care Problems of the Homeless Population

Some health problems such as acquired immunodeficiency syndrome, mental illness, and substance abuse may put individuals at increased risk for homelessness. Other health problems occur as a result of the conditions associated with being homeless. Examples of such problems are dependent edema, skin ulcerations and cellulitis, parasitic illnesses, infestations, trauma, sexual assault, hypothermia, respiratory illness, tuberculosis, and malnutrition. The treatment and care required for some health problems are complicated by the circumstances of homelessness. It is difficult to manage care for the mentally ill or for the diabetic person who is homeless or for a person who requires bed rest or antihypertensive medications. Consider the problems of a homeless person who is diabetic, for example, and needs to have daily access to insulin and a sterile syringe and needle, to protect insulin from deterioration from temperature changes, to manage an appropriate dietary regimen, and to ensure care of the extremities, especially the feet. The dietary and pharmacologic management of any acute or chronic disease is more challenging for homeless individuals. In many places, homeless individuals have great difficulty obtaining health care (Brickner et al., 1986). Frequently the emergency room becomes the only entry for access to health care.

Until Brickner and colleagues (1985) described data collected from homeless patients seen in a New York City free clinic, very little information about the health problems of the homeless was available. In addition to psychiatric disorders, Brickner and colleagues (1986) identified the following as occurring more commonly in homeless persons: trauma; respiratory disease, including tuberculosis; parasitic infestations; and peripheral vascular disease. Because of the severe pruritus caused by scabies and lice infestations, secondary problems such as infection result from the scratching. Respiratory disease and infestations (e.g., scakes lice) are more easily transmitted because of the living and environmental conditions of the homeless. Peripheral vascular problems also occur as a result of living conditions; edema develops when homeless people are not able to lie down and their legs remain dependent.

This leads to cellulitis, ulceration, and infection. In cold weather, frostbite is another problem that contributes to peripheral vascular disease.

Homeless children experience delays in getting immunizations; they have a higher rate of chronic physical problems such as anemia and asthma than do children in the general population (Acker et al., 1987; Wright & Weber; 1987). They also have serious emotional, developmental, and learning problems (Bassuk et al., 1986; 1987; 1988). Homeless adolescents have a higher prevalence of substance abuse, sexually transmitted diseases, and pregnancy than the general adolescent population (Wright & Weber, 1987). Because of age and length of time spent on the streets, the health status of homeless youths may be better than that of homeless adults. However, in addition to mental illness, homeless children suffer problems similar to those of homeless adults, such as inadequate nutrition, exposure to the elements, lack of facilities for routine hygiene, and victimization. The more commonly reported physical health care problems in children from 16 of the Robert Wood Johnson Foundation-Pew Memorial Trust Homeless Health Care programs were upper respiratory tract infections, skin disorders, and gastrointestinal tract problems (Wright & Weber, 1987).

Homeless women suffer from pregnancy-related problems and as victims of physical assault (Brickner et al., 1985; Wright et al., 1987). Homeless women who are pregnant experience poor nutrition, delays in receiving or a lack of prenatal care, and a higher incidence of having low birth weight infants.

## *Mental Illness*

Provision of care for the deinstitutionalized or never institutionalized mentally ill population who are homeless is complicated by the lack of community-based treatment facilities and the lack of adequate housing or shelter for these individuals. Wright and Weber (1987) estimated that 30 to 40 percent of those homeless seeking health care had psychiatric disorders. Brickner and colleagues (1985) previously identified alcoholism and psychiatric disorders as the top two common health problems occurring in the homeless patients to whom primary care was provided.

Fischer and colleagues (1986) compared the mental health status of a sample of 51 homeless mission users with a sample of 1338 domiciled men in the same community. The homeless men were found to have a higher prevalence rate in all the DIS/DSM III diagnostic categories and to have higher rates of hospitalization for both physical and mental health problems. Studies of the prevalence of psychiatric disorders in the homeless population are summarized in the Institute of Medicine (1988) report. A greater percentage of homeless women than men are mentally ill (Aiken, 1987). In a study of 80 homeless mothers and 151 children living in shelters in Massachusetts, Bassuk and colleagues (1986) found that a large percentage of the mothers had personality disorders and lacked any major supportive relationships. About half the children manifested difficulties such as developmental lags and learning problems and experienced anxiety and depression. It was determined that about half the children needed further psychiatric evaluation.

## Alcohol Abuse

Current estimates for homeless men suggest that 25 to 40 percent have serious alcohol problems (Institute of Medicine, 1988). In comparison to the general population, this is a considerably higher rate. Homeless individuals with alcohol problems are more likely to seek health care because they experience more physical disabilities than homeless people who do not have alcohol problems (Fischer & Breakey, 1987; Koegel & Burnam, 1987). Wright and Weber (1987) found that homeless alcoholics experience trauma, severe upper respiratory infections, serious skin problems, active tuberculosis, hypertension, and cardiac disease more frequently than do nonalcoholic homeless people. It is difficult for alcohol abusers to find shelter because many emergency shelters will not accept homeless people who have been drinking. There is an acknowledged lack of alcohol detoxification and rehabilitation programs. For some with serious physical and mental health problems, alcohol withdrawal may require hospitalization. Following detoxification, these patients need treatment programs and specialized supportive housing accommodations in an alcohol-free environment.

## Drug Abuse

Scant information is available about the number of homeless people who are drug abusers; however, an annotated bibliography covering articles on alcohol and drug abuse among the homeless is available (U.S. Department of Health and Human Services, 1988). Wright and Weber (1987) reported a rate of 10 percent for the 16 foundation-sponsored projects. Younger age was associated with illicit drug use; this is in contrast to the association of alcohol abuse with older age. Homeless drug abusers more frequently had a diagnosis of acquired immunodeficiency syndrome, liver disease, peripheral venous stasis, and cardiac disease than did homeless non–drug abusers. Many homeless people who are seeking health care have dual or multiple diagnoses, including drug and alcohol abuse and mental illness. This presents additional problems in the provision of health care for this population because treatments and treatment systems for these diagnoses are specific and often separate; frequently those with a secondary diagnosis are excluded. There is a need for treatment programs that are designed to address these dual and multiple diagnoses (Institute of Medicine, 1988).

## Barriers to Access to Health Care

Sutherland (1988) gives an overview of the problems encountered in the provision of health care to homeless people, including flaws in coverage by Medicare and the difficulties experienced in accessing services. The Institute of Medicine report (1988) acknowledges many problems with the current system of eligibility for benefits for health care. In addition to the inability to pay for health care, other barriers to access to care among the homeless include a lack of or difficulty in obtaining transportation to health care services, cultural differences between the providers and the clients, and in some communities, insufficient or lack of health care services. If the need is greater than the number of services available, delays in getting seen and a long waiting time for appointments all contribute to decreasing access for homeless individuals. Some homeless people do not trust the health care system or the providers and fear the institutions. In some instances the system is very difficult to negotiate, and substance abusers and mentally ill homeless people may be unable to access the system. For homeless women with children, it may be impossible to get through the system without provision of child care. The requirement of having an appointment may be a barrier to access for some homeless. Behaviors of homeless people also may create barriers to accessing health care. Because they lack adequate facilities for daily hygiene, their appearance and other noncompliant behaviors may cause health care providers to avoid them. Negative attitudes conveyed by providers also may be a barrier to access to health care for homeless individuals.

## Initiatives Taken

Since 1982, when the U.S. Conference of Mayors brought national attention to the shortage of emergency services (shelter, food, and income maintenance), this conference has continued to report on homelessness, hunger, and poverty. Its annual reports have provided information about how cities have responded to the problems, and it has also identified required national responses (U.S. Conference of Mayors, 1987a, b).

The Robert Wood Johnson Foundation-Pew Memorial Trust Health Care for the Homeless Program was the initial attempt to address the problem of providing health care to homeless individuals. A national effort carried out in selected large cities, the program was cosponsored by the U.S. Conference of Mayors. Fifty cities were eligible to apply for a grant; 18 were funded for four years (1985 to 1988) under this program, and an additional city was funded by special arrangement. Proposals had to include development of a program to provide health care to homeless people, efforts to improve their access to other services and entitlements, and a plan for continuation of the program following termination of the grant. Prior to this large-scale demonstration, there was a question of whether the homeless would use health care and social services if they were provided in areas easily accessible to them and were free. The homeless did use the services and did return for additional service (Lindsey, 1989; Wright & Weber, 1987). Another unknown element was whether these health care services had to be provided separately from services that already existed for nonhomeless people. The varied approaches used by the 19 funded projects to provide health care are summarized in the Institute of Medicine report (1988). Some used outreach and case management, some used mobile vans, others located clinics in existing shelters, and some had freestanding clinics. Client accessibility to a range of health care services was considered an essential component for a successful program. Examples of the range of services are prenatal care, alcohol treatment programs, dental care, mental health programs, provision for x-ray and other diagnostic services, and social services. Because of the circumstances associated with homelessness, the need for specialized housing arrangements was acknowledged particularly for severely physically ill or mentally ill homeless people.

Indicators of interest in the homeless by federal policy makers are the more than 30 bills concerned with homelessness that were introduced into the 100th Congress. The resulting Stewart B. McKinney Homeless Assistance Act, signed into law in the summer of 1987, now provides federal funding to cities where grant applications for support services and primary health care services for the homeless have been successful. In addition to health care, there is provision of funding for food, shelter, and education programs. However, in this era of great attention on reducing the federal budget deficit, the level of funding and even continuation of federal support are not assured.

Nurses have been involved in addressing issues associated with the homeless populations. The National Institute of Mental Health funded a small invitational workshop to address the role of nurses in meeting the health and mental health needs of the homeless (U.S. Department of Health and Human Services, 1986). Recommendations from this workshop addressed education and training needs of nurses to care for this population and changes in the current health and social service systems necessary to meet the diverse needs of this group. They also recommended that nurses advocate a coordinated, comprehensive response to the needs of homeless people, and they proposed that nursing research develop a data base on the homeless, establish demonstration projects for service delivery, and evaluate service models for their effectiveness in providing care to the homeless. There is a continuing need for a larger segment of nurses to discuss these issues and to act on these recommendations.

There is a poignant account of the establishment of a nurses' clinic at Pine Street Inn in Boston in 1972 (Reilly & McInnis, 1985). The Inn provides 300 beds for homeless men and 50 beds for homeless women as an emergency shelter. Nurses from Boston City Hospital, after a month of studying the health needs of the Pine Street Inn inhabitants, decided that nursing interventions were appropriate for the health care problems identified. This nurses' clinic has changed during the past 18 years from being part time and voluntary to becoming a fully staffed clinic that includes nursing staff assigned from the Boston Health and Hospitals Department and the Massachusetts Department of Mental Health. The Pine Street Inn clinic nurses also have documented that the most common health problems experienced by the homeless individuals include respiratory diseases, infestations of scabies and lice, stasis ulcers, and cardiovascular disorders (Reilly & McInnis, 1985). Because of the northeastern Massachusetts climate, frostbite and hypothermia also were problems for this homeless population. An early focus of the nurses' clinic work was testing and follow-up for those with symptoms of tuberculosis; as a result, the numbers of active cases and deaths from tuberculosis have been reduced in the Pine Street Inn inhabitants.

There now are several other nurse-managed clinics that serve homeless populations. These include the University of California, Los Angeles School of Nursing Health Centers located in the skid row area of downtown Los Angeles (Lindsey, 1989); the University of Kentucky School of Nursing Clinic in Lexington; the Nurse Clinic for the Homeless managed by the College of Nursing, Medical University of

South Carolina; the Homeless Project at the State University of New York at Buffalo; and the Nurse-Managed Clinic for the Homeless at Pace University in Pleasantville, New York. Using nurse-managed clinics as a model for providing primary health care to homeless individuals has worked. Often these clinics are located in facilities that provide other services to the homeless populations, and thus they have been established outside the mainstream of health care delivery systems.

The development, staffing, financing, and work done by one of the Universities of California, Los Angeles School of Nursing Health Centers are described briefly as an example of what nurses have contributed in providing primary health care for a homeless population. Nurse practitioner faculty at the University of California, Los Angeles School of Nursing in 1983 took the opportunity to begin providing primary health care to homeless individuals on a part-time basis in a large room of a shelter in the skid row area of downtown Los Angeles. This activity resulted in a site for faculty practice, a placement for students, and a population for research, and it provided a greatly needed service to the community. From such a meager beginning, the School now operates two nurse-managed health centers for homeless adults and children in downtown Los Angeles. These health centers are licensed as community clinics and are now open full time (5 days a week) and are staffed with full and part-time salaried employees. A director of clinic services, a master's degree–prepared nurse practitioner, provides for the clinical administration of the centers. Primary health care also is provided almost exclusively by master's degree–prepared nurse practitioners; a licensed vocational nurse is employed in one clinic. Physicians are employed on a limited part-time basis, e.g., four hours per week; one remains available on call. Some additional assistance is provided by personnel (non-health care) employed by the facilities in which the clinics are located and by the School of Nursing. A social worker has been part of the employed staff of the first health center, and one is available at the second center through the facility services. Linking social services and health care is a critical element. For the first few years of operation, an outreach worker was employed. However, more clients continued to arrive at the clinic than could be seen, and the small staff and the relatively small space precluded caring for the number of homeless who sought care. Certainly an outreach worker or team can be extremely helpful in locating homeless who need care, but it also is critical to have the staff and services available when the homeless arrive. The health centers primarily see clients on a drop-in basis because it is difficult for homeless individuals to make appointments and to keep them. Nurse practitioners diagnose the health care problems, furnish medications based on approved protocols, provide wound care, and perform other procedures as determined necessary. They do screening for tuberculosis, including administration and reading of skin tests. They attempt to teach homeless individuals about their health care problems and the pertinent self-care activities necessary for managing these problems, such as lice infestations or dependent edema or leg ulcerations. Clients with mental illness, those with chronic unstable problems, and those who are acutely ill are all referred and in some cases transported to the appropriate county facility.

These School of Nursing Health Centers have been established in areas of Los Angeles where homeless people congregate and are outside the regular established health care delivery systems. However, some support to operate the centers is provided by mainstream systems. For example, a local hospital provides for some laboratory tests, and the county has provided for a full-time licensed visiting nurse and continues to provide supplies and medications. Contractual arrangements were made with the facilities in which the health centers are located; one is a shelter, the Union Rescue Mission, and the other is a religious center that assists indigent and homeless individuals and families, the St. Francis Center. Both of these agencies cover the expenses for the clinic space and utilities. The major financing has been and continues to be through grants and donations. The School's first health center was originally funded for 4 years under the Robert Wood Johnson Foundation-Pew Memorial Trust Health Care for the Homeless Program. Subsequently, it has continued to be funded as one of the seven Los Angeles sites now covered under the Stewart B. McKinney Homeless Assistance Act. Support also has been received form the "comic relief events" held to raise money for health care for the homeless. The second health center was initiated through a grant received from the Division of Nursing, Department of Health and Human Services. In addition to this funding, by expanding the number of homeless served, the health centers became eligible for and have obtained state money that recently was made available for clinics providing health care to the homeless in California. All of the grant funding is used to employ personnel to staff the health centers and to manage patient records. It is very unlikely that the clinics would ever be self-supporting from Medicaid because the great majority of the homeless seen are not eligible for such payments. It is more likely that some of the cost of care will be recovered from benefits for services provided by the second health center because more children and women are seen there. There is considerable contribution by school administration and interested faculty in the management and continued operation of these clinics.

The centers represent a difficult but important initiative, and nurses have a major contribution to make in this arena. For example, between March, 1985, and June, 1989, 34,706 visits were recorded for the initial health center; of these, 26,878 were for health care and the remaining 7828 were for social services or transportation to other agencies. The 26,878 health care visits were made by 8675 clients; more than half (53 percent) the clients visited the clinic more than once. Additional information about the diagnoses and services provided has been reported elsewhere (Brecht, Lindsey, & Stuart, 1990). It is clear that homeless individuals have health care problems and that they will seek health care when it is free and easily accessible to them and when they can trust the providers and are treated with dignity. From our experience and that of others, a nurse-managed clinic is one cost-effective approach for providing primary health care to this very needy population.

## Issues and Implications

It has been stated that homelessness "represents a social problem that no system of social services has yet been designed to meet" (Holden, 1986, p. 570). Homelessness is a manifestation of extreme poverty, lack of some type of a stable residence, and disaffiliation from friends and family. The word homeless suggests that the solution is to provide housing for the increasing number of these disenfranchised individuals. This would be of tremendous help, but homelessness is a much more complicated phenomenon; the homeless as a population are not a homogeneous group. Because of these differences, there is need for a spectrum of housing options. Those who are temporarily or situationally without housing need options that are different from those who are episodically homeless and those who are chronically without a stable residence. Since approximately one third have mental illness, there is a need for housing with different levels of supervision. Other homeless people are chronically ill and may never be able to be reintegrated into society and to function independently. For a time, one solution to the increasing number of homeless people was to establish more shelters. Both public and private organizations established and continue to support emergency shelters. However, although shelters have provided for emergency temporary sleeping and in some cases for feeding arrangements, they are not a short- or long-term solution. Bassuk acknowledges that "shelters have been saddled with the impossible task of replacing not only the almshouses of the past but also the large state mental institutions" (Bassuk, 1984, p. 40). Providing shelter is also a major economic problem; for example, New York City houses about 10,000 homeless individuals and 5000 homeless families each night (Lockhead, 1988b). The New York City budget for the homeless increased from 6.8 million dollars in 1978 to 312 million dollars in 1988. To house a family of four in a welfare hotel, the city spends $1900 a month, with half the support coming from federal dollars (Lockhead, 1988b). Some homeless people receive general relief support, but in most urban areas, the level of benefits received is not sufficient for them to obtain stable housing. A major question for communities and governments is how the economic burdens are to be carried and distributed. The homeless populations are not as transient as once believed; many have become homeless in the communities in which they have lived for a number of years, and they have remained as homeless in their communities. Not all communities are committed to providing short-term assistance and planning for long-term solutions.

Homelessness has created hostilities among different factions in communities. For example, there are those advocates who want to provide shelter and food, and those who want the homeless to be removed from the area. There are those who think services should be provided but who say not in my neighborhood or not in my backyard (the NIMBY factor). There are those who say that if you provide services for the homeless, more will gather in the areas where these services are provided. Then there are those who say, if you do not provide services where the homeless congregate, these services will not be accessible to them. If you provide services and more homeless people avail themselves of them, the costs for the providers and the communities offering the services will increase. Ultimately, the question of who is to pay surfaces.

Other ethical, political, and economic issues to consider include the questions: (1) does personal freedom of homeless individuals supersede the involuntary commitment or institutionalization of those who are mentally ill; (2) does personal freedom of the homeless individual supersede public health and safety; (3) does personal freedom of the homeless individual supersede the personal freedom of individuals who own homes or businesses in communities where homeless people are congregating; (4) does every individual have a right to housing; (5) what obligations does or should society have for the children of homeless families; and (6) who should provide health care to the homeless, where should it be provided, and how should it be financed? These few questions suggest only a fraction of the magnitude of the very complicated, growing social phenomenon of homelessness.

Consider homeless children as an example; these children lack adequate nutritional intake, which influences their growth, development, and general health. If they are hungry, they have problems with concentration and learning, and given their environmental living conditions, they may lack sleep as well. They may have no place to do school work. Homelessness also affects children's attendance at school. Families move from shelter and shelter and transportation from a shelter to schools may not exist. These circumstances lead to irregular attendance, or moving from one school to another, or absence from school altogether. Reports from schools that have homeless children indicate the chaos and disruption that occur as a result of the status of these children. They have behavioral, emotional, and developmental problems and experience academic failures. The consequences that result from these circumstances have long-term effects for the individual children and for the nation. Urgent consideration must be given to decrease homelessness of families with children.

The Institute of Medicine (1988) report describes the extreme variability and complexities associated with Medicaid coverage across communities and states. An example given is that "27 states provide Aid to Families with Dependent Children, or AFDC (and thus, automatically Medicaid), to two-parent households with children in which the principal wage earner is unemployed and 23 states in which such households are ineligible for Medicaid" (Institute of Medicine, 1988, p. 83). The report further notes that because of eligibility differences, at any point in time, slightly over half of those with an income 150 percent below poverty level have Medicaid coverage. Wright and Weber (1987) reported that of the homeless people for whom the benefit status was known and who were seen more than once by 16 of the Robert Wood Johnson Foundation-Pew Memorial Trust funded homeless projects, only 21 percent had Medicaid. Only about half of those seen were receiving some type of benefit; the range of those homeless receiving benefits across the 16 projects was 22 to 82 percent. This can be accounted for both by differences in eligibility requirements across states and in composition of the homeless populations served (e.g., families with children versus single men and women). Individuals who are single and who have no children and no certified disabilities are not eligible for Medicaid; thus many homeless are excluded from Medicaid eligibility. The expansion of Medicaid and its decoupling from other entitlement programs are recommendations supported by the Institute of Medicine (1988). At least for the federally supported entitlement programs, the eligibility requirement of having a fixed address has been removed. Benefits for treatment of mental illness are not adequate. Not all states have Medicaid programs that include funding for mental health care and in those that do, the coverage for inpatient treatment is frequently limited to 30 days (Institute of Medicine, 1988). The U.S. Conference of Mayors' report (1987b) on local responses to needs of mentally ill homeless persons identified the need for a broad range of services. These included mental health services, health care, rehabilitation services, income support, opportunities for social interaction, and assistance in accessing services and obtaining housing, which includes supportive services. There is a need to develop new approaches for service delivery to this special population. Examples of day drop-in centers and outreach services to engage the isolated, disaffiliated homeless person were given as case studies.

There is a necessity for coordination of services with mental health, alcohol, and drug abuse programs because as many as two thirds of the homeless have one of these disorders, and as many as one fourth may have two or more of these problems (Wright & Weber, 1987). Some of the current problems include the delays in getting into drug and alcohol rehabilitation programs and the unavailability or insufficiency of critically needed after-care or transitional facilities. Comprehensive community mental health services and specialized services for substance abusers are requisite in helping homeless persons. The facilities must be available, must be staffed with professionals skilled in working with homeless people, and the provision for long-term support must be part of the rehabilitation programs. Because of scarce resources, priorities have not always included provision of health care for the homeless.

The need to link treatment, supervision, rehabilitation programs, and special housing for some homeless individuals is paramount. Some subpopulations of homeless people require specific approaches and targeted programs; for example, people with acquired immunodeficiency syndrome who become homeless, particularly as the disease progresses, single-parent homeless families, pregnant homeless adolescents, teenage or adult alcoholics who are homeless, and the chronically mentally ill homeless.

Health care providers, particularly private practitioners, are not abundant in low-income communities; this has forced a shift in the provision of care for the poor and homeless to hospitals, especially public hospitals. This, in turn, has resulted in a tremendous burden to the hospital system, where a large percentage of uncompensated care is provided. In large urban areas, emergency, trauma, and maternity services and outpatient departments are heavily utilized by the poor. Many public hospitals have budget deficits. The Institute of Medicine (1988) study concluded that "uninsured homeless individuals are, in a sense, competing with the growing numbers of other uninsured domiciled people for the relatively scarce resource of subsidized hospital services, especially because the homeless population is concentrated in those areas where the demands on hospitals are greatest" (Institute of Medicine, 1988, p. 92).

Freestanding clinics, including nurse-managed clinics, also provide health care to homeless and indigent people. These clinics are more variable in terms of funding support, location, and services provided. Coordination and provision of a range of required services may be problematic. There are barriers to access to health care for homeless people, and frequently the care is incomplete and fragmentary. Whether or not an outreach effort is used and who functions as the outreach worker or team of workers depend on multiple factors, including the safety of the environment and the availability and adequacy of services to provide care once homeless individuals who have health care needs are identified. Outreach efforts can range from having a fully equipped, supplied, and professionally staffed mobile van to a single (non-health care professional) person operation. A nurse can serve in this capacity; however, major considerations include the scope of services to be provided in outreach, the level of preparation of the nurse, and the cost-effectiveness of using a nurse.

Although an outreach effort certainly can uncover homeless people in need of care, it may be more efficacious to develop a clinic that is permanently and easily accessible to the homeless. Establishing an outreach effort can assist in linking homeless individuals with health care and social services; what is important, however, is that these services be available. Although a nurse-managed clinic provides one level of care, it is not sufficient to manage the entire range of health care problems experienced by homeless people. Similar to managing the needs of the general population, a range of provider services must be available and accessible to homeless people. This means that in addition to the use of clinics for primary health care, there must be a way to integrate homeless individuals into the mainstream of health care delivery systems or a way to make such services available to this population. To make this work may require use of facilities for showers and provision of clean clothes and socks and shoes; it may require transportation to a provider agency or institution and a return trip. A case manager may need to be used to ensure adherence to a treatment regimen and for follow-up appointments or referrals. If bed rest is advised, for example, special shelter arrangements need to be made. This very brief description only highlights some of the more obvious circumstances. One additional major consideration is how this care and other services are to be reimbursed. This requires discussion of reforms that are beyond the scope of this chapter. However, until this issue is resolved, provision of an adequate range of health care to this population is unlikely to occur. For example, dental care and eye care are virtually unavailable in many places. Frequently there is a long wait for an appointment for prenatal care, and thus pregnant homeless women may get prenatal care only in their third trimester.

Because the prevalence of active tuberculosis and asymptomatic tuberculosis infection has been reported to be more than 100 times higher in some homeless populations than for the general population, the Centers for Disease Control developed recommendations in 1987 to be taken as preventive measures against an increase in tuberculosis (Centers for Disease Control Division of Tuberculosis Control, 1987). The first task is to determine who among the homeless population has tuberculosis and where they stay. Programs for educating shelter workers about tuberculosis and screening for homeless people to help in case finding are essential. Provision of housing and supervision for homeless individuals with active tuberculosis, and if necessary, hospitalization are recommended. An intensive multidrug regimen carried out under supervision may be necessary. Homeless individuals with active disease need to be isolated until the treatment renders them noninfectious. In addition to the health of the individual, such a program is critical to prevent spread of the disease to others.

The changing composition of the homeless population to include more women and children, the prevalence of mental illness in this population, and the incidence of tuberculosis all have far-reaching implications for the provision of health care for these people. Clearly, resources are skimpy and services are fragmented and uncoordinated and frequently insufficient for the increasing number of homeless individuals who need assistance. At the very least, they need food, shelter, and health care. Beyond this, programs of long-term support, for detoxification, and for after care and rehabilitation are essential. Homeless individuals are alone, without the usual affiliations and support systems. They need long-term assistance to help them rejoin and reintegrate into the community. In addition, effective strategies and interventions to prevent or decrease first-time homelessness are imperative.

All these factors create the overarching context that influences the availability of and the delivery of health care to the homeless populations. Health care for homeless individuals has been provided in facilities established outside the regular health care systems (examples include the clinics set up in shelters) as well as within the routine delivery systems. Experience suggests that it is important to have the services available in areas where homeless people congregate. Availability, ease of access, no cost, and sufficient numbers of and coordination of services are the issues that must be addressed. These services must be staffed with professionals who are skilled in assisting homeless people. To enlarge the number of professionals who have these skills, students enrolled in health- and social service–related professional schools must have learning opportunities in working with homeless populations. Clearly, there is a need for a change in current systems dealing with homeless individuals and in resolving the many complexities of homelessness, including the delivery of health care.

This brings us back to the social, political, and ethical issues of who should provide health care to the homeless, where should it be provided, and how should it be financed. And finally, we must grapple with the issue of how health care ranks in relation to other priorities, such as food, shelter, clothing, social services, rehabilitation, long-term transition programs, job training, psychiatric counseling, education for the growing population of homeless children, and permanent housing. Homelessness has emerged as a major and complex phenomenon; how to provide health care to this population is only one of the extenuating problems. However, we do not need to accept those resources that currently exist.

## REFERENCES

Acker, P.J., Fierman, A.H., & Dreyer, B.P. (1987). An assessment of parameters of health care and nutrition in homeless children. *American Journal of Diseases of Children, 141*(4), 388.

Aiken, L.H. (1987). Unmet needs of the chronically mentally ill: Will nursing respond? *Image: Journal of Nursing Scholarship, 19*(3), 121–125.

Alliance Housing Council (1988). *Housing and homelessness.* Washington, DC: National Alliance to End Homelessness.

Bassuk, E.L. (1984). The homeless problem. *Scientific American, 251*(1), 40–45.

Bassuk, E.L., & Rosenberg, L. (1988). Why does family homelessness occur? A case-control study. *American Journal of Public Health, 78*(7), 783–788.

Bassuk, E.L., & Rubin, L. (1987). Homeless children: A neglected population. *American Journal of Orthopsychiatry, 5*(2), 1–9.

Bassuk, E.L., Rubin, L., & Lauriat, A. (1986, September). Characteristics of sheltered homeless families. *American Journal of Public Health, 76,* 1097–1101.

Berne, A.S., Dato, C., Mason, D.J., & Rafferty, M. (1990). A nursing model for addressing the health needs of homeless families. *Image: Journal of Nursing Scholarship, 22*(1), 8–13.

Boondas, J. (1985). The despair of the homeless aged. *Journal of Gerontological Nursing, 11*(4), 8–10, 12–13, 36.

Bowdler, J.E. (1989). Health problems of the homeless in America. *Nurse Practitioner, 14*(7), 44–51.

Breakey, W.R., Fischer, P.J., Kramer, M., Nestadt, G., Romanoski, A.J., Ross, A., Royall, R.M., & Stine, O.C. (1989). Health and mental health problems of homeless men and women in Baltimore. *Journal of American Medical Association, 262*(10), 1352–1357.

Brecht, L., Lindsey, A.M., & Stuart, I. (1990). *Health care needs of the homeless.* Berkeley, CA: California Policy Seminar.

Brickner, P., Scanlan, B., Conanan, B., Elvy, A., McAdam, J., Scharer, L., & Vicic, W. (1986). Homeless persons and health care. *Annals of Internal Medicine, 104,* 405–409.

Brickner, P.W., Scharer, L., Conanan, B., Elvy, A., & Savarese, M. (Eds.) (1985). *Health care of homeless people.* New York: Springer Publishing Co.

Burt, M.R., & Cohen, B.E. (1989). Differences among homeless single women, women with children, and single men. *Social Problems, 36*(5), 508–523.

Centers for Disease Control Division of Tuberculosis Control (1987, May 8). Tuberculosis control among homeless populations. *Morbidity and Mortality Weekly Report, 36*(17), 257–260.

Chafetz, L. (1988). Perspectives for psychiatric nurses on homelessness. *Issues in Mental Health Nursing, 9,* 325–335.

Chavkin, W., Kristal, A., Seabron, C., & Guigli, P. (1987). The reproductive experience of women living in hotels for the homeless in NYC. *New York State Journal of Medicine, 371,* 10–13.

Council on Scientific Affairs (1989). Health care needs of homeless and runaway youths. *Journal of American Medical Association, 262*(10), 1358–1361.

Damrosch, S., & Strasser, J.A. (1988). The homeless elderly in America. *Journal of Gerontological Nursing, 14*(10), 26–29.

Doolin, J. (1986). Planning for the special needs of the homeless elderly. *The Gerontologist, 26*(3), 229–231.

Farr, R.K., Koegel, P., & Burnam, A. (1986). *A study of homelessness and mental illness in the skid row area of Los Angeles.* Los Angeles: Los Angeles County Department of Mental Health.

Fischer, P.J., & Breakey, W.R. (1986). Homelessness and mental health: An overview. *International Journal of Mental Health, 14*(4), 6–14.

Fischer, P.J., & Breakey, W.R. (1987). Profile of Baltimore homeless with alcohol problems. *Alcohol, Health and Research World, 11*(3), 36–37.

Fischer, P.J., Shapiro, S., Breakey, W.R., Anthony, J.C., & Kramer, M. (1986). Mental health and social characteristics of the homeless: A survey of mission users. *American Journal of Public Health, 76*(5), 519–524.

Francis, M.B. (1987). Long-term approaches to end homelessness. *Public Health Nursing, 4*(4), 230–235.

Holden, C. (1986). Homelessness: Experts differ on root causes. *Science, 232,* 569–570.

Holden, C. (1988). Health problems of the homeless. *Science, 242,* 188–189.

Hu, D.J., Covell, R.M., Morgan, J., & Arcia, J. (1989). Health care needs for children of the recently homeless. *Journal of Community Health, 14*(1), 1–8.

Institute of Medicine (1988). *Homelessness, health and human needs*. Washington, DC: National Academy Press.

Koegel, P., & Burnam, M.A. (1987). Traditional and nontraditional homeless alcoholics. *Alcohol, Health, and Research World, 11*(3), 28–35.

Lewis, M.R., & Meyers, A.F. (1989). The growth and development status of homeless children entering shelters in Boston. *Public Health Reports, 104*(3), 247–250.

Lindsey, A.M. (1989). Health care for the homeless. *Nursing Outlook, 37*(2), 78–81.

Lockhead, C. (1988a, May 16). Nowhere to go, always in sight. *Insight on the News,* 8–11.

Lockhead, C. (1988b, May 16). All alone with no home. *Insight on the News,* 12–15.

Lockhead, C. (1988c, May 16). Door opening to dignity. *Insight on the News,* 16–18.

McDonald, D.D. (1986). Health care and cost containment for the homeless: Curricular implications. *Journal of Nursing Education, 25*(6), 261–264.

Nyamathi, A., & Shuler, P. (1989). Factors affecting prescribed medication compliance of the urban homeless adult. *Nurse Practitioner, 14*(8), 47–54.

Piliavin, I., Westerfelt, H., & Elliott, E. (1989). Estimating mental illness among the homeless: The effects of choice-based sampling. *Social Problems, 36*(5), 525–531.

Reilly, E., & McInnis, B.N. (1985). Boston, Massachusetts: The Pine Street Inn Nurses' Clinic and Tuberculosis Program. In P.W. Breckner, L.K. Scharer, B. Conanan, A. Elvy, & M. Savarese (Eds.), *Health care of homeless people* (pp. 291–299). New York: Springer Publishing Company.

Ropers, R.H., & Boyer, R. (1987). Perceived health status among the new urban homeless. *Social Science Medicine, 24*(8), 669–678.

Rossi, P.H., Wright, J.D., Fisher, G.A., & Willis, G. (1987). The urban homeless: Estimating composition and size. *Science, 235,* 1336–1341.

Salem, D.A., & Levine, I.S. (1989). Enhancing mental health services for homeless persons: State proposals under the MHSH Block Grant Program. *Public Health Reports, 104*(3), 241–246.

Satin, K.P., Frerichs, R.R., & Sloss, E.M. (1982). Three-dimensional computer mapping of disease in Los Angeles County. *Public Health Reports, 97*(5), 470–475.

Slavinsky, A.T., & Cousins, A. (1982). Homeless women. *Nursing Outlook, 30,* 358–362.

Snow, D.A., Baker, S.G., & Anderson, L. (1989). Criminality and homeless men: An empirical assessment. *Social Problems, 36*(5), 532–549.

Strasser, J.A. (1978, December). Urban transient women. *American Journal of Nursing, 78,* 2076–2079.

Sutherland, A.R. (1988, Fall). Health care for the homeless. *Issues in Science and Technology, 5*(1), 79–86.

Tucker, W. (1987, September 25). Where do the homeless come from? *National Review,* 32–35, 40–43.

U.S. Conference of Mayors (1986). *The continued growth of hunger, homelessness and poverty in America's cities: 1986. A 25-city survey*. Washington, DC: U.S. Conference of Mayors.

U.S. Conference of Mayors (1987a). *A status report on homeless families in America's cities: A 29-city survey*. Washington, DC: U.S. Conference of Mayors.

U.S. Conference of Mayors (1987b). *Local responses to the needs of homeless mentally ill persons*. Washington, DC: U.S. Conference of Mayors.

U.S. Conference of Mayors (1988). *A status report on hunger and homelessness in America's cities: 1988. A 27-city survey*. Washington, DC: U.S. Conference of Mayors.

U.S. Conference of Mayors (1989). *A status report on hunger and homelessness in America's cities: 1989. A 27-city survey.* Washington, DC: U.S. Conference of Mayors.

United States Department of Health and Human Services (1988). *Alcohol and other drug abuse among homeless individuals: An annotated bibliography.* Rockville, MD: National Institute on Alcohol Abuse and Alcoholism.

U.S. Department of Health and Human Services (1986). *The role of nurses in meeting the health/mental health needs of the homeless.* Washington, DC: National Institute of Mental Health, Office of the Assistant Secretary for Health.

U.S. Department of Housing and Urban Development (1984). *A report to the secretary on the homeless and emergency shelters.* Washington, DC: Office of Policy Development and Research.

U.S. House of Representatives Select Committee on Children, Youth, and Families (1987). *The crisis in homelessness: Effects on children and families. (Hearing held on February 24, 1987.)* Washington, DC: U.S. Government Printing Office (#72-237).

Vladeck, B. (1988, Fall). A national scandal. *Issues in Science and Technology,* 5(1), 86–87.

Whitman, D. (1988, February 29). Hope for the homeless. *U.S. News and World Report,* 25–28; 31; 34–35.

Wright, J.D. (1989). *Address unknown: The homeless in America.* New York: Aldine de Gruyter.

Wright, J.D., & Weber, E. (1987). *Homelessness and health.* Washington, DC: McGraw-Hill.

Wright, J.D., Weber-Burdin, E., Knight, J.W., & Lam, J.A. (1987). The National Health Care for the Homeless Program. University of Massachusetts, Amherst: The First Year Report prepared by the Social and Demographic Research Institute.

## Chapter 25

# The Nursing Challenges of Acquired Immunodeficiency Syndrome

GWEN VAN SERVELLEN

$T$HE FIRST CASE of acquired immunodeficiency syndrome (AIDS) was diagnosed in the United States in 1981. The human immunodeficiency virus (HIV), which attacks and destroys the body's immune system, has infected about 1 million persons in the United States. The number of cases of full-blown AIDS, representing about 10 percent of those people currently infected, is expected to continue to increase. As of July 1991, more than 182,834 cases of AIDS have been reported to the Centers for Disease Control (Centers for Disease Control, 1991).

Earlier predictions of the prevalence of HIV infection were influenced in part by a change in reported AIDS incidence in 1987, when the slowing of the rapid upward trend in rate of increase occurring among nonintravenous drug-using homosexual/bisexual men engendered some hope that the prospect of control, over time, was within reach.

One can look to the slowing trend in cases found among homosexual and bisexual men as evidence that prevention and public educational efforts worked to decrease the incidence of HIV infection in the early 1980s. Other factors, however, resulted in this trend. The use of antiviral and other therapies by mid-1987 led to a lengthening of the incubation period from infection with HIV to AIDS, and possible decreases in the completeness and timeliness of reporting are believed to have affected the rate of increase–decline (Centers for Disease Control, 1989a). For this reason, undue optimism about significant changes needs to be held in check.

New cases diagnosed at high rates continue to place demands on existing health services. Persons with AIDS are being seen and treated in a variety of settings. Although most prefer to be at home and receive help from friends or visiting nurses' associations, a portion are at home with no outside help. Others are hospitalized in acute inpatient medical units or acute psychiatric units. A small proportion are in hospices and skilled nursing facilities. An unknown but rapidly growing number utilize a combination of AIDS residential facilities and emergency or temporary housing; others are homeless. It is clear that the number of cases of AIDS will continue to increase and will tax the health care delivery systems in new and significant ways, making it imperative for all health and social services and for nurses, in particular, to respond to the challenge.

Problems in lobbying for responsive health delivery systems are in part a consequence of the uneven distribution of cases of AIDS across the country. The United States accounts for 40 percent of the world's reported AIDS cases. Yet, it should be understood that a small number of cities within a select number of states account for the majority of these cases. The picture of HIV infection and AIDS cases as it is geographically distributed across the United States has not changed a great deal since 1981. The Centers for Disease Control annual incidence rates per 100,000 people consistently show the states of New York, New Jersey, Florida, and California to be high ranking. With the exception of the addition of Puerto Rico, now ranking highest with 41.4 cases per 100,000 people, the rank order of states reporting cases of AIDS per 100,000 people has not changed. The Centers for Disease Control's July 1989 figures indicate that New York, with 23,424 cases, and California, with 20,478 cases, made up a little less than half (43 percent) of the cumulative total of AIDS cases reported to the Centers for Disease Control. One reason why it has been difficult to capture the attention of Congress is that far many more states have very small numbers of cases.

## Distribution of Acquired Immunodeficiency Syndrome Across Principal Transmission Categories

The reporting system of the Centers for Disease Control identifies key classifications of those at risk of HIV infection by means of specific modes of transmission. Prevalence reports are based on these classifications. These classification systems differ according to age grouping. Modes of transmission for adolescents and adults are different from those for children (age 13 and younger).

Modes of transmission of AIDS among adults and adolescents consist of seven basic categories:

1. male homosexual/bisexual contact,
2. intravenous drug use (female and heterosexual male),
3. male homosexual/bisexual contact and intravenous drug use,
4. hemophilia/coagulation disorder,
5. heterosexual contact,
6. recipient of blood transfusion, blood components, or tissues, and
7. other/undetermined.

The last category may refer to either health care workers or patients whose source of transmission remains undetermined.

Modes of transmission of AIDS among children (ages 13 and younger) usually fit one of three basic categories:

1. hemophilia/coagulation disorder,
2. born of a mother with or at risk for AIDS/HIV infection, or
3. a recipient of a blood transfusion, blood components, or tissue.

The cumulative total of AIDS cases in the United States among adults and adolescents indicates that male homosexual/bisexual practices are responsible for 57 percent of the total number of AIDS cases in this age group through June 1991. Intravenous drug use (among males or females) accounts for only 19 percent of the cumulative cases of AIDS illness. Despite the decline in rate of increase in diagnosed AIDS cases among nonintravenous drug–using homosexual/bisexual men in 1987, AIDS cases continue to be a problem.

Of continually growing concern is the forecast for HIV infection and subsequent AIDS illness among other groups: intravenous drug users, heterosexuals, and newborns (children of female intravenous drug users). Among children (13 years and younger), the highest proportion of AIDS cases has occurred in those whose mothers were infected with HIV through the use of intravenous drugs (Centers for Disease Control, 1989d).

The majority of AIDS cases occur in adults and adolescents, at the rate of 100 times that for pediatric cases. Nonetheless, the fear of increased prevalence among children, primarily because of the increase in AIDS in female intravenous drug users, is justified. It should be noted that although the total number of AIDS cases is significantly less than that for adults and adolescents practicing high risk behaviors, the ability of children to survive AIDS is no better than that of their older counterparts. The case fatality rate for children is no different from that for adults and adolescents. Therefore, children seem to have no better or worse chance of surviving AIDS illness (Centers for Disease Control, 1989b). The disease does exert a significant impact on young adult mortality. In 1987, for example, AIDS deaths accounted for 11 percent of all deaths in men 25 to 34 years of age. For women in this same age group, AIDS accounted for only 3 percent of all deaths.

## Current Conceptual and Operational Definitions of AIDS

Historically, AIDS was viewed in largely pessimistic ways, as a "death penalty" or "a tragic deadly illness" like "the plague"—a serious epidemic that had far-reaching implications for the survival of humankind. These notions of AIDS reflected in part the fear and hysteria that were associated with a disease that had no cure, was fatal, and afflicted the heretofore healthy, young, and productive male population in ways that were difficult to accept and comprehend. Without a doubt, all those afflicted would die; at the time, the survival period from initial diagnosis of AIDS illness to death was thought to be about 18 months but could be as short as six months and rarely lasted two years. Since the mid-1980s, however, several advances have occurred that have added both optimism and objectivity to health providers' views of AIDS and are reflected in the current conceptualization of HIV disease.

The AIDS problem has been reconceptualized as HIV/AIDS disease. Human immunodeficiency virus disease has been described in two classification systems (Vlahov, 1989). Essentially, what these systems do is provide further sophistication in looking at AIDS as a disease process. One is the Centers for Disease Control's four-group classification system, and the second and less commonly used paradigm is the Walter Reed Staging Classification System. The Centers for Disease Control's classification consists of (1) Group I—Acute Infection, (2) Group II—Asymptomatic Infection, (3) Group III—Persistent Generalized Lymphodenopathy, and (4) Group IV—Other Diseases. The Centers for Disease Control's classification identifies critical diagnostic parameters that help distinguish AIDS illness from HIV symptomatic and asymptomatic infection. Although the Centers for Disease Control's framework is useful, it has certain shortcomings in surveillance studies. It does not reveal a great deal about an individual's condition, nor is it precise about immune status. What is known is only that the individual's immune status is compromised sufficiently to result in specific opportunistic infections and/or malignancies.

In contrast, the Walter Reed System is more complex and takes into consideration several additional clinical indicators that depict the level of immune compromise present in the person infected. The Walter Reed System is a seven-stage classification system that is intended to yield prognostic significance when applied to individual cases. The Reed System, devised in 1985, was to accomplish two things: (1) it would provide a prognostic framework for patients; and (2) it would provide a meaningful stratification system around which to evaluate new therapeutic interventions, e.g., new drug trials. The major difference in the two systems is that the Walter Reed System uses T-helper cell count markers, whereas the Centers for Disease Control's does not. Because the health of persons infected with the virus is highly influenced by T-cell counts, the clinical interest in such a classification system is obvious, especially if optimal treatment impact can be linked with one's classification.

In addition to important advances in classifying HIV disease, the reports of infection with HIV's not being a near fatal disease have contributed to some optimism. The Centers for Disease Control report that the median interval between infection with HIV and onset of AIDS is nearly 10 years (Centers for Disease Control, 1989c).

At least in one study the average incubation period for those getting AIDS through sexual transmission was approximately seven to eight years (Lifson, Rutherford, & Jaffe, 1988). Those at risk by way of blood transfusion, however, fare much worse, according to this study. For those infected through blood transfusion, the median time from point of exposure to development of symptoms was just 46 months. The second most critical issue is the estimated survival time once one is diagnosed with AIDS. Impressive numbers of survivors have been observed to live as many as five to 15 years after diagnosis with AIDS. Additionally, recent advances in the treatment of persons with AIDS and those infected with the virus suggest that treatment with azidothymidine and other antiviral agents, immune modulators, and surface active agents significantly prolongs life or improves the quality of life while the patient is under treatment.

There is increasing impetus to support the idea that AIDS is a chronic controllable disease. Despite researchers' desires to move in this direction, the evidence to validate this shift needs bolstering. The following facts outline the major challenges to be addressed in supporting the trend to define AIDS as a chronic controllable disease and not a fatal terminal illness.

There is as yet no vaccine to prevent or reduce the risk of acquiring HIV infection. All patients diagnosed with AIDS eventually do die; they have limited ability to alter the quality of their lives once they are diagnosed with AIDS. Although the virus can exist in individuals in a latent state for long periods of time, the ultimate outcome once the disease surfaces is still bleak. In a large sample of patients in New York City, the result was profound immunosuppression in 85 percent of the diagnosed patients within five years (Rotherberg et al., 1987). A recent HIV/AIDS surveillance report (Centers for Disease Control, 1991) showed a positive trend downward in the case-fatality rates since 1988. Still, conclusions about the impact of treatment on prolonging life in patients are made with caution.

## Practice Issues Related to the Care of Individuals with Human Immunodeficiency Virus/Acquired Immunodeficiency Syndrome

Human immunodeficiency virus infection is a disease that affects multiple body systems. Its physiologic presentation offers multiple challenges in the areas of nutrition, elimination, and pain management. However, psychological adaptation to the disease is of considerable importance to the health of the individual. Whether viewed as a problem around managing treatment or as an integral part of the condition, the psychological impact of HIV infection should receive thoughtful consideration. Additionally, both HIV infection and AIDS have been shown to have significant social, political, familial, and economic consequences. These ramifications and those neurologic and psychological sequelae associated with HIV disease present a unique and complex problem to the health delivery system.

The following is an overview of the nursing care problems involved in caring for those persons who are affected by or infected with HIV.

For purposes of discussion and in keeping with the notion that HIV infection should be viewed on a disease continuum, the following care categories were formulated: (1) "the worried well," those who are at risk but whose HIV status is not confirmed and those whose HIV status is positive but who are currently asymptomatic, (2) those who are HIV-positive and symptomatic but who do not have AIDS, and (3) those at various stages of AIDS illness. Within each category are specific health care delivery issues confronting nursing care to these individuals, and these will be addressed as well.

### The Worried Well

Until HIV status is confirmed through HIV antibody testing, it is presumed that an individual is HIV-negative. This is in spite of the fact that certain individuals may practice high-risk behaviors and are likely candidates to develop HIV disease. HIV-positive individuals who are currently asymptomatic are those whose HIV status has been confirmed through antibody testing but who do not demonstrate any symptoms indicative of AIDS-related complex (ARC).

The problems of those individuals who are not yet infected with HIV and those who are are not altogether different, with the exception that HIV-positive asymptomatic individuals may be on clinical trials with experimental drugs such as azidothymidine (Retrovir). However, this is not commonplace, and many asymptomatic HIV-positive persons do not have the opportunity to receive treatment.

The nursing care problems related to this category of persons are largely psychosocial and educational. Knowledge deficits, anxiety, and stress are major problems afflicting this group, and these problems sometimes combine to produce poorly informed anxious individuals who lack proper support systems to adequately cope. Controlling stress and anxiety is paramount. Managing stress through support groups, maintaining a healthy lifestyle, and improving one's support network are important. Sometimes anxiety gets so acute as to require formal therapy and the temporary use of antianxiety and/or antidepression medication.

Educating these individuals about HIV disease is critical. Information about the course of disease, treatment options, how and when to be enrolled in a drug trial, and how to act responsibly in reducing exposure to others must be provided. Even individuals at this stage of the disease need health care providers who are experienced and knowledgeable in HIV disease and are sensitive to the needs of the worried well. Although several informal AIDS networks are available and for the most part provide accurate information, these persons will benefit from a personal relationship with a health care provider whom they trust and who can be a reliable treatment source at some later date. In most cases the burden of intervention lies with the primary care provider. Adequate health care services for "the worried well" are severely lacking. This is for several reasons. First, the needs of these individuals are largely unrecognized and, therefore, neglected by health care providers. Second, services that would address their needs, e.g., psychoeducational interventions, are regarded as preventive in nature and, unless an acute anxiety or depressive episode results, are not covered by insurance. Also, even if services were available and clients were reimbursed for treatment, sufficient denial exists in this group to negatively influence appropriate use of whatever resources were available. Last, adequate numbers of competent primary care providers are lacking.

## Human Immunodeficiency Virus–Positive Symptomatic Individuals

This category of disease, sometimes referred to as AIDS-related complex (ARC) is a stage in HIV infection in which a variety of signs and symptoms or even diseases occur but not to the degree to warrant a diagnosis of AIDS. A symptomatic HIV-positive status is not the worse scenario in the continuum of HIV disease, but it is sufficiently serious to remind those infected with HIV that they are at the mercy of a potentially devastating life-threatening disease. Since HIV infection can affect every organ system of the body, the precise nursing care needs of individuals at this stage may vary greatly, depending on the infections incurred and the body systems affected. HIV disease can affect the peripheral and central nervous systems, alter blood cell composition, and produce malignancies.

At the least, if he or she is symptomatic, the individual usually experiences fever and generalized malaise. The cluster of signs and symptoms most frequently associated with ARC include fever, night sweats, thrush, weight loss, persistent diarrhea, malaise, chronic fatigue, and persistent generalized lymphadenopathy.

Individuals who have acute symptomatic HIV disease (i.e., with ARC) can be assisted with prophylactic treatments of azidothymidine. The use of azidothymidine has been shown to decrease the frequency of infections, improve the functional status of individuals, and promote weight gain. It is being studied for its overall effect on increasing life span in persons with either AIDS or ARC. This treatment is not easy to obtain and is expensive. It is the principal governmentally approved antiviral treatment that can be used to treat HIV infection at any stage—whether asymptomatic or symptomatic infection. Azidothymidine can produce major side effects, including anemia and neutropenia.

Nursing care problems associated with HIV symptomatic individuals depend a great deal on the presenting symptoms. Interventions designed to relieve fatigue and malaise, anorexia, fevers, and diarrhea and to treat thrush infection are indicated.

Because the symptomatic stage, which is accompanied by clear signs of immune suppression, prevents the patient from denying the possibility of a downward course, several psychological responses may occur that need to be addressed. These include anxiety, fear, and depression related to declining health status and any beginning doubts related to treatment efficacy. Fears and concerns about death and dying may appear, but problems related to maintenance of a productive work and personal lifestyle may prevail. Common questions at this stage are: How long will I remain well enough to work? When will I need additional help, e.g., financial and social support sufficient to maintain myself at home and in my community? There is substance for worry, and it is this category of individuals who can be significantly helped with community-based volunteer services. The major problem in providing health services of this kind is that they are available in large AIDS epicenters but are virtually absent in geographical areas where there is a lack of information, expertise, compassion, and concern and/or a well-organized system. Even community-based medical and voluntary services in large epicenters must contend with several problems, e.g., (1) the wide variety of needs, (2) training of semiprofessionals and/or volunteers, and (3) significant budget limitations. The proliferation of volunteer support services to help symptomatic persons is suggestive of the fact that (1) a single organization cannot meet all those demands of infected individuals for education, symptomatic treatment, and psychosocial support, and (2) some people prefer to experiment with a variety of traditional and/or nontraditional services.

## Those Diagnosed with Acquired Immunodeficiency Syndrome

The diagnosis of AIDS is reported on the basis of laboratory confirmation of cellular immune deficiency without known cause and the diagnosis of specific opportunistic infections and/or secondary cancers. In 1985 and then again in 1987, the

Centers for Disease Control extended the definition to include other conditions if HIV infection was concomitantly confirmed. These diseases included disseminated histoplasmosis, chronic isosporiasis, certain non-Hodgkin's lymphomas (1985 revision), extrapulmonary tuberculosis, HIV encephalopathy, HIV wasting syndrome, and other presumptively diagnosed indicator diseases (1987 revision).

Most nursing diagnoses identified for HIV-infected persons are appropriate for both HIV symptomatic individuals and persons whose status meets the criteria for full-blown AIDS. Current outlines of AIDS-related symptoms and/or client needs are provided in several nursing reviews (Laskin, 1988; Meisenhelder & LaCharita, 1989; Nily, 1988; Pomerantz & Harrison, 1990a; Taravella, 1989). Essentially these outlines are comprehensive and sometimes quite detailed in addressing specific conditions, e.g., those related to *Pneumocystis carinii* pneumonia or Kaposi's sarcoma.

Actual or potential problems are associated with the disease itself, medication side effects, and/or complications related to secondary infections. Although hospitalization was previously a consideration for general problems related to AIDS illness and to initiate a new treatment, inpatient services are now more judiciously employed. Hospitalizations are likely to occur for such problems as side effects of drug therapy and neurologic work-ups. Nonetheless, uncontrolled symptom management for one or more problems, especially pneumonia, continues to be a reason for hospitalizing persons with AIDS.

Potential nursing diagnoses and/or patient needs include the following problem areas:

1. Altered skin integrity due to disease process, immobility, poor nutritional status, incontinence
2. Impaired nutritional status frequently accompanied by
3. Alteration in elimination-diarrhea incontinence
4. Alteration in mental status and impaired cognitive functioning due to disease process, opportunistic infections, and/or medications
5. Respiratory distress, including shortness of breath, dyspnea, tachypnea, cough, cyanosis
6. Anxiety, depression, anger, and fear associated with diagnosis, self-image role changes, guilt, and prognosis death and dying
7. Fatigue and malaise associated with stage of disease, change in nutritional status medications
8. Inadequate resistance to infection due to neutropenia and disease process
9. Fevers associated with disease process, infection, or drug reaction, anorexia, nausea, vomiting, diarrhea
10. Bleeding due to disease process and/or medications
11. Pain due to disease process
12. Local and systemic reactions to medications
13. Injury due to potential falling
14. Need for education of patient, significant or supportive others, and/or family regarding disease process, care at home or hospital, medications,

and treatments. Clarification of resuscitation status, will, and power of attorney
15. Moderate to severe self-care deficit with impaired home management
16. Ineffective coping of patient, significant/supportive others, and/or family
17. Social isolation due to impaired mobility, ineffective coping of patient and supportive others.

All of these problems or needs may not be observed in each and every patient, and the magnitude of the problem and/or response to intervention are also variable. End-stage terminal patients usually exhibit more problems. These include nausea and vomiting, diarrhea, dehydration, urinary incontinence, cough, hypoxemia, and respiratory pain, decubitus ulcers, pain, delirium, dementia, and weight loss. Fear, anxiety, and depression may also prevail as these patients face the prospect of impending death and concerns for the welfare of their supportive significant others (Pomerantz & Harrison, 1990a). The exact clustering of patient problems over time, once they have been diagnosed with AIDS, is highly dependent on several factors. These include overall immune status compromise, particular opportunistic diseases, and level of supportive services available. At times they may feel well enough to carry on everyday activities, maintain social activities, and even continue some level of employment. At other times they are very sick, require hospitalization, or become homebound and less able to care for themselves.

Persons with AIDS may be on drug protocol studies that involve consistent monitoring from primary care clinicians, and when they are hospitalized they need expert, compassionate nursing and medical care. Even if homebound, they will benefit from daily care, sometimes 24-hour care, from persons with knowledge and/or experience with AIDS treatment. Hospice or home care nursing services are needed to plan and supervise care and to treat various patient problems, including administration of intravenous drugs and treatments. In some but not all instances, home health aides may be used to provide care. However, because these aides are not always available or recognized in some states, more often than not, care of the AIDS patient in the home is managed by the patient's friends or family and minimally assisted by nurses. Hospital care is costly and not preferable to most patients. On the other hand, hospice care is often not available despite the fact that it is more appropriate for end-stage patients than is hospitalization.

There is considerable debate over the wisdom and feasibility of establishing dedicated hospital and/or hospice units for persons with AIDS. In a survey conducted by Modern Health Care, 40 American hospitals were reported to operate dedicated inpatient acute care AIDS units, representing 750 beds in 10 states and Puerto Rico. Of these beds, 49 percent were available at private not-for-profit hospitals, 20 percent at public hospitals, and 21 percent at investor-owned facilities (Taravella, 1989). It was predicted that the numbers of dedicated units would increase significantly in 1989 as a result of the creation of new units and the expansion of existing ones. Activities of these kinds reported in this survey revealed that the total number of dedicated AIDS beds available at United States hospitals may increase in 1989 to 936 beds at 48 facilities (Taravella, 1989). This projection was derived from a survey of 42 health associations and almost 200 hospitals nationally, principally in states with 10 percent or more of the nation's total AIDS cases.

Several reasons for establishing dedicated units have been cited that appeal to both cost and/or quality of care issues.

Essentially, the following features characterize a dedicated unit:

1. Beds on the unit are exclusively reserved for HIV-infected patients.
2. A multidisciplinary team approach is utilized that may include social workers, clinical nurse specialists, infectious disease specialists, psychologists, psychiatrists, neurologists, nutritionists, community volunteers, and ministerial services.
3. Nursing staff members are selected to work on the unit with full knowledge of and commitment to the care of HIV-infected persons.
4. Units frequently work closely with community-based AIDS organizations to coordinate volunteer services.

These units have been associated with a number of positive outcomes, most of which seem plausible if not fully documented: (1) more effective care owing to more highly trained, committed staff, including in some cases, "reverse prejudice"—a staff that is less fearful, more sympathetic, and more interested in learning than staff elsewhere in the hospital; (2) sophisticated and compassionate nursing care; (3) physicians and nurses who are specialized in AIDS care and therefore are more likely to order fewer tests, arrange shorter stays, and keep patients out of the hospital as much as possible; (4) the possibility of reduced incidents of accidental exposure owing to needle sticks and other forms of transmission in a health care setting because staff are more aware and specially trained; and (5) inspired health team work, the spirit and support of which is calming to patients (Pomerantz & Harrison, 1990b).

In sum, those who support the dedicated unit approach claim that it improves coordination of services, provides a better psychosocial environment for patients and their significant others, and promotes AIDS expertise among staff, increasing staff opportunities to develop specialized expertise in HIV infection and the medications, treatments, and investigational drugs used to treat the disease.

There is very little actual evidence to support establishing AIDS dedicated units as compared with using a scattered approach. Much of the information to date relies on testimonial statements and/or impressionistic summaries made by those hospitals that have dedicated units coupled with patient endorsements. One study of the relative differences in dedicated units compared with general medical units housing patients of mixed diagnoses found that patients on special care units reported fewer hospital stress factors. These differences were found to be significant in areas of important care dimensions such as ambiguity about one's care and condition and feelings of abandonment and impersonal treatment. However, patients' levels of distress with various hospital stressors were generally low on both kinds of units (van Servellen, Lewis, & Leake, 1990). When these patients were compared with oncology patients on dedicated units and to oncology patients using the scattered bed approach (using general medical patients as controls), unit type did have some predictive value. Diagnostic category alone did not predict level of stress. It is important to point out that stresses related to absence of supportive family networks, adverse physical environment, and uncertainty and unpredictability of the future were experienced by over half the study's total sample. These stressors were experienced less by general medical patients when compared with AIDS and oncology patients. Additionally, stress scores in these categories were higher for oncology patients than for AIDS patients.

The survey conducted by *Modern Health Care* reported several reasons why some hospitals were not willing to establish dedicated units:

1. physical renovation would be needed and this would prove costly,
2. nurses might be hard to find because of the emotional stress and fear,
3. the hospital could become identified as an "AIDS hospital" and that would discourage non-AIDS patients from seeking care at that institution,
4. patients might be stigmatized,
5. administrative processes might be disrupted, and
6. the special dedicated unit might become too "independent" (a hospital within a hospital).

To date there are insufficient data to support any or all conclusions surrounding the advantages and disadvantages of dedicated units. However, experience with special care units in other areas, e.g., oncology and burn care, supports the dedicated unit approach.

A major over-riding issue in the care and treatment of patients with AIDS is expense, coupled with inadequacies in the care delivery system. It has been estimated that the cumulative costs of treating all persons in the United States who have AIDS from time of diagnosis to death may reach 7.8 billion dollars by 1993 (Agency for Health Care Policy and Research, 1990). Additionally, the average lifetime cost of treating a person with AIDS (previously estimated to be $75,000) has risen. This increase reflects greater use of drugs, e.g., azidothymidine and aerosol pentamidine, over longer survival periods. Lifetime costs are also based on 1.6 hospital admissions per year per patient and an average hospital stay of 15.8 days.

The lifetime costs of treating patients with HIV/AIDS are also dependent upon proper utilization of services for individual patients and in accordance with their course of illness. What is known is that lifetime costs per patient can be quite variable and reflect the state of the art and public response in any given region of the country. For example, physician's level of expertise and ability to treat patients as outpatients, advances in treatment that sustain patients in the home, and the increase in coordinated systems of care in the community frequently make a difference in both whether a patient will be hospitalized and the length of the hospitalization.

The very sick patient needs skilled and often continuous care. Sometimes intensive care inpatient settings are appropriate. But for end-stage patients, hospital care is not appropriate or necessary. Additionally, care in the home, or hospice, is less costly than hospital care. The average cost per patient per day who receives home or hospice care is estimated to be less than $100; this has been compared with hospital costs of at least ten times this amount per day (Arno, 1986; Burda & Powills, 1986; Martin-Parker, 1986). Home care and/or hospice services are not available to the extent needed. The palliative orientation of the traditional hospice approach would seem to run counter to the more active orientation of some AIDS hospice services. Although this issue raises concerns, as yet there are no data-based studies to document this conflict or any inherent negative outcomes for patients in securing appropriate care. If these cases are too therapy-intensive to fit the hospice ideology, which is generally palliative in nature, some change may be in order. It is unlikely that hospices will want to deny patients sophisticated drug therapies to treat opportunistic infections, which are the leading cause of death in these patients. What proportion of AIDS care is truly palliative? If care is not totally palliative, should AIDS patients really be treated in hospices? The problem of provision of services will not be quickly remedied. Although most of the care could be done on an outpatient basis, services to meet the current and increasing needs are not in place. And of growing concern are the number of homeless patients roaming the streets who are either infected with HIV or have full-blown AIDS. Homeless missions, shelters, subway stations, and the streets, especially in AIDS epicenters, are showing distressingly larger numbers of persons for whom little to no service is provided. Up to this point, social services have dealt with AIDS and homelessness as separate problems. This situation is extremely critical and must be addressed in any federal response to the needs of the homeless.

## *Education of Health Providers for Provision of Quality Care to Individuals Infected with Human Immunodeficiency Virus*

The need for widespread AIDS education of health providers is quite evident. With the spread of HIV infection, increasing numbers of health care professionals are becoming involved in the care and treatment of HIV-infected persons at all stages. Second, the spread of the disease beyond current AIDS epicenters has resulted in more individuals with only minimal information who need a better baseline working knowledge of the disease. Finally, the reluctance of many health care professionals to care for HIV-infected individuals, along with already existing staff shortages, makes the provision of responsive educational programs even more important.

The aim of many organized efforts to educate health care professionals about HIV infection has been to launch major baseline information training programs. These programs have largely provided foundational information covering the epidemiology of HIV, the diseases associated with it, and the psychosocial aspects of AIDS. Explanations of guidelines of the Centers for Disease Control for universal prevention are always included. Although didactic information provided in lecture and/or slide presentation format has been used, a variety of enhancement activities, e.g., audiotapes, panel, trigger tapes, and break-out discussion groups, have also been endorsed and utilized, particularly to alter any negative attitudes that prevail among providers.

Several important considerations in the design of these programs should be addressed. First is the absence of education of any significance. Second is the level of education and method used. Third is the attention to patient outcomes and their measurement as a factor of the education and/or training provided.

The status of nursing education in HIV infection reveals that some important work needs to be accomplished. Essentially, there is no minimum standard curriculum regarding HIV infection or AIDS at any level of nursing education. Very few schools of nursing provide HIV/AIDS content; and when it is provided, this content can vary a great deal. Also, in most instances it is presented didactically. For this reason, service agencies may be unsure of what to expect of their staff. And this uncertainty would result in the need for in-service education, some of which would be unnecessary for some individuals. Some important events have occurred to improve the status of HIV education. First, a position paper published by the Oncology Nursing Society in 1988 provided a guide for nursing practice in HIV disease (Halloran, Hughes, & Mayer, 1988). Content about HIV disease that could be included at various levels of education was identified. Additionally, the National League for Nursing has submitted guidelines to be used by schools of nursing in incorporating HIV/AIDS–related content in curricula. Also, test material developed by the National League for Nursing on caring for persons with AIDS is available to schools that wish to test for basic knowledge and attitudes prerequisite to delivering care to HIV-infected persons (National League for Nursing, 1988).

Initial generalizations about insufficient knowledge and fears surrounding the care of HIV-infected persons within and across provider groups have been well documented. Reluctance of providers, especially nurses and physicians, to treat persons with AIDS or those suspected to be at risk received a great deal of attention because of the need to ensure an adequate responsive cadre of caregivers. Reports of reluctance and fear were revealed in various studies (Blumfield et al., 1987; Douglas et al., 1985; Kelly et al., 1988; Lewis et al., 1987; Royse & Birge, 1987; Searle, 1987; van Servellen et al., 1988).

Several studies also looked at the absence of baseline knowledge among practitioners (Searle, 1987; Lewis, Freeman, & Corey, 1987; van Servellen et al., 1988). These studies of baseline knowledge largely concerned themselves with the issue of whether diagnostic, history-taking, and risk reduction counseling expertise as well as general awareness of infection precautions existed among those in line to give direct care and counsel to HIV-infected persons.

Level of knowledge was identified as a critical variable affecting attitudes and willingness to provide care (Imperato et al., 1988; Kelly et al., 1988; Lewis et al., 1987). And yet, attitudes and negativity cannot be divorced from desire to learn about AIDS. The intensity of negativity toward persons whose behavior places them at risk may actually present a significant barrier to learning about AIDS and becoming prepared to care for these patients. This is not as true for the aspect of learning basic information about infection control, since those facts may be seen as personal preparation to care for AIDS patients. However, learning about the specific treatment and psychosocial needs of these patients who require commitment and investment is different.

Evidence about the effects of AIDS educational programs on health providers' knowledge and willingness to care for HIV-infected persons is relatively limited.

The major evaluative component consists of measuring program efficacy and/or effort, e.g., the number in attendance. Some case studies and larger regional educational efforts have been evaluated for their impact on knowledge and attitudes. There has been some research to show that educational programs presented to practicing health providers improve basic knowledge and can shift negativity.

Conclusions about these educational evaluation studies are difficult to make because few studies go into detail about baseline preparation and/or readiness of participants to receive information, the program content and design, and the standards and measures to evaluate the success of the program and to determine significant changes. For these reasons, it is also difficult to sort through the meaning of conflicting results because willingness to care may or may not be affected by baseline generic educational programs.

Perhaps the most challenging feature of education for the health provider is knowing when to use what approach. Although the initial efforts in provider education were directed at providing as many as possible with basic information, this aim has shifted dramatically in the last few years. Advanced education and training for role competency and the need to accelerate nursing research in HIV infection are at the forefront. With changing technology in AIDS care, the absence of advanced skill and knowledge becomes a liability. Absence of advanced knowledge and skill may actually affect willingness to care. This deficit could soon become more critical in undermining a shortage of providers than fears and negative feelings toward those who are HIV infected or those whose behaviors place them at risk of infection.

## Nursing Research Priorities for the Advancement of Quality Care in Human Immunodeficiency Virus Disease

Nursing research efforts in support of advancing quality care to HIV-infected individuals are increasing in numbers and significance. Much still needs to be accomplished. The following discussion summarizes various gaps and some limited progress in the last decade.

A recent report of the literature in nursing on AIDS revealed that during a 52-month period from January 1983 through April 1987, nine articles on AIDS or HIV infection were reported in the nursing journals (Larson, 1988). The majority of these articles were not research articles, but discussed issues such as care concerns, care delivery, and what to teach. In an analysis of articles published from May 1987 through December 1988, Larson (1988) found some improvement but indicated that not enough focus was placed on nursing care research. Over 20 months, 20 research or data-based articles were identified. The majority focused on attitudes, fears, and knowledge of nurses about AIDS and HIV. Five were directly or indirectly related to prevention and/or treatment. One was concerned with costs of care, and one focused on the informational needs of HIV-infected individuals, highlighting the mental health needs of HIV symptomatic and asymptomatic individuals. The lack of clinical research as it related to the physiologic impairment and psychosocial management of HIV-infected persons was quite evident from this analysis.

During the period August 1988 through April 1989, the National Center for

Nursing Research approved and funded nine research grants focusing on AIDS. These studies included the following topic areas: pediatric AIDS, nursing needs and persons with AIDS across different settings, HIV antibody testing in cases of sexual abuse, quality of nursing care for People with AIDS (PWAs), self-care nursing approaches to AIDS/ARC via computer network, ethical problems experienced by PWAs, and parental acceptance and care of gay men dying of AIDS.

The problems associated with nursing research to date are not unlike those in other disciplines. They span the entire research process from the stage of conceptualization to problems in methodology and include these problems: (1) on the whole, simplistic conceptual approaches have been used, (2) a negligible amount of work has been done to predict nursing care problems over time, and (3) few qualitative studies have been launched that would increase the depth of our knowledge of the complexity of certain nursing care problems, e.g., changing high-risk behavior, coping with psychological distress and mental impairment, and choice of coping responses in response to fear and denial.

The applicability of other research to studies in HIV infection is uncertain. Implications cannot always be extrapolated from studies of other populations with terminal and/or chronic yet fatal illness because of certain distinct features of HIV disease. The rapid decline in health heretofore seen in AIDS, the younger average age, the ethnic and sexual proclivities of patients with the disease, and the complex interplay of social stigma and psychosocial management issues are unique. Also, this disease is not only chronic and fatal but also infectious. The stress and risk to providers and the certainty of a fatal prognosis must inform analyses of care delivery issues.

HIV research is problematic because of methodologic and ethical concerns. These include problems surrounding access to subjects and concerns for protecting the confidentiality of subjects' health status as well as protecting the confidentiality of provider attitudes and opinions. Moreover, data collection instruments are not always sensitive to AIDS issues.

The overall aim of nursing research in the care and treatment of HIV-infected persons should encompass prevention, care delivery systems, and clinical nursing measures to treat the actual and potential responses to HIV infections considered as a disease continuum. Those infected and those affected by AIDS are the appropriate subjects of this research effort. With this in mind, an over-riding goal should be identification and testing practices and creating systems of care delivery that enhance high quality and cost-efficient care for HIV-infected individuals and facilitate effective participation of their caregivers, whether they are nonprofessional or professional providers.

## Summary

A great deal of hope lies in the fact that over the last 5 years, in particular, medical science has made major advances in understanding the HIV virus, in developing drugs to fight HIV infection at all stages, and in treating the illnesses associated with infection. Nonetheless, the demands on the health care system are likely to increase and to create new problems. In the epicenters, AIDS could surpass all other major illness-related deaths among those under age 65. Educational efforts to stop the spread of the infection have not been as effective as had been hoped. Human immunodeficiency infection among drug users and their sexual partners and infants is increasing. The number of HIV-positive babies continues to grow in all AIDS epicenters. The widespread fear of AIDS still affects societal responses to those at risk. Unnecessary restrictions on those who have the disease or who practice at risk behaviors must continually be countered with policies and legislation to help the afflicted and to avoid discriminatory practices (Gottlieb & Hartman, 1990).

Initiatives to increase access for AIDS patients to multiple settings, including outpatient respiratory care, and to a wider range of facilities, including hospices, are important. Provision of support for home and community-based services when otherwise patients would require institutional care should receive priority. The provision of specialized services for children who are HIV-positive, including foster family homes, also needs attention.

There is a tremendous opportunity for nursing to impact the course of HIV disease and the design of the delivery system that will emerge to meet the rising burden of this illness. These opportunities are highly dependent on advances in nursing research and education. Research is needed to develop effective nursing interventions for the problems of the infected; to determine how nurses should provide assistance to informed caregivers who bear much of the day-to-day burden; to evaluate the cost-effectiveness of nursing service delivery models; and to prevent the spread of the disease. Providing widespread and appropriate levels of education to nurses will better ensure a pool of responsive and knowledgeable practitioners to meet the demands of HIV infection in its second decade.

REFERENCES

Agency for Health Care Policy and Research (1990, February). Cumulative costs of treating AIDS are estimated in *Research Activities*. U.S. Department of Health and Human Services, *126*, 5.

Arno, P. (1986). The non-profit doctor's response to the AIDS epidemic. *American Journal of Public Health, 76*(11), 1325–1330.

Blumfield, M., Smith, P.J., Milazzo, J., Seropian, S., & Wormser, G.P. (1987). Survey of attitudes of nurses working with AIDS patients. *General Hospital Psychiatry, 9*, 58–63.

Burda, D., & Powills, S. (1986). AIDS: A time bomb at hospital's door. *Hospitals, 60*(1), 54–61.

Centers for Disease Control (1989a). Update: AIDS and human immunodeficiency virus infection in the United States. *Morbidity and Mortality Weekly Report, 38*, 1.

Centers for Disease Control (1989b). Update: AIDS and human immunodeficiency virus infection in the United States. *Morbidity and Mortality Weekly Report, 38*, 3.

Centers for Disease Control (1989c, August). HIV/AIDS surveillance: AIDS cases reported through July, 1989. U.S. Department of Health and Human Services, p. 1.

Centers for Disease Control (1989d, August). HIV/AIDS surveillance: AIDS cases reported through July, 1989. U.S. Department of Health and Human Services, p. 7.

Centers for Disease Control (1991, July). HIV/AIDS surveillance report, pp 1–18.

Douglas, C.J., Kalman, C.M., & Kalman, T.P. (1985). Homophobia among physicians and nurses: An empirical study. *Hospital Community Psychiatry, 36*(12), 1309–1311.

Gottlieb, M., & Hartman, S. (1990, February). Challenging AIDS: The second decade. *AIDS Patient Care, 4*(1), 3–7.

Halloran, J., Hughes, A., & Mayer, D.K. (1988). Oncology nursing society position paper on HIV-related issues. *Oncology Nursing Forum, 15*(2), 206–216.

Imperato, P.J., Feldman, J.G., Nayeri, K., & Dehovitz, J.A. (1988). Medical students' attitudes toward caring for patients with AIDS in a high incidence area. *New York State Journal of Medicine, 88,* 223–227.

Kelly, J.A., St. Lawrence, J.S., Hood, H.B., Smith, S., & Cook, D.J. (1988). Nurses' attitudes towards AIDS. *The Journal of Continuing Education in Nursing, 19*(2), 78–83.

Larson, E. (1988). Nursing research and AIDS. *Nursing Research, 37*(1), 60–62.

Laskin, M. (1988). Pain management in the patient with AIDS. *Journal of Advanced Medical Surgical Nursing, 1*(1), 37–43.

Lewis, C.E., Freeman, H.E., & Corey, C.R. (1987). AIDS-related competence of California's primary care physicians. *American Journal of Public Health, 77,* 795–799.

Lifson, A.R., Rutherford, G.W., & Jaffe, H.W. (1988). The natural history of human immunodeficiency virus infection. *Journal of Infectious Disease, 158,* 1360–1367.

Martin-Parker, J. (1986). Ensuring quality hospice care for the person with AIDS. *Quality Review Bulletin, 12*(10), 353–358.

Meisenhelder, J.B., & LaCharita, C.L. (1989). *Comfort in caring—nursing the person with HIV infection.* Chicago: Scott, Foresman/Little Brown.

National League for Nursing (1988). *AIDS guidelines for schools of nursing.* New York: National League for Nursing.

Nily, G. (1988). AIDS: Opportunistic diseases and their physical assessment. *Journal of Advanced Medical Surgical Nursing, 1*(1), 27–36.

Pomerantz, S., & Harrison, E. (1990a, February). End-stage symptom management. *AIDS Patient Care, 4*(1), 18–20.

Pomerantz, S., & Harrison, E. (1990b, February). End-stage symptom management. *AIDS Patient Care, 4*(1), 36–37.

Rotherberg, R., Woelfel, M., Stoneburner, R., Milberg, B.A., Parker, R., & Truman, B. (1987). Survival with the immunodeficiency syndrome: Experience with 5833 cases in New York City. *New England Journal of Medicine, 317,* 1297–1302.

Royse, D., & Birge, B. (1987). Homophobia and attitudes towards AIDS patients among medical, nursing and paramedical students. *Psychological Reports, 61,* 867–870.

Searle, E.S. (1987, January 3). Knowledge, attitude and behaviour of health professionals in relation to AIDS. *Lancet, 1*(8523), 26–28.

Taravella, S. (1989, February). Reserving a place to treat AIDS patients in the hospital. *Modern Health Care, 19*(6), 34.

van Servellen, G.M., Lewis, C.E., & Leake, B. (1988). Nurses' knowledge, attitudes and fears about AIDS. *Journal of Nursing Science and Practice, 1*(3), 1–7.

van Servellen, G.M., Lewis, C.E., & Leake, B. (1991). The stresses of hospitalization in the AIDS patient. *International Journal of Nursing Studies, 27*(3), 235–247.

Vlahov, D. (1989). AIDS: Overview, immunology, virology, and informational needs. *Seminars in Oncology Nursing, 5*(4), 232.

Chapter 26

# Breaking New Ground in Elder Care: Practice, Research, and Education

NEVILLE E. STRUMPF
CATHERINE M. STEVENSON

"Wish not so much to live long as to live well."
—*Benjamin Franklin*

*I*N ANY DISCUSSION of nursing and health policy in the 1990s, it is impossible to ignore an established demographic shift to an aging society, and the costs, responsibilities, and ethical requirements of living in that transformed world. These changes are occurring not only in the United States but also throughout Western Europe and all industrialized nations, many of which have markedly declining fertility rates. Among the most urgent of issues for elder health care in the United States will be reform of or alternatives to the existing system of long-term care. At present, this system satisfies almost no one: burdens are heavy on those needing extensive care and on their families; costs are rising rapidly and competition is stiff for shrinking public funds; access to care is often limited; and a system of reimbursement for comprehensive care across a continuum, including institutional and community services, is piecemeal if it exists at all (Rivlin & Wiener, 1988).

In this chaotic atmosphere, nursing still remains a potentially powerful force in the planning and humane implementation of care for older people. Following a description of demographics, this chapter reviews a decade of progress by gerontologic nurses in caring for the elderly, with special emphasis on practice exemplars, clinical care issues and related research, implications for future development of geriatric and gerontologic nursing services, and educational trends of the future. Since other chapters in this text are specifically devoted to the organization and financing of long-term care services and also to nursing homes, the discussion here considers clinical practice in hospitals and the community.

## Who Are "the Old?"

When the Republic of the United States was founded, a newborn child could expect to live until the age of 35. In 1900, only 4.1 percent of the population was 65 or older, and in 1950 it was 7.7 percent. Now, with 30,000,000 persons in this country

419

above the age of 65, the proportion is 12 percent, and by 2020, it will reach 17.3 percent. The most rapid increase is expected between the years 2010 and 2030, when the "baby boomers" reach 65. Currently, in a grayer America, the median age is 33. Today, Americans can and are living well into their 90s; the fastest growing segment of the United States population is the group 85 and over. Each year, 30,000 people in the United States celebrate their 100th birthday; by the year 2000, 100,000 persons will do so annually (American Association of Retired Persons, 1986; U.S. Senate Special Committee on Aging, 1987–88).

Examination of life expectancy reveals that, on average, females can expect to live longer than males (78.2 years versus 71.2 years), with white females having the longest life expectancy (78.7), followed by black females (73.7), white males (71.8), and black males (65.3) (U.S. Senate Special Committee on Aging, 1987–88). Among the aging, females form a noticeable majority, 147 women for every 100 men over 65. Science has yet to provide an adequate explanation of the gender gap, which is seen throughout the industrialized or industrializing world and varies from about four years in Greece to ten years in the Soviet Union; in the United States, women live approximately seven years longer than men ("Need to bridge," 1987). Beginning research points to genetic, immunologic, hormonal, and psychological explanations for these differences (Holden, 1987).

The length and quality of life depend, in part, on heredity. The chance to blow out 85 candles increases with each parent or grandparent who reached that milestone. The single greatest contributor to the gender gap in life expectancy is heart disease, which accounts for as much as 40 percent of the sex differential ("Need to bridge," 1987). Other social and behavioral factors affecting health and life span are type of work, use of alcohol and cigarettes, degree of stress, amount of exercise, and adequacy of nutrition. Feelings of self-reliance and optimism may contribute to better health and a longer life (Sagan, 1987). "Successful" aging quite possibly is linked to personal habits and environmental influences.

Other characteristics of a large and diverse aging population are worthy of consideration. Most older people live in noninstitutional settings; only 5 percent of those 65 and older live in nursing homes, about 1.5 million people (American Association of Retired Persons, 1986). Obviously, very advanced age, physical and mental frailty, and lack of family or social support are significant contributors to nursing home placement. Nearly one third of all noninstitutionalized older persons live alone; because of female longevity, many in this group are widows (Wise & Hurd, 1987). Despite a prevailing mythology that children in the United States abandon their elders, most older Americans residing in communities see at least one child on a regular basis. Over two million caregivers provide unpaid assistance to 1.2 million noninstitutionalized frail, older persons nationwide (American Association of Retired Persons, 1986). Of great significance is the stress this creates for the "sandwich generation," who are attending to the needs of their own children on the one hand, and the needs of their aging parents on the other (Silverstone & Hyman, 1989).

According to a survey by the American Association of Retired Persons, growing numbers of older Americans want to remain in their homes until the end of their lives (Schogol, 1990). About half of persons 65 and older live in just eight states.

California, New York, and Florida have over 2 million elderly persons each, followed by more than a million persons each in Illinois, Michigan, Pennsylvania, and Texas. Eleven states have 13 percent or more of the population in the 65+ group, and these include Florida (17.6 percent) and Pennsylvania (14.3 percent). Older people are less likely to live in metropolitan areas than younger people and less likely than other groups to change residence (American Association of Retired Persons, 1986).

Despite a great deal of publicity about how well off older Americans are, and it is indeed true that genuine progress toward economic well-being for this group has been made in the last two decades, about 12 percent of persons 65 and older still have incomes below the poverty level, with the poorest of those being 85 years of age or more, women, and minorities (American Association of Retired Persons, 1986; Older Women's League, 1990). A major source of income for older people remains Social Security, with older households also more likely than younger ones to have members covered by Medicaid (American Association of Retired Persons, 1986).

Feeling good in one's later years is partially related to perceptions of health. Currently, seven of ten older persons describe their health as "good" or "excellent" compared with others their age (U.S. Senate Special Committee on Aging, 1987–88). Not until age 85 and older does about half the population report limitations in activities because of chronic illness. Most of the noninstitutionalized population over 65 are able to manage their daily needs. Nevertheless, at least one chronic health problem is typical, and multiple conditions are commonplace. Heart disease, cancer, and stroke are the usual causes of death.

In addition, mental health problems are significantly more frequent in later life and can greatly influence the course of physical illness. Alzheimer's disease and other organic mental disorders affect more than 6 percent of adults 65 and over, and cognitive impairment, whether from Alzheimer's or other causes, is one of the principal reasons for institutionalization. Recent findings by Evans and associates (Evans et al., 1989) concerning the prevalence of Alzheimer's disease with increasing age (42 percent among those 85 and older) are a serious concern given the rising elderly population.

As we contemplate the nature of health services now and in the future, the implications of an aging population are these: more people above the age of 75, a growing number of whom will experience functional disability or debilitating illness; large numbers of elderly women, many of whom are compromised by poverty levels higher than their male counterparts; and increasing pressures at both community and institutional levels to handle older, frailer patients, particularly as family members become unable to manage the burdens of care. Thus, for obvious reasons, the need is tremendous to promote the maintenance of functional ability and independence among the elderly population for as long as possible and also to provide community-based and institutional supports that are high in quality, economically feasible, and equally accessible. Although the current system of long-term care falls far short of these ideals, the contribution of expertise from gerontologic nursing suggests the efficacy of certain approaches in delivery of services and improvement of outcomes.

## Advanced Practice in Gerontologic Nursing

We will assume the merits of the clinician/practitioner or clinical specialist holding, at a minimum, a master's degree in gerontologic nursing. As put forward by the American Nurses' Association (1987) in *Standards and Scope of Gerontological Nursing Practice*, specialists have the knowledge and skills to do the following:

1. Demonstrate an in-depth understanding of the many interacting pathophysiologic and psychosocial changes of aging as well as the interventions necessary for management of these alterations in health status experienced by older adults.

2. Employ clinical reasoning as a basis for distinctions between customary and unusual findings, judgments concerning functional status, and decisions regarding management of the health status of an older person.

3. Provide comprehensive gerontologic nursing services independently, cooperatively with other caregivers, or collaboratively with an interdisciplinary team.

4. Develop, offer, and evaluate services of a variety of institutional and community settings that promote healthy aging, prevent development or exacerbation of health problems, and support the strengths of the older person.

5. Participate with professional colleagues, older persons, and families in mutually defining, exploring, and resolving as much as possible the ethical dilemmas that arise in the care of individuals with the complex problems associated with age.

6. Provide consultation, education, or supervision as warranted to other professionals, to other individuals with responsibility for care, and to any person or group offering health and social services for older persons and their families.

7. Provide leadership and advocacy for older persons and their families in obtaining the health, legal, social, and community services they require.

8. Collaborate in, use, and disseminate research that develops the body of knowledge in gerontologic nursing and advances the health care of older persons.

9. Provide professional leadership regarding gerontologic nursing standards and services to consumers, other health care professionals, and policy makers.

10. Participate in continuing education, national and state nursing organizations, the process of certification, and the ongoing evaluation of the standards of gerontologic nursing practice.

Although specialization in gerontologic nursing has been recognized by the American Nurses' Association since the 1960s, growth in the number of nurses choosing the field has been slow, and graduate programs in gerontology, compared with those in other specialties, are few. As of January, 1990, 9000 nurses held an American Nurses' Association certification in gerontology: 8109 as gerontologic nurses; 1210 as gerontologic nurse practitioners; and 127 as clinical specialists in gerontologic nursing ("Need grows," 1990). More than 2000 registered nurses took certification examinations in gerontology in October of 1989; therefore a significant increase in these figures is likely, although even then they are extremely modest given national demographic trends.

Incorporation of the specialized gerontologic nurse into emerging models of practice is, thus, a slow process, with little in the literature to date detailing roles, outcomes, and costs. Nevertheless, a survey of 82 graduates from the Gerontological

Nurse Clinician Program at the University of Pennsylvania (1982 to 1989) confirms that unique positions in long-term care are being created as the result of shifts in the customary functions of hospitals, nursing homes, and community agencies. In ambulatory settings, the roles include case management and referral, especially with problems such as urinary incontinence, dementia, elder abuse, and stroke. Other innovative uses of the primary care skills of gerontologic specialists are in geropsychiatric consultation, home care, day care, managed care systems, health maintenance organizations, continuing care retirement communities, and area agencies on aging. In hospitals, new models of practice in gerontology include nurse-to-nurse consultation, discharge planning, geriatric assessment teams and units, and geriatric nurse specialists for hospital-based skilled nursing facilities (SNFs) and nursing home placement units. The following section highlights several of these emerging models of advanced clinical practice.

## "Practice Exemplars" in the Community

"Caring the On Lok Way" may be the ideal, at the start of this decade, in pairing "innovative services with creative financing to keep nursing home eligible elders living in their own homes" (O'Malley & Brooks, 1990, p. 64). On Lok, Chinese for happy, peaceful abode, is a community-based, long-term care organization that applies the principles of health maintenance organizations to frail elders 55 years and older who live in parts of San Francisco. Like a home maintenance organization, On Lok is financed through capitation payments, in this case, through special waivers from Medicare and Medicaid for services needed by participants (Ansak & Zawadski, 1983). Most services are delivered by On Lok staff in day health centers, although services are also available in the home through a home health program. The multidisciplinary team is integral to On Lok's comprehensive range of services (e.g., primary care, skilled nursing, physical/occupational/speech therapy, social services, nutrition), but professional nurses are key members of the day health and home health programs. Two gerontologic nurse practitioners (GNPs) at On Lok provide primary care services to 30 percent of the program participants (Morishita & Hansen, 1986). Among the many things On Lok means to its more than 300 enrollees is a chance, even under circumstances of considerable frailty and disability, to remain where they want to be, living at home while receiving the necessary skilled care.

The On Lok model is an excellent example of the role played by professional nurses, and especially GNPs, in ambulatory care. As gatekeepers, these practitioners find themselves caring for patients who are difficult to treat because of age, social problems, and number of complex health problems (Diers, 1983). In a comparison of the clinical practice of a geriatric nurse practitioner and two internists (McDowell, Martin, Snustad, & Flynn, 1986), the GNPs were especially successful in keeping patients in the community rather than having them placed in institutions. The authors concluded that GNPs offer effective, cost-efficient, high-quality health care for the frail and vulnerable elderly. Other studies of nurse practitioners in community-based practice suggest favorable outcomes, e.g., dramatic improvements in hypertension, blood glucose levels, and duration of hospitalization in persons with selected chronic diseases (Runyan, 1975) as well as maintenance of health and prevention of reinstitutionalization of developmentally disabled persons, including those who are elderly (Ziring et al., 1988). It is perhaps the nurse practitioner's approach to symptoms, comfort, and comprehensiveness that explains such success (Diers, Hamman, & Molde, 1986).

Home health services, defined as those services provided to individuals and families in their place of residence for the purpose of promoting, maintaining, or restoring health and minimizing the effects of illness and disability (Stewart, 1979), clearly represent a new avenue for creative, exemplary practice with older adults. Because the patients often encountered in home care have usually been discharged "quicker and sicker" from hospitals and are frequently beset by multiple problems, the expertise of an interdisciplinary geriatric team is desirable. La Vizzo-Mourey (1989) puts forward the idea of a traveling team approach using home health agencies. The core members of the team include a nurse practitioner, a physician, and a social worker, and like the efforts of teams in rehabilitation and acute and long-term care, it is reasonable to assume similar successes in the accuracy and completeness of diagnosis, assessment and enhancement of function, reduction in nursing home placement, decrease in medications, and improvement in cognition. The potential for Medicare reimbursement of a diverse mix of skilled in-home services clearly makes feasible the idea of a traveling team on which all the personnel with the exception of the physician are employees of one or more home health agencies. This is a model still to be fully realized, especially since acute care needs immediately following hospitalization are the ones most likely to receive reimbursement. One example of a broader approach to such reimbursement is the Rural Health Clinics Services Act, which not only provides reimbursement for primary care in rural clinics but also authorizes some home health care by clinic staff for patients served by the program (Mundinger, 1983). In addition, many hospital-based home care programs operated by Veterans Administration Medical Centers use copractice models with physicians and GNPs (Capezuti, 1985), with some provision for home visits by the "team."

These models of ambulatory practice are characterized by inconsistent mechanisms of financing; often they are highly indigenous products of particular regions, with special populations and specific opportunities for funding. Few would challenge the intrinsic value of the services rendered or the quality of outcomes achieved. Whether they are site-specific, as in a day hospital program (a model that has achieved great success in the United Kingdom) or home-based (On Lok combines both), the improvement in function and decrease in institutionalization are noticeable. Components of these models are evident in the use of nurse practitioners to manage residential and skilled nursing services in continuing care retirement communities (Butler, 1986) and in a small but definitely increasing number of specialized nurse-managed programs such as poststroke consultation, and a continence clinic at the University of Pennsylvania, and an elder abuse prevention and dementia evaluation and care center at the University of Medicine and Dentistry of New Jersey in Stratford.

## "Practice Exemplars" in the Hospital

Prospective payment brought dramatic changes to American hospitals in the 1980s. Admission patterns and patient mix were altered; shorter stays became increasingly common; and the number of community and rural hospitals declined, along with general reductions in the number of beds, emergency rooms, and trauma centers. Despite these changes, geriatric patients are admitted more frequently, stay longer, are likely to be readmitted, and undergo many more diagnostic procedures than younger patients. More than ever, hospital-based models of practice employing GNPs could play a significant role in facilitation of in-patient evaluation and management, therapy aimed at minimizing functional decline and at decreasing the chances of rehospitalization, and a well-planned, timely discharge.

As hospitals increasingly use in-patient nurse practitioners, the benefits of a Geriatric Consultation Service are being explored and documented. Usually, such consultation services are composed of an interdisciplinary team of specialists from nursing, medicine, social work, and psychiatry. At the University of Pennsylvania, comprehensive geriatric evaluations are conducted as part of an outpatient program and on inpatient units in the acute care hospital (Sullivan, 1986). As the GNP's role in the acute care setting has evolved, it is most evident that areas of greatest concern to staff nurses are management of patient confusion, pharmacologic problems, and planning for discharge under the pressure to shorten length of stay as much as possible.

The literature suggests that the effectiveness of the geriatric team is greater than the sum of its parts, especially its strength to uncover potentially reversible problems and to suggest useful alternative therapies (Blumenfield, Morris, & Sherman, 1982). The comprehensiveness of assessment and management of the older patient in the United Kingdom is an admirable one, and in many ways, emerging geriatric consultation teams in this country emulate the approach of the British.

In 1982, geriatric consultation teams (consisting of physician, nurse, and social worker) were introduced into six acute care hospitals in Monroe County, New York (1) to reduce the number of elderly patients backed up in the community's acute care hospital beds, and (2) to document barriers in the hospital to maintaining or restoring independence of function and appropriate discharge of these patients (Barker et al., 1985). Four "system issues" were identified as potentially correctable obstacles to maintaining function and achieving expeditious discharge: remediable psychosocial problems, discontinuation of essential services because of lack of Medicare coverage, deficient coordination between hospital and community-based personnel, and delays in determining eligibility for Medicaid. Those patients judged at risk for prolonged hospitalization were followed by the team, with significant declines in length of stay attributed to a variety of medical, rehabilitative, and social interventions. It was the conclusion of the Geriatric Consultation Team Project that such services implemented elsewhere could be expected to reduce the problem of prolonged hospital stays by catalyzing the prompt use of appropriate hospital-based and community-based services.

Unlike the more broadly based modality of a consultation team, the specialized geriatric evaluation unit, also patterned after models developed in the United Kingdom, has as its goals "increasing the patient's levels of functioning, improving diagnosis and treatment, achieving more appropriate placement, reducing the use of institutional services, and generally increasing the overall quality of care delivered to elderly patients" (Rubenstein et al., 1984, p. 1664) using a team of physicians, nurses, and a social worker. In their clinical trial, Rubenstein and colleagues were able to demonstrate "substantial positive effects on a targeted subgroup of frail elderly inpatients, beyond the benefits of usual medical care," including "longer survival and less use of acute-care and long-term institutional services after one year of follow-up than similar patients receiving the usual hospital inpatient and outpatient services" (p. 1669). The investigators also noted improvements in functional status and morale, all at costs recovered over 12 months through savings in other services, such as acute hospitalization and nursing home care.

An acute care geriatric unit established at Park Ridge Hospital in Rochester, New York, specifically to provide rehabilitative care to geriatric patients with acute medical and/or surgical diagnoses and using gerontologic nurse specialists, also demonstrated substantial positive effects on both elderly patients (functional status) and cost (length of stay) (Boyer, Chuang, & Gipner, 1986).

The limited but striking evidence for the efficacy of hospital-based strategies to improve outcomes for older patients, while simultaneously containing costs, needs much further investigation. Yet both consultation teams and geriatric units employing the services of a nurse practitioner or specialist suggest an exemplary approach, especially in view of the central role American hospitals are still likely to play in the future. Such strategies, which could also include the use of nurse practitioners as discharge coordinators or managing other specialized units (e.g., rehabilitation or skilled nursing), are appropriate models from many perspectives—those of the patient, the provider, and the system itself. Among the greatest challenges in these beleaguered times for health care in the United States will be documentation of outcomes, determination of costs, and creative solutions to our frequently misguided, often tangled mechanism of reimbursement.

## Gerontologic Nursing Research

The *Social Policy Statement* of the American Nurses' Association (1980) emphasizes that "The future of nursing practice and . . . health care depends on nursing research designed to . . . generate an up-to-date organized body of nursing knowledge" (p. 1). As models for the clinical practice of gerontologic nursing have become more firmly established, the need for a sound research base is increasingly obvious. Although early research efforts were rather limited, notable contributions to that body of knowledge have been made in the last decade and several lines of inquiry are now securely in place.

The first major effort to describe the state of the art in gerontologic nursing was undertaken by Basson in 1967. Basson (1967) found little research emanating from a theoretical base; she noted especially the need for information that could be applied to a range of problems encountered in practice with older adults. Certainly a landmark in the latter category was the earliest gerontologic research undertaken by an American nurse, a study of the elderly ambulatory patient by Schwartz and others (1964).

A decade later, Gunter and Miller (1977) analyzed studies published in *Nursing Research* from 1952 to 1976, concluding that gerontologic nursing research reflected minimal attention to the integration of biologic, psychological, and sociological knowledge. Later, Robinson (1981) conducted a systematic review of gerontologic nursing research and, like her predecessors, found little reference to an underlying theoretical framework and many studies that focused on attitudes and opinions. At the same time, a review of the major nursing journals publishing gerontologic research led Kayser-Jones (1981) to recommend conducting more clinical studies, especially in the areas of incontinence, confusion, immobility, and the problems produced by drug interactions and reactions. Other recommendations included the need for longitudinal studies and investigations of mental health care needs of the aged.

Building on these earlier reviews, Burnside (1986) conducted a survey of gerontologic nursing research from 1975 to 1984, producing a list of 113 studies, the majority on nursing activities (23) and attitudes (21) concerning care of the elderly. Attention to clinical problems was meager (e.g., six articles on accidents and falls, two on sleep). She did note a growing reliance on a theoretical framework, cluster studies of particular phenomena, and a consistent pattern of adding to the body of psychosocial research (e.g., reality orientation). Nevertheless, Burnside identified 28 problems needing much greater study, including abuse, Alzheimer's disease and care, cost-effective deliveries or therapies, delirium and dementia, depression, exercise and mobility, incontinence, infection control, nutrition, restraints, sundown syndrome (nocturnal confusion) and wandering. In the most recent survey of gerontologic nursing research, Haight (1989) focused on long-term care facilities from 1984 to 1988. In a list of 66 studies, more clinical problems emerged, including eight studies on incontinence. Using the suggestions of Burnside and the results of her own review, Haight proposed a gerontologic research agenda for nursing in the 1990s focused on the environment, health promotion and clinical problems, disease prevention, personnel required, costs, patient and family issues, and nursing practice. Currently, the National Center for Nursing Research, National Institutes of Health, has named Priority Expert Panel C for Long-Term Care for Older Adults to refine that agenda and make recommendations for future funding.

Although a thorough review of the latest clinical research in gerontologic nursing is beyond the scope of this chapter, great strides are now evident, including studies of problems noted by Burnside and in the areas identified by Haight. Without question, information from research focused on genuine clinical problems is the essential tool of the gerontologic nurse practitioner.

The significance of some of these clinical advances has been chronicled in two issues of *Geriatric Nursing*, May/June and July/August of 1990, as part of the journal's tenth anniversary. In an accompanying editorial, Huey (1990) writes, "We could think of no more fitting way to celebrate . . . than to ask a few of the . . .

pioneers . . . to tell us how practice has changed" (p. 107). Most apparent in the work that follows by acknowledged investigators is the relationship of their research to clinical practice:

1. *Alzheimer's disease:* Abraham and Neundorfer (1990) note the contribution of nurses and other health care professionals in designing and implementing services and investigating their effectiveness, including improvements in physical activities (e.g., eating), therapeutic environments, accuracy of assessment tools, and management of specific problems (e.g., wandering).

2. *Restraints:* Strumpf and colleagues (1990), who began 5 years ago to study the routine use of mechanical restraints for older persons in hospitals and nursing homes, describe a scientific base that seriously questions the practice. They propose a set of alternatives to physical restraint, including physical (positioning, evaluation of drugs, toileting, comfort, pain relief, change in treatment, massage, sensory aids, and hydration); psychosocial (authorization of "no restraint" from resident/family, provision of sense of security, attention to resident's agenda, active listening); activities (daily physical therapy/ambulation, gait training, distraction, recreation, exercise); and environmental (contoured chairs, low beds, alarm systems, background music, camouflage, noise reduction, controlled lighting, and personal space).

3. *Incontinence:* As Wells (1990) notes, few areas have moved so dramatically from resigned suffering to rigorous assessment and intervention. Most significant was the research on therapeutic alternatives (prompted voiding, pelvic muscle exercise, and biofeedback) for stress incontinence. In addition, research has led to the development of more appropriate disposable garments and incontinence devices.

4. *Acute confusion:* A decade of nursing research has expanded understanding, recognition, and management of acute confusion, especially during hospitalization (Forman, 1990). Factors now known to be associated with acute confusion are irreversible changes in neural structure, physiologic alterations such as fluid and electrolyte imbalances, and sensory deficits. With better diagnosis and treatment, it is estimated that lengths of stay for acutely confused hospitalized elders could be reduced, at considerable savings to Medicare.

5. *Family caregiving:* Systematic investigations reveal that the stresses of caregiving are complex, with the nature and extent of caregiving tasks, not necessarily the level of elder function, being the most important variables (Baldwin, 1990). With an increasing number of impaired elders living at home, strategies for caregivers are critical, as well as documentation of the need for respite, support services, and appropriate reimbursement.

6. *Pain:* A few lessons from the research: Pain is not normal with aging; chronic pain can lead to depression; elderly patients are more sensitive to analgesic drugs, often requiring lower doses than younger adults; and a combination of drug and nondrug treatments (transcutaneous nerve stimulation; heat, cold, and massage; biofeedback, hypnosis, and relaxation; distraction) for pain relief often works well with the elderly (Ferrell & Ferrell, 1990).

7. *Depression:* Buckwalter (1990) states the case plainly and forthrightly: "Being 'old and sad' isn't normal" (p. 179). Depression is a serious yet highly treatable problem, one that may be brought on by the many drugs used to treat illnesses common in the elderly. Drugs with fewer adverse side effects are now available,

electroconvulsive therapy can be safe and effective for selected patients, group therapy for the cognitively intact elderly person is potentially useful and cost-effective, and fostering perceptions of control can lead to positive outcomes.

8. *Pressure ulcers:* According to Braden and Bryant (1990), "The 80's brought refinements in assessment, plus a wave of new products and techniques" (p. 182). Among the most significant contributions of nurse researchers has been the development of tools permitting accurate identification of those at risk for pressure ulcers as well as proper staging so that the appropriate wound care product can be selected and used correctly. A great deal is now known from clinical trials on the uses of topical solutions and gels; wound cleansers, antiseptics, and antimicrobials; growth factors; electrical stimulation and hyperbaric oxygen; and new techniques of debridement using carbon dioxide lasers.

Obviously, the above list represents only a small portion of the clinical research related to the problems encountered in gerontologic nursing. Yet, it is impressive in its relevance to practice and its contribution to quality care at reasonable cost. In so many cases, the knowledge based on this research figures prominently in reducing suffering, decreasing hospitalization, postponing institutionalization, and using limited numbers of personnel as efficiently as possible.

## *Education for the Future*

In a classic article on the gerontologic nursing specialty, Davis (1983) speculated on the future, predicting that all undergraduate schools of nursing would require separate theory and clinical experiences in gerontologic nursing; state boards of nursing would test knowledge of gerontologic nursing; master's-degree prepared specialists would be paid for private services from fiscal intermediaries; large numbers of graduate programs—master's and doctoral—would be preparing specialists in gerontology; certification for gerontologic nursing would be available through the American Nurses' Association; general hospitals would have specialized units for the aged; and a national health plan assuring preventive health care to all older people would be in place. Except for state board testing and a national health plan, one could argue that we are moving toward achievement of these goals at the beginning of the 1990s.

At the University of Pennsylvania, all undergraduate students *are required* to take a theory and clinical course on care of the older adult during their junior year. Our experience to date suggests that treating gerontologic nursing like any other course in the curriculum has a positive impact on knowledge, enthusiasm, and acceptance. We have deliberately focused the course on the acute needs of the hospitalized elder, leaving until the senior year the complex problems encountered in the home or long-term care facility or involving case management. As we remember who the patients are in the majority of settings where nurses do their work, it is essential that gerontology be a part of every nurse's basic education and that teaching include a thorough understanding of the problems of older people in hospitals or receiving long-term care services at home or in a specialized facility.

Given the size of the older population and the challenges associated with caring for the sickest among them, preparation for advanced practice through graduate education deserves continued support and development. Although more geronto-logic nurse clinicians, practitioners, and specialists are in the field than ten years ago, the statistics cited earlier are meager indeed when compared with demand. Our experience also suggests that the most successful mechanism for managing the gerontologic enterprise in a school of nursing is to link faculty to both undergraduate and graduate programs in order to encourage undergraduates to submatriculate to the master's program; to demonstrate exemplary practice at clinical sites using gradu-ates of the master's program; to connect faculty research to problems germane to practice; and to foster among the clinical experts a desire to engage in doctoral or even postdoctoral study.

Again, referring to Davis' predictions, certification through the American Nurses' Association is a reality, and some state Boards of Nursing, as in Pennsylvania, deter-mine other criteria for advanced practice in gerontology. The preceding examples of practice models suggest a valuable role for hospital-based geriatric units and services, and if national health is not yet a reality, limited reimbursement from Medicare and Medicaid for services performed by nurse practitioners is available. Davis' predictions can become a standard by the year 2000 if we concentrate now on development of clinical models known for quality, efficiency, and cost-effectiveness; documentation of the outcomes of these clinical approaches using research that is rigorously designed; and through education, creation of a larger supply of nurses who are knowledgeable and articulate about the care of older people.

## Conclusion

This review of contributions by specialists in gerontologic nursing conveys a sense of optimism concerning the changes occurring in care of older Americans. Indeed, as the demographic patterns clearly suggest, a large population is in need of services, despite the overall improvements in well-being and longevity. As it has become clearer both to nursing and other health professions that standards based on practice, education, and research are integral to geriatrics, models of care, still few in number but significant because of successful outcomes, have appeared around the country. Repeatedly, these "practice exemplars," as described here, demonstrate several things in common: interdisciplinary teams that include one or more nurses with advanced preparation in gerontology; emphasis on assessment and maintenance of function, with a goal of community care for as long as possible; and creative strategies for financing, with an understanding that certain investments "up front" may reap dividends later through savings accrued by reduced stays in hospitals and nursing homes. Above all, emerging models of care in the community and in the hospital suggest the gains to be had when an expanding knowledge base concerning older adults is applied to the physical, psychological, and social problems so common in this population. Although reform of the long-term care system in the United States is as yet an unrealized dream, it is through such compelling evidence that we can indeed look forward to "breaking new ground in elder care" in the 1990s.

REFERENCES

Abraham, I.L., & Neundorfer, M.M. (1990). Alzheimer's: A decade of progress, a future of nursing challenges. *Geriatric Nursing, 11,* 116–119.

American Association of Retired Persons (1986). *Profile of older Americans.* Washington, DC: American Association of Retired Persons.

American Nurses' Association (1980). *A social policy statement.* Kansas City, MO: American Nurses' Association.

American Nurses' Association (1987). *Standards and scope of gerontological nursing practice.* Kansas City, MO: American Nurses' Association.

Ansak, M.L., & Zawadski, R.T. (1983). On Lok CCO-DA: A consolidated model. *Home Health Services Quarterly, 4,* 147–170.

Baldwin, B.A. (1990). Family caregiving: Trends and forecasts. *Geriatric Nursing, 11,* 172–174.

Barker, W.H., Williams, T.F., Zimmer, J.G., Van Buren, C., Vincent, S.J., & Pickrel, S.G. (1985). Geriatric consultation teams in acute hospitals: Impact on back-up of elderly patients. *Journal of the American Geriatrics Society, 33,* 422–428.

Basson, P.H. (1967). The gerontological nursing literature search: Study and results. *Nursing Research, 16,* 267–272.

Blumenfield, S., Morris, J., & Sherman, F.T. (1982). The geriatric team in the acute care hospital: An educational and consultation modality. *Journal of the American Geriatrics Society, 30,* 660–664.

Boyer, N., Chuang, J.C., & Gipner, D. (1986). An acute care geriatric unit. *Nursing Management, 17,* 22–25.

Braden, B.J., & Bryant, R. (1990). Innovations to prevent and treat pressure ulcers. *Geriatric Nursing, 11,* 182–186.

Buckwalter, K.C. (1990). How to unmask depression. *Geriatric Nursing, 11,* 179–181.

Burnside, I. (1986). Gerontological nursing research: 1975 to 1984. In National League for Nursing, *Overcoming the bias of ageism in long-term care.* New York: National League for Nursing.

Butler, J.K. (1986). Life care community practice. In M.D. Mezey & D.O. McGivern (Eds.), *Nurses, nurse practitioners: The evolution of primary care.* Boston: Little, Brown.

Capezuti, E. (1985). Geriatric nurse practitioners: Their education, experience, and future in home health care. *Pride Institute Journal of Long-Term Home Health Care, 4,* 9–14.

Davis, B.A. (1983). The gerontological nursing specialty. *Journal of Gerontological Nursing, 9,* 527–532.

Diers, D. (1983). Nurses in primary care—the new gatekeepers? *American Journal of Nursing, 83,* 742–745.

Diers, D., Hamman, A., & Molde, S. (1986). Complexity of ambulatory care: Nurse practitioner and physician caseloads. *Nursing Research, 35,* 310–314.

Evans, D.A., Funkenstein, H.H., Albert, M.S., Scherr, P.A., Cook, N.R., Chown, M.J., Hebert, L.E., Hennekens, C.H., & Taylor, J.O. (1989). Prevalence of Alzheimer's disease in a community population of older persons. *Journal of the American Medical Association, 262,* 2551–2556.

Ferrell, B.R., & Ferrell, B.A. (1990). Easing the pain. *Geriatric Nursing, 11,* 175–178.

Forman, M.D. (1990). Complexities of acute confusion. *Geriatric Nursing, 11,* 136–139.

Gunter, L.M., & Miller, J.C. (1977). Toward a nursing gerontology. *Nursing Research, 26,* 208–221.

Haight, B.K. (1989). Update on research in long-term care: 1984–1988. In National League for Nursing, *Indices of quality in long-term care: Research and practice.* New York: National League for Nursing.

Holden, C. (1987). Why do women live longer than men? *Science, 238,* 158–160.

Huey, F.L. (1990). Clinical advances, political setbacks. *Geriatric Nursing, 11,* 107.

Kayser-Jones, J. (1981). Gerontological nursing research revisited. *Journal of Gerontological Nursing, 1,* 217–223.

LaVizzo-Mourey, R. (1989). The home team. In R. LaVizzo-Mourey, S.C. Day, D. Diserens, & J.A. Grisso (Eds.), *Practicing prevention for the elderly.* Philadelphia: Hanley & Belfus.

McDowell, B.J., Martin, D.C., Snustad, D.G., & Flynn, W. (1986). Comparison of the clinical practice of a geriatric nurse practitioner and two internists. *Public Health Nursing, 3,* 140–146.

Morishita, L., & Hansen, J.C. (1986). GNP and the LTC team. *Journal of Gerontological Nursing, 12,* 15–20.

Mundinger, M.O. (1983). *Home care controversy.* Rockville, MD: Aspen Systems.

Need grows for gero nurses (1990, April). *American Nurse, 22*(4), 14.

Need to bridge gap between biology, social sciences to find explanation for gender gap (1987, September 28). *Aging Research and Training News, 10*(9), 107.

Older Women's League (1991). *Heading for hardship: Retirement income for American women in the next century.* Washington, DC: Older Women's League.

O'Malley, K., & Brooks, S. (1990). Caring the On Lok way. *Geriatric Nursing, 11,* 64–66.

Rivlin, A.M., & Wiener, J.M. (1988). *Caring for the disabled elderly.* Washington, DC: Brookings Institution.

Robinson, L. (1981). Gerontological nursing research. In I. Burnside (Ed.), *Nursing and the aged* (2nd ed.). New York: McGraw-Hill.

Rubenstein, L.Z., Josephson, K.R., Wieland, G.D., English, P.A., Sayre, J.A., & Kane, R.A. (1984). Effectiveness of a geriatric evaluation unit. *New England Journal of Medicine, 311,* 1664–1670.

Runyan, J.W. (1975). The Memphis chronic disease program: Comparisons in outcome and the nurse's extended role. *Journal of the American Medical Association, 231,* 264–267.

Sagan, L.A. (1987). *The health of nations: True causes of sickness and well-being.* New York: Basic Books.

Schwartz, D., Henley, B., & Zietz, L. (1964). *The elderly, ambulatory patient.* New York: Macmillan.

Schogol, M. (1990, April 24). Aging at home. *Philadelphia Inquirer.*

Silverstone, B., & Hyman, H.K. (1989). *You and your aging parents* (3rd ed.). New York: Pantheon.

Stewart, J.E. (1979). *Home health care.* St. Louis: C.V. Mosby Company.

Strumpf, N.E., Evans, L.K., & Schwartz, D. (1990). Restraint-free care: From dream to reality. *Geriatric Nursing, 11,* 122–124.

Sullivan, E. (1986). Tertiary care centers: A role for the geriatric nurse clinician. *Oasis, 3,* 1, 3.

U.S. Senate Special Committee on Aging (1987–1988). *Aging America: Trends and projections.* Washington, DC: U.S. Department of Health and Human Services.

Wells, T. (1990). Conquering incontinence. *Geriatric Nursing, 11,* 133–135.

Wise, D., & Hurd, M. (1987). *Elderly people living alone: Aging and the prospects of poverty.* Baltimore: Commonwealth Fund.

Ziring, P.R., Kastner, T., Friedman, D.L., Pond, W.S., Barnett, M.L., Sonnenberg, E.M., & Strassburger, K. (1988). Provisions of health care for persons with developmental disabilities living in the community. *Journal of the American Medical Association, 260,* 1439–1444.

# PART V

Shaping the Future

## Chapter 27

# Nursing's History: Looking Backward and Seeing Forward

JOAN LYNAUGH

$S$OREN KIERKEGAARD, the 19th century Danish philosopher and theologian, assayed a pragmatic but common justification for studying history with this aphorism: . . . life can only be understood backwards, but, it must be lived forwards. In that spirit this essay offers a historical interpretation of American nursing as we find it now. It is hoped that it will provide a useful framework for conceptualizing the shape of our discipline and its place in our society for the rest of this decade and beyond.

## Creating American Nursing

Human beings know that sickness, injury, birth, and aging are inevitable, unavoidable human experiences. To preserve individual lives and social stability, caregivers are charged with the work of helping others through these periods of dependency. For all of recorded time, this caring work has been primarily a function of the family, the basic structural unit of social life. In some cultures, certain aspects of the caring work has fallen to persons outside the family, usually religious or benevolent groups. We do not find the beginnings of formalized, secular nursing—that is, systematic, widespread delegation of nursing work to nonfamily workers—until the 19th century. Beginning in the 1830s and then with more conviction in subsequent decades, people began to consider total reliance on family caregivers in times of sickness to be dysfunctional. Clearest expression of this new thinking was found in the urban and increasingly secular societies of the Western world. Between 1860 and 1880, the idea of moving some part of the work of caring from the domestic setting of the family to the nurse and the hospital finally took root, spawning new institutions and new occupations.

Influential experiments in modern nursing first appeared in Germany, then in England, France, the United States, and Canada (Hampton, 1949; Poplin, 1988;

435

Woodham-Smith, 1951). Rapidly industrializing economies in Europe, England, and America, which needed their workers gathered together in factories, mines, and shops, proved a fertile environment for change. As the people of these industrializing countries left rural farms and villages and moved to cities, their traditional communities, their way of life, and their methods for coping with the exigencies of daily experience, including sickness and childbirth, were forever altered. Thus industrialization, combined with urbanization, helped set the stage for the "invention" of nursing as we know it today.

Nineteenth-century American nurses watched over hospital patients, gave them food, bathed them, kept order in the wards, and dispensed medicine. They collaborated with hospital board members to reform the hospital so as to match the idealized middle class home, that is, a place of safety, cleanliness, and respectability where healing would be possible. Nurses established routines in hospitals that made the execution of medical regimens feasible; thus they persuaded physicians to send patients to hospitals instead of relying on family care at home. The hospital and nurse training school guaranteed their constituents that care would be available to them when needed and that the hospital could safely substitute for home in times of sickness (Long & Golden, 1989).

Nursing was reformist, not revolutionary; it accommodated both traditional and novel views of women's social role. For about 30 years, the idea of nursing as "every woman's work" coexisted with the idea of nursing as a specialized social task requiring a defined education. The classic example of this duality is Florence Nightingale's influential book, *Notes on Nursing*, published in 1860 in the United States. Addressing not nurses but a general audience of literate women, Nightingale argued that all women of intelligence needed to understand basic nursing principles. Similarly, the first Philadelphia training school for nurses, organized by physician Ann Preston at Woman's Hospital in 1861 and financed by Philadelphia benefactor Pauline Henry, opened its nurses' classes to all women of Philadelphia who wished greater proficiency in their domestic responsibilities (O'Brien, 1987).

Hospital nursing caught on quickly; it became a durable new strategy to deal with social dislocation and upheaval of custom in work and family life. By the 1890s, we find the phrase "trained nursing" integrated into the language of American life. The nurse, whether depicted in a "Gibson girl" profile or as serenely vigilant at the bedside, symbolized an optimistic modern response to the problems of caring for dependent members of society. Equally important, she did it within existing boundaries of domestic propriety so that middle class Americans could accept and support her new work.

Nursing, a distinct occupation requiring specified skills and knowledge, carved out its niche in the world of work outside the domestic sphere and attracted women to its hospital training schools for several reasons. It was a respectable, interesting occupation that seemed to fit the ideal of individual productivity espoused by a growing middle class. Further, nursing as paid work was economic salvation for many women. It offered a way to make a living to women who found themselves redundant and unemployed in an industrializing economy. And it merged easily with a wide range of late 19th century moral and progressive philosophies that stressed "usefulness" for women as a modern substitute for piety and commitment to family (Baer, 1985; Vicinus, 1985).

Nursing's assignment, that is, caring for dependent, sick Americans, could hardly have been carried out without significant social and political change. Gradual erosion of 19th century laissez-faire political attitudes toward dependency and poverty allowed a few new social services to emerge at the beginning of this century. Lillian Wald and Lavinia Dock are the best remembered of many nurses who worked to change the social agenda through public health, education, school and industrial health, and settlement house work. The Children's Bureau, protective labor legislation, venereal disease programs, the antituberculosis campaign, and the progressive income tax were products of progressive and populist activists trying to ameliorate some of the harsher aspects of our capitalist system through political change.

Nursing, now redefined as an occupation based on formal training (instead of "every woman's work"), developed at the same time as teaching, library science, engineering, forestry, dentistry, veterinary medicine, accounting, telegraphy, history, and many more specialized occupations. Some of these occupations metamorphosed into professions, some became extinct, and some, like nursing, are still self-consciously debating questions of entry to the work, standards of practice, and professional status. The point is that nursing, among many other occupations, evolved in an industrial, urban context that supported, and indeed required, specialization of work and workers.

Nursing leaders were energized by a variety of motivations. For some, like Linda Richards, it was religious commitment; for others, like Lillian Wald, it was the opportunity for real reform; and for many, it was the excitement of learning new things and doing important, paid work in careers that freed them from traditional domestic, family dependence.

In the early years of the 20th century these new nurses focused on solving the patient care problems confronting them and on sustaining their schools in the face of extreme financial hardship (Nutting, 1984). They banded together into alumnae associations to counteract the loneliness of a practice life isolated by private duty nursing in their patients' homes. Later, thousands joined the American Red Cross and went off to World War I. If they married, their nursing careers usually stopped, not to resume unless they were widowed or otherwise thrown back on their own resources.

Nursing education and practice took direction from sweeping intellectual changes in science and medicine. Radical change in 19th century medical thinking eventually altered the way the general public conceived of disease. Theories of specificity of cause and treatment of disease drove out earlier concepts of general causation based on compatibility or incompatibility between the person and environment. These ideas of specific causation and the search for specific treatments became even more popular when late 19th century revelations based on the germ theory led to the discovery of specific pathogens such as the tubercle bacillus. Confidence in medicine, inspired by these new achievements, helped fuel the growth of hospitals and nursing (Rosenberg, 1987).

## Hospitals, Nurses, and the Health Marketplace

Nurses were enthusiastic about 20th century scientific and technologic strategies for dealing with sickness. Indeed, nursing made the remarkable proliferation of community hospitals possible. Their patients' requirements for intensive personal care, combined with new technology that both saved and created labor, served to shape the work of nurses. The operating rooms, the new x-ray machines, the laboratories, the scientific diet kitchens, and the pharmacies—all were managed by nurses. They also washed the patients, the beds, the floors and walls, and all the equipment—anything that might carry infection, the still dreaded, although better understood, bane of the hospital experience. The amount of physical labor required to conduct the hospital of 1900 was prodigious. By then, hospitals had electricity, telephones, flush toilets, and elevators. Desperately ill, febrile patients needed to be bathed and fed, however. Every surgical item was sterilized and wrapped by nurses' hands, nurses mixed and poured every medication, and they folded and stored every piece of linen.

By 1910 nearly every community in the United States had at least one hospital and probably more, depending on the size and ethnic and/or religious composition of the population. All these hospitals (the number peaked near 7000 in 1920) needed nurses. What emerged between 1890 and 1940 was a collection of small, local enterprises operating in the private sector. The majority of these were organized as voluntary charities, somewhat competitive along ethnic, religious, and local lines, but because they were charitable projects, they were not governed either by public authority or by marketplace rules (Long & Golden, 1989).

What many of these hospitals did have in common was cheap help—the student nurses in the training schools. The availability and persistence of exploitative student labor, a system created and sustained by the problems of underfinanced hospitals, corrupted the education of nurses. American procrastination in solving this problem also undermined hospitals' early promise as purveyors of general health care to their communities. One can argue that the reliance of hospitals on cheap student labor not only prevented Americans from facing the real personnel costs of institutional care but stunted the development of broad-based community services. The use of untrained and constantly changing pupils made it necessary to centralize patient care so that the pupils could be closely supervised by a small number of experienced nurses. Notwithstanding pupils' limitations, for the hospital managers it was essential that a constantly renewed supply of low cost general workers compensate for institutional dependence on uncertain charity and variable revenues from paying patients (Lynaugh, 1989b; Rosner, 1982).

Hospital popularity among the American middle class coincided, at the turn of the 20th century, with educational decisions that called for eight years of universal public education for all children. Communities taxed themselves to support public education, but Americans chose not to make general care of the sick a tax-funded service. People who sought professional health care for themselves or their families expected to pay cash to both physicians and hospitals. If they could not pay, they cared for themselves. If that became impossible, they were forced to seek charity, either from local hospitals or from other benevolent groups in their communities. For a variety of cultural and economic reasons, the idea of any level of personal health care as a tax-supported right did not take root during the period of rapid hospital development.

Instead, Americans restricted government responsibility for health to marginal care of the desperate poor, the insane, those with dangerous infectious disease, and later to childhood immunization against contagious disease. Except for scattered public health service hospitals and military installations, the federal government played no role at all in health care. Insane asylums, city and county hospitals for the sick poor, and tuberculosis hospitals were supported by local or state revenues.

Hospital expansion went forward in an environment of economic uncertainty. Voluntary hospitals, the vast majority of successful community hospitals, depended on patient fees, benefactors, and local donations for their entire income; importantly, after the turn of the century they did get special tax relief in most communities. Nevertheless, many failed when benefactor generosity and stringent management did not keep up with costs. The local, religious, and ethnic segmentation that characterized hospital development guaranteed that many hospitals would be small and, therefore, vulnerable to financial exigencies (Lynaugh, 1989b).

Even though the American market-oriented economic system seemed poorly suited and even hostile to financing and delivering social services, we managed to build a complicated structure of voluntary hospitals and agencies. These coped, as best they could, with the fundamental incompatibility between demanded health services and unfettered free enterprise (Stevens, 1989). It seems clear that Americans wanted and needed hospitals in their communities, even though they could not solve the problem of how to make hospitals fit into normal ways of doing business.

Most American nurses were introduced to their life's work in the voluntary, local hospital system; thus, the first 60 years of nursing history were dominated by private values and local custom. Decisions about nursing practice and education were essentially insulated from public debate. Even compliance with early 20th century registration laws regulating nursing practice in the states was voluntary (Tomes, 1983).

It would be decades before Americans grappled with the immutable fact that sick people run out of money, cannot work, and cannot pay their bills for health care or anything else. Americans could not reach a consensus on European ideas of public spending for general health care. The debate over universal access to health care began around 1915 in the United States. It was set aside with the advent of World War I but raised repeatedly in subsequent years, and the argument continues today.

The first major move toward collective responsibility for health and social services came in Franklin Roosevelt's administration with the Social Security Act of 1935. National health insurance was part of the original Social Security proposals, but it was abandoned when Roosevelt concluded that the American Medical Association's opposition to "socialized medicine" could scuttle the whole idea of Social Security. Nevertheless, the 1935 legislation signaled that Americans would support social programs. Although Social Security relied on an insurance concept, it was a firm step toward some measure of collective responsibility for individual welfare. In the meantime, also in the 1930s, Americans began to buy individual hospital insurance in the form of locally controlled Blue Cross and Blue Shield plans and a variety of commercial insurance plans.

After 1900, voluntary community hospitals began to use their beds mostly for surgical patients and for those with acute medical illnesses; they also opened wards for maternity patients and children. Throughout these years hospital boards came to believe that if they filled their beds with people who could not pay and the chronically ill who would not get better, the resulting losses would ruin their institutions. As one hospital board member from a voluntary hospital in Kansas City remarked in 1917, "[we must] develop this institution to a high plane of efficiency; taking it away from the invalid home idea; also from the [image of a] high class boarding house for chronic cases" (Lynaugh, 1989b).

Visiting nurses and public health nurses were influenced by the American enthusiasm for community hospitals. Their practice in the neighborhoods of cities and towns and in rural counties, which had been accelerated by the social reform climate early in the 20th century, was independent of hospitals. But as Karen Buhler-Wilkerson has shown, their work eventually was affected by the growing dominance of hospitals in the American health care system (Buhler-Wilkerson, 1989). In fact, the success of hospitals in garnering the major production of new dollars through health insurance in the late 1930s may have undermined the earlier potential of visiting nurse and public health services to ameliorate gaps in health services, especially for the poor and chronically ill.

Many nurses, physicians, and other health care leaders understood the folly of limiting hospital responsibility to short-term, treatable ills. Interest in the chronically ill and the aged as well as efforts to improve general health among the population continued throughout the first four decades of this century. Experiments with neighborhood health centers and expanded health department services found some support. Public enthusiasm and medical confidence, however, combined to focus more and more attention and money on scientific medicine and the search for cures. In the decades after World War I, planners visualized the hospital as the institutional center from which health services would assuage the ills of each community.

However, since the insurance plans devised in 1930s were designed to cover only acute care services, the chronically ill and the aged, who were not protected by insurance coverage, found themselves outside of community hospital interests. The poor remained the responsibility of local government or private charity. Hospitals, in Charles Rosenberg's cogent phrase, clung to their "inward vision" of scientifically based, curative medicine (Rosenberg, 1979).

## Recreating American Nursing

American confidence in health and health care underwent profound alteration in the general economic depression of the 1930s, followed by worldwide war in the 1940s. These cataclysmic events marked our gradual turning away from reliance on highly localized, private approaches to health care. World War II was a watershed event for nursing, for the general social and world consciousness of Americans, and for the health care system.

Nursing leaders in the 1940s deliberately exploited the war emergency to seek a new deal for nursing. They pushed for better education, better standards of nursing service, and better pay. They merged five weak national nursing organizations into two stronger units, and they gained some accrediting control over the nursing education system. The National Nursing Council for War Service, a voluntary committee of nursing leaders, collaborated with nurses in the United States Public Health Service; they used foresight and political acumen to lever nursing out of its isolated and fragmented localism (Goostray, 1969; Lynaugh, 1990).

The problem for nursing before World War II was how to improve nursing education within impoverished hospitals and deliver safe nursing care using mostly student caregivers. The problem after the war was how to create both a new nursing education system outside the hospital and a safe nursing care system using mostly paid caregivers.

Focusing the history of the first 60 years of nursing this sharply is not intended to deny the existence of university nursing education before World War II. However, the impact of collegiate programs and graduates was small. Nor should the importance of visiting and public health nurses and the reforms in which they participated be diminished. Rather, emphasis is placed here on the dominance of hospitals in 20th century nursing history. Delivering safe nursing care in hospitals and relocating nursing education away from hospitals into colleges and universities, two linked problems, absorbed the energies of postwar nurses.

## Delivering Safe Nursing Care

Delivering safe care using paid staff instead of an all student work force was very much complicated by the postwar expansion of hospitals. Demand for hospital services was up, partly because of successful labor negotiations for better health insurance in America's burgeoning postwar economy. The Hill-Burton Act of 1946 financed new hospitals and the reconstruction of old hospitals. New hospitals and more beds helped to exacerbate the already existing severe shortage of nurses after the war. Intregrating nurses' aides, practical nurses, and student nurses into teams led by professional nurses (team nursing) was the strategy of the day. But because of the protracted shortage of professional nurses and increasing demand for hospital beds, team nursing often degenerated into an assembly line type of functional hospital nursing care system. Head nurses and supervisors with prewar experience and limited educational preparation were accustomed to relying on student workers in large numbers. Students were getting scarcer for two reasons—the rising operating expenses of hospital schools and restrictions on exploiting student labor by accrediting agencies.

Care of patients inside hospitals clearly needed redesign to cope with different caregiver personnel and rising acute illnesses among hospital patients. It took about 15 years of struggle and readjustment through the 1950s before staff nursing by graduate nurses replaced reliance on students and broke away from the rigid, novice-oriented assignment systems of prewar hospitals. Imitating the 1940s idea of the postoperative recovery room, geographic clusters of the sickest patients were created to try to use professional nurses more efficiently and better guarantee the safe care of patients.

Nurses and hospital administrators altered traditional uses of space, i.e., wards and private rooms, to cope with the influx of seriously ill people and the intensive postoperative care problems created by more invasive surgical procedures. They put certain types of less physiologically stable patients into intensive care units and changed staffing patterns to improve the patient-nurse ratio. New treatments and new technologies were spurred by popular concern about heart disease, a leading cause of death. Federal funding in the 1960s assured that patients with coronary artery disease got special attention in coronary care units. A few years later, passage of the 1965 Medicare/Medicaid legislation ensured a constant flow of patients and dollars into hospitals.

The motive for reorganization of nursing practice was to conserve nurses and assure hospital patients of protection from neglect. And, in fact, anecdotal evidence suggests that the problem of poor care for unstable hospital patients (i.e., patients being left alone with signs and symptoms unattended) is much less severe 30 years later.

But there is a history lesson here—the lesson of the unintended outcome. The intensive or special care unit, which was devised to conserve the number of nurses needed to care for the most seriously ill patients and to put the "best" nurses with the sickest patients, did accomplish the latter goal. However, the strategy increased rather than decreased the demand for nurses. At the risk of oversimplifying a complex series of events, what seems to have happened is that the intensive care unit, instead of reducing the total number of nurses needed to staff hospitals, proved to be a breeding ground for experts. Expert nursing in intensive care units made it possible to deploy technology successfully and to try more vigorous treatments, and more progressive therapy made nurses even more in demand as well as more expert (Lynaugh & Fairman, 1990).

Our experience with critical care nursing, as it is now called, is reflective of the history of all of nursing. The advent of trained nurses made hospitals possible—made it feasible to cluster the sick in large numbers and care for them safely and efficiently. One hundred years later, the advent of critical care nurses made it possible to create and expand intensive care units—made it feasible to cluster extremely sick people and care for them more effectively.

In both cases—the 19th century hospital and the 1960s intensive care unit—we instituted change to solve specific problems. We could not foresee where those changes would lead us. Creation of intensive care units led to complete renovation of the interior of hospitals. Patients now are grouped according to the stability of their physiologic condition. No longer are they assigned a bed by 1950s categories such as sex, ability to pay, or the identity of the admitting physician.

The hierarchy of nursing changed as well. Specialized clinical nursing expertise now ranks with or above administrative position as a measure of professional status. The clinical nurse specialist in many institutions either supersedes the head nurse or supervisor or shares the same status.

Paralleling this massive investment in high technology and intensive care in the 1960s and 1970s was a strong movement to enable all Americans to have access to ordinary medical care under its new rubric—primary health care. Proponents for primary health care argued that each person should be able to obtain service from a general health care provider without restriction owing to income or place of residence.

It became evident to primary health care advocates that no such policy could be implemented if the credential for all primary health care providers remained a medical degree. The idea of the nurse practitioner and the physician's assistant was born, along with an effort to restore the general medical practitioner, renamed the family physician. The nurse practitioner movement of the 1970s became an avenue to advanced clinical expertise for nurses working with the chronically ill and with children as well as those providing care in the areas of minor illness, public health, and health education.

The political promise of access to care for all proved ephemeral in the political and economic turmoil of the late 1970s and the 1980s. Nevertheless, nurse practitioner practice evolved successfully and encompassed responsibility for delivering health services to a wide spectrum of the population. Growing dependence on nurse practitioners is verified by their success in winning direct reimbursement for their services, thus breaking through the monopoly on insurance payment for direct patient care enjoyed by physicians since the 1930s.

These two practice arenas, critical care and primary health care, exemplify the responsiveness of nursing to societal demands for certain services. Although some nurse leaders argue that nursing is altogether too responsive to social pressure, critical care nurses and primary care nurse practitioners are just the most recent examples of an occupation willing and able to change itself as its environment changes. Seen in this light, these recent movements are logically correlative with the renaissance of American midwifery under nursing's auspices and turn of the century public health nursing.

## Creating a New Educational System

Creating a new nursing education system outside the hospital proved just as difficult as restructuring nursing practice. The associate degree nursing education strategy was proposed in 1950 by nurse educator Mildred Montag to prepare "technical" nurses in the rapidly expanding community colleges of the nation. Planners expected that graduates from associate degree nursing programs would replace hospital school graduates. Other new nurses would come from the expanding baccalaureate nursing programs. In the original concept outlined by Montag and others (Montag, 1951; Montag, 1959) baccalaureate nursing graduates would be accountable for patient care and would direct the work of the nurse technician. That is not what happened.

Hospitals were starved for nurses; neither they nor state boards of nursing made distinctions between graduates of associate degree, baccalaureate, or diploma programs. It was easier for hospitals and state regulators to assume that all nurses were the same in terms of registration, assignments, pay, and advancement. Inability to differentiate levels of nursing practice responsibilities on the basis of educational preparation or any other abstract standard has proved to be one of the most intractable problems of 20th century nursing.

Although it is beyond the scope of this chapter to detail the problems of nurse supply, demand, and quality in our current health care system, it is possible to outline the debate for the last 50 years. Historically, there are at least two and possibly three sets of enduring conflicts. First, nurse leaders' efforts to upgrade preparation for practice and to restrict numbers often conflict with social desires to contain cost in providing nursing care. Second, differentiation of nursing practice to improve quality through specialization conflicts with institutional needs for flexible generalist nursing staffs. And finally, nurse-controlled practice and differentiated practice, such as that of nurse practitioners and nurse midwives, creates competitive fears among physicians.

Redesigning nursing practice and nursing education during the three decades after World War II dominated nursing's attention. In the background, however, a dramatic, slow-moving shift changed the context of the education debate. More and more nurses were going to college. Nurse veterans coming out of service went to college on the GI Bill; later, other nurses found support for higher education under the federal Nurse Training Acts of the 1960s.

The postwar revolution in American higher education—i.e., access of the middle and working classes to college—finally enabled nursing, with its members largely drawn from those classes, to realize its long-standing educational agenda. Nurses began to earn baccalaureate degrees, master's degrees, and doctoral degrees in substantial numbers.

The tuition dollars these nurses paid were lifesaving for small, struggling nurse education programs in colleges and universities. From 1964, when federal funding for nursing education stood at $9,900,000, through and beyond the peak year of 1973, when $160,000,000 was appropriated, nurse education programs in colleges and universities grew at an unprecedented rate. Once those nursing schools in colleges and universities attained a viable size through the influx of financially aided students, they could begin to attend to the training of clinical specialists, well-prepared faculty, and researchers. Direct federal aid for students leveled off in the 1970s, but the infusion of funds in the decades following World War II proved crucial to the movement of nursing education out of hospitals and into mainstream higher education.

In the United States, higher education is one proxy for class. In our polyglot, immigrant society, we use college education and accumulated wealth to substitute for inherited status. Of course, there always had been nurses of middle class and even upper middle class origins. From the beginning, daughters of clergy, bankers, wealthier physicians, and university professors made their careers in nursing. But the majority of nurses were from the working class; their hospital training gave them a new opportunity to make a living but did not change their class status.

Under the double handicap of gender and class, it is somewhat surprising that nurses have been able to control the fate of nursing as much as they have. Part of nurses' social authority stemmed from the essential and intimate nature of the work and their complex relationships with patients. Nurses are taught to adopt a "nursing character," to use Susan Reverby's phrase, which allows them to transcend class barriers in the care relationship (Reverby, 1987b). This means that in the nurse-patient relationship the nurse is able to keep control of the encounter even when differences in class, gender, or race might suggest otherwise. But when nurses operated outside the care relationship, e.g., in negotiations with hospital boards, university presidents, or physicians, their "nursing character" lost its effectiveness. To be in the places where health policy decisions were made meant breaking through class barriers. Before the educational revolution of the second half of this century, class handicaps, along with gender, prevented all but a few nurses from attaining sufficient social authority to be full participants in the negotiations that determined and managed the fate of their profession.

In addition to gaining access to higher education, nurses benefited from the civil rights achievements of the 1960s women's movement. Lavinia Dock and women's rights advocates of the pre-World War I era constantly reiterated one basic tenet: nurses' rights and women's rights are inextricably linked. Present-day nurses, although still socially conservative, seem much more in tune with women's rights than were Dock's colleagues during the first women's rights campaign. Nursing, in its relationship with society, is more pragmatic and confrontational and less deferential and altruistic than it used to be. In that sense nursing is now more integrated and less isolated from the larger society.

## Conclusion

When sick, injured, and dependent people first gathered together in hospitals, chaos resulted because clustering the sick in hospitals elevated ordinary domestic and medical problems to herculean proportions. Nursing, practiced at a relatively simple but resolute level, reduced chaos to order as nurses, to again use a Reverby phrase, were "ordered to care" and they did (Reverby, 1987b). At the same time, a peculiar hospital-based nursing education system helped subsidize the rapid growth of America's hospital system.

Beginning in the 1930s and resuming after World War II, a protracted and sometimes stumbling effort to change the staffing system in hospitals ultimately produced a safe, responsive level of nursing practice using fully trained nurses. It is clear, however, that constant reconceptualization and revamping are required to deliver safe nursing care both inside and outside institutions.

Nursing education is no longer dominated by hospitals, but it is still tightly linked to nursing practice. With all its problems, the nursing education system is remarkably well developed, although it is chronically underfunded. Nursing still faces thorny issues of licensure and credentialing of its basic practitioners and specialists as well as severe disadvantages in reimbursement. Probably the most difficult educational problem for nurses will be to agree on and plan for an appropriate mix of levels of nursing personnel.

Since the beginning of nursing history, leaders in nursing have been slow or unwilling to acknowledge and take responsibility for aides, attendants, and similarly trained personnel. These auxiliary personnel are often feared as threats to quality of care or as competitive to nurses. Moreover, nursing educators who teach at different levels such as master's, baccalaureate, associate degree, practical nursing, and in continuing education communicate with each other with difficulty and rarely plan together. Possibly, as nurses become more certain of the nature of advanced practice and more confident about nursing's research and place among the professions, they may be able to cope effectively with demands for more basically trained caregivers.

The major deficit in the American health care system continues to be citizens' access to health care services. Access problems range from lack of insurance, which excludes needy persons from acute care, to a preponderance of low quality, high-cost nursing home care. These problems persist in spite of enormous expenditures (600 billion dollars in 1990) and unrelenting political attention. What Americans want is what we seem to have always wanted—a responsive community of health-related services. A significant proportion of demanded services today is nursing's responsibility. Given this country's history of restless, short-term problem solving, it is going to be extremely difficult for Americans to rethink health care, but it seems likely that inexorable pressure for fiscal reform and renewed concern about problems such as high rates of infant mortality and the crisis of acquired immunodeficiency syndrome will drive change.

The issues remain much the same as they were when nursing was invented: how, where, and how much care should be given when people cannot care for themselves; how should care be paid for; how will the work of care be divided; where will caregivers come from; and how much knowledge and skill should caregivers have?

As we search for answers to these questions, we should not forget one important difference between the 19th century and now. Nursing is very much with us, with its expertise in devising care systems, its holistic care orientation complementing medicine's specificity, its flexibility and resilience, and its two million members. Although born in the 19th century, nursing grew to maturity in the tumult of the 20th century. We can hope that our experience, seasoned knowledge, and commitment will be sufficient to the task of restructuring American health care for the 21st century.

## REFERENCES

Baer, E. (1985). Nursing's divided house—An historical view. *Nursing Research, 34*, 32–38.

Buhler-Wilkerson, K. (1989). *False dawn: The rise and decline of public health nursing 1900–1930.* New York: Garland Publishing, Inc.

Goostray, S. (1969). *Memoirs: Half a century in nursing.* Boston: Nursing Archive.

Hampton, I. (1949). *Nursing of the sick 1893.* Reprint. New York: McGraw-Hill Book Company.

Long, D., & Golden, J. (Eds.) (1989). *The American general hospital: Communities and social context.* Ithaca & London: Cornell University Press.

Lynaugh, J. (1989a). *The community hospitals of Kansas City, Missouri, 1870–1915.* New York: Garland Publishing, Inc.

Lynaugh, J. (1989b). From respectable domesticity to medical efficiency: The changing Kansas City Hospital, 1875–1920. In D. Long & J. Golden (Eds.), *The American general hospital: Communities and social contexts* (pp. 21–39). Ithaca & London: Cornell University Press.

Lynaugh, J. (1990). Stepping in. *Nursing Research, 39*, 126–127.

Lynaugh, J., & Fairman, J. (1990). History of care of the critically ill since 1940. Unpublished data.

Montag, M. (1951). *The education of nurse technicians.* New York: G.P. Putnam's Sons.

Montag, M. (1959). *Community college education for nurses.* New York: McGraw-Hill Book Co.

Nutting, A. (1984). *A sound economic basis for schools of nursing and other addresses.* Reprint. New York: Garland Publishing, Inc.

O'Brien, P. (1987). "All a woman's life can bring:" The domestic roots of nursing in Philadelphia, 1830–1885. *Nursing Research, 36,* 12–17.

Poplin, I. (1988). *A study of the Kaiserswerth Deaconess Institute's Nurse Training School in 1850–1851: Purposes and curriculum.* Unpublished doctoral dissertation, University of Texas at Austin.

Reverby, S. (1987a). A caring dilemma: Womanhood and nursing in historical perspective. *Nursing Research, 36,* 5–11.

Reverby, S. (1987b). *Ordered to care: The dilemma of American Nursing, 1850–1945.* Cambridge: Cambridge University Press.

Rosenberg, C.E. (1979). Inward vision and outward glance: The shaping of the American hospital, 1880–1914. *Bulletin of the History of Medicine, 53*(3), 346–391.

Rosenberg, C.E. (1987). *The care of strangers: The rise of America's hospital system.* New York: Basic Books, Inc.

Rosner, D. (1982). *A once charitable enterprise: Hospitals and health care in Brooklyn and New York, 1885–1915.* Cambridge: Cambridge University Press.

Stevens, R. (1989). *In sickness and in wealth: American hospitals in the twentieth century.* New York: Basic Books, Inc.

Tomes, N. (1983). The silent battle: Nurse registration in New York State, 1903–1920. In E. Lagemann (Ed.), *Nursing history, new perspectives, new possibilities* (pp. 107–132). New York: Teachers' College Press.

Vicinus, M. (1985). *Independent women: Work and community for single women, 1850–1920.* Chicago & London: University of Chicago Press.

Woodham-Smith, C. (1951). *Florence Nightingale 1820–1910.* London & Glasgow: Fontana Books.

## Chapter 28

# Physician Payment Reform: Implications for Nursing

CAROL ANN LOCKHART

$C$ONCERN ABOUT HOW much Americans pay for health care and what they receive for their money stimulated public debate and action during the 1980s and continues to do so in the 1990s. The rate of increase in the portion of the Medicare budget paid to physicians has made physician fees a focus in that public debate.

Current physician payment methods are dominated by a fee-for-service approach. The approach encourages high utilization (high volume) of services and increased use of procedures and technology, since such activities are paid at a higher rate than nonprocedural or low technology services.

Fee-for-service payments have resulted in disparities in income across medical specialties, with surgical and technical specialties more highly rewarded than other specialties, such as family practice. It has also influenced and unbalanced physician choices of specialty and location of practice. Physicians tend to choose those areas and specialties in which reimbursements are highest. Stated more broadly, fee-for-service payment methodology has distorted the market for physician services.

In order to correct these imbalances, the federal Medicare program is redesigning its physician payment policies. The policies will seek to simulate a "perfect market," where supply of services and types and quantities of specialists are influenced by demand for services at a given price. The price, however, will no longer be set by the physician but according to a new methodology adopted by the federal government. This chapter discusses the new payment policies and evaluates their implications for nurses.

### Context for Reform (1965 to 1990)

Over 32 million elderly and disabled individuals receive their health care through Medicare. Those over 65 account for approximately 12 percent of the United States population, and their numbers are increasing by between 1 and 2 percent per year. By the year 2000 they will account for 13 percent and by 2050 a total of 22 percent of the population. This means that nearly 65 million people will be eligible for Medicare, more than double the number currently served (U.S. Congress, Senate, Special Committee on Aging, 1987–1988).

Among Medicare recipients, those over 75 will make up over 50 percent of the eligible population by the year 2000. "Elderly persons use more health services than other age groups. They account for 30 percent of all hospital discharges, 20 percent of all doctor visits, and one-third of the country's personal health care expenditures even though they constitute only 12 percent of the population. When they are hospitalized they stay about 50 percent longer than the general population" (Physician Payment Review Commission, 1989, pp. 17, 18). The implication is that more people will require more care as they live longer and have more serious and chronic health needs.

Medicare Part B, the Supplementary Medical Insurance program, provides coverage for physician services, outpatient hospital care, laboratory tests, durable medical equipment, and certain other selected services. To participate in Part B, a person must already participate in the Part A Hospital Insurance Program and pay a monthly Part B premium. Ninety-seven percent of the Part A beneficiaries who are eligible for Part B have enrolled in the program (Physician Payment Review Commission, 1989, chap. 1).

Although the Part A Hospital Insurance Trust Fund is funded primarily through Social Security payroll taxes, beneficiary premiums for Part B services must, by law, provide 25 percent of the revenues needed for the Part B (Supplementary Medical Insurance) Trust Fund. Over 70 percent of the remaining funds are drawn from the general tax revenues of the federal government, whereas a very small percentage is raised through interest on the trust fund itself.

As the demands on the Medicare program increase owing to increased numbers of beneficiaries and services, the allocation of funds to the program becomes problematic. Since most of the outlays for Part B services come from tax revenues, any growth in costs or related services will require tax dollars and place Medicare in direct competition with other programs and services that might otherwise be funded by the federal government.

This concern about expenditure growth sharpened because between 1980 and 1988 Medicare outlays increased, on average, 13.1 percent per year. Part B grew at an average rate of 17 percent per year between 1980 and 1988. The 1988 expenditures totaled 88 billion dollars, with 35 billion dollars going for Part B services. Physician services account for 72 percent of the Part B expenditures (Physician Payment Review Commission, 1989, p. 12).

Studies suggest that the majority of the increases are attributable to growth in volume of services per beneficiary and the substitution of more expensive and largely technical procedures for less expensive services (Mitchell et al., 1989; McMenamin et al., 1988). With the expenditure increases already experienced and the anticipated increases from escalating costs, volume of services, technology, and aging of the population, the Congress and others have identified Medicare Part B as a target for policy reform.

## Medicare Physician Payment Policy (1965 to 1990)

For the most part, physicians are independent entrepreneurs. The charges they establish may be paid in full or modified by a third party (insurance or government) paying the fee. Once a reimbursement price is offered, a physician may or may not accept it as payment in full. If it is not accepted, the patient may be billed for any difference or "balance" (balance bill) left between the third-party payment and the physician's charges, unless this is prohibited by law or contract. Although other approaches to physician payment such as capitation arrangements and salaries do exist, the fee-for-service approach is the most common and widely used.

When Congress enacted Medicare, it agreed to adopt the existing fee-for-service approach for medical care and to pay "reasonable charges." The term reasonable charges is used to mean whatever charge a physician bills as long as the charge does not exceed the "customary" charges he or she billed for the previous year for the same service, or the "prevailing" charges used by other physicians in the same area for that service. This approach to deciding the rate of payment came to be called "customary, prevailing and reasonable" (CPR). Since each physician's and region's pattern of charges varies, payment schedules for medical services differ significantly from one area of the country to another (Physician Payment Review Commission, 1987, chap. 2).

This CPR fee-for-service approach provides an incentive for physicians to establish a relatively high pattern of charges, since the maximum charge allowed is based on the individual physician's own pattern of charges and those of other practitioners in the area. The higher the charge pattern, the higher the permissible reimbursement level. Payment is made for services delivered; hence, the more services delivered, the more fees paid. There are no incentives to limit the number of services provided or the use of new technology, since all but a few services are reimbursable.

The result is that Medicare physician payments reward or penalize certain styles of medical practice, specialties, services (e.g., procedures and surgery versus evaluative or cognitive services), and locations for services (e.g., urban versus rural). This disparity between payments for procedures in different locations and facilities and payments for different specialties cannot be explained by the different costs physicians experience in operating their practices (Physician Payment Review Commission, 1987, p. ix).

Limited efforts at control of the annual rate of increase in payment rates to physicians, prospective review of services utilized, and limitations on physician balance billing were instituted in the 1980s but were unable to hold expenditure increases in check. Congress and those attentive to public policy came to accept that the underlying physician payment method was flawed (as was the hospital payment method in 1983) and must be changed if there was to be reasonable control over medical expenditures.

## Medicare Physician Payment Reform

Responding to the need for control on expenditures for physician services, the 101st Congress made physician payment reform a part of the Omnibus Budget Reconciliation Act of 1989 (OBRA 89; Public Law 101-239). The law established

1. the structure to create a national Medicare schedule of fees (Medicare fee schedule);
2. limits on the balance a physician can bill a beneficiary;
3. a formula for specifying the rate at which the volume of services provided is allowed to increase (Medicare volume performance standards); and
4. federal support for defining what is effective medical care and practice.

The reforms are the result of study and research Congress initiated in 1985. Many are based on work done by the Physician Payment Review Commission created by Congress in 1986. The Commission's annual recommendations to the Congress address ". . . adjustments to the reasonable charge levels for physicians' services . . . and changes in the methodology for determining the rates of payment, and for making payment for physicians' services . . ." under Part B of the Medicare program (Physician Payment Review Commission, 1987).

In its first report to Congress (March 1, 1987), the Commission identified a series of goals it would use to guide decisions on payment reform. The changes enacted in 1989 reflect goals that seek to (1) ensure access to care for beneficiaries; (2) maintain or improve the quality of care provided; (3) provide financial protection for beneficiaries to ensure that the level of their responsibility is not so high as to prevent access to care or cause economic hardship; (4) ensure equity of payment among physicians so that similar payments are made for similar services among similarly qualified physicians; (5) slow the growth in outlays from the Supplementary Medical Insurance Trust Fund; (6) ensure that the payment method used is understandable to the beneficiary, physician, and general public; (7) ensure orderly change from one payment method to another; and (8) provide pluralistic approaches that can accommodate the various ways health services are organized so as not to exclude both fee-for-service and capitation approaches. (Physician Payment Review Commission, 1987).

Refinements to the reasonable charge (CPR) approach, payment for packages of related services, and capitation were considered as options and remain options for future action. Although each option has attractive features, a predetermined schedule or listing of the fees to be paid by Medicare was deemed the most appropriate and easily implemented approach. Years of experience with fee-for-service payments by the over one-half million American physicians was a primary reason for the decision. The ability to exercise controls on expenditures without changing the payment mechanism itself, only the pricing structure, made a fee schedule an attractive option.

A comparison of key features of existing Medicare physician payment policies

**TABLE 28–1   A Comparison of Medicare Physician Payment Policies**

| Reasonable Charge Policies | Medicare Fee Schedule Policies |
|---|---|
| 1. Fee-for-service | 1. Fee-for-service |
| 2. Physician-determined fees | 2. Medicare-determined fees |
| 3. Wide variations in fees for same services | 3. Same fee for same service |
| 4. Specialists paid higher fee for a service | 4. Same fee for same service (no specialty differential) |
| 5. Fees based on physician and community pattern | 5. Fees based on resources required to provide service |
| 6. Relative value of one procedure to another physician determined | 6. Relative value of one procedure to another based on resource costs |
| 7. Procedural/technical services given greater value than evaluation and management services | 7. Services valued according to resource costs—values more consistent across types of services |
| 8. Beneficiary and physician unsure of payment level by Medicare | 8. Beneficiary and physician aware of Medicare payment prior to service |
| 9. Medicare payment varies by physician and area of the country | 9. Medicare payment consistent by service and region (slight adjustment for geographic cost variation) |
| 10. Beneficiary can be billed for portion not paid by Medicare | 10. Limits on beneficiary liability for portion of bill not paid by Medicare |
| 11. Utilization (volume) controlled in minor ways | 11. Volume performance standard set for each year |

with those created under the 1989 legislation is presented in Table 28–1. The comparison highlights the scope of the changes under way in Medicare and the discussion in this chapter.

## Resource-Based Relative Value Scale

In 1985, in anticipation of physician payment reform, Congress directed the Health Care Financing Administration (the agency that administers the Medicare program) to conduct a study to develop a resource-based relative value scale reflecting the value of the services physicians provide (Consolidated Omnibus Budget Reconciliation Act of 1985 [C]OBRA85: P.IL. 99-272). The Health Care Financing Administration funded William Hsiao and colleagues at Harvard University in a major study of the relative resources needed to produce one physician service as compared with another. The research, which previously had been done on a limited scale, was to objectively determine value based on resource requirements (Hsiao et al., 1988a, 1988b).

Introduction of a Medicare fee schedule based on resources is an effort at estimating the price of medical services given a "perfect" theoretical health care market rather than the reality of one in which competing and conflicting influences distort the price, supply, and demand for services. As Hsiao notes: "The RBRVS [resource-based relative value scale] study uses a rational and systematic process to derive the relative prices that would have emerged from a reasonably competitive market" (Hsiao, 1989). And as a Physician Payment Review Commission report states, "A resource-cost basis would reflect estimates of what relative values would be under a hypothetical market that functions perfectly. Under such a market, competition derives relative prices to reflect the relative cost of efficient producers" (Physician Payment Review Commission, 1989, chap. 3).

The resource-based relative value scale developed from Hsiao's work is the cornerstone of the development of the Medicare fee schedule. Although other resource components and weighting of the components affect the formula for the relative value scale, on average, slightly more than one half of the value is attributable to the value of physicians' work as defined by Hsiao. Of the remaining one half, most is attributable to practice expense, with a small percentage assigned to the cost of malpractice insurance (Physician Payment Review Commission, 1990).

Hsiao's study provided estimates of the amount of physician time, mental effort and judgment, technical skill, physical effort (intensity), and stress involved in performing a medical service. Physician work is divided into (1) preservice work (e.g., review of chart and laboratory reports before seeing the patient); (2) intraservices work (services given on a face-to-face basis); and (3) postservice work (e.g., scheduling surgery, ordering and reviewing diagnostic tests). The estimates of the work are developed from vignettes describing patient characteristics and the physician service or procedure to be provided. The vignette is assigned a service or procedure code from the common procedural terminology nomenclature used by Medicare for reporting services; therefore, each total work value that is developed is associated with a common procedural terminology code (Hsiao, Braun, Dunn, & Becker, 1988). This ongoing study and refinements to the study by the Physician Payment Review Commission and the Health Care Financing Administration will result in the assignment of a value to a physician service.

The second major component of the resource-based relative value scale estimated costs (which is not taken from the work by Hsiao) is practice costs or the cost of nonphysician input necessary to provide physician services. These costs represent about 48 percent of the average physician's total revenue (Gonzalez & Emmons, 1988). Practice costs include salaries for personnel (nurses, technicians, and receptionists) plus the cost of office space (e.g., utilities), nonmedical supplies and equipment (e.g., furniture), medical supplies, and administrative expenses.

Malpractice costs are usually included in practice costs. In the Medicare relative value scale, however, they will be pulled out of the overall costs and addressed separately in order to clearly identify their impact on the cost of services. Such costs vary significantly by specialty and will be adjusted to reflect that difference. They will also be adjusted to ensure that there is no financial incentive to order or perform one procedure over another and thereby receive a higher reimbursement than is necessary for the malpractice portion of practice costs.

A last consideration in the development of the resource-based relative value scale will be a geographic practice cost index. This index will reflect the differences experienced in maintaining practices in different geographic areas of the country, with adjustments made to factor out high cost amenities that are not necessary to the practice. Once completed, the resource-based relative value scale will be reviewed and revised by the Health Care Financing Administration at least every five years.

## Medicare Fee Schedule

The fee schedule will be developed by multiplying the resource-based relative value scale times a dollar conversion factor (specified by Congress) and an adjustment factor for geographic fee differences between one locality and another. No allowance will be made for physician specialists. Instead, practice costs will consider only the cost of the services provided, not the specialty designation of the provider. In other words, two physicians performing the same procedure and therefore expending the same resources will be rewarded in the same manner, even if one is a specialist and the other is not.

The Medicare fee schedule will be phased in over five years (1992 to 1996). Since it is based primarily on resource costs, the fees to be paid will be different from reasonable charges. The fees per unit of time for invasive procedures, imaging, and laboratory procedures are higher under the CPR approach but will be lower under a cost-based fee schedule. Fees per unit of time for evaluation and management services will increase. The changes will, in general, reflect an increase in "value" for "hands-on" care by primary care and general practice physicians and reduced "value" for technical procedures and surgery.

Because of the difference in the payment methodology used in the Medicare fee schedule, some physicians are seen as winners (general and family practitioners and internists), whereas others are deemed the losers (surgeons and some specialists). The "losers," however, have been and will remain some of the most highly reimbursed practitioners under Medicare, since their services are still highly valued, even under the resource-based relative value scale.

Modifications to fees that seek to bring practitioners in line with the values defined under the resource-based relative value scale will begin in 1992. The Medicare fees offered in 1996 will be based totally on the resource-based relative value scale. During this phase-in period, changes to coding will be implemented to make reporting of services consistent with the scale and consistent between regions of the country. Eventually, coding reforms will attempt to capture information on the severity of illness of the person receiving services, information that is not now available.

## Medicare Volume Performance Standards

Implementation of a Medicare fee schedule moves the Medicare payment methodology toward a more rational market approach to purchasing physician services. Even so, it does nothing to control the volume of services used under Medicare.

An annual Medicare volume performance standard will attempt to control utilization of services by defining a targeted level of increase beyond which the program should not grow in any one year.

The volume performance standard will be set by calculating an allowance for (1) medical cost increases and inflation (as measured by a Medical Economic Index); (2) growth and aging in the eligible population; and (3) a comparison between the prior year's change in expenditures and a previously designated standard for expenditure change. The hope is that the volume of services will not exceed the current year's standard, which will be set to allow utilization to remain within the allocation of the current year's funding.

Congress will make annual decisions on both the performance standard and the fee update for the following year. The decisions will consider advice from the Health Care Financing Administration and the Physician Payment Review Commission. Should Congress fail to act, the legislation specifies a "default" formula or what percentage of change should be used in the absence of any specific action by Congress.

If the volume of services in a given year is less than or equal to the standard, the next year's fee updates should allow for reasonable inflation in prices and volume. If, however, the volume performance standard is exceeded, the allowable inflation or growth in volume of services will be held to a lower level. Thus, if physicians are unable to stay within the standard for volume and exceed expected expenditures during one year, the next year limitations are placed on their fees.

The pressure to control the volume of services offered by physicians will be applied at a national rather than a local or regional level. (The Physician Payment Review Commission will continue to study how other than a national volume performance standard might be implemented.) A national volume performance standard may not offer a clear enough connection to individual physician orders to result in a diminished volume of services under Medicare. In addition, since Medicare accounts for an average of only 33 percent of physicians' annual revenue, any constraints will apply to only a portion of most physicians' incomes (Physician Payment Review Commission, 1989).

Without a leveling off or decline in the volume of services used, expenditures may remain beyond those deemed acceptable to Congress. If that occurs, more stringent volume performance standard requirements at a regional or local level may be instituted in order to increase physician awareness of and response to the controls. Since Medicare is only one payer, another way to increase the pressure for volume control would be to encourage other payers to adopt the same approaches used by Medicare or some version of them. Should that occur, physicians would be faced with the same incentives and constraints in all areas of their practice.

Whether the Medicare volume performance standards will succeed in providing incentives strong enough for physicians to control their use of resources is unclear.

> The Volume Performance Standard System provides a collective incentive to the physician community to slow the growth of expenditures to Medicare beneficiaries. It is intended that this be accomplished by reducing services that provide little or no benefit to patients rather than by holding down physician fees . . . the rate of growth of expenditures can be reduced over the next several years while maintaining access and quality of care. This challenge and the work required to meet it will fall primarily to the medical profession. Only they can identify and reduce services of little or no benefit.

Recent efforts of medical organizations to begin or to accelerate the development and use of practice guidelines show that the medical profession is already at work (Lee, 1990).

## Practice Guidelines

Practice guidelines, outcomes, and effectiveness research are to assist physicians in determining the best medical approach to care and the most effective use of resources. It is the expectation and hope that as guidelines are developed, physicians will be able to remain within targeted volumes and expenditures because of their improved ability to appropriately choose and utilize resources.

Development of the guidelines is seen as a five- to ten-year process. To aid in their development, Congress created an Agency for Health Care Policy and Research. The Agency is ". . . to enhance the quality, appropriateness, and effectiveness of health care services, and access to such services, through the establishment of a broad base of scientific research and through the promotion of improvements in clinical practice and in the organization, financing, and delivery of health care services." It will ". . . conduct and support research, demonstration projects, evaluations, training, guidelines development, and the dissemination of information, on health care services and on systems for the delivery of such services . . ." (Omnibus Budget Reconciliation Act, 1989).

Data collection, research on outcomes, dissemination of information, and development of guidelines will be the focus of much activity in the research community. However, the excitement about the research potential is tempered by the realization that if physicians cannot or do not respond in time, the perceived need for implementing controls on Medicare expenditures will overshadow the measured approach to volume control envisioned by the use of practice guidelines.

Within the reforms of physician payment is a subtle threat. If physicians do not define and appropriately use guidelines quickly, they will see their income from Medicare decline as congressional controls on volume and inflation begin to limit their fees.

## Limits on Physician Income

One reform that directly limits physicians' incomes (and reduces beneficiary out-of-pocket costs) is the imposition of limits on the amount a physician may balance bill a patient. If a physician does not accept Medicare payment as payment in full (accept assignment), he or she bills the patient for the difference between what is charged and what Medicare will pay. Under payment reform, physicians will be limited in the amount they can charge the Medicare beneficiary above the Medicare fee schedule amount. The limits will be phased in, with 115 percent being the limit by 1993 and thereafter.

As with the practice guidelines, however, there is a subtle threat in the policy. Congress might yet require physicians participating in Medicare to accept its fees as payment in full (mandatory assignment), particularly in areas where beneficiaries have little or no choice of provider (e.g., radiology, pathology, anesthesiology, and emergency services). If such a policy were instituted, however, the fear is that physicians might refuse to participate as Medicare providers. Whether this would happen is questionable, since in 1988 over 60 percent of the physicians in Medicare were already in a participating and supplier program in which they agreed to accept Medicare payment as payment in full (Physician Payment Review Commission, 1990, p. 15).

Physicians are wary of the payment reforms that have been initiated. Their concern is justified because the policies already created and those to be created will modify the operating incentives and rewards present in medicine. If other payers follow Medicare's lead, change will occur even more rapidly and broadly. By the year 2000, the practice of medicine will have been directly and subtly changed by the payment reforms initiated in 1990.

## Nurses and Medicare Payment Policy

The congressional choice of reforms of physician payment is intended to create a self-regulating system (market). These reforms are one more effort at ". . . seeking automatic, technical solutions to political problems" (Rodwin, 1989).

How these choices for reform will impact nurses is still unclear. Nursing services were not considered a significant issue in the development of the reforms. Although the need to consider such services has been discussed, the Physician Payment Review Commission has interpreted its responsibilities to Congress to be limited almost exclusively to consideration of physician-related issues. Requests by nurses and other nonphysician providers to be included in the research have not stimulated the interest of the Physician Payment Review Commission or the Health Care Financing Administration thus far.

For this reason, organized nursing lobbied for inclusion of language in the Omnibus Budget Reconciliation Act 1989 legislation that requires the Physician Payment Review Commission to study the implications of the Medicare fee schedule on payment to nonphysician practitioners. That work, however, is of only a few months' duration. When compared with the years of research and millions of dollars already invested in the work of Hsiao and the Physician Payment Review Commission, it is evident that there will need to be more invested in defining nursing's value within medicine and health.

What is the resource-based "value" of nursing services? If a nurse does the same work as a physician, is the work of the same value? If the outcomes are the same, should the payment be the same? Should services billed directly by nurses under Medicare be included in the Medicare volume performance standard? These are questions to which there are as yet no clear answers. If nurses wish to receive direct payment from Medicare for their services, these questions will have to be answered or nursing services will not fit within the payment scheme of Medicare.

Answering such questions, however, will be difficult. A significant amount of the data necessary to conduct the research is not available and, as yet, has not been addressed by the coding reforms under way. Even where nurse-specific data are coded using Medicare common procedural technology, such data are not collected or reported. In many cases the nurse's services are simply coded under the employing physician's identification number, thereby making the service and its impact unidentifiable.

### Payment to Nurses Under Medicare

Nursing services under Medicare are figured as part of the cost of doing business. In the hospital setting, nursing services are calculated as part of the "market basket" of services a hospital must buy to operate. Under the Medicare fee schedule, nursing is included in nonphysician inputs to a physician service. Nursing is part of the cost of practicing medicine.

Relatively few providers other than physicians directly bill Medicare for their services. Chiropractors, dentists, podiatrists, and osteopaths can bill as physicians under Medicare. The range of services they offer is somewhat limited, however, and does not represent a major portion of the Part B payment outlays. Nurses, like psychologists, are designated as nonphysician providers and represent only a very small percentage of the direct services billed under Medicare Part B.

Nurse practitioners, certified nurse midwives, nurse anesthetists, and certified nurse specialists have all sought direct reimbursement from Medicare and other third-party payers. They have had some success, but even when they are paid directly, the price is often set below that for physicians or limited in some other manner. Physician assistants have not sought direct payment for their services but instead receive payments indirectly by billing through the employing physician or institution. This indirect method of payment is also the most common payment method used to reimburse nurses (U.S. Congress, Office of Technology Assessment, 1986).

Direct payment to nonphysician providers is seen as an unattractive option in light of the escalation in costs and volume experienced with physicians. The fear of insurers is that extending direct reimbursement to additional providers will add to total health care expenditures.

Most groups seeking direct reimbursement argue that they can deliver care at a lower cost than physician providers. Nonphysician providers rarely act as substitutes for physician services but more often become added providers receiving payment for added services. Under the resource-based fee schedule, however, options might be explored that could include nonphysician providers and additional services within a Medicare framework that is presumed to have rational price and volume control mechanisms. Nurses seeking direct reimbursement could then be required to live within the price and service constraints created for physician providers.

Another concern expressed is whether nonphysician providers can offer the same medical services as physicians. Using practice guidelines, it may be possible to minimize or do away with such an argument if nonphysician providers agree to use physician guidelines for those same services which they perform. Nurses could continue to provide specific nursing services but at the same time be reimbursed for doing those services that are the same as those provided by physicians.

Nurses and other nonphysician providers need to determine in what areas their work is the same as that of physicians. The resource-based approach to defining "value" for a service can assist in doing that. Once this is completed, the debate can turn to whether the nonphysician provider should be paid equally for the work. The fee can be made less than that of a physician simply by using a different (lower) conversion factor when translating the relative value scale into a fee schedule. But, the work itself need not be "devalued." Throughout the health care system, hospitals and physicians are negotiating differing and discounted rates with payers. They are not, however, saying that what they produce is not of the same value, whatever price they finally accept.

Nursing organizations and individual nurses do not all agree on whether the best strategy for achieving direct reimbursement for nurses is to seek equal pay for equal work or to offer nursing services as a lower cost alternative to physician care. Improved information about the resource costs and "equality" of physician and nurse work can help nurses work through their decision making about direct reimbursement and the prices they set. Nurses can decide to charge less because they choose to or because it is politically expedient. They need not deny the equality of their work in order to receive payment.

Whatever nurses achieve in third-party payment will come from competition and conflict with physicians and cooperation among nurses. Payments to nurses will be drawn from the same sources as payments to physicians. Even though expenditures by Medicare and other payers could be increased to accommodate new services and nonphysician providers, it is unlikely that this will happen. The result is and will continue to be competition among providers for the same dollar. Nurses have had only limited success in this competition to date. To succeed, they must work cooperatively on an agreed-upon agenda.

## Influencing Medicare Payment Policy

The Physician Payment Review Commission describes a four-step process for updating the fees under the Medicare fee schedule. It entails ". . . a formula approach linking the conversion factor to an index of physicians' practice expenses; the existing regulatory rulemaking process of the Department of Health and Human Services; an independent commission charged with providing technical information and advice to Congress; and negotiation between physicians and the federal government" (Physician Payment Review Commission, 1989, p. 174).

The negotiations surrounding Medicare provider payment policy will be dictated by the political process and lobbying by individuals, physician's organizations, and other professional groups, such as the American Nurses' Association. No single group will be charged with responsibility for negotiating payments, as is done in Canada and some European countries.

This fragmented process, although confusing, is part of the checks and balances of our American political system. It also permits individuals and groups to intervene at various points in the process. Nursing must intervene. To date, however, nursing and other nonphysician providers have been singularly unsuccessful in influencing the process. The reforms are still new, and over the next five years nurses must define and claim a role in the process or nurse-provided services will continue to be calculated as a "cost of doing business."

The development of practice guidelines and outcomes research offers nurses another opportunity to influence the character of Medicare policy. Although the guidelines are to determine the effectiveness and appropriateness of care, the focus of the work is on defining ineffective and inappropriate care. Nurses must participate in these definitions of care and show how nursing is a significant component of any positive (or negative) outcome of medical care. The Agency for Health Care Policy and Research can serve as an important source of funding for needed nursing research.

Nurses are advocates for the patient. The effect of the Medicare fee schedule on the Medicare beneficiary is a major unknown in physician payment reform. Careful study and oversight will be required for nurses and others to be sure that patients do not find their access to care or the quality of their care limited directly or indirectly (or unpredictably) by the policies enacted in an effort to control health care expenditures.

## Conclusion

Nurse practitioners have been seeking direct fee-for-service payment from third-party payers. The assumptions that have guided these efforts, however, must be re-examined in light of the policy changes under way within Medicare. Extensive research is needed to define where nurses substitute for physician-provided care and nursing's "value" within the framework of the new Medicare payment policies. Nurses can then pursue direct payment for services, whether at a full or discounted price.

When physician payment reforms are fully implemented, Medicare and the nation will still not have changed the medical delivery system. Medicare will still be a program that focuses on acute medical services, almost to the exclusion of the other services necessary for the well-being of an elderly and increasingly aging population. The reforms will have addressed how much we pay for health care, not what it is we receive for that money or whether what we receive is what we need to remain healthy as individuals or as a nation. Assessment and subsequent reform of the health care system will remain a part of the nation's public policy agenda.

REFERENCES

Gonzalez, M.L., & Emmons, D.W. (Eds.) (1988). *Socioeconomic characteristics of medical practice, 1988.* Chicago: American Medical Association.
Hsiao, W.C. (1989, Winter). Objective research and physician payment: A response from Harvard. *Health Affairs, 8*(4), 72–75.

Hsiao, W.C., Braun, P., Dunn, D., & Becker, E.R. (1988, October 28). Resource-based relative values: An overview. *Journal of the American Medical Association, 260*(16), 2347–2353.

Hsiao, W.C., Braun, P., Becker, E., Causino, N., Couch, N.P., De Nicola, M., Dunn, D., Kelly, N.L., Ketcham, T., Sobol, A., Verrilli, D., & Yntema, D.B. (1988a, September 27). *A national study of resource-based relative value scales for physician services: Final report.*

Hsiao, W.C., Braun, P., Becker, E., Causino, N., Couch, N.P., De Nicola, M., Dunn, D., Kelly, N.L., Ketchum, T., Sobol, A., Verilli, D., & Yntema, D.B. (1988b, December). *A national study of resource-based relative value scales for physician services: Supplemental report.* Cambridge, MA: Harvard University, Department of Health Policy and Management, Harvard School of Public Health and the Department of Psychology.

Lee, P. (1990, May 3). Testimony before the Subcommittee on Health, Committee on Ways and Means. Washington, DC: U.S. Congress.

McMenamin, P., West, H., & Marcus, L. (1988, October). *Changes in Medicare Part B physician charges: Final report.* Springfield, VA: Mandex, Inc.

Mitchell, J.B., Wedig, G., & Cromwell, J. (1989, Spring). The Medicare physician fee freeze. *Health Affairs, 8*(1), 21–33.

Omnibus Budget Reconciliation Act of 1989 (OBRA 89: Public Law 101-239).

Physician Payment Review Commission (1987). *Annual report to Congress.* Washington, DC: Physician Payment Review Commission.

Physician Payment Review Commission (1989). *Annual report to Congress.* Washington, DC: Physician Payment Review Commission.

Physician Payment Review Commission (1990). *Annual report to Congress.* Washington, DC: Physician Payment Review Commission.

Rodwin, V.G. (1989, Winter). Physician payment reform: Lessons from abroad. *Health Affairs, 8*(4), 76–83.

U.S. Congress, Office of Technology Assessment (1986, December). *Nurse practitioners, physician assistants, and certified nurse-midwives: A policy analysis (Health Technology Case Study 37), Office of Technology Assessment-HCS-37.* Washington, DC: U.S. Government Printing Office.

U.S. Congress, Senate, Special Committee on Aging: American Association of Retired Persons; Federal Council on the Aging; and U.S. Department of Health and Human Services, Administration on Aging (1987–1988). *Aging America: Trends and projections,* Washington, DC: U.S. Government Printing Office.

## Chapter 29

# *Nursing Education: Shaping the Future*

MYRTLE K. AYDELOTTE

*T*HE SYSTEM OF nursing education in the United States has developed from the interplay of policies, programs, and standards adopted and implemented by nursing faculties as they respond to the expectations and health care needs of society and to advances in knowledge, science, and technology. Decisions made by nursing faculties as they react to these forces have more than an impact upon the immediate situation. The impact is long range. For this reason, policy decisions about nursing education must include a forecast of health care delivery and society of the future as well as consideration of the current social context in which nursing finds itself. Also underlying the considerations about the nursing program is the changing role of a profession as it renegotiates its social mandate with society. Hence, a proposal for change of policy is based on a set of complex factors.

The influence and impact of nursing education on future nursing services in this country and worldwide are not to be underestimated. Nursing education is the foundation upon which the quality of nursing care rests and from which the knowledge base for practice evolves. It also provides the perspective from which nursing research questions and their exploration are viewed, and the framework upon which the systems of nursing care delivery are designed. The future of these four elements is dependent upon the characteristics and the strength of nursing education as it is constructed and conducted.

Since the establishment of the first schools of nursing in the United States, nursing has made great progress. Standards of practice have been elevated, large numbers of nurses have been educated, and the quality of nursing care has risen. The growth of nursing knowledge through research has been phenomenal, and nursing delivery systems have greatly improved and are more innovative than in prior years. As it moves into the last decade of this century, the nursing profession can reflect and build on its successes (Elliott, 1987).

As nursing moves through the nineties, the nursing profession debates continuing problems that have their origins in nursing's history and culture and the society in which nursing finds itself. Nursing's educational system remains truncated (Stuart,

1981), the result of unplanned and undirected evolution, compromise, timidity, and lost opportunity. The control of nursing has been external to rather than self-directed by the profession (Schlotfeldt, 1988). The public image of nursing continues to be that of a feminine occupation (Fagin & Diers, 1983), highly technical in nature, physically very demanding (Aydelotte, 1988a), oppressed, subordinate to medicine, and offering little promise of prestige and status compared with other professions open to women. In spite of the presence of the largest number of well-prepared nurses in the history of nursing, the process of professionalization of the occupation is slow. The demand for nursing services has exceeded the supply of nurses, chiefly because of the way nurses are rewarded and utilized in the current delivery system. The number of applicants to nursing schools is fewer than in prior years, although there was a slight increase in admissions in 1988 over 1987 (Nursing enrollments, 1990), and the quality of those applicants is of serious concern (Farrell, 1988; Rosenfeld, 1987).

These problems are compounded by demographic and social changes in the population, changes in the work force, limited financial resources for health care, the pressures for cost containment of health and medical care, and the demands for innovation placed on the health care delivery system in this country. Thus, how will the nursing profession build upon its successes and mount the task of meeting its social obligation to provide nursing care for the vast number of our citizens who will need it in the future? How will the nursing education system respond to the expectations placed upon it? What are the national policies that need to be put into place?

The literature of the 1980s is replete with publications identifying issues in nursing and the need for change in nursing education and practice. Among these are the reports of the National Commission on Nursing Implementation Project (Aydelotte, 1990); *The Seventh Report to the President and Congress on the Status of Health Personnel* (U.S. Department of Health and Human Services, Public Health Service, Health Resources and Service Administration, 1990); *Curriculum Revolution: Mandate for Change* and *Curriculum Revolution: Reconceptualizing Nursing Education*, both published by the National League for Nursing (Aydelotte, 1988b; 1989b) and two publications of the American Association of Colleges of Nursing, *Essentials of College and University Education for Professional Nursing* (Aydelotte, 1986) and *Alternate Conceptions of Work and Society: Implications for Professional Nursing* (Lindeman, 1988). The underlying theme of all these publications and much of the other literature is change.

Although the recent literature presents persuasive arguments that problems do exist, offers explanations of the dilemmas and paradoxes facing nursing, and proposes ideas for resolution, there is no one common thread appearing throughout it as to how to resolve the dilemmas and paradoxes. Further, except for data about a few specialist groups, such as nurse practitioners and nurse midwives, there are limited quantitative data describing the impact of many of the programs on the quality and cost-effectiveness of the care provided by the graduates of the various programs. Also missing are hard data regarding the characteristics of the applicants to many of the programs, the modifications that are taking place within programs, and the rationale for changes. No comprehensive evaluation studies of programs were found in the literature. Anecdotal information and rumor lead one to believe that changes

**TABLE 29–1 Nursing Education Programs Leading to First Professional Degree (1987) by Number and Size of Enrollment***

| Type of Program | Number | Student Enrollment |
|---|---|---|
| Baccalaureate | 467 | 73,621 |
| Associate | 789 | 90,399 |
| Diploma | 209 | 18,927 |
| Master's† | 6 | NA |
| Doctoral† | 2 | NA |

* Source: Aydelotte, M.K. (1989). *Nursing data review 1988*. New York: National League for Nursing.

† Source: Martin, C.E. (1989). Alternatives for students with life experiences: Reconceptualizing nursing education. In Aydelotte, M.K. *Curriculum revolution: Reconceptualizing nursing education* (p. 106). New York: National League for Nursing.

are occurring but these changes have not been documented, except for the 1987 survey of 26 programs conducted by the National Commission on Nursing Implementation Project (Aydelotte, 1987). In this survey, only 15 programs responded. Six diploma programs were making the transition to baccalaureate programs; seven diploma programs were changing to the associate degree type; and one combined diploma and associate degree program was changing to baccalaureate education. One practical nursing program was becoming an associate degree program.

The discussions in the literature continue the diversity, flexibility, and the lack of standardization of the educational base for nursing practice. No one article or combination of papers proposes what the system of nursing education of the future should be. Will the present proliferation of schools and programs and the resulting great diversity of graduates continue? What type of planned action is needed to give order to the system so that the public will have an understanding of the nature of the nursing care they will receive and prospective students will know what kind of practice they will be prepared for by their education?

In this chapter, the current system of nursing education is described, the merits of the various nursing programs are commented on, the issues confronting educators are discussed, and directions for the future are proposed.

## The Current System of Nursing Education Leading to the First Professional Degree

Five different educational programs prepare individuals for entry into professional nursing practice. The graduates of all programs are eligible to sit for the same examination, which if passed, authorizes them to practice as *professional nurses* and permits them to use that title. These programs are diploma programs, operated by hospitals; associate degree programs, operated by community colleges and senior colleges and universities; baccalaureate programs, operated by institutions of higher learning; and graduate programs at the master's and doctoral degree levels, also operated by senior colleges and universities. Currently, there are 1473 programs at all levels (Table 29-1).

On February 3, 1990, the National League for Nursing released preliminary data on nursing school enrollments and graduations. There was a slight increase in enrollments in 1988 for associate and baccalaureate programs (Aydelotte, 1990).

These programs vary in admission requirements, length and content of curricula, faculty requirements, and standards for graduation. The standards to be met for national accreditation of the programs are set by the councils within the National League for Nursing, which serves as the national accrediting agency. At the state level, a regulatory body approves the operation of the program. There is no one set of standards that must be met by all *five* programs.

The fact that all five programs lead to eligibility to write the same licensing examination and, upon passing it, to use the same title, *professional nurse*, adds to confusion about the abilities and the differences of the graduates. The diversity of education and the lack of a universally accepted minimum content base make it "almost impossible to generalize about a nurse's abilities, codify colleagueships with other types of care providers, or set meaningful standards for nursing practice" (Christman, 1979, p. 21).

It is difficult for the public, prospective students, and some nurses themselves to differentiate the purpose and mission of these educational programs, although the official statement indicates that the graduates of the programs differ in knowledge, practice application, and accountability (Murphy, 1983). The focus of baccalaureate and higher degree programs is considered to be broader, enriched by liberal arts content, and the curriculum is stated to encompass more in leadership, research, public health, and health teaching. However, the differences in clinical content, skill development, and outcome competencies among the programs are difficult to identify.

The master's degree program leading to entry to professional nursing practice, admission to which is available to college graduates possessing a degree in a discipline other than nursing, usually features preparation for a nursing specialty as a major component along with the preparation for general practice. Two programs at the doctoral level lead to the first professional degree, entitled the nursing doctorate. These programs are available to those who have previously earned a degree in another field. These programs are often misinterpreted as advanced preparation in a nursing specialty or a research degree in nursing.

## Less than Baccalaureate Programs

Diploma nursing education programs have some severe limitations. The lack of a larger academic environment in which nursing students can associate with students in other majors is obvious. Although some students in hospital diploma programs enroll in community or liberal arts colleges for related courses, usually in the first year, in many respects they are quite isolated from interaction with other types of students. The clinical nursing experiences are also somewhat narrow, primarily within one institution, and they are illness-oriented. In large part, the curricula follow a model borrowed from medicine or a behavioral-mechanistic model (Bevis, 1988). If the graduates were perceived as having a single focus, as technicians or technologists and not as professionals, the narrowness of focus and selection of the model would be more acceptable.

Since their establishment, the associate degree programs have had the greatest growth of all programs. This growth was stimulated by federal funding and early recognition by the leadership of the community colleges that there was a population of individuals who wished to be educated in a short-term program in order to begin earning a salary quickly. The investment of time by the individual was a prime consideration. The associate degree program has served a social mobility purpose that is commendable, but it has contributed to problems in the nursing occupation and for the graduate as well. Although many faculty members would agree that the focus of the associate degree is narrow and technical in scope, employers and the graduates themselves view the preparation as professional, especially in light of the title accorded them following passage of the licensing examination. This perception creates severe problems of image and, in nursing services, leads to the placement of all graduates regardless of educational preparation in similar positions. The majority of graduates of all programs enter nursing practice as staff nurses.

Discussions with directors of nursing and individuals in clinical leadership positions indicate that the content of the associate degree curriculum is too thin and diffuse for the professional nursing practice for which the graduate is licensed to practice and for technical practice as well. The curriculum covers content from liberal arts and science too broadly and does not select the content that is critical to technical practice and apply it in a synthesized form, so that the student develops the knowledge and skills required of a well-prepared technician. The current associate degree programs are designed to prepare a general technician rather than one who can perform well in the care of specific populations, such as those requiring long-term care, or children and adults with acute conditions, or the aging. Unpublished anecdotal information also indicates that some of the associate degree programs are beginning to select a specific focus in order to give the graduate a higher level of skill in the care of selected populations, such as those requiring long-term care or those who are acutely ill.

## Baccalaureate Nursing Programs

The purpose of the baccalaureate nursing program is to prepare professional nurse general practitioners who are competent to practice in a wide variety of settings with highly diverse populations. These programs are usually four academic years in length, with approximately half the program spent in liberal arts and supporting courses, a pattern that was established in the mid-1950s. Since that time, the growth of knowledge about health, illness, human development and behavior, pathologic conditions, and nursing has been tremendous. The complexity of nursing care has increased many fold.

Although individuals entering nursing programs today are slightly older than in prior years, it can be questioned whether or not the majority of baccalaureate students are prepared to confront the expectations in the nursing program and to handle difficult clinical situations. The complexity of the course content, the time required to develop generalizations, critical judgment, and higher intellectual skills, and the amount of the practice involved in selecting and executing nursing interventions challenge the present organization of the curriculum and its implementation and the amount of time allotted for such education.*

Of greatest importance, however, is the question of whether or not the student is given the opportunity to develop into the type of professional needed today to care for people. Nursing encompasses an art, a humanistic orientation, a feeling for the value of the individual, and an intuitive sense of ethics and of the appropriateness of action taken. It embodies more than an objective-rational and behavioral approach to problems of health and illness. The nature of the practice requires more than the comprehension of complex information; it requires the development of values, maturity, and ethics. Watson (1988) points out that time is required to introduce and cultivate these qualities.

Change in baccalaureate nursing education, which has been called for, is based on the opinion that the current models on which nursing curricula are based add to confusion regarding the outcomes. Bevis (1988) proposes that the Tyler model of the nursing curriculum, based on behavioral learning theory, which was introduced in the 1950s and continues today, is no longer appropriate for professional nursing, since it stresses mechanistic and technical abilities with little emphasis on intellectual skills, fundamental and essential attitudes, and values. The different perspectives proposed by nursing theorists likewise create problems when used as models for curricular design. Fawcett (1984) points out that a wide range of perspectives are now applied in viewing nursing and proposes a metaparadigm that could be considered as a model; however, as Brodie (1984) remarked in her commentary, there is no universal acceptance of the meaning of the concepts that are used in the various theories. The use of various models, including those developed by nurse theorists, those constructed from the nursing process and from the behavioral field, and those borrowed from medicine, adds to the confusion and loss of consistency of the content.

Weaknesses in the baccalaureate program content are as follows:

- The content is insufficient to provide students with the knowledge and skills to deal with the vast range of human experiences they will encounter in professional general nursing practice.
- Understanding of the economics of health care is lacking, and the relationship between clinical nursing decisions and financial cost is not made explicit.
- The nature of the technology with which the nurse must deal, including computerization, informatics, and decision making, is complex and not adequately treated.

---

* Although data are missing and the source of the information is informal, it has been stated by others that some baccalaureate programs have chosen to select a focus such as health or illness care or an elective of a nursing specialty in order to meet the problem of content. These programs may not be meeting their responsibility for preparing a beginning general practitioner, unless the curriculum is changed markedly and the time frame for the curriculum is extended. The student is not receiving adequate exposure to the total range of knowledge essential to general practice.

- Insufficient attention is given to the development of ethics, values, intellectual skills, and socialization as a professional.
- The curriculum does not prepare a professional who can interact with other health care professionals as an equal and who can participate in the redesign of the delivery of care. Decisions are required at the point of delivery as well as at the executive level.

## Master's and Doctoral Degree Programs

The master's and doctoral degree programs for entry into professional nursing practice differ from the baccalaureate programs in that the student is usually older and is a non-nursing college graduate. The focus in the master's programs is entry into practice and practice in some aspect of nursing specialization. Currently only six such programs are reported in the literature. Diers (1987) refers to this type of program as a combined program. The course is three years in length and no baccalaureate degree is granted at any point. In her description of four of the six programs, Diers points out that all but one are in private universities, have small and limited enrollments, and have highly selective admissions policies. The number of nursing specialties from which students may select a major ranges from one in one school to a high of six in another. Diers reports that there has been a decline in applications to these combined programs since 1983, and she attributes this to a number of factors. She points out in particular the lack of funding for students, the environment in which nursing is practiced, and the lack of adequate financial rewards for the work.

Although the older student is more self-directed and able to handle the complexity of the information and situations more easily, it can be assumed that the problem of the adequacy of the range and depth of content for competence in both general and specialty practice arises. The question of the balance between the theory basic to nursing practice and theory for role functioning is also puzzling and could present difficulties in interpreting the placement of the graduate. No follow-up studies of these graduates were found in the literature. Since their degree includes preparation for a nursing specialty, it could be expected that their impact would be included among nursing specialists who are prepared at the master's degree level, and the weaknesses of the program would not be unlike those of the programs preparing nurses for specialization.

Currently, the literature reports only two doctoral programs leading to the first professional degree (Fitzpatrick & Modly, 1990), although others are under consideration (Watson & Bevis, 1990). A preliminary evaluation of the Doctor of Nursing Program at Case Western Reserve University revealed that these graduates differed from baccalaureate graduates in nursing from the same university on selected demographic variables, held higher state board scores, and sought nontraditional roles (Fitzpatrick, Boyle, & Anderson, 1986). Fitzpatrick and Modly report that there are 200 Doctor of Nursing graduates of the Case Western Reserve University program currently practicing. Longitudinal studies indicate that these graduates demonstrate a strong professional career commitment, are leaders and professionals, have moved into clinical practice positions, and have been interested in furthering their education and careers. They have progressed more rapidly in the nursing field than baccalaureate graduates of the school. The Doctors of Nursing portray careers that are reflective of practice.

These two authors identify the problems associated with the Doctor of Nursing program as it has developed. The problems are mainly related to the perception of the program by others: the goals of the program are not understood, and the purpose of the Doctor of Nursing program as distinct from other doctoral programs in nursing, such as the Ph.D., D.N.S., and D.N.Sc., are not perceived. The authors state that understanding the nature of professional education in general is a problem for others. Future plans for the program "lead to an even clearer distinction between ND [Doctor of Nursing] graduates and graduates of other educational programs" (Fitzpatrick & Modly, 1990, p. 98). Also of concern is the marketing of the newly graduated Doctor of Nursing, in that employers expect the individual, as an entry level practitioner, to perform in traditional roles. The program places emphasis on clinical practice, scientific inquiry, and professional socialization. The graduate is a generalist in professional nursing practice.

A review of the literature indicates that nursing education leading to the first professional degree has accomplished five goals:

- Nursing education has become a distinct and legitimate part of colleges and universities (Moccia, 1988). The academic nature of nursing is challenged infrequently.
- Nurses are also recognized as having more power, in the sense that more nurses are filling leadership positions in the community, institutions, and government.
- Nursing education, particularly the associate degree programs, has contributed to the growth of a very large work force. This growth in nurse supply has been accompanied by a better prepared leadership group in nursing.
- Many of those receiving the first professional degree have gone on to advanced study.
- Last and very important, the graduates of nursing programs are demonstrating the ability to provide a reliable quality of care to those whom they serve.

These gains are balanced against a number of deficits and limitations in addition to those discussed earlier. First, the models used in the undergraduate educational programs are inappropriate (Bevis, 1988; Curtin, 1984; Diekelmann, 1989). There is too much emphasis on behavioral objectives. Values, ethics, and morality are neglected in the socialization of students (Lynn, McCain, & Boss, 1989), partly the result of a compartmentalization and separation of factual knowledge from knowledge that leads to wisdom and the sense of being a professional. The content presented is irrelevant to the current emerging society, the public's need for care, and the revamping of the health care system. The education is directed toward the preparation for a "job" rather than for a life as a professional. The nursing process, purported to be a logic underlying nursing practice, ignores the role of intuition, pattern recognition, and the sense of salience (Benner, 1984; Miller & Rew, 1989; Tanner, 1988).

Second, some faculty members view themselves as information givers (Bevis, 1988; Clayton, 1989) rather than as individuals who encourage, promote, and foster the students into the role of a professional (Watson, 1988). The faculty members themselves are not models of excellent professional practitioners.

Third, the majority of baccalaureate programs use models that are technical in nature or lacking conceptual focus. These models also lack the teaching of compassion and healing behaviors; they are based on rule-governed behavior rather than behavior that arises from syntactical, contextual, and inquiry learning (Bevis, 1989). The baccalaureate programs lack the content essential to professional practice in today's world and that of the future.

Fourth, the master's degree programs are different in that they lead to specialization in nursing as an emphasis rather than general practice. Data are lacking to indicate whether these graduates move into positions that test their general knowledge or whether they become generalists after a period of specialty practice or vice versa.

Fifth, the difficulties encountered by the first Doctor of Nursing degree program relate to the understanding held by nurses and other health groups about the nature of education for professional practice. Apparently, individuals in nursing and the health field have been unable to distinguish and accept differences between the baccalaureate nursing graduate and the graduate holding a professional practice doctorate. They also confuse the graduate with a professional practice doctorate and the nurse holding a doctoral degree that prepares her for a research or nurse scientist career. Likewise, they do not differentiate between the professional doctorate graduate and the nurse with a doctorate representing advanced clinical specialization, in which clinical investigation and scholarship are the goals. Limitations are also imposed by the readiness of the nursing and health communities to accept general professional nursing knowledge as meriting a practice doctorate and the willingness of institutions to restructure and resign nursing delivery systems to utilize the talents of the professional doctorate graduate.

## Issues Related to Preparation for the First Professional Degree

The complexity of the issues surrounding nursing education preparation for the first professional degree is almost overwhelming. The variation in programs and the modifications in curricular content are many, leading to confusion and misperception of what the graduate of a program really is. The issues relate to the nature, scope, and functions of nursing practice; how professional nursing practice differs from lay nursing, medicine, and other professions (Orlando, 1987); questions relating to faculty practice; the selection of content and teaching strategies; the difference between preparation for a specialty and for general practice at entry level and the desirability of that preparation; and the desirability or undesirability of articulation between and among programs.

The faculty's use of the current published statements regarding professional nursing as the base for the structure of the curriculum is of questionable merit. Statements regarding the nature of professional nursing are too global and broad to be used in interpreting nursing to the general public, to the prospective student, and to employers. The American Nurses' Association's document, *Nursing: A Social Policy Statement* (Aydelotte, 1980) does not state the purpose, role, and function of nursing clearly, concretely, and precisely enough so that its meaning and the differences from lay nursing, other provider services, and technologic services are readily apparent (Orlando & Dugan, 1989). This is an issue the nursing profession must address.

The issues of the role of faculty and the inclusion of practice as an integral part of faculty have been under active discussion in the nursing profession for years (Lambert & Lambert, 1988). In spite of all the attention given to the subject, the issue continues to be debated by nurse educators (de Tornyay, 1987). The issue is how the role should be defined, whether or not certain modes of nursing care delivery are a legitimate part of the role, how nursing practice can be integrated into the faculty role, the part it plays in promotion and tenure, and how the necessary structural arrangements can be put into place. Apparently, many nursing faculty members have adopted as the model for their faculty role the one carried out by faculty members in colleges of liberal arts and education rather than the role of the faculties of professional colleges, such as dentistry, medicine, pharmacy, clinical psychology, and law. The lack of active practice on the part of nursing faculty contributes to problems of credibility, socialization of students, development and testing of knowledge, utilization of research, and interprofessional and intraprofessional conflict.

## The Issue of Educational Mobility

The current system of nursing education for entry into professional nursing practice is characterized by a proliferation of programs and diversity. The practice of educational mobility contributes to that character. Graduates of diploma and associate nursing programs have the opportunity to matriculate into baccalaureate and master's degree programs, many receiving credit gained through course work and experience through advanced placement examinations. The practice has been defended as an appropriate response to the changing needs of society and is seen as desirable action to implement the resolution on entry to practice passed by the American Nurses' Association House of Delegates in 1965.

In 1986 to 1987, there were 603 baccalaureate programs accepting registered nurses holding a diploma or an associate degree and 156 baccalaureate programs designed exclusively for registered nurses (Aydelotte, 1989c). These programs graduated a total of 10,714 students in 1986 to 1987, 39 percent of whom were from the special programs. The number of these kinds of registered nurses returning for baccalaureate degrees stabilized in 1987.

Educational mobility continues as a political issue despite the thought, time, and energy already devoted to the subject since 1960 (Waters, 1989) and the promulgation of the concept of an open curriculum. Although the practice of admitting registered nurse students and the use of advanced placement examinations are well established in the educational systems, many nursing programs prohibit challenge examinations for courses that include professional nursing practice content, nursing research, leadership and management, community nursing, and advanced nursing (Arlton & Miller, 1987).

Rapson (1990) and Reed (1983) identify the two issues of educational mobility: (1) educational access versus quality control of programs, and (2) educational mobility versus career or job mobility. These authors view career mobility and job mobility as different, the latter being a change in the same position level, whereas the former implies movement along a career trajectory. The two issues are highly emotional and have resulted in mandating of educational mobility in three states.

In other professions, such as law, medicine, pharmacy, dentistry, and veterinary medicine, the educational process preparing paraprofessionals is different from that preparing professionals and does not serve as the base for the professional education curriculum. If they qualify for admission, technicians or technologists may enter the curriculum that prepares professionals and generally do not receive credit for courses that are the equivalents of courses in the professional program. Experience is rarely credited.

The current practice of educational mobility in nursing has contributed to the increase in the number of baccalaureate and master's degree graduates in nursing, and in that respect, the practice has merit. With changes in education designed to produce professionals in nursing for the future, the practice of educational mobility through advanced placement will undoubtedly continue because of the principle of individual differences, but if preparation for the first professional degree in nursing moves into a graduate program, the impact of prior course credit may diminish. Greater differentiation of the practice and the educational programs will emerge if this change occurs.

## Higher Degree Nursing Education

Nursing education programs offered to students holding a license to practice and leading to a master's or doctoral degree are highly diverse. The programs vary in their admission requirements, length, number and content of courses, amount of credit to be earned, identification of majors, and degree conferred.

*Master's Programs.* Admission requirements to master's programs are set by each school. Thus, depending on the school, the degree required for admission to the program may be one or more of four degrees: diploma, associate, baccalaureate, or master's. In 1987, there were 194 master's programs in nursing, which represents a 66 percent growth in numbers of programs over the last decade. In 1987, these programs had an enrollment of 6113 full-time students and 15,082 part-time students, a gain in enrollment of 17 percent over the last 5 years. The greatest number of students are enrolled in advanced clinical nursing (over two thirds), which includes nurse practitioners. This number is followed by those in nursing administration and management, and then those in teaching (Aydelotte, 1989c).

In a 1985 survey of master's programs, Forni (1987) found that of the 132 schools that responded, many different models were being used to structure the program. The length of the master's programs varied from 9 to 28 months, with approximately one third requiring two full academic years (Snyder, 1990). The focus of the master's program is on aspects of specialty nursing practice and on aspects of the functional role.

Many issues are related to the master's program in nursing. Hoeffler and Murphy (1984) give an excellent overview and historical perspective of the development of specialization in nursing and identify many problems. Among these are multiple paths of entry; the use of multiple titles for the roles that master's degree graduates fill; the great variety of expectations of the graduates; the lack of uniform core content or common nursing phenomena; the great diversity of types of specialization; and the narrowness of the subject matter. Snyder (1990) points out that the specialization focuses on delivery of care and not on areas of knowledge that lead to the development of the discipline. The balance between preparation for advanced clinical nursing practice and for the functional role remains a serious issue.

Styles (1989) analyzed graduate programs listed by the National League of Nursing in 1985 in order to find patterns of specialization. She found that the descriptions fall into a variety of categories and that the random development of specialization in nursing has not led to a recognized hierarchy of arrangement of content.

Although viewed as responsive to societal needs and having contributed to improvement in nursing care, nursing education programs at the master's level have a number of weaknesses. Major gaps exist between the needs of practice and the preparation of nurses for the practice (Martin et al., 1989; Salmon, 1989). The majors in these programs are designed to prepare students for positions (jobs) rather than prepare individuals who are generalist-specialist professionals with knowledge of nursing phenomena underlying specialty practice. The multiple admission standards and the great variety of curricula lead to confusion regarding the nursing knowledge base and competencies of the graduates. The lack of a schema for specialization contributes to the problem of curricular design in that similarities and dissimilarities of content are not identified.

*Doctoral Education.*    Doctoral education in nursing is expanding rapidly. As of October 1988, there were 52 programs (*Doctoral Programs in Nursing,* 1989). The growth from six programs that were open in 1968 to the 45 reported in 1987 (Aydelotte, 1988b) represents an increase of 650 percent over the 20-year period. The number of students enrolled in doctoral programs has increased by 170 percent in the past decade. The number increased by 9.4 percent during the year 1986. Nine new programs opened in 1986 and three in 1988 and three in 1989.

Several articles give excellent reviews of the historical development and growth of doctoral education (Forni, 1989; Grace, 1990; Hart, 1989; Lenz, 1990; Meleis, 1988). Grace points out the diverse points of view and orientation regarding the content of doctoral education and the divergence of opinion about its desired ends in nursing. In her 1983 review of the research on doctoral education, Murphy (1985) found little differentiation between the professional and research degrees and little agreement on the scientific basis of practice; the focus of the research was found to be dependent on the particular faculty member's interest, and the philosophical position of the graduate school was the prime determinant of the conceptual nature of the doctoral program. Lash (1987) reconfirmed these findings. Lenz (1990) reports change in some of these findings. Of the 45 programs that she studied, 33 lead to a Doctor of Philosophy degree and 13 to the professional degree. The enrollments varied widely, from five to 350. The range in amount of credit required by the program was wide, from zero to over 70 postmaster's credits. Some core content is common to all programs, but the nature of the nursing specialties content is very diverse, as is the diversity within the program itself. Some believe that the specialties should be based on faculty strength; others believe it should be determined by the students.

Review of the recent literature relating to doctoral education identifies several problem areas, concerns, and issues. Concern is expressed over the proliferation of academic doctoral programs that may lack institutional and school capability to carry the program (Amos, 1974), the lack of research strengths and scholarly productivity of the faculty, the lack of agreement regarding the scientific base for nursing practice, and the emphasis on structure and regulation (Downs, 1988). Individuals differ in their preference of the degree to be conferred. Little agreement exists on the concept of specialization and the degree to which specialization beyond the master's degree level is an integral part of doctoral education. Contrary to the normal concept of specialization in other disciplines, which move from a general base to increasing depth of specialization in the field through the doctorate, nursing tends to favor an hourglass approach—general-specialized-general.

An analysis of the literature suggests that

- There is a lack of agreement about the object and the nature of doctoral education in nursing.
- There is a lack of agreement about the roles for which doctoral graduates are prepared. Are they prepared primarily for academic work, or to practice as researchers or clinical scientists, or for leadership positions in education and practice settings? Little recognition is given to the differences in individual career trajectory and the fact that the graduate may move from one type of career to another.
- The content of the courses and the number of credits in the programs vary greatly.
- Concern has been expressed over the quality of the faculty, in particular their scholarliness, and the quality of the research being carried out.
- The relationship of specialization courses to other more generalized courses remains unclear.

Some of these issues are being addressed through conferences on doctoral education and the issuance of statements of quality, but the quality of the doctoral programs has been studied very little. Holzemer and Chambers (1986) studied the growth and quality of doctoral education programs from 1979 to 1984. They assessed four variables: quality of the faculty, the academic program itself, students and alumni, and available resources. They added a time dimension of three intervals, and included items in the questionnaire relating to the academic and social environments. The sample consisted of the 14 programs that had participated in the 1979 evaluation project and also were a part of the 1984 project. The results indicated that, over time, faculty had increased their commitment to both research and scholarly activities. Students with higher grade point averages than those in prior years were being admitted to the programs. The students' perceptions of the quality of the teaching had increased significantly, and both student and faculty perceptions of the scholarly excellence of their respective programs also had increased significantly. Holzemer and Chambers stated that the findings suggest an increase in overall quality of these 14 programs. However, recognition must be given to the fact that undoubtedly the composition of each of the two groups (the students and the faculty), both of which had contributed to the program scores, had changed over the five-year period.

Further studies of the doctoral programs and their graduates are much needed. Of particular significance are longitudinal studies of the graduates and the nature of faculty productivity and contributions.

## Future Directions: Shaping the Future

In nursing education, the issues consolidate themselves into two that have been unresolved over the years. Both are highly sensitive. The first is the issue of differentiation. The profession has failed to recognize that the use of differences can be advantageous to all. The issue of differentiation deals with the preparation, roles, and relationship between professionals and paraprofessionals, the characteristics of each, and the need for both; the difference and interplay between generalists and specialists; the difference between careers and jobs; and the difference in the motivation of individuals and the career paths they choose.

The second issue deals with the models observed in higher education. Nursing has chosen the academic model as the pattern to follow in designing its education, undoubtedly as a reaction to its historical roots in medicine and hospitals and its early move into departments of education for advanced study. For decades, nursing has rejected its identification as a practice discipline and has not modeled its education after the practice professions of law, medicine, dentistry, and veterinary medicine. Instead, it has chosen models from engineering, education, and the liberal arts and sciences. The time has come for nursing to announce itself as a practice profession and to model its education after the established practice professions. Further, education in nursing at the doctoral level after entry differs from that of other scientific disciplines. In other scientific disciplines, the progression is from the most general knowledge base at the basic level to increasing specialization throughout graduate study. In nursing, the pattern is general preparation at the basic level also, but the individual becomes "highly specialized in a clinical specialty at the master's level, and [moves] again into general perspective at the beginning [of] doctoral study before research specialization" (Grace, 1990, p. 152).

The seriousness of the issues and concerns relating to nursing education calls for a major overhauling of the system. The changing demographics of the population, the changing work environment, and the changing student body call for a restructuring of nursing education (Conway-Welch, 1990). Nurses are needed who can introduce changes in nursing practice and in the organization of a resource-driven health care system, can add to the knowledge of nursing science, and can influence and shape national and local health policies. These goals call for an upgrading of professional nursing education and the construction of an educational system that makes sense.

The character and quality of a professional service are determined largely by the character, quality, and usefulness of the education the practitioner has received. Professional nursing is characterized by diversity. Professional nurses practice in a diversity of settings. They serve a diversity of patients and clients. They deal with a great diversity of knowledge, information, technology, and human conditions. They engage in exchange with a diversity of other workers. The common knowledge and skills required in professional general nursing practice to meet this great diversity are vast. Differentiated or additional knowledge is required if the nurse chooses to practice a specialty, and other roles, such as faculty roles, research and clinical scientist roles, and executive roles, require different and more extensive knowledge.

In order for the nursing educational system to be efficient, economic, effective, readily understood by the public, and responsive to societal changes, it must be built so that the foundation, that educational base for entry into professional nursing practice, is sound and comprehensive enough to meet the diversity that is inherent in the nursing practice of the current period. It must be flexible enough to accommodate quickly to new knowledge and technology and to projected changes in the future. The base should also enable economical acquisition of differentiated and additional knowledge if the nurse chooses a career requiring additional formal study. Thus, professional nursing education should be directed toward preparing a careerist in nursing who possesses a solid base for general professional nursing practice. The individual is socialized as a professional and has a philosophic and value system that is compatible with this role.

Several courses of action should be considered in building such a system of nursing education. First, the current system of preparing individuals for the first professional degree should be rejected outright, one of the choices proposed in the preface of the National League for Nursing's publication *Curriculum Revolution: Mandate for Change* (Aydelotte, 1988b). This proposal will lead to a "Transformation in nurses themselves, and thus of nursing."

Four options for change in the educational programs leading to the first professional degree are possible:

1. Redesign the baccalaureate curriculum and its implementation to accommodate the new knowledge, skills, and socialization experiences that are needed to produce a professional who is a general practitioner. This will require a substantial increase in the length of the program. The credential will remain the baccalaureate degree.

2. Recognize that the above option is not feasible because of the time required for the student to complete the program, the necessary preparation of the faculty, and the current market and work environment. Reduce the expectation to prepare a professional and produce a "minispecialist" who is currently highly marketable. This action will limit the graduate's opportunity in career development, since the general base in both the liberal arts and professional nursing is absent. The graduate will be a nursing specialty technician, and the credential will be the baccalaureate degree. The graduate will need additional education to become a professional in the

true sense. Problems of differentiating between this graduate and the current master's level specialist may arise.

3. Adopt the master's degree as the credential for entry into professional practice. Increase the amount of liberal arts content in the baccalaureate curriculum, add new nursing knowledge and skills, and provide for the socialization experiences and philosophic base. This decision may create confusion because the current master's degree is heavily identified as a nursing specialty practice degree.

4. Adopt the professional doctorate as the credential for entry into professional practice. Redesign the program with a liberal arts base and course work for general professional practice, emphasizing a strong clinical focus and practice features. Provide for socialization as a professional.

This author's preferred program is that leading to a Doctor of Nursing as the first professional degree, built on at least 3 years and preferably 4 of liberal arts education. The rationale for the proposal is voiced by Aydelotte (1989d), Watson and Bevis (1990), and Duffy (1990). This choice is not based on the experience of the two doctoral programs currently in existence. Both of these are in private universities, and the concept has not been tested in public universities. One university has clearly identified the problems in the implementation of the idea. The program is perceived as controversial and is being changed. Reported as influential in bringing about the change are the financial cost of the program to the student, the difficulty of arranging different clinical experiences for the student, the fact that the expectations of the graduates are not being met in the current workplace, and the fact that employers do not understand the difference between the preparation of the Doctor of Nursing graduate and the baccalaureate graduate. However, in spite of this one school's experience, the concept of entry into professional practice in a profession based on doctoral preparation has merit. The concept is not new. The pharmacy profession is currently undergoing debate regarding a change in this direction (Manasse & Giblin, 1984; Study Commission on Pharmacy, 1979). The professions of medicine and law have undergone the move from baccalaureate education to that of the professional doctorate.

The argument put forth here for a universal nursing doctorate as the degree for entry into professional nursing practice includes the following:

- The content for professional nursing practice and socialization for the role merit doctoral preparation.
- A nursing doctorate would eliminate the current fragmentation and confusion regarding multiple levels of education for the first professional degree.
- The differentiation between the technical and professional programs will increase and become more distinct.
- The differentiation between professional and technical roles that is currently taking place will become even more marked and less confused. The surveys conducted by the National Commission on Nursing Implementation Project demonstrate that differentiation is now taking place.
- The professional nurse will be on an educational level with other health professionals with fewer educational and social distinctions. The doctoral

degree will be an asset to the nurse in relationships with others, since in our society, credentials are important.

- Systems of health care need revamping. Nurses who are prepared to participate in making these changes, who are articulate, and who command attention because of their knowledge base and skill are needed to assist in the reorganization of the delivery of care.
- Marked changes in the delivery system of health care and the reorganization of roles and relationships are predicted in the restructuring for the future. New roles, new staffing configurations, new relationships, and new expectations will result. Improved utilization of all personnel is the desired objective. Fewer truly professional nurses may be needed. Knowledgeable clinical nurses who are innovative and who can implement these changes are required.
- There is evidence that a pool of non-nursing college graduates and individuals seeking second career choices is available. There are 18 National League for Nursing accredited nursing education programs designed for non-nurse college graduates, only one of which is at a public university (Aydelotte, 1989a). References are made in the literature to other nursing schools with enrollments that include non-nurse college graduates. The one Doctor of Nursing program that opened in the fall of 1990 reported no problem in recruitment, and the other Doctor of Nursing program reported the same experience.
- Career choices and select positions are currently available for doctorally prepared nurses. Anderson and coworkers (1985) found that 5678 doctorates were designed for faculty positions, and for 169 health service agencies, 502 doctorates were identified as needed within the next five years. If professional nurses enter practice with a doctorate and with experience and maturity, some of the clinical positions in agencies could be filled by them.

Preparation for specialty nursing practice would follow the Doctor of Nursing degree, a pattern that is used in other professions such as dentistry and law. Restructuring of nursing education is needed to ensure a fit between theory, research, and practice. The master's program may be combined with cognate fields and lead to dual master's degree preparation. Admission to the specialization area in master's programs should be standardized in that individuals entering the program should hold a first professional degree in nursing, not only a license to practice. Further, master's programs need to be comparable from one institution to another. The lack of consistency in course content, the narrowness of some of the content, and the multiple entry levels add to the confusion about the competencies of the graduates. The problem of educating for specialty nursing practice is a complex one because of the haphazard evolution of specialization. A special group commissioned by the Tri-Council of Nursing should be asked to study and adopt a schema that simplifies the present classification and identifies the content of the specialties and subspecialties. Styles' (1989) study clearly identifies the disarray in specialization and the need for delineating the knowledge base of the specialties and subspecialties.

Doctoral study beyond the professional practice doctorate (Doctor of Nursing) would lead to the Doctor of Philosophy degree, a practice not uncommon in other professions. Faculty engaged in doctoral education leading to the degree beyond the first professional degree is showing a preference toward that degree. Grace (1990) proposes both the research doctorate and the clinical or applied research doctorate, a proposal that makes sense in view of the fact that the career trajectory of individuals varies (Chaska, 1990). Since nursing is preoccupied with image and prestige, the degree granted at the end of the dual track program will probably be the same. The important feature is the careful planning of the total program as a whole, not piece-meal or dependent upon obtaining a master's degree in a specialty prior to admission to the doctoral program. Chaska suggests that both tracks require core courses in selected subject matter. Since nursing has not yet developed its own divisions of knowledge through research, the areas of concentration in the doctoral program could focus on areas of clinical practice or selected nursing phenomena that cut across several populations, with a gradual narrowing and deepening of the concentration as the student progresses through the program. As nursing knowledge develops, changes can be introduced in the area of concentration.

Consideration of support of professional nurses who wish to take graduate studies in other disciplines is timely. The arguments presented by Tschudin (1966) and Schlotfeldt (1966) are still persuasive. Nursing knowledge has developed, but the progress is due, in part, to the fine nurse scientists who were produced when that program was in place. As selected nurses study in the basic sciences, strong connections should be maintained with the faculty of nursing. After their degrees, these nurse scientists can audit or enroll in nursing courses offered by their colleagues, as needed, to fill in any gaps in their nursing knowledge. The growth in collaborative research, the development of emerging fields of knowledge in the sciences, the study of nursing phenomena that cuts across several fields, and the need to learn methodologies used by other disciplines warrant the support of individual nurses engaging in doctoral study in the basic sciences.

The second course of action deals with the associate degree programs. First, because of the recent attention given to the nurse shortage, enrollments in the technical programs (associate degree) will probably remain steady. Emphasis should be placed on the preparation of fine, skilled nursing technicians who can assist professional nurses in their work. Education programs should maintain consistency in the standards of competence expected of each graduate. The relationship between the professionals and these technicians, who are in a true sense paraprofessionals, should be made explicit to both the graduates and their employers. Further, the knowledge base of the technicians is a "spin-off" of that once held by the professional; consequently, the professional body determines the content of that knowledge. In this sense, the knowledge base is different from that held by the professional.

Attention should be directed toward the restructuring of the education for the nurse technician. Evolution of the technical role will continue as reorganization of nursing delivery systems unfolds. Individuals who are highly knowledgeable about the restructuring within service institutions and agencies need to promote dialogue with the political leadership in the community colleges where existing programs for registered nurses are conducted. The community college leadership is encouraged to become aware of the trends that are shaping the future of these community college graduates and the opportunities that will be present for well-trained technicians.

A sudden and sharp change in policy creates anxiety and fosters debate and argument. The major argument against the above proposals for change in policy will center on maintaining a sufficient number of nurses in the work force. The second argument concerns the cost of the education and the quality of the educational offerings.

Harris (1990) and Widnall (1988) offer information regarding recruitment that is useful to nursing. Harris predicts that in the 21st century, one third to one half of college students will be students of color. This is a pool from which nursing should draw. In her study of women in the sciences and engineering, Widnall found two points in the students' life plans that were critical—the choice of career and during graduate study. Nursing should concentrate its efforts on attracting and retaining students at these times using marketing strategies appearing in the literature. The rapid rise of women in law, medicine, dentistry, veterinary medicine, and graduate business schools indicates that women are interested in the professions. Nursing must present a positive image of the work and the satisfactions inherent in it rather than the negative outlook that has characterized its presentations. Changes are occurring in the work environment and in its economic conditions. Of particular significance in recruitment is the fact that as the health care system changes, new roles for professional nurses will emerge. We need nurses capable of designing and filling them.

New federal initiatives in nursing should seek financial assistance for students who are candidates for the proposed doctoral program in addition to funds for specialty training. Partnerships among institutions of higher learning, health care institutions, and community services are needed in order to pool the human resources needed to provide the education. Consortia are in order. Some baccalaureate schools may change goals and offer nurse technician programs leading to a baccalaureate degree, or they may close or become linked to larger schools. Larger and fewer schools may result, which in the end may be less costly (Morton, 1983). Combining smaller programs of nursing with a university school and academic health center could result in improvements and general upgrading of programs. The various school faculties could be combined into one, and practice professionals as adjunct faculty could be pooled to provide the education and practice arrangements. Library and laboratory resources and technologic equipment could be merged. Students would gain by having access to a wider social and cultural environment and a greater variety of practice settings and cultures. Economies of scale could be achieved, resulting in better use of both human and financial resources. Multiple programs within the same school are expensive, and schools should focus their efforts or combine programs into larger entities. Collaboration between faculties and expert practitioners will be imperative in order to meet the task.

Basic to the implementation of such programs is the need for planned and directed change, a relatively new concept to nursing. Nursing needs a National Center for Nursing Education to guide its reformulation of a new educational system. Chaska (1990) proposes a general framework for such an entity. The purpose of the Center would be to test out new designs, implement replication of successful ones, and ensure consistency of programs and outcomes while accommodating to innovation and regional differences. Confusion and overproliferation of programs should be avoided.

Placement of a National Center for Nursing Education and its funding presents dilemmas in view of the several groups interested in influencing and controlling nursing education. Nurses are a national resource, but placement of nursing within a government agency runs the risk of political influence and control, a risk most professions avoid. The National Commission on Nursing Implementation Project, funded by the W.K. Kellogg Foundation, has functioned well because of the design of the governing body and its funding. An arrangement by which the Tri-Council of Nursing takes the initiative and seeks funding may serve nursing and society well.

A new policy is desperately needed. Out of the current chaos must come order based upon vision and a look into the future. Nursing will not meet its social mandate if action is delayed. The action on a new policy will require a willingness to accept change, boldness, courage, and forthright leadership. This is no time for hesitation or timidity.

## REFERENCES

Amos, L.K. (1985). Issues in doctoral preparation in nursing: Current perspectives and future directions. *Journal of Professional Nursing, 1*(2), 101–108.

Anderson, E., Roth, P., & Palmer, I.S. (1985). A national survey of doctorally prepared nurses in academic settings and health service agencies. *Journal of Professional Nursing, 1*(1), 23–33.

Arlton, D.M., & Miller, M.E. (1987). RN to BSN: Advanced placement policies. *Nurse Educator, 12*(6), 11–14.

Aydelotte, M.K. (1980). *Nursing: A social policy statement.* Kansas City, MO: American Nurses' Association.

Aydelotte, M.K. (1986). *Essentials of colleges and university education for professional nursing.* Washington, DC: American Association of Colleges of Nursing.

Aydelotte, M.K. (1987). *Schools of nursing that have changed from one type of program or from one type of credential to another.* Summary. Work group I. Xeroxed. Milwaukee: National Commission on Nursing Implementation Project.

Aydelotte, M.K. (1988a). *Attitudes, values and beliefs of the public in Indiana toward nursing as a career: A study to enhance recruitment into nursing.* Indianapolis: Sigma Theta Tau.

Aydelotte, M.K. (1988b). *Curriculum revolution: Mandate for change.* New York: National League for Nursing.

Aydelotte, M.K. (1989a). *Accredited nursing education programs for the non-nurse college graduate.* Xeroxed. New York: National League for Nursing, Division of Education and Accreditation Services.

Aydelotte, M.K. (1989b). *Curriculum revolution: Reconceptualizing nursing education.* New York: National League for Nursing.

Aydelotte, M.K. (1989c). *Nursing data review 1988.* New York: National League for Nursing, Division of Research.

Aydelotte, M.K. (1989d). *Nursing—the future: A profession or a technological occupation?* Indianapolis: Sigma Theta Tau International.

Aydelotte, M.K. (1990). *News from NLN: NLN's exclusive data projects a nursing shortage in 1990's.* New York: National League for Nursing.

Benner, P. (1984). *From novice to expert.* Menlo Park, CA: Addison-Wesley.

Bevis, E.O. (1988). New directions for a new age. In National League for Nursing, *Curriculum revolution: Mandate for change* (pp. 27–52). New York: National League for Nursing.

Bevis, E.O. (1989). The curriculum consequences: Aftermath of revolution. In National League for Nursing, *Curriculum revolution: Reconceptualizing nursing education* (pp. 115–134). New York: National League for Nursing.

Brodie, J.N. (1984). A response to Dr. J. Fawcett's paper: "The metaparadigm of nursing: Present status and future refinements." *Image: Journal of Nursing Scholarship,* 16(3), 87–89.

Chaska, N.L. (1990). The kaleidoscope of nursing. In N.L. Chaska (Ed.), *The nursing profession: Turning points* (pp. 645–685). St. Louis: C.V. Mosby.

Christman, L. (1979). Professional nurse responsibility and accountability. In American Academy of Nursing, *Nursing's influence on health policy for the eighties* (pp. 21–23). Kansas City, MO: American Academy of Nursing.

Clayton, G.M. (1989). Curriculum revolution: Defining the components. *Journal of Professional Nursing,* 5(1), 6–55.

Conway-Welch, C. (1990). Emerging models of post-baccalaureate nursing education. In J.C. McCloskey & H.K. Grace (Eds.), *Current issues in nursing* (3rd ed.) (pp. 137–141). St. Louis: C.V. Mosby.

Curtin, L. (1984). Editorial opinion: Who or why or which or what? *Nursing Management,* 15(11), 7–8.

Diekelmann, N. (1989). Curriculum revolution: A theoretical and philosophical mandate for change. In National League for Nursing, *Curriculum revolution: Reconceptualizing nursing education* (pp. 25–42). New York: National League for Nursing.

Diers, D. (1987). When college grads choose nursing. *American Journal of Nursing,* 87(12), 1631–1637.

de Tornyay, R. (1987). Toward faculty practice. *Journal of Nursing Education,* 26(4), 137.

*Doctoral programs in nursing* (1989). Mimeographed. Distributed at National Doctoral Forum, June 1989. Indianapolis: University of Indiana.

Downs, F.S. (1988). Doctoral education: Our claim to the future. *Nursing Outlook,* 36(1), 18–20.

Duffy, M.E. (1990). Needed: New models for professional nursing education. In N.L. Chaska (Ed.), *The nursing profession: Turning points* (pp. 84–91). St. Louis: C.V. Mosby.

Elliott, J.E. (1987). Nursing education and nursing practice: The need for consensus. *Journal of Professional Nursing,* 3(4), 194–198.

Fagin, C., & Diers, D. (1983). Nursing as metaphor. *American Journal of Nursing,* 83(9), 1362.

Farrell, J. (1988). The changing pool of candidates for nursing. *Journal of Professional Nursing,* 4(3), 145, 230.

Fawcett, J. (1984). The metaparadigm of nursing: Present status and future refinements. *Image: Journal of Nursing Scholarship,* 16(3), 84–87.

Fitzpatrick, J.J., Boyle, K.K., & Anderson, R.M. (1986). Evaluation of doctor of nursing (ND) program: Preliminary findings. *Journal of Professional Nursing,* 2(6), 365–372.

Fitzpatrick, J.J., & Modly, D.M. (1990). The first doctor of nursing (ND) program. In N.L. Chaska (Ed.), *The nursing profession: Turning points* (pp. 93–99). St. Louis: C.V. Mosby.

Forni, P.R. (1989). Models for doctoral programs: First professional degree or terminal degree? *Nursing and Health Care,* 10(8), 429–434.

Forni, P.R. (1987). Nursing's diverse master's programs: The state of the art. *Nursing and Health Care, 8*(2), 71–75.

Grace, H.K. (1990). Issues in doctoral education in nursing. In J.C. McCloskey & H.K. Grace (Eds.), *Current issues in nursing* (3rd ed.) (pp. 151–155). St. Louis: C.V. Mosby.

Harris, R.L. (1990). Recruiting Afro-Americans into the graduate school pipeline. *Perspectives, 28*(1), 6, 11–12.

Hart, S.E. (1989). *Doctoral education in nursing: History, process, and outcome.* New York: National League for Nursing.

Hoeffler, B., & Murphy, S.A. (1984). Specialization in nursing practice. In American Nurses' Association, *Issues in professional nursing practice*, No. 2 (pp. 1–13). Kansas City, MO: American Nurses' Association.

Holzemer, W.L., & Chambers, D.B. (1986). Healthy nursing doctoral programs: Relationship between perceptions of the academic environment and productivity of faculty and alumni. *Research in Nursing and Health, 9,* 299–307.

Lambert, C.E., & Lambert, V.A. (1988). Faculty practice: Unifier of nursing education and nursing service? *Journal of Professional Nursing, 4*(5), 346–355.

Lash, A.A. (1987). The nature of the doctor of philosophy degree: Evolving conceptions. *Journal of Professional Nursing, 3*(2), 92–101.

Lenz, E.R. (1990). Doctoral education: Present views, future directions. In N.L. Chaska (Ed.), *The nursing profession: Turning points* (pp. 114–121). St. Louis: C.V. Mosby.

Lindeman, C.A. (Ed.) (1988). *Alternate conceptions of work and society: Implications for professional nursing.* Washington, DC: American Colleges of Nursing.

Lynn, M.R., McCain, N.L., & Boss, B.J. (1989). Socialization of RN to BSN. *Image: Journal of Nursing Scholarship, 21*(4), 232–237.

Manasse, H.R., & Giblin, P.W. (1984). Commitments for the future of pharmacy: A review and opinion of the Pharm. D. curricular debate. *Drug Intelligence and Clinical Pharmacy, 18,* 420–427.

Martin, C.E. (1989). Alternatives for students with life experiences: Reconceptualizing nursing education. In National League for Nursing, *Curriculum revolution: Reconceptualizing nursing education* (pp. 101–115). New York: National League for Nursing.

Martin, J.E., White, J.E., & Hansen, M.M. (1989). Preparing students to shape health policy. *Nursing Outlook, 37*(2), 89–93.

Meleis, A.I. (1988). Doctoral education in nursing: Its present and its future. *Journal of Professional Nursing, 4*(6), 436–446.

Miller, G., & Rew, L. (1989). Analysis and intuition: The need for both in nursing education. *Journal of Nursing Education, 28*(2), 84–86.

Moccia, P. (1988). Curriculum revolution: An agenda for change. In National League for Nursing, *Curriculum revolution: Mandate for change* (pp. 53–64). New York: National League for Nursing.

Morton, P.G. (1983). The financial distress of higher education: Impact on nursing. *Image: Journal of Nursing Scholarship, 5*(4), 102–106.

Murphy, E. (1983). Competencies of graduates of nursing programs: Readdressed and reaffirmed. In National League for Nursing, *Perspectives in nursing 1983–1985* (pp. 186–196). New York: National League for Nursing.

Murphy, J.F. (1985). Doctoral education of nursing: Historical development, programs, and graduates. In H.H. Werley & J.J. Fitzpatrick (Eds.), *Annual Review of Nursing Research* (vol. 3) (pp. 171–189). New York: Springer Publishing Co.

National Commission on Nursing Implementation Project (1990). *Nursing's vital signs: Shaping the profession for the 1990s.* Battle Creek, MI: W.K. Kellogg Foundation.

Nursing enrollments rebound across nation [news] (1990). *American Journal of Nursing, 90*(1), 119, 126.

Orlando, I.J. (1987). Nursing in the 21st century: Alternate paths. *Journal of Advanced Nursing, 12*(4), 405–412.

Orlando, I.J., & Dugan, A.B. (1989). Independent and dependent paths: The fundamental issue for the profession. *Nursing and Health Care, 10*(2), 77–80.

Rapson, M.F. (1990). Educational mobility: The right of passage for the RN. In N.L. Chaska (Ed.), *The nursing profession: Turning points* (pp. 69–76). St. Louis: C.V. Mosby Co.

Reed, S.B. (1983). Educational mobility: From concept to reality. In National League for Nursing, *Perspectives in nursing 1983–1985* (pp. 157–165). New York: National League for Nursing.

Rosenfeld, P. (1987). Nursing education in crisis: A look at recruitment and retention. *Nursing and Health Care, 8*(5), 282–286.

Salmon, M.E. (1989). Public health nursing: The neglected specialty. *Nursing Outlook, 37*(5), 226–229.

Schlotfeldt, R. (1966). Doctoral study in basic disciplines—a choice for nurses. *Nursing Forum, 5*(2), 68–74.

Schlotfeldt, R. (1988). The scholarly nursing practitioner. In C.A. Lindeman (Ed.), *Alternate conceptions of work and society: Implications for professional nursing* (pp. 15–29). Washington, DC: American Association of Colleges of Nursing.

Snyder, M. (1990). Specialization in nursing: Logic or chaos? In N.L. Chaska (Ed.), *The nursing profession: Turning points* (pp. 107–113). St. Louis: C.V. Mosby.

Stuart, G.W. (1981). How professionalized is nursing? *Image: Journal of Nursing Scholarship, 13*(1), 18–23.

Study Commission on Pharmacy (1979). *Pharmacist for the future: The report of the study commission on pharmacy.* Ann Arbor: Health Administration Press.

Styles, G. (1989). *On specialization in nursing: Toward a new empowerment.* Kansas City, MO: American Nurses' Foundation.

Tanner, C. (1988). Curriculum mandate: The practice revolution. In National League for Nursing, *Curriculum revolution: Mandate for change* (pp. 201–215). New York: National League for Nursing.

Tschudin, M.S. (1966). Doctoral preparation in other disciplines with a minor in nursing. *Nursing Forum, 5*(2), 51–56.

United States Department of Human Services, Public Health Service, Health Resources and Services Administration (March, 1990). *Seventh Report to the President and Congress on the status of health personnel in the United States* (Department of Health and Human Services Publication No. HRS-P-OD-90-1). Washington, DC: U.S. Government Printing Office.

Waters, V. (1989). Transforming barriers in nursing education. In National League for Nursing, *Curriculum revolution: Reconceptualizing nursing education* (pp. 91–100). New York: National League for Nursing.

Watson, J. (1988). A case study: Curriculum in transition. In National League for Nursing, *Curriculum revolution: Mandate for change* (pp. 1–8). New York: National League for Nursing.

Watson, J., & Bevis, E.O. (1990). Nursing education: Coming of age for a new age. In N.L. Chaska (Ed.), *The nursing profession: Turning points* (pp. 100–106). St. Louis: C.V. Mosby.

Widnall, S.E. (1988). AAAS presidential lecture; voices from the pipeline. *Science, 241,* 1740–1745.

*Chapter 30*

# Nursing Research: Weaving the Past and the Future

ADA SUE HINSHAW

$N$URSING RESEARCH IS facing a future of exciting opportunities and important challenges. The foundations for handling this future with sensitivity and vision are well established. The profession's progress with nursing research and the development of nursing science needs to be celebrated. A growing body of knowledge is evident to guide practice, the research programs are in the mainstream of science, and the infrastructure to facilitate nursing research is available in multiple academic and health care systems. These accomplishments are the beginning of an exciting movement to systematically create a science reflecting a nursing perspective interfacing with multiple related bodies of knowledge.

Numerous leaders have noted the need for the profession's research programs to identify the information required to guide the practice of nursing (Hinshaw, 1988a; Meleis, 1987; Stevenson, 1987). The opportunity to create such a body of knowledge is enhanced by the "mainstreaming" of nursing research in an interactive environment with other biologic, social science, and health care disciplines. The establishment of a visible structure and force for nursing research at the national level within the prestigious National Institutes of Health (NIH), which supports other biomedical and behavioral research in the United States, was an important advance. The National Center for Nursing Research promotes the interaction of nursing research programs with programs of other health care disciplines. Studying nursing questions within interdisciplinary research teams in order to handle the complexity of the issues involved in such investigations has also contributed to the mainstreaming of the discipline's research programs. Nursing's ability to contribute to science in general as well as ensure the excellence or currency of its knowledge base depends on maintaining a position in the center of health care science.

The development of foundations for facilitating systematic inquiry was the primary focus of earlier years in nursing research (Stevenson, 1987) and has consumed major resources in terms of federal and organizational support. Several infrastructures are clearly established. For example, more than at any other point in nursing history, centers or offices for research and research facilitation are an integral part

485

of academic and clinical settings, doctoral and postdoctoral students are being supported in educational programs with research-intensive environments, research and clinical journals are reporting research and research utilization endeavors, and research communities for nursing investigators are evident at international, national, regional, and state levels of the profession. Facilitating the communication of research, supporting research through small grants, and defining research priorities have become central to numerous general and specialty nursing professional organizations. In order to continue to promote nursing research and the development of knowledge to guide practice, it is valuable to examine the past in relation to future priorities and directions.

## Examining the Past

The foundations that are the basis of the current strong momentum in nursing research provide evidence of the individual, professional, institutional, and federal commitments to nursing research. Foundations are defined as the conceptual and operational underpinnings required to sustain long-term, fully developed research programs in nursing research. Such foundations include:

- Establishing the value of research and the critical nature of its relationship to nursing practice,
- Building the research resources and structures needed to facilitate full-scale research programs, and
- Developing the commitment to generate the body of knowledge required to guide nursing practice.

### Establishing the Value of Research in Practice

Today the natural partnership that exists between nursing practice and research is taken for granted. The basic premise of making complex clinical, administrative, and educational decisions in nursing practice is an accurate, reliable body of knowledge from which relatively predictable outcomes can be achieved (Hinshaw, 1988a). As Schlotfeldt (1977, pg. 5) noted, "empirical evidence concerning nursing's contributions to promoting the well-being and recovery of persons who experienced illnesses and injuries has become firmly established in the nation's folk wisdom." The basic value of research's contribution to nursing practice has been generated and cultivated over an extended period of time. Early leaders, such as Nightingale (1860), Dock (1900), Robb (1906), Nutting (1912, 1926), Goodrich (1932), Stewart (1943), Wald (1915), and Roberts (1954), identified the breadth and scope of nursing practice and education and valued the need for empirical observation and accurate information to support professional decisions.

The founding of nursing education within institutions of higher learning for both graduate and undergraduate degrees assisted in generating a value system for research. The establishment of a graduate course and later undergraduate programs for nurses at Teachers College, Columbia University, in 1899 opened new opportunities for nursing; which the profession was quick to develop. By the mid-1930s, a number of both undergraduate and graduate programs had been established within universities and institutions of higher education (Gortner & Nahm, 1977). In this country, institutions of higher education have the societal mandate and responsibility for the discovery and transmission of new knowledge. Infrastructures to facilitate the scientific inquiry processes through which knowledge is generated are an integral part of such institutions. With the integration of nursing into higher education, the role of discoverer and researcher was a natural acquisition. However, as the value of research became apparent for both educational and practice purposes, the need for research development strategies to establish a cadre of nurse scientists and the infrastructures needed to facilitate the research programs of the discipline became evident.

## Building the Structures and Resources for Nursing Research

The structures and resources needed for the foundation of nursing's research programs were developed in several arenas: professional organizations, institutions of higher learning, and the federal government. Multiple strategies were implemented to establish the necessary structures: the development of a cadre of prepared nurse scientists; establishment of offices and centers for nursing research within academic and clinical settings; and evolution of nursing scientific communities at institutional, regional, national, and international levels. Many of these strategies were supported initially by federal programs for nursing research and research training.

*Federal Programs for Nursing Research and Research Training.* The leadership provided by colleagues administering the federal programs for nursing research and research training from 1954 to 1986 is to be applauded. Even in an atmosphere of limited resources and cost containment, the strategies used to facilitate nursing inquiry were widely selected and helped to build the foundations needed for strong research and research training programs.

The first federal structure for nursing research was the Research Grants and Fellowship Branch established in 1955 within the Division of Nursing Resources, started in 1949 under the Public Health Service Act of 1944. Initially, the Division was a section of the Bureau of Medical Services, the precursor to the National Institute of General Medical Sciences at the National Institutes of Health (Gortner, 1973). With increasing pressure from nurses requesting consultation on research design and grantsmanship, the Division was congressionally mandated to begin an extramural research program in research support and research training with a budget of $625,000 ($500,000 for the support of research and $125,000 for research training). An intramural program was part of the Division of Nursing Resources (National Advisory Council for Nursing Research, 1989).

The Division of Nursing Resources combined with the Division of Public Health Nursing in 1960 and was renamed the Division of Nursing. The Research Grant and Fellowship Program was then a branch within the new Division, and it was ultimately moved from the National Institutes of Health to the agency responsible for the manpower and clinical training/educational programs of the health care professions, currently known as Health Resources and Services Administration (HRSA).

In April 1986, after a unified effort by the nursing community, the National Center for Nursing Research was established at the National Institutes of Health as a freestanding, legislatively mandated, structure responsible for the support of basic and clinical research as well as research training related to nursing practice and patient care. The importance of the National Center for Nursing Research was that it signified the move of nursing research back into the mainstream of health care science that is traditionally supported at the National Institutes of Health. The National Center for Nursing Research also provided the visible structure needed in the federal government to focus programs and resources on support of the research required for nursing practice and patient care. The establishment of the National Center for Nursing Research provided a surge of energy for the growing momentum for nursing research, propelling the field into another era of development.

*Cadre of Nurse Researchers.*     In the late 1950s and early 1960s, several nursing leaders addressed the need for nurses prepared in research, among them McManus (1960, 1961a, 1961b) and Mereness (1964), who discussed the need for doctoral preparation of nurses. The major intent of the professional thrust for doctoral education for nurses was to prepare leaders needed to facilitate nursing scholarship and to amass the critical cadre of scientists needed to generate and test a body of knowledge for the discipline. Federal support for the research training of nurses began formally in 1955 with the Special Predoctoral and Postdoctoral Research Fellowship Program (National Center for Nursing Research, 1988). This fellowship was individually initiated for a doctorate in nursing or a related discipline. The program was started with approximately $125,000 for awards, administered by the Research Grants and Fellowship Branch at the Division of Nursing Research (Abdellah, 1987). In the early years, many of the awards went to nurses obtaining doctoral degrees in related biologic, behavioral, and allied fields because of the limited number of doctoral programs that were available in nursing.

In order to prepare larger numbers of individuals for faculty roles in the developing doctoral programs in nursing, the Nursing Scientist Graduate Training Program was established in 1964. Nurse researchers were trained in a variety of basic sciences, e.g., biology, physiology, psychology, sociology, and anthropology. Ten years later in 1974, the National Research Service Award Act provided both institutional and individual predoctoral and postdoctoral awards, to aspiring scientists in multiple health care disciplines and related sciences. In nursing, individual fellowships were awarded primarily until 1987, when substantially increased research resources were available and more schools of nursing had research-intensive environments that could support institutional research training awards.

With the establishment of the National Center for Nursing Research in 1986, the concept of a research career trajectory was advanced (National Center for Nursing Research, 1988). In order to continue to sustain a cadre of nurse researchers committed to excellence in science, the profession had to develop a career orientation to research and research training. The basic premise was that to be current in a research field and its methodologies requires updating and retraining throughout the research career. A series of award mechanisms (including predoctoral, postdoctoral, midcareer development, and senior investigator fellowships) were made available to implement the concept of a research career trajectory.

Additional National Center for Nursing Research objectives for facilitating research training are (1) increasing the number of individuals in research training, (2) increasing the number of postdoctoral fellows supported, and (3) increasing the number of institutional National Research Service Award Act awards to research-intensive environments. A multi-year projection of the number of trainees to be supported will culminate in 320 traineeships and fellowships being awarded per year by approximately 1993 as compared with 146 supported in 1986. These predictions were made in 1985 on the basis of the recommendations of the National Academy of Sciences, Committee on National Needs for Biomedical and Behavioral Research Personnel. The percentage of postdoctoral fellows has increased from 8 percent in 1986 to 18 percent in 1989. The proportion is expected to increase to 25 to 30 percent by the mid-1990s. The institutional awards have increased from two in 1986 to 14 in 1990 and are expected to continue to gradually increase.

One of the major foundations for an active research program in a discipline is a well-prepared cadre of scientists. Maintaining such a cadre and providing mechanisms by which the individuals can remain on the cutting edge of science is critical to the rapidly evolving body of nursing knowledge.

*Offices and Centers for Nursing Research.* One of the most productive strategies for facilitating research of faculty and clinicians in academic and clinical agencies has been the establishment of offices and centers for nursing research. Although the specific responsibilities of these offices and centers vary, their primary purpose is the enhancement of research productivity through consultation, proposal review, networking with other colleagues, administration of small grant programs for pilot studies, and providing communication channels for the nursing research being conducted within the institution (e.g., planning of seminars, conferences, and publication of newsletters). The first center for nursing research and education was established in 1953 at Teachers College, Columbia University, in order to "strengthen and improve education for Nursing by conducting research on nursing and nursing education problems and disseminating the results, and by preparing nurses to do research" (Notter & Hott, 1988, p. 9). According to Stevenson (1987), the first center for nursing research and practice issues, founded to facilitate the development of science basic to the nursing discipline, was at Wayne State University under the leadership of Dr. Harriet Werley. The first privately funded Center for Nursing Research was established at the University of Pennsylvania in 1980, funded by the Pew Charitable Trusts.

Since the establishment of these early centers, a number of others have been developed in the most research-intensive institutions. The last 15 to 20 years have also marked the development of such structures in clinical agencies as well as in academia. The existence of such offices/centers in both types of agencies is related to higher research productivity, e.g., increased numbers of doctorally prepared faculty and staff and more extramurally funded research and publications (Dienemann, 1987; Batey, 1985).

Two federal programs initially were activated to enhance the development of research-intensive environments within the institutions. The original program (1958 to 1966) focused on the development of faculty within academic institutions (Faculty Research Development Grant). The institutional awards primarily went to midcareer faculty who were interested in incorporating the research role into their faculty responsibilities but either did not have doctoral preparation or were a number of years past obtaining their earned doctorates (Stevenson, 1987; Gortner, 1973). According to Gortner, the initial objectives for this program were achieved by 1966. The second program focused on research development rather than faculty development and provided the funds for the establishment of many of the early offices and centers for nursing research in the institutions. The offices and centers were judged so successful in terms of facilitating research productivity that numerous others were developed. A recent study suggests that 51 percent of a sample of 49 offices and centers were supported by institutional hard money, 24 percent by a combination of hard money and grant funds, and only 22 percent by only grant monies (McArt, 1987).

The offices and centers have provided a visible structure within academic and clinical agencies for funneling resources to nursing research, just as the National Center for Nursing Research serves this purpose federally. The visibility sensitizes faculty and students to their responsibility for scholarship and science as well as educates colleagues in other disciplines about the importance nursing places on research. The offices and centers also have many operational benefits: effective use of resources, coordination of consultation services, and serving as a focal point for the administration of small grant funds for pilot studies. Thus, they have become a major force in facilitating the research programs of the profession.

*Nursing Scientific Community.* The development of a scientific community for nurse researchers is another important cornerstone that has been put in place in building the structures and resources for nursing research. Refinement of the values, policies, and procedures of the community will occur over time; however, the basic structure is in place. The community has been differentiated on the institutional, regional, national, and international levels.

A scientific community is characterized by three factors—communality, colleagueship, and constructive competition (Gortner, 1983; Gortner & Schultz, 1988; Hinshaw, 1986). Communality refers to sharing research ideas and findings and providing critiques of each other's research endeavors in order to enhance the rigor of the conceptual and methodologic issues. Critically examining each other's scholarly efforts stimulates additional ideas and helps to refine current projects. Colleagueship is defined as constructing the supportive environment within which ideas can be challenged and individuals are willing to risk sharing their scholarly endeavors. Such an environment is conducive to promoting the discovery process and enhancing creativity, which are the cornerstones of scientific breakthroughs. Constructive competition is valuable in that it provides a strong motivator for creating ideas; however, such competition needs to be monitored by the scientific community in order to block negative repercussions.

Several strategies have facilitated the development of nursing's scientific community. One strategy was the opening of communication channels for sharing and

critiquing research and for dissemination of the findings of nursing research programs. Conferences and professional and scholarly journals are basic tools for the
communication of the research. Many of the early conferences were supported by
the federal research programs as these were developed on the national and regional
levels. In 1959, the American Nurses' Association, supported by Division of Nursing
funds, launched the first of nine research conferences extending until 1968. The
Council of Nurse Researchers of the American Nurses' Association has continued to
sponsor national research conferences on a biennial basis. In the same time period,
the Western Commission for Higher Education in Nursing began the first of the
regional research conferences entitled Communicating Nursing Research. In 1992,
the Western Society for Research in Nursing will celebrate its 25th annual conference, the first six of which were funded by the Division of Nursing. Currently, in
1990, all of the five nursing regions sponsor annual research conferences. Other
major organizations such as the Veterans' Administration and the military also sponsor research conferences. In 1983, Sigma Theta Tau held the first international
nursing research conference in Madrid, Spain. These conferences are held bienni-
ally. In addition, international conferences are sponsored by the American Nurses'
Association Council of Nurse Researchers and by several of the specialty organizations in nursing, such as the Oncology Nursing Society (Stevenson, 1987).

Professional journals have been created for the scientific reporting of the findings
of the research programs and for the review and application of the results. The first
journal, *Nursing Research*, was started in 1952, with two other journals being initiated a number of years later: *Research in Nursing and Health* (1978) and the *Western
Journal of Nursing Research* (1979). The *Annual Review of Nursing Research* originated in 1983 and represented a major advancement in the critique and review of
the research programs of the discipline. Several journals and newsletters have also
been created to disseminate research findings: e.g. *Applied Nursing Research* and
*Research Reviews: Studies for Nursing Practice.*

Many of the general and specialized professional organizations have sections
devoted to the development of research and research policy. They may issue statements, develop formal research agendas, administer small grant programs, and coordinate research activities such as conferences. These activities provide major support
to the scientific communities in the profession. Nursing research agendas have been
formalized by a number of professional organizations, e.g., American Nurses' Association, *Directions for Nursing Research: Toward the Twenty-First Century* (1985),
and the American Organization of Nurse Executives, *Final Report of the Ad Hoc
Committee in Nursing Administration Research* (1987). These research agendas are
important in allocating resources and determining priorities for research. The American Nurses' Foundation and Sigma Theta Tau administer small grant programs that
provide funds for pilot studies. These programs are very important in providing the
pilot data needed for successfully competing for federal funds. A number of the
specialty organizations also provide small grant awards to their membership, e.g.,
Oncology Nursing Society, American Association for Critical Care Nurses, and Association of Operating Room Nurses.

Thus, a number of strategies have been used to facilitate the creation and maintenance of scientific communities in nursing. These communities are critical to promot-

ing excellence in the science of nursing, since they stimulate creativity coupled with examining the scientific rigor and clinical relevance of the profession's research programs.

## Developing a Commitment to Generate Knowledge for Nursing Practice

The new or current era of nursing research focuses on generating knowledge for nursing practice. Since the 1920s, clinical studies have been conducted by nurses questioning their practice, e.g., Broadhurst's study of hand washing in 1927 and Ryan and Miller's investigation of disinfecting thermometers (1932). However, the clinical studies were sparse and rarely replicated. During the era from 1940 to 1965, nursing research primarily focused on educational curriculum questions or investigations of nursing personnel in relation to organizational variables (Gortner & Nahm, 1977). During the early 1960s, the research programs refocused on investigating the role of nursing and the nursing process. According to Gortner and Nahm (1977), there were still only a limited number of nurse-researchers prepared to assume the principal investigator position during this period.

In the decade between 1965 and 1975, a major expansion of clinical research programs occurred that were particularly focused on health care problems confronting special, vulnerable, at-risk populations (Gortner & Nahm, 1977). Studies of nursing systems as these influenced the delivery of quality nursing care were the second major focus of the research programs. As of about 1977, an increased number of studies were reflective of major clinical questions and practice issues. A series of intervention studies was evident (Johnson & Rice, 1973; Johnson et al., 1978); however, most of these investigations were descriptive in nature.

Between 1975 and the mid-1980s, the profession was developing a definitive and more refined definition of nursing research. A number of priority statements were issued by the general and specialty organizations of the profession. Isolated policy statements by these organizations were evident in the earlier time frame (e.g., American Nurses' Association, 1962); however, never had the number of priority statements been as great. With this renewed understanding of the opportunities for nursing research, the pressure increased to access additional resources in a stable fiscal environment that would facilitate the rapid growth of the knowledge base that had been outlined in the numerous priority statements. This unified organizational pressure, combined with the professional organizations' growing ability to influence health care policy at the national level, resulted in the establishment of the National Center for Nursing Research at the National Institutes of Health. With the move of nursing research to the National Institutes of Health, the resources for research programs stabilized and increased appreciably. However, nursing's response to the opportunity to develop the research programs of the discipline rendered even the sizable increase in funds minimal in terms of the research that could be conducted.

The challenge of the current era of nursing research is to generate knowledge that is clinically relevant and scientifically rigorous in order to contribute to the health care of the public. The challenge in generating the knowledge base will be to develop a "passion for substance" (Meleis, 1987). The new vision of knowledge creation for the discipline focuses on the development and testing of information that is basic to the practice of the profession. In this vision, a number of nursing scholars (Ellis, 1970, 1982; Fitzpatrick, 1988; Hinshaw, 1989; Meleis, 1987; Stevenson, 1988) suggest that the priority of the current era is to identify the major clinical phenomena and questions involved in the profession's practice.

Facilitating the development of substantiated bodies of information in relation to clinical phenomena and questions is critical to promoting excellence in nursing's knowledge base. This basic premise has motivated the generation of nursing research priorities by many organizations in order to provide direction for the critical areas that need to be studied. The movement to promote clusters of studies through priority setting has to be balanced against the need to facilitate creativity for the nurse scientist.

Research programs are also basic to achieving substantiated bodies of knowledge in a specifically defined area of study. Such programs as Brooten's team investigation of early discharge under the care of clinical nurse specialists (Brooten et al., 1986) are proliferating in the nurse researcher community as the concept of a research program is understood and the resources are available to support the programs. In the past, several avant garde researchers engaged in programs of research, such as Johnson's studies on the relationship of sensory information to individual distress responses in traumatic events (1973, 1978) and Pender and colleagues' work with the health promotion model (Pender, Walker, Sechrist, & Stromborg, 1988).

The exciting challenge in developing knowledge for nursing science will be to do so in a manner that enhances the creativity and process of discovery. It is an innovative endeavor linked with rigor and discipline. Examining the past provides an understanding of the major foundations that have been built to support research and a vantage point from which to respond to the challenge of developing knowledge for nursing practice.

## Future Opportunities and Directions for Research

The opportunities for nursing research are endless and exciting. This is both a time of celebration for what has been accomplished in nursing research and a time to confront the future challenges with creativity, responsibility, and scientific rigor. The momentum exists for expanding the basic and clinical body of knowledge for the discipline, given the profession's pressure for identifying nursing research priorities and the increasing resources available for the support of the research programs.

A number of directions can be predicted for future nursing research programs. These are both substantive and methodologic in nature.

### Future Directions for Substantive Research Areas

*National Nursing Research Agenda.*     The long-term strategic plan of the National Center for Nursing Research, the National Nursing Research Agenda, identifies the research priorities to be developed nationally for the next five years. The purpose of the National Nursing Research Agenda is to promote depth in developing a knowledge base for nursing practice, to provide structure for selecting scientific opportunities and initiatives, and to provide direction for nursing research within the discipline (Hinshaw, 1988b). The priorities outline the substantive areas around which clusters of projects will be supported. The priorities identified in the National Nursing Research Agenda are selected by the nursing community and organized in a time frame that permits their refinement, communication to the community in the form of program initiatives, and publication of a "state of the science" monograph for the priority area. The criteria for selecting the priorities include a critical area of health care concern to the American public; a practice area in which nursing as a profession can make an impact; an area that is on the cutting edge of science; an area that is costly in terms of the health care burden to the public; and an area in which nurse scientists are available in adequate numbers to conduct the research (Bloch, 1990). The seven priorities identified are as follows (Hinshaw, Heinrich, & Bloch, 1989):

- Low birth weight—Mothers and infants
- Human immunodeficiency virus infection: prevention and care
- Long-term care for older persons
- Symptom management
- Information systems to improve nursing care
- Health promotion for adolescents
- Technology dependency across the lifespan

Resources will be devoted to these seven priority areas in a time frame that covers five years of initial program initiatives. Such a long-term strategic plan facilitates the nurse researcher's ability to plan for the "window of opportunity" for funding with the priorities and prepare for the application process. An updating process with the nursing community will provide for the addition of new priorities or the refinement of the original seven in future years.

*Discipline Priorities.*   A number of other priorities will be developed for nursing science. These will include areas such as the study of bioethical concerns in nursing practice, delineating the concept of promoting health within various populations and age cohorts, describing and testing the relationship of self-care to multiple facilitative factors and outcomes, defining and identifying nursing-sensitive outcomes, and testing the relationship of the cost of health care to the quality of care provided.

BIOETHICS AND CLINICAL PRACTICE.   The field of research in bioethics and clinical practice is rapidly expanding. As Fry (1989) notes, the development of bioethics as a field of study is expected to differ from other health care disciplines for nursing in terms of the practice variables and relationships. For nursing, the research is expected to focus on critical clinical questions faced by clients, families, and health care providers. The studies will be based on the appropriate philosophic theories but will include an empiric, methodologic approach to the questions raised. Jameton and Fowler (1989) have explored many of the issues integral to the concept of ethical inquiry and empiricism and conclude that morality can be studied with empirical research methods. A recent workshop on Bioethics and Clinical Practice predicted that the resolution of bioethical dilemmas will mushroom as a field of study, particularly in relation to increasing the empiric data needed to guide crucial practice decisions (Moritz, 1990).

HEALTH PROMOTION FOR CLIENTS, FAMILIES, AND COMMUNI-TIES. The American Nurses' Association policy statement for nursing research, *Directions for Nursing Research: Toward the Twenty-First Century* (1985), listed as the first priority for research "promoting health, well-being, and ability to care for oneself among all age, social, and cultural groups." The health promotion priority of the National Nursing Research Agenda will initially focus on healthy behaviors for adolescents and young people. Health promotion for other clients or for families and communities can be expected to increase in terms of research programs. Given nursing's orientation to health rather than illness, this is a natural area of study for the discipline.

Several specific areas of interest are obvious for health promotion. One, health promotion for the elderly population, is of major concern to health care providers in general. There is a shift toward maintaining health in the older individuals for as long as possible. For example, reducing frailty in the elderly in terms of muscle strength, balance, and gait for walking and making the home more "user friendly" are the targets of a cluster of studies across the country supported by the National Institute on Aging and the National Center for Nursing Research. References in the literature to the prevention of urinary incontinence, decubitus ulcers, and osteoporosis reflect nursing's concern with the prevention of such clinical conditions rather than their treatment (Adams, 1986; Brower & Crist, 1985; Wells, 1983).

A second area of interest is the promotion of health within illness, a concept to which nursing seems particularly sensitive (National Center for Nursing Research, 1990a). Chronic illness is expected to be of increasing concern in the future (Callahan, 1985). Nursing research will focus on client and family adaptation to chronic conditions, as is evident in current research programs, for example, Norbeck's (1988) study of social support is often within the context of a strategy that promotes functional adaptation to chronic illnesses. As chronic illnesses escalate as a societal issue, nursing research will focus not just on the adaptation to the chronic conditions but also on the promotion of health within the illness context. This area of study will be particularly important because it will enhance the individual's and the family's ability to remain optimally functional and independent.

QUALITY OF LIFE. Quality of life research will become increasingly important given the shift toward chronic illnesses as the central concern of health care. Thus far, quality of life research has focused most on cancer (Grant et al., 1983; Lewis, 1982; Padilla et al., 1983), end-stage renal disease (Deniston, Carpentier-Alting, Kneisley, Hawthorne, & Port, 1989), and other chronic illnesses. Germino (1987) is studying quality of life in relation to symptom distress. This whole area of research can be expected to expand significantly in relation to patients with acquired immunodeficiency syndrome and their families. Part of the research programs will focus on the psychometric issues involved with developing specific measures for quality of life, given different illnesses and clinical conditions (Greenwald, 1987).

SELF-CARE RESEARCH. During the past several years, increasing attention has been given to the concept of self-care, particularly within the context of Orem's model of nursing (1985). Nursing has contributed significantly already to the science involved with self-care (Gast et al., 1989) but has the potential to provide further understanding of individuals' self-care abilities or actions and how these relate to other major factors, such as cognitive structure regarding health (Neeves, 1980), motivators for self-care (Riesch & Hauck, 1988), or the age of the individual enacting self-care (Hungelmann, 1984). Woods (1989, p. 1) outlines an additional field of study with self-care—its relationship to health. She suggests that "Linking self-care explicitly to a perspective of health can help delineate more clearly the nature of self-care, its consequences, and areas deserving further study."

NURSING-SENSITIVE OUTCOMES.    The area of outcome research has a long history in nursing and in health services research. Donabedian's (1966) early work with a process, structure, and outcomes model provided guidance for numerous acute care and long-term care agencies' quality assurance programs in the 1970s. The current resurgence of this area of research is related to the federal government's new agency and agenda focused on medical effectiveness and the development of guidelines for health care practices regarding specific illnesses or clinical conditions (Agency for Health Care Policy and Research, 1990a).

For nursing, a recent task force of the profession's researchers in nursing systems recommended to the National Center for Nursing Research that future research initiatives need to focus on identifying and defining "nursing sensitive patient outcomes" (National Center for Nursing Research, 1990b). Since a number of the patient outcome indicators are relatively gross, such as length of stay and mortality and morbidity rates, the measures often are not sensitive to nursing interventions. Research in this area will encompass conceptual identification as well as psychometric development of measures for indexing the nursing-sensitive outcomes. The outcomes and measures will be developed primarily for clinical conditions that are central to the practice of nursing, such as pain, urinary incontinence, confusion, and fatigue (Agency for Health Care Policy and Research, 1990b). In addition, research programs will probably focus on relating nursing-sensitive outcomes to nursing interventions used under certain defined clinical conditions or illnesses. The profession's interest in this area of study was underscored by the 1990 conference sponsored by the American Nurses' Association and cosponsored by the Agency of Health Care Policy and Research, the Division of Nursing, and the National Center for Nursing Research on "Effectiveness and Outcomes of Health Care Services: Implications for Nursing."

COST AND QUALITY OF CARE BALANCE.    Nursing research has a long history of interfacing quality of care and cost factors in research programs (Fagin & Jacobsen, 1985). This long-standing interest in the suitable balance or ratio between the cost of health care and the quality delivered can be predicted to increase with society's continuing concern with the rising costs of health care. In general, the studies to date have been descriptive in nature, with relatively simple measures of cost (Fagin, 1982). Analyzing the factors involved in the relationship of cost to the quality of care will require extensive study in addition to testing models of care balanced against cost. Methodologically, the challenge will be to devise more sensitive measures for the quality of care and cost factors of interest; this is not unlike the research that must occur with the nursing-sensitive outcomes. Research in this area is important to nursing administrators and clinicians in order to deal more predictably with prospective payment systems, cost containment measures, and increased competitiveness in the health care delivery systems (McCloskey, Gardner, Johnson, & Maas, 1988; see also Chapter 2).

*Congressional and Societal Priorities* Congressional priorities for health care research, which reflect specific societal issues, will also motivate research programs for the discipline. Health care societal issues provide a major thrust for research programs. For example, society's concern with human immunodeficiency virus infection and acquired immunodeficiency syndrome has motivated a number of researchers to transfer their research programs into this area of study. In 1990, Congress' growing concern with the lack or shortage of health care in rural areas motivated a number of program initiatives from federal agencies.

In 1991, considerable dialogue has occurred about the need for an increasing body of research centered around women's health issues. Nursing has a solid body of research in progress that studies women's health from various perspectives. The studies are in several areas: midlife health problems such as the relationship of menopausal changes to sleep pattern and gastrointestinal functional disturbances and to risk factors for illnesses such as osteoporosis and cardiac conditions; caregiver issues such as the burden of care, quality of the caregiving relationship, and morbidity consequences; pregnancy risks, including predictors of postpartum depression symptoms and predictors of health outcomes for single-mother families; and other issues such as psychobiologic correlates of perimenstrual symptoms and the recovery of older women following hip fractures or myocardial infarction. These areas of research will increase substantially if nursing's current investment in this area is any indicator of interest.

As other societal issues evolve, additional areas of study will also develop in relation to the public's health care concerns.

## Future Directions for Methodologic Issues

Possible future directions for several methodologic issues will be considered. These directions are important if nursing science is to realize its potential for contributing to health care.

*A Biopsychosocial Interface for Nursing Research.* A number of scholars have suggested that nursing science needs to reflect the richness obtained by interfacing knowledge from multiple disciplines within a nursing perspective, framework, and set of values (Gortner, 1983; Hinshaw, 1987; Shaver, 1985). According to Shaver (1985, p. 186), nursing care and thus nursing research "must encompass all factors that act, either singly or in combination, on human health." This is a model that operationalizes the concept of holism and acknowledges the complexity of clinical practice and the research programs needed.

In order to represent adequately the different sciences required for nursing practice, the biologic science dimension of the research programs needs to be strengthened (Bond & Heitkemper, 1987). This was the considered judgment of a National Center for Nursing Research ad hoc task force of nurse researchers with a specialty in the biologic sciences. The intent of the recommendation was to facilitate research and research training, which enhances the interface of nursing science and the biologic sciences. A characteristic of several nursing research programs is the concurrent use of biologic and psychosocial measures of certain concepts, e.g., Nakagawa-Kogan and her colleagues' study of stress using biologic and psychosocial indicators (Nakagawa-Kogan, Garber, Egan, Jarrett, & Hendershot, 1988). Strength in the biologic aspects of nursing research needs to be balanced with the obvious current strength in the social sciences in order to ensure that the multiple dimensions essential to understanding health and illness are interactive in the developing knowledge base for the discipline (Hinshaw, 1988c).

*Testing of Therapeutic Actions.*   In the near future, the descriptive research of the discipline will provide the base needed to move to the next stage in the research programs, the testing of therapeutic actions or nursing interventions. Gortner (1990) argues for encouraging an acceptance of diversified philosophies for nursing science and thus the legitimization of multiple methodologic approaches. She is particularly concerned that nursing be able to utilize experimental and other methods that allow for the testing of the existence and directionality of relationships among the factors under study. Such relationships are basic to guiding decisions in practice situations that require relatively predictable outcomes. Several studies analyzing the methods used in nursing research have noted a limited number of intervention studies (Ganong, 1987; Moody et al., 1988). As the state of the science develops, the testing of theories and the relationships among interventions and outcomes within the context of the theories will be more prevalent.

*Basic Science Studies.*   An increase can be expected in the number of basic science studies in nursing research. Many of the current clinical research programs require a basic science component. For example, Frantz and Xakellis' investigation of the effect of transcutaneous nerve stimulation on the healing of decubitus ulcers suggests that the intervention is effective owing to increased circulation to the healing wound site (Frantz & Xakellis, 1989). This basic premise needs to be studied. Gill, Anderson and colleagues (1988) have shown that non-nutritive sucking stimulates growth for premature infants—why? What is the basic explanatory mechanism for such a relationship? As more clinical intervention-outcome relationships such as these evolve, nurse researchers will begin to ask the basic science as well as clinical science questions needed to refine the clinical interventions.

*Philosophic and Methodologic Diversity.*   During the last three years, a shift toward viewing diversity as a strength has become evident in the conceptual positions taken in the literature; a variety of methodologic approaches and their underlying philosophies about science have been given a high value. Multiple philosophic stances (Dzurec, 1989; Kidd & Morrison, 1988; Whall, 1988) and methodologic approaches (Moccia, 1988; Myers & Haase, 1989) are suggested to provide a rich repertoire from which to develop nursing knowledge. Many articles recommend resolving the classic qualitative versus quantitative dilemma by integrating the two within studies or using each as appropriate to the research questions and the state of the science for the areas being studied (Myers & Haase, 1989; Porter, 1989). This theme is endorsed by Meleis (1987) in her plea to turn from concentrating on the philosophic and methodologic dilemmas involved with nursing research to focusing instead on identifying the substance of nursing practice. Viewing philosophic and methodologic diversity as a strength can be expected to continue with future deliberations.

*Collaboration in Nursing Research.*   Intradisciplinary and interdisciplinary research teams will proliferate in the future because of the complexity of the research questions and the study designs. Given the complexity of the research questions, different types of expertise are needed to adequately address the issues involved.

Intradisciplinary research teams of clinicians and nurse researchers provide a rich mixture of expertise that can protect the practice significance and scientific credibility of a study during the research process. In addition, such teams bridge the gap between theory, research, and practice (Zelauskas, Howes, Christmyer, & Dennis, 1988). Often these teams serve as links between academia and clinical settings (Hinshaw, Chance, & Atwood, 1985). Researchers functioning in clinical settings facilitate the formation of intradisciplinary teams and serve as team members as well. These teams also facilitate the dissemination of findings from the research programs into clinical as well as scientific forums as a result of the different primary role identities of the various members of the team. The clinicians assist in disseminating information to their colleagues in practice, whereas the researchers share the research in the scientific arenas.

Interdisciplinary teams are productive because various types of knowledge can be interfaced through the interaction of team members who represent multiple disciplines. These teams provide a rich base for the study of nursing questions but also enhance other disciplines' understanding of nursing research (Oberst, 1980). Interdisciplinary research is one strategy for integrating nursing research into the mainstream of the broader research community.

*Dissemination and Utilization of Research Findings.*   With the strong momentum to generate nursing knowledge in last several years, less has been noted on the dissemination and utilization of the information gained from the research programs. Prior to 1985, several models for dissemination and utilization were studied, e.g., the conduct and utilization of research in nursing (Horsley, Crane, Crabtree, & Wood, 1983) and the Western Commission for Higher Education in Nursing project, which applied the Lewin model of social change to the issues involved in implementing or utilizing research findings (Krueger, Nelson, & Wolanin, 1978). These issues will become prominent as the research programs from the past several years come to completion and substantiated findings need to be transferred into practice.

## Conclusion

As the discipline's research programs come to fruition, the profession has positioned itself to be able to use the findings to influence health care policy. Identifying clear, significant priorities for study, striving for excellence in the evolving knowledge base, and ensuring substantiation of the study findings will provide a creditable scientific position from which to address societal health care issues.

Weaving the past and the future together for nursing research has resulted in an analysis of the foundations currently underpinning the discipline's scientific endeavors. The strengths and trends seen in these foundations have led to a number of predictions about the future directions for nursing research, directions that will lead to many challenging adventures for expanding the science required to guide nursing practice.

## REFERENCES

Abdellah, F.G. (1987, February). Remarks to the National Advisory Council, National Center for Nursing Research. Bethesda, MD: National Institutes of Health.

Adams, M. (1986). Aging: Gerontological nursing research. In H.H. Werley, J.J. Fitzpatrick, & R.L. Taunton (Eds.). *Annual Review of Nursing Research*, Vol. 4 (pp. 77–103). New York: Springer Publishing Company.

Agency for Health Care Policy and Research (March 1990a). *Medical treatment effectiveness research*. Rockville, MD: Department of Health and Human Services, Public Health Service, AHCPR.

Agency for Health Care Policy and Research (February 1990b). *Nursing Advisory Panel for Guideline Development: Summary*. Rockville, MD: Department of Health and Human Services, Public Health Service, ACHPR.

American Nurses' Association (1962). ANA blueprint for research in nursing. *American Journal of Nursing, 62*(8), 69–71.

American Nurses' Association Cabinet on Nursing Research (1985). *Directions for nursing research: Toward the twenty-first century*. Kansas City, MO: American Nurses' Association.

American Organization of Nurse Executives (1987). *Final report of the ad hoc committee on nursing administration research*. Chicago: American Hospital Association.

Anderson, G. (1986). Pacifiers: The positive side. *Maternal Child Nursing, 11*(2), 122–124.

Batey, M.V. (1985). Nursing research productivity: The University of Washington experience. *Western Journal of Nursing Research, 7*(4), 489–493.

Bloch, D. (1990). Strategies for setting and implementing the National Center for Nursing Research priorities. *Applied Nursing Research, 3*(1), 2–6.

Bond, E.F., & Heitkemper, M.M. (1987). Importance of basic physiologic research in nursing science. *Heart & Lung, 16*(4), 347–349.

Broadhurst, J., Rang, G.C., & Schoening, E. (1927, October). Hand brush suggestions for visiting nurses. *The Public Health Nursing, 29*, 487–489.

Brooten, D., Kumar, S., Brown, L.P., Butts, P., Finkler, S.A., Bakewell-Sachs, S., Gibbons, A., & Delivoria-Papadopoulos, M. (1986). A randomized clinical trial of early hospital discharge and home follow-up of very-low-birth-weight infants. *New England Journal of Medicine, 315*, 934–939.

Brower, H.T., & Crist, M.A. (1985). Research priorities in gerontologic nursing for long-term care. *Image: Journal of Nursing Scholarship, 27*(1), 22–27.

Callahan, D. (1985). Ethics and health care: The next twenty years. *American Journal of Hospital Pharmacy, 42*, 1053–1057.

Committee on National Needs for Biomedical and Behavioral Research Personnel (1985). *1985 Report: Personnel needs and training for biomedical and behavioral research*. Washington, DC: National Academy of Sciences.

Deniston, O.L., Carpentier-Alting, P., Kneisley, J., Hawthorne, V.M., & Port, F.K. (1989). Assessment of quality of life in end-stage renal disease. *Health Services Research, 24*(4), 555–578.

Dienemann, J. (1987). Nursing research centers: A survey of their prevalence, functions and school characteristics. *International Journal of Nursing Studies, 24*(1), 35–44.

Dock, L.L. (1900, October). What we may expect from the law. *American Journal of Nursing, 1*, 8–12.

Donabedian, A. (1966). Evaluating the quality of medical care. *Milbank Memorial Fund Quarterly, 44*(3, Part 2), 166–206.

Dzurec, L.C. (1989). The necessity for and evolution of multiple paradigms for nursing research: A poststructuralist perspective. *Advances in Nursing Science, 11*(4), 69–77.

Ellis, R. (1970). Values and vicissitudes of the scientist nurse. *Nursing Research, 19*, 440–445.

Ellis, R. (1982). Conceptual issues in nursing. *Nursing Outlook, 30,* 406–410.

Fagin, C. (1982). The economic value of nursing research. *American Journal of Nursing, 82,* 1844–1849.

Fagin, C., & Jacobsen, B.S. (1985). Cost-effectiveness analysis in nursing research. In H.H. Werley & J.J. Fitzpatrick (Eds.), *Annual Review of Nursing Research,* Vol. 3 (pp. 215–238). New York: Springer.

Fitzpatrick, J.J. (1988). How can we enhance nursing knowledge and practice? *Nursing and Health Care, 9*(9), 517–521.

Frantz, R.A., & Xakellis, G.C. (1989). Characteristics of skin blood flow over the trochanter under constant, prolonged pressure. *American Journal of Physical Medicine & Rehabilitation, 68*(6), 272–276.

Fry, S.T. (1989). Toward a theory of nursing ethics. *Advances in Nursing Science, 11*(4), 9–22.

Ganong, L.W. (1987). Integrative reviews of nursing research. *Research in Nursing & Health, 10,* 1–11.

Gast, H.L., Denyes, M.J., Campbell, J.C., Hartweg, D.L., Schott-Baer, D., & Isenberg, M. (1989). Self-care agency: Conceptualizations and operationalizations. *Advances in Nursing Science, 12*(1), 26–38.

Germino, B.B. (1987). Symptom distress and quality of life. *Seminars in Oncology Nursing, 3*(4), 299–302.

Gill, N.E., Behnke, M., Conlon, M., McNeeley, J.B., & Anderson, G.C. (1988). Effect of nonnutritive sucking on behavioral state in preterm infants before feeding. *Nursing Research, 37*(6), 347–350.

Goodrich, A.W. (1932). *The social and ethical significance of nursing: A series of addresses.* New York: Macmillan.

Gortner, S.R. (1973). Research in nursing: The federal interest and grant program. *American Journal of Nursing, 73*(6), 1052–1055.

Gortner, S.R. (1983). The history and philosophy of nursing science and research. *Advances in Nursing Science, 5*(1), 1–8.

Gortner, S.R. (1990). Nursing values and science: Toward a science philosophy. *Image: Journal of Nursing Scholarship, 22*(2), 101–105.

Gortner, S.R., & Nahm, H. (1977). An overview of nursing research in the United States. *Nursing Research, 26*(1), 10–33.

Gortner, S.R., & Schultz, P.R. (1988). Approaches to nursing science methods. *Image: Journal of Nursing Scholarship, 20*(1), 22–27.

Grant, M.M., Padilla, G.V., Presant, C., Lipsett, J., & Runa, P.L. (1983). Cancer patients and quality of life. *Proceedings of the Fourth National Conference on Cancer Nursing* (pp. 2–11). Atlanta: American Cancer Society.

Greenwald, H.P. (1987). The specificity of quality-of-life measures among the seriously ill. *Medical Care, 25*(7), 642–651.

Hinshaw, A.S. (1986, December). The tao of nursing research: The creative principle order nursing science and research. Keynote address: Sixth Annual Research Conference of the Southern Council on Collegiate Education for Nursing, Shreveport, LA.

Hinshaw, A.S. (1987, November). Integrating the sciences and humanities in health care. Elizabeth Sterling Soule Lecture, University of Washington, Seattle.

Hinshaw, A.S. (1988a). Practice, research are natural partners. *The American Nurse, 20*(6), 4.

Hinshaw, A.S. (1988b). The National Center for Nursing Research: Challenges and initiatives. *Nursing Outlook, 36*(2), 54, 56.

Hinshaw, A.S. (1988c, October). *A national agenda for nursing research.* Unpublished paper presented at the University of Minnesota, Minneapolis, MN.

Hinshaw, A.S. (1989). Nursing science: The challenge to develop knowledge. *Nursing Science Quarterly, 2*(4), 162–171.

Hinshaw, A.S., Chance, H.C., & Atwood, J.R. (1985). Testing a theoretical model for job satisfaction and anticipated turnover of nursing staff. *Nursing Research, 34*(6), 384.

Hinshaw, A.S., Heinrich, J., & Bloch, D. (1989). Evolving clinical nursing research priorities: A national endeavor. *Journal of Professional Nursing, 4*(6), 398, 458–459.

Horsley, J.A., Crane, J., Crabtree, M.K., & Wood, D.J. (1983). *Using research to improve nursing practice: A guide.* Orlando, FL: Grune & Stratton.

Hungelmann, J. (1984). Components of self-care abilities of older persons with chronic disease. *Dissertation Abstracts International, 45,* 1731B.

Jameton, A., & Fowler, M.D.M. (1989). Ethical inquiry and the concept of research. *Advances in Nursing Science, 11*(3), 11–24.

Johnson, J.E., & Rice, V.H. (1973). Sensory and distress components of pain: Implication for the study of clinical pain. *Nursing Research, 23*(4), 203–209.

Johnson, J.E., Rice, V.H., Fuller, S.S., & Endress, M.P. (1978). Sensory information, instruction in a coping strategy, and recovery from surgery. *Research in Nursing and Health, 1*(1), 4–17.

Kidd, P., & Morrison, E.F. (1988). The progression of knowledge in nursing: A search for meaning. *Image: Journal of Nursing Scholarship, 20*(4), 222–224.

Krueger, J.C., Nelson, A.H., & Wolanin, M.O. (1978). *Nursing research: Development, collaboration, and utilization.* Germantown, MD: Aspen Systems.

Lewis, F.M. (1982). Experienced personal control and quality of life in late stage cancer patients. *Nursing Research, 31,* 113–119.

McArt, E.W. (1987). Research facilitation in academic and practice settings. *Journal of Professional Nursing, 3*(2), 84–91.

McCloskey, J.C., Gardner, D., Johnson, M., & Maas, M. (1988). What is the study of nursing service administration? *Journal of Professional Nursing, 4*(2), 92–98.

McManus, R.L. (1960). Doctoral evaluation nursing. *Nursing Outlook, 8,* 543–546.

McManus, R.L. (1961a, April). Nursing research—its evolution. *American Journal of Nursing, 61,* 76–79.

McManus, R.L. (1961b, May). Today and tomorrow in nursing research. *American Journal of Nursing, 61,* 68–71.

Meleis, A.F. (1987). Revisions in knowledge development: A passion for substance. *Scholarly Inquiry for Nursing Practice, 1*(1), 5–19.

Mereness, D. (1964, September). Preparing the nurse researcher. *American Journal of Nursing, 64,* 78–80.

Moccia, P. (1988). A critique of compromise: Beyond the methods debate. *Advances in Nursing Science, 10*(4), 1–9.

Moody, L.E., Wilson, M.E., Smyth, K., Schwartz, R., Tittle, M., & Van Cott, M.L. (1988). Analysis of a decade of nursing practice research: 1977–1986. *Nursing Research, 37*(6), 374–379.

Moritz, P. (Ed.). (1990). *Bioethics and clinical practice: Examining research outcome and methods* (Proceedings of the Workshop, January 12–13, 1989). Bethesda, MD: National Center for Nursing Research, National Institutes of Health (NIH Publication No. 90-1579).

Myers, S.T., & Haase, J.E. (1989). Guidelines for integration of quantitative and qualitative approaches. *Nursing Research, 38*(5), 299–301.

Nakagawa-Kogan, H., Garber, A., Egan, K., Jarrett, M., & Hendershot, S. (1988). Hypertension self-regulation: Predictors of success in diastolic blood pressure reduction. *Research in Nursing and Health, 11,* 105–115.

National Advisory Council for Nursing Research (1989). *Biennial report to the Congress, 1987–1988.* Bethesda, MD: National Institutes of Health.

National Center for Nursing Research (1988). *Trajectory for research training and career development: A position paper.* Unpublished document.

National Center for Nursing Research (1990a, June). *Health promotion/disease prevention branch: Report to the National Advisory Council for Nursing Research.* Unpublished document.

National Center for Nursing Research (1990b, June). *Report on task force on patient outcomes measures.* Unpublished document.

Neeves, E. (1980). The relationship of hospitalized individuals' cognitive structure regarding health to their health self-care behaviors. *Dissertation Abstracts International, 44,* 3039B.

Nightingale, F. (1860). *Notes on nursing: What it is and what it is not.* London: Harrison.

Norbeck, J.S. (1988). Social support. In H.H. Werley, J.J. Fitzpatrick, & R.L. Taunton (Eds.), *Annual Review of Nursing Research,* Vol. 6 (pp. 85–109). New York: Springer Publishing Company.

Notter, L.E., & Hott, J.R. (1988). Evolution of the research movement in nursing. *Essentials of nursing research* (4th ed.). New York: Springer Publishing Co.

Nutting, M.A. (1912). *Educational status of nursing.* Washington, DC: U.S. Government Printing Office (U.S. Bureau of Education Bulletin #7).

Nutting, M.A. (1926). *A sound economic basis for schools of nursing and other addresses.* New York: Putnam.

Oberst, M.T. (1980). Nursing research: New definitions, collegial approaches. *Cancer Nursing, 3*(6), 459.

Orem, D. (1985). *Nursing: Concepts of practice* (3rd ed.). New York: McGraw-Hill.

Padilla, G.V., Presant, C., Grant, M., Metter, G., Lipsett, J., & Heide, F. (1983). Quality of life index for patients with cancer. *Research in Nursing and Health, 6,* 117–126.

Pender, N.J., Walker, S.N., Sechrist, K.R., & Stromborg, M.F. (1988). Development and testing on the health promotion model. *Cardiovascular Nursing, 24*(6), 41–43.

Porter, E.J. (1989). The qualitative-quantitative dualism. Image: Journal of Nursing Scholarship, *21*(2), 98–102.

Riesch, S., & Hauck, R. (1988). The exercise of self-care agency: An analysis of construct and discriminant validity. *Research in Nursing and Health, 11,* 245–255.

Robb, I.H. (1906). *Nursing: Its principles and practice for hospitals and private use* (3rd ed.). Cleveland: E.C. Koeckert.

Roberts, M.M. (1954). *American nursing: History and interpretation.* New York: Macmillan.

Ryan, V., & Miller, V.B. (1932). Disinfection of clinical thermometers: Bacteriological study and estimated costs. *American Journal of Nursing, 32,* 197–206.

Schlotfeldt, R.M. (1987). Structuring nursing knowledge: A priority for creating nursing's future. *Nursing Science Quarterly, 1*(1), 35–38.

Shaver, J.F. (1985). A biopsychosocial view of human health. *Nursing Outlook, 33*(4), 186–191.

Stevenson, J.S. (1987). Forging a research discipline. *Nursing Research, 36*(1), 60–64.

Stevenson, J.S. (1988). Nursing knowledge development: Into era II. *Journal of Professional Nursing, 4*(3), 152–162.

Stewart, I.M. (1943). *The education of nurses.* New York: Macmillan.

Wald, L.D. (1915). *House on Henry Street.* New York: Henry Holt & Co.

Wells, T.J. (1983). "Hmmm," "huh," and "ahha!" Gerontological nursing research. *Journal of Gerontological Nursing, 9*(7), 372–377.

Whall, A.L. (1988). State of the art and science. *Journal of Gerontological Nursing, 14*(9), 6–7.

Woods, N. (1989). Conceptualizations of self-care: Toward health-oriented models. *Advances in Nursing Science, 12*(1), 1–13.

Zelauskas, B.A., Howes, D.G., Christmyer, C.S., & Dennis, K.E. (1988). Bridging the gap: Theory to practice—part II, research applications. *Nursing Management, 19*(9), 50–52.

## Chapter 31

# The Nurses' National Health Plan

PAMELA MARALDO
CLAIRE M. FAGIN

*D*AILY ACCOUNTS IN the media exhort policy makers to rectify the ills of a health care system that is failing. Many "influentials" in the nation (Califano, 1989; Enthoven, 1989; Freudenheim, 1989; Schroeder et al., 1989) have become increasingly outspoken about the growing inability of our elaborate system of medical care to meet the health needs of our society. Public criticism of American hospitals has become more and more prominently featured in the popular press. For instance, in the past few years, *Board Room Reports Newsletter* (1989), which is widely read by corporate executive officers of the Fortune 500 companies, cautioned readers to stay out of hospitals; *American Health* (Cohn, 1987), with a readership of over one million, ran a feature story stressing the dangers of hospitals and warning that they should be avoided at all costs and only used as places of last resort; and *Glamour Magazine* (Health Care in America, 1988) published the results of a survey of 1006 readers in which 35 percent of respondents said that they believed they have had grounds for malpractice suits against physicians.

Many leading health care experts attribute the growing public dissatisfaction with health care to the increasing use of invasive medical technology for what are often considered marginal returns. Criticizing the current state of our biomedical enterprise, Califano (1989) pointed out that a large share of Medicare funds are spent on life-sustaining technology for individuals over 80 years of age in their last year of life. He acknowledges the great strides made in reducing deaths from cardiovascular disease, but he indicates that much of the success is attributable to changes in lifestyle, dietary habits, and smoking.

The record does not permit us to say that Americans are receiving better health care as a result of our exorbitant health care expenditures. There is a growing consensus that approximately half of the surgeries and procedures performed annually in the United States are unnecessary (Brook & Kahn, 1988). The sentiments expressed by Lynaugh and Fagin (1988) capture these opinions:

. . . as the 20th century draws to a close, these acute-care, interventionist models and disease-focused designs for payment for care seem to have become a problem. They fail to correspond in a functional way with our increasingly perceived need for providing care for children, the old, the chronically ill and the dying. There is heightening concern that these needs are in competition with each other for declining resources.

The preservation and prolongation of life have resulted in an increase in the incidence of chronic conditions of the population at all ages. Most are not amenable to cure but require interventions that enhance or stabilize functional capacities. Steps must be taken in the not too distant future to shift the emphasis of the American health system from acute, episodic care to prevention, primary care, and long-term care.

As the health care dilemmas in our country today are explored, the key policy issues that emerge are cost, access, and quality. Other chapters have considered specific aspects of these issues. A more general approach is taken here and the problems in these areas are highlighted. A health care solution that addresses these issues, meets the nation's emergent needs, and makes appropriate use of nurses is proposed.

## Cost

Every administration since Richard Nixon's has sought to bring health care inflation under control. Medicare continues to be one of the most rapidly rising components of the federal budget despite the introduction of diagnosis-related groups. American spending on health care not only continues to increase but also remains higher than in other industrialized countries. Health care inflation continues to outpace the overall inflation rate by a substantial margin. Even though hospital use has decreased (close to 40 percent of the nation's hospital beds are empty), potential savings have been diluted by steadily increasing prices for hospital care.

Savings from inpatient hospital care have also been offset by rapidly growing expenditures for outpatient care and the growth in volume of services provided under Medicare Part B. There is every reason to expect the Congress and the administration to continue their efforts to restrain health care spending. Spending on Medicare has risen more than tenfold since 1970, with the fastest rising component of health cost becoming Medicare Part B physician payments.

Industry has every reason to be concerned about the rising cost of care. Medical care costs are running at 5 to 10 percent of payroll, and with 20, 25, or 30 percent annual increases, employers "can project that number out four or five years and that percentage [of payroll] will double" (Lamm, 1989). Thus, managers are increasing their efforts to hold down costs by encouraging employees to become better shoppers of health care. Establishing higher deductibles and co-payments, second opinion plans, utilization review, and the encouragement of less costly outpatient options are all strategies to motivate consumers to make informed decisions about their care.

Some employers have moved aggressively toward managed care options, requiring employees to use a health maintenance organization* or preferred provider organization. In the midst of the increasing cost constrained climate, labor disputes involving health care benefits emerged as a major reason for work stoppage and labor walkouts in 1989. A case in point was the much publicized Bell Telephone strike.

Numerous national polls have been conducted recently, attesting to increasing dissatisfaction on the part of employers with health care costs (Hart, 1990; McQueen, 1991). In a recent poll of 50 large corporations and 50 major union leaders, Metropolitan Life Insurance Company found that half the labor leaders regarded limiting what employers call health cost sharing as a top contract priority, ahead of wages and other issues. About 38 percent of the executives reported that their two biggest negotiating priorities are health cost sharing and job security. And 90 percent of 400 employers surveyed recently said they plan to sharply restrict medical benefits for employees' families by the year 2000 (Karr & Carnevale, 1989). In 1985 the average medical insurance premium per employee was $1671; by 1989, it had increased to $3117 (*Health costs soaring*, 1989).

## Access

Some 37 million people in the United States have no health insurance and thus limited access to health care. In addition to the uninsured, there is a growing perception that more Americans are having difficulty gaining access to appropriate care when they need it. Between 1976 and 1987, the number of Americans reporting that there were times in the past year when they did not have money to pay for care increased from 15 to 21 percent (Health Insurance Association of America, 1988).

One approach to problems of access is expanding Medicaid coverage to pregnant women, infants, and children. Clearly this is a step in the right direction. Yet, even with increased coverage, it is ". . . difficult for pregnant women and children covered by Medicaid to find a physician who will treat them, because Medicaid physician reimbursement is so low" (Wagner, 1989).

Access to care is also severely limited for people who have "uninsurable" conditions such as cancer, diabetes, heart disease, and acquired immunodeficiency syndrome. Although "risk pools" are designed to increase the availability of health insurance for people with "pre-existing" conditions who can afford private coverage, the 42,000 people currently enrolled in such pools "are only a tiny fraction of the uninsured" (Burda, 1989). The number of medically uninsurable persons is estimated to be between 1 and 2 million.

Lack of access to services such as home care, day treatment centers, and nursing home care is a problem for most of the population, since a very small percentage has long-term care insurance covering these services. The financing of home care services has been severely limited because of fears that home care will supplement

---

* Although costs of health maintenance organizations have also risen, the assumption is that higher enrollments will lead to more health maintenance organizations and stabilized or reduced costs.

rather than substitute for nursing home and hospital care, thus increasing aggregate health costs.

Nurse practitioners have been instrumental in providing care to underserved populations and populations at risk (Office of Technology Assessment, 1987). Legislative initiatives such as the Rural Health Clinics Act and reimbursement of nurse midwives under Medicaid represent important steps in making nursing care more available to those in need. However, limitations on reimbursement of nurses still severely restrict the potential for nursing to contribute significantly to improved access to care.

## Quality

Health care in the United States is increasingly fragmented, too highly specialized, and insensitive to the range of needs of many patients. Infant mortality and other measures of health for the United States lag behind those of comparable countries like England, Canada, and the countries of Western Europe. These poorer health indicators are attributable, in part, to the heterogeneous nature of the United States population and the problems of access mentioned earlier.

However, poor outcomes may be the result, at least in part, of financial incentives in our current health care system. For example, some types of surgical procedures are profitable to hospitals under current financial arrangements. As a result, some hospitals that perform complex procedures, such as open heart surgery, do not do the minimum number of operations required to maintain proficiency, as defined by the American College of Surgeons. "In 1986, one hospital [in California] did 68 such heart bypass operations and had a death rate of 17.6 percent. The best hospitals, however, typically did several hundred cases and had death rates between one and four percent" (Enthoven, 1989).

Numerous studies have documented that much surgery is unnecessary and that risks to patients often outweigh the possible benefits (Eddy, 1986; Medical Benefits, 1987; Meyers & Gleicher, 1988; National Leadership Commission on Health Care, 1989). For example, 44 percent of coronary artery bypass surgeries have been estimated to be unwarranted or of questionable value. For cardiac pacemaker implants, 20 percent of procedures were judged not to be necessary and another 36 percent were ambiguous. Approximately 32 percent of carotid endarterectomies were done without sufficient justification (*How doctors have ruined health care*, 1990). Robert Brook of the RAND Corporation, who studied the appropriateness of medical care, concluded that "One-fourth of hospital stays, one-fourth of hospital days, one-fourth of procedures and two-fifths of medications could be done without. Almost every study that has seriously looked for hospital overuse has found it, and virtually every time at least double-digit overuse has been found" (Brook & Kahn, 1988).

Concerns over quality are growing in all sectors of health care, not just hospitals. Not long ago, congressional representatives held hearings on the quality—or lack of quality—in home health agencies, referring to home health as the "black box" of quality. A study by the Institute of Medicine (1986) found that quality in nursing homes was substandard and made major recommendations for change, including requirements for increases in nursing staff.

The Medicare and Medicaid programs are the building blocks of a nursing agenda for the nation's health in the future. These programs now provide 40 percent of the nation's health care funding. Moreover, as public policies governing these programs change, private insurers covering the rest of the population usually quickly follow suit.

## Nursing's National Health Plan

The question of universal health insurance is of the first order of importance at this time as problems of cost, quality, and access to health care are examined. Various forms of national health coverage are being discussed seriously by many groups. Some policy makers are predicting that a plan may be enacted within the next five years. Corporate leaders and unions agree that the government must step in, and the pressure for change has indeed become formidable.

The leadership of the Democratic party has taken the initiative to shape a national health plan that would encourage the use of managed care options to control costs and improve access. Although the plan has been criticized for not going far enough (to control costs), many are pleased that the party leadership has taken the initiative to at least begin to address the problem (Frankel, 1991).

The White House, on the other hand, has been seriously rebuked for a lack of attention to domestic policy in general, and health policy in particular. For instance, Senator Bill Bradley publicly chastised President Bush for advocating a billion dollar aid package to the Soviet Union in the face of serious problems in providing basic health services that threaten to destroy the very social fabric of the nation.

Seasoned policy makers predict that during presidential campaigns health care is too politically volatile to touch. Substantial reform to rectify existing problems almost inevitably will mean that someone's political ox will be gored. In any event, the Democrats are determined to place health care high on the list of campaign priorities. Thus the debate over health care reforms is destined to be on the national policy agenda for the foreseeable future.

Nursing organizations have historically been supportive of universal health insurance. Now, for the first time ever, a nursing-sponsored national health plan that would provide access to needed services and emphasize the economic advantages of direct reimbursement for nursing, both outpatient and inpatient, and the specific designation of nurses as providers for certain services has been developed by the National League for Nursing (NLN) and the American Nurses Association (ANA). This plan has since been endorsed by nearly 1 million nurses.

For nursing's part in the national health debate, endorsement or development of a proposal should depend, in part, on whether the proposal would promote the utilization of nurses, because the evidence is overwhelming that greater access to nurses is in the public interest. It is important for nurses to identify and support others seeking the changes they endorse and then provide policy makers with the facts and figures that will advance the potential for their inclusion in any national plan under discussion.

In our view, nursing has taken the preferable course of action to fashion its own national health plan, setting forth something more substantial and visible than the measured response nursing has previously offered to the national debate. As policy makers and key representatives from special interest groups ask nursing spokespersons the inevitable question in health policy discussions, "What is nursing's agenda? What is nursing doing about important health care problems?" Nursing leaders can now say with certainty what that agenda is. And they proceed to point to a litany of examples.

For whatever reasons in the past, nursing's responses did not stand out in the public's mind. Other interest groups, such as the insurers and the employers, who have been uninformed about nursing's position on key health policy matters, will now begin to get a clear understanding of nursing's unique perspective.

For the first time, nursing has given clear expression to nursing's own principles and ideals by advancing nursing's own national health plan and positioning nurses and nursing care as mainstream providers of cost-effective, high-quality care. Because the health care climate is ripe for change and because policy makers are looking for new solutions, there is likely to be substantial receptiveness to nursing's themes and messages.

What are the key provisions of nursing's plan? Nursing's priorities and the main tenets of a nursing-sponsored national health proposal are as follows:

1. Every American would have health insurance.
2. Health insurance must provide coverage for a broader range of services than those typically covered in acute care policies i.e., managed care arrangements, home and community based care.
3. Financial incentives should be shifted to encourage managed care, including the provision of preventive, primary care, and long-term care services.
4. Consumers would have freedom of choice and access to a variety of providers, including nurses, for the most appropriate health care services.
5. Standards of quality should be outcome-oriented and tied to reimbursement policies.

Since United States health policy has traditionally been of an incremental nature and national health insurance may not be politically possible in the short run, the following should be nursing priorities in the near term.

## Access to Primary and Preventive Health Care Services for Pregnant Women and Young Children.

Providing care to pregnant women and young children would go a long way toward closing the gap in access to health services. It is estimated that one fourth of the uninsured are children (Wagner, 1989). Any incremental expansion of public programs probably will start by covering more low-income pregnant women, infants, and children because of the strong evidence of the effectiveness of such interventions.

*Prenatal Care.*   It is estimated that low birth weight infants could be reduced by 15 percent among whites and 12 percent among blacks if all women began prenatal care in the first trimester of pregnancy and continued to receive it throughout pregnancy (Institute of Medicine, 1985). The Office of Technology Assessment (1988) estimates that early prenatal care saved the United States health care system between $14,000 and $30,000 per low birth weight infant in newborn hospitalization and rehospitalization in the first year of life.

Approximately 75 percent of pregnant women have normal pregnancies and births that could be handled by nurse-midwives (Lubic, 1988). If even 25 percent of the 3.6 million pregnant American women used birthing centers, 717 million to 3.3 billion dollars could be saved.

The recent study of women in a rural area near Elmira, New York (Olds, Henderson, Tatelbaum, & Chamberlin, 1988), showed that home visits by nurses to low-income women during and after pregnancy to teach them the basics of child rearing resulted in less child abuse, healthier babies, and better employment and educational achievements by the mothers.

Some progress has been made toward the goal of improving access to care for pregnant women and young children with the federally mandated extension of Medicaid coverage for all pregnant women with incomes of 133 percent of the federal poverty level and their children up to 6 years of age. Additionally, states may exercise the option of extending coverage to women with incomes under 185 percent of the federal poverty level. Essentials of such plans must include continuous and immediate enrollment, referral protocols for high-risk patients, quality control measures, and adequate funding to provide comprehensive services, including health education.

*Child Care.*   Every child should have access to primary care. Well baby programs are essential, as are school health programs in which nurses provide primary health care and health education. A national demonstration and evaluation of the impact of school health programs (Meeker, 1988) showed that school nurse practitioners were able to handle 87 percent of the health care problems presented in a school context with 96 percent resolution, no duplication of services, and at one quarter of the cost of conventional care.

## Access to Long-Term Community and Home Care

Expanded coverage for long-term care in community and home settings must be included in a national health plan. The majority of care needed by the elderly does not fall into the realm of acute care; rather, most of the elderly suffer from chronic illnesses, which largely require nursing care (*There's No Place Like Home*, 1989). Consumer surveys indicate a preference for care in the home, and home care has been demonstrated to be cost saving when it substitutes for more costly care in hospitals. A nursing-sponsored national health program would establish home care and community-based care as the mainstays of health care delivery while utilizing hospitals for trauma and treatment of acute illnesses.

It is essential to modify the existing gatekeeper role of physicians with regard to utilization of primary care and long-term care in community settings. Physicians are the appropriate gatekeepers and referral source for hospital services and the diagnosis and treatment of acute illness. Physicians are not the appropriate gatekeepers for access to nursing care in home and community-bound settings. They have neither the expertise nor the interest to control access to nursing care, as is currently required to obtain reimbursement for home nursing care.

Nursing home care must also be substantially improved. The evaluation of the Robert Wood Johnson Teaching Nursing Home program offers important insights (Shaughnessy, Kramer, & Hittle, 1988). The evaluators of this experiment found that the teaching nursing home approach, which used nurses in expanded roles, reduced hospitalization rates for nursing home patients, fostered an environment conducive to maximizing patients' physical and cognitive functioning, and reduced total costs. The evaluators specifically recommended Medicare and Medicaid reimbursement for the cost of nurse clinicians, education for aides, and selected educational programs, since these resulted in lower hospitalization rates for teaching nursing home patients as compared with those in control sample nursing homes.

### Nurses as Gatekeepers in a Managed Care Environment

As the costs of health insurance have escalated, employers have adopted systems of managed care as a strategy to buy the most efficient package of services at the best price. Managed care offers unprecedented opportunities for nurses to function as gatekeepers to improve quality and continuity of care as well as containing cost, and a nursing-sponsored national health plan should position nurses in this role. Nurses are the most appropriate providers to serve as case managers, coordinating care across settings. We have already discussed the appropriateness of the nurse provider in relation to pregnant women and young children. The evidence suggests that nurses are ideal providers to determine the need for home care, nursing home care, and care in a community setting, since so many of the problems clients experience have to do with activities of daily living. As indicated earlier, the tight group of physicians at the gate to health care services must be altered. Expert nurses know the needs of the family requiring care and the appropriate focus and method of care. Further, for managed care to result in improved outcomes for clients, as contrasted with cost savings for insurance companies or corporations, nurses must have the authority to allocate resources devoted to that care.

## Nursing: In the Public Interest

A national health plan that provides the public with access to nurses practicing at their optimal capacity would be extremely important in advancing the nation's health, in increasing consumers' satisfaction with their care, and as a tool to reduce costs. Nurses' knowledge about the health problems of people throughout the life cycle and their understanding of and focus on individuals and families' experiences of illness give them the capacity to assist the ill and disabled in managing their own health and in living life as productively as possible. Nurses are able to establish better communication with patients, to provide more effective counseling, and a faster health recovery than other providers (Office of Technology Assessment, 1987). In addition, nurses include clients in the decision-making process about their own plan of care, a factor that influences care outcomes and consumer satisfaction.

The issue of soaring health costs is a complicated one involving a complex array of factors. Policy makers are well aware of nursing's potential primary health care services at costs below those of physician-managed care. But there is concern as to whether expanded reimbursement for nurses will lower health costs in the aggregate or increase them. Policy makers contend that health care is an economic anomaly in which increased supply tends to drive up demand, and the increased demand permits providers to command higher prices. Thus, some policy analysts argue that reimbursing nurses would constitute an "add-on" to health care costs. However, this is a specious argument.

If nurses were permitted to practice within their areas of competence and expertise, the additional costs of increasing the number of providers would be offset by the substantial cost savings resulting from different utilization patterns of patients. It is well known that nurses use less unnecessary technology and are less likely to recommend institutional care than are physicians. Consider all the "add-ons" that will be needed if care is to be provided to the 37 million uninsured people under existing arrangements. Expanding insurance coverage based on the present inefficient arrangements would be a foolish step for the state or federal government to take when nurse providers are able to offer excellent primary and first-line care at lower costs. Psychologists, physical therapists, chiropractors, and others—convinced of the worth of their services—have all overcome the add-on argument (which has been advanced for over a decade) with fewer supporting data than nursing has collected but with strong political pressure.

Within recent years, policy makers have become more receptive to nursing's cost containment potential for a number of reasons. First, the dollar comparisons in the case of nurse-midwives versus obstetricians and nurse anesthetists versus anesthesiologists are striking. When congressional representatives became convinced that nurse midwives would follow a mother's progress prenatally, deliver the baby, and continue to monitor the mother through the postpartum period at substantially lower rates than those of obstetricians, they enacted a proposal to reimburse nurse-midwives under Medicaid. Private insurers have also increased their coverage of nurse midwifery services, and consumers in large numbers have elected nurse midwives as their caregivers in pregnancy and for primary gynecologic care. Similarly, legislation enacted in 1986 provided direct reimbursement for certified registered nurse anesthetists under Medicare, and nurses have served the public well in this role.

For nursing to be successful in achieving Medicare Part B reimbursement, eligibility must be carefully defined to include the subset of nurses who provide care that substitutes for that of other providers. Thus, we are recommending direct reimbursement to nurse practitioners and clinical nurse specialists with formal credentials for advanced nursing practice. This would include but not be limited to pediatric nurse specialists, nurse midwives, gerontologic nurse specialists, and family or women's health practitioners and nurse specialists in advanced practice in the care of persons with acquired immunodeficiency syndrome and other chronic health problems. To restrict the numbers involved and ensure quality, legislation could mandate certification and master's degree preparation. The maximum number of such nurses is no more than 60,000 at this time; all are involved with the most vulnerable populations, and numerous studies have already shown that they are performing cost-effectively.

The notion of nurses' involvement in a national health insurance system probably will draw comments of "a two-tiered system of health care." It is even possible that we will hear recommendations for the use of nurses for the bottom tier and of physicians for the same interventions at higher tiers of cost. When consumers have a choice, however, a substantial proportion use nurse providers. The growing number of health maintenance organization enrollees choosing nurse-midwives evidence that the public does not consider nursing care second class. However, the public should be given the opportunity to choose nursing care without financial penalty.

To summarize, nursing's strategy for the future should include the following interrelated elements:

- *Provide universal access* to primary and preventive health services. A phased-in approach could provide care to pregnant women and children first.
- *Expand coverage* of community-based systems of care substantially by introducing incentives for greater utilization of home care and community nursing center services. Here, too, a phased-in approach would provide home and community care to the frail elderly first through expansion of Medicare and Medicaid options, with cost sharing depending on economic status.
- *Long-term care* coverage is seriously deficient for the nation's elderly and chronically ill (Merrill & Somers, 1989). A plan that would provide basic benefits for long-term care and a continuous case management system across payers is essential.
- *Cost control.* Nurses as primary care providers would offer the distinguishing cost control feature in the plan. In addition, short- and long-term home care, care in community settings, and nursing home care would be offered with built-in incentives to select the least expensive appropriate option.
- *Substantially increase research* on new models of health care delivery to measure their effectiveness, quality, and cost compared with existing systems.
- *Encourage researchers* to improve clinical interventions that enhance function.

## Conclusion

In an era in which cost, quality, and access present increasingly difficult problems, nurses are an extremely valuable and untapped resource. As high-quality, cost-effective providers, nurses are prepared to make a vital contribution to addressing the problems in health delivery for the future. Nurses must be active participants in the major decisions affecting the organization and financing of health care. Perceptions of the problems in the current health care system, proposals for solutions, and nursing's special position in these solutions have been explored. Focus has been on shaping a nursing agenda—a nursing-sponsored national health plan—that would utilize nurses as cost-saving providers in areas of greatest need: prenatal care and primary and long-term care. The essential nature of including nurses in public program reimbursement in order to provide access to nursing services to people and populations in need, for both the present and the future, has been stressed. Care of the chronically ill, prenatal care, care of women and children, elder care offered in the community, the home, and the nursing home, through fee-for-service or managed care, are appropriate areas for nurses, operating independently and interdependently.

Societal trends have converged in recent years to create a demand for the very knowledge and skills that nursing has to offer. The shift in focus from a health care system centered on "cure" to one that must "care" for the increasing numbers of chronically ill, coupled with the major issues facing us in health care—cost, access, and quality—are issues for which the nursing profession could provide solutions. The nursing profession has the right and responsibility to advance these new initiatives and achievable health care reforms to improve the health of the American public.

## REFERENCES

Brook, R., & Kahn, K.L. (1988, December). Interpreting hospital mortality data. *Journal of the American Medical Association, 260*(24), 3625.

Burda, E. (1989, August). The evolution of alternative health care delivery systems. Washington, DC: *EBRI Issue Brief, 93*(1).

Califano, J., Jr. (1989, April). Billions blown on health. *New York Times*, p. 9.

Chambliss, L., & Reier, S. (1990, January 9). How doctors have ruined health care. *Financial World*, pp. 23–24.

Cohn, V. (1987, March). How to survive a hospital. *American Health*, 98–99.

Eddy, D. (1986, September 4). Variations in the use of medical and surgical services. *New England Journal of Medicine, 315*(10), 650–651.

Enthoven, A. (1989, July 13). A cost-unconscious medical system. *New York Times*, p. A23.

Freudenheim, M. (1989, May 8). A health-care taboo is broken. [Business Day]. *New York Times*, p. D1.

Health care in America: A reader survey (1988, August). *Glamour Magazine*, pp. 25–26.

Health costs soaring (1989, August). *Philadelphia Inquirer*, p. .

Health Insurance Association of America (1988). Health and health insurance: The public's view. HIAA Report, 1976–1988.

Institute of Medicine (1985). *Preventing low birthweight*. Committee to Study the Prevention of Low Birthweight, Division of Health Promotion and Disease Prevention. Washington, DC: National Academy Press, 1.

Institute of Medicine (1986). *Improving the quality of care in nursing homes*. Washington, DC: National Academy Press.

Karr, A.R., & Carnevale, M.L. (1989, August 11). Facing off over health-benefits: Emotional side of issue makes bargaining hard [Marketplace]. *Wall Street Journal,* p. B1.

Koska, M.T. (1989, February 5). Quality—thy name is nursing care, CEO's say. *Hospitals,* p. 32.

Lamm, R. (1989, August). Saving a few sacrificing many at great cost. *New York Times,* p. 17.

Lubic, R.W. (1983). Childbirthing centers: Delivering more for less. *American Journal of Nursing, 88*(7), 1054–1056.

Lynaugh, J.E., & Fagin, C.M. (1988). Nursing comes of age. *Image: Journal of Nursing Scholarship, 20*(4), 184–189.

McQueen, M. (1991, June 28). Voters, sick of the current health care system, want Federal Government to prescribe remedy [Politics & Policy]. *Wall Street Journal,* p. A14.

Meeker, R.J. (1988). A comprehensive school health initiative. *Image: Journal of Nursing Scholarship, 18*(86), 86–91.

Merrill, J.C., & Somers, S.A. (1989). Long-term care: The great debate on the wrong issue. *Inquiry, 26,* 317–320.

Meyers, S., & Gleicher, N. (1988, December 8). A successful program to lower Caesarian section rates. *New England Journal of Medicine, 319*(23), 1512–1516.

Office of Technology Assessment (1987). *Nurse practitioners, physician assistants, and certified nurse-midwives: A policy analysis.* Health Technology Case Study No. 37.

Office of Technology Assessment (1988). *Healthy children: Investing in the future.* Washington, DC: U.S. Government Printing Office.

Olds, D.L., Henderson, C., Tatelbaum, R., & Chamberlin, R. (1988). Improving the life-course development of socially disadvantaged mothers: A randomized trial of nurse home visitation. *American Journal of Public Health, 78,* 1436–1445.

Report of the National Leadership Commission on Health Care (1989). *For the health of the nation: A shared responsibility.* Ann Arbor, MI: Health Administration Press.

*Results of second opinion program for coronary artery bypass graft surgery* (1987, October 31). Medical Benefits.

Schroeder, S., Zones, J.S., & Showstack, J.A. (1989). Academic medicine as a public trust. *New England Journal of Medicine, 262*(6), 803–811.

Shaughnessy, P.W., Kramer, A.M., Hittle, D.F. (1988, December). *The teaching nursing home experiment: Its effects and implications.* Study Paper 6. Denver: Center for Health Services Research, University of Colorado Health Sciences Center, 47.

There's no place like home. (1989, January). *U.S. News & World Report,* p. 42.

Wagner, L. (1989, July). Access for all people. *Modern Health Care, 28*(33), 17.

# Index

Page numbers followed by a "t" refer to tables; page numbers followed by an "f" refer to figures.

517